PROGRESS IN BRAIN RESEARCH

VOLUME 140

THE BRAIN'S EYE:
NEUROBIOLOGICAL AND CLINICAL ASPECTS
OF OCULOMOTOR RESEARCH

Other volumes in PROGRESS IN BRAIN RESEARCH

Volume 112: Extrageniculostriate Mechanisms Underlying Visually-Guided Orientation Behavior, by M. Norita, T. Bando and B.E. Stein (Eds.) – 1996, ISBN 0-444-82347-6.
Volume 113: The Polymodal Receptor: A Gateway to Pathological Pain, by T. Kumazawa, L. Kruger and K. Mizumura (Eds.) – 1996, ISBN 0-444-82473-1.
Volume 114: The Cerebellum: From Structure to Control, by C.I. de Zeeuw, P. Strata and J. Voogd (Eds.) – 1997, ISBN 0-444-82313-1.
Volume 115: Brain Function in Hot Environment, by H.S. Sharma and J. Westman (Eds.) – 1998, ISBN 0-444-82377-8.
Volume 116: The Glutamate Synapse as a Therapeutical Target: Molecular Organization and Pathology of the Glutamate Synapse, by O.P. Ottersen, I.A. Langmoen and L. Gjerstad (Eds.) – 1998, ISBN 0-444-82754-4.
Volume 117: Neuronal Degeneration and Regeneration: From Basic Mechanisms to Prospects for Therapy, by F.W. van Leeuwen, A. Salehi, R.J. Giger, A.J.G.D. Holtmaat and J. Verhaagen (Eds.) – 1998, ISBN 0-444-82817-6.
Volume 118: Nitric Oxide in Brain Development, Plasticity and Disease, by R.R. Mize, T.M. Dawson, V.L. Dawson and M.J. Friedlander (Eds.) – 1998, ISBN 0-444-82885-0.
Volume 119: Advances in Brain Vasopressin, by I.J.A. Urban, J.P.H. Burbach and D. De Wied (Eds.) – 1999, ISBN 0-444-50080-4.
Volume 120: Nucleotides and their Receptors in the Nervous System, by P. Illes and H. Zimmermann (Eds.) – 1999, ISBN 0-444-50082-0.
Volume 121: Disorders of Brain, Behavior and Cognition: The Neurocomputational Perspective, by J.A. Reggia, E. Ruppin and D. Glanzman (Eds.) – 1999, ISBN 0-444-50175-4.
Volume 122: The Biological Basis for Mind Body Interactions, by E.A. Mayer and C.B. Saper (Eds.) – 1999, ISBN 0-444-50049-9.
Volume 123: Peripheral and Spinal Mechanisms in the Neural Control of Movement, by M.D. Binder (Ed.) – 1999, ISBN 0-444-50288-2.
Volume 124: Cerebellar Modules: Molecules, Morphology and Function, by N.M. Gerrits, T.J.H. Ruigrok and C.E. De Zeeuw (Eds.) – 2000, ISBN 0-444-50108-8.
Volume 125: Volume Transmission Revisited, by L.F. Agnati, K. Fuxe, C. Nicholson and E. Syková (Eds.) – 2000, ISBN 0-444-50314-5.
Volume 126: Cognition, Emotion and Autonomic Responses: The Integrative Role of the Prefrontal Cortex and Limbic Structures, by H.B.M. Uylings, C.G. Van Eden, J.P.C. De Bruin, M.G.P. Feenstra and C.M.A. Pennartz (Eds.) – 2000, ISBN 0-444-50332-3.
Volume 127: Neural Transplantation II. Novel Cell Therapies for CNS Disorders, by S.B. Dunnett and A. Björklund (Eds.) – 2000, ISBN 0-444-50109-6.
Volume 128: Neural Plasticity and Regeneration, by F.J. Seil (Ed.) – 2000, ISBN 0-444-50209-2.
Volume 129: Nervous System Plasticity and Chronic Pain, by J. Sandkühler, B. Bromm and G.F. Gebhart (Eds.) – 2000, ISBN 0-444-50509-1.
Volume 130: Advances in Neural Population Coding, by M.A.L. Nicolelis (Ed.) – 2001, ISBN 0-444-50110-X.
Volume 131: Concepts and Challenges in Retinal Biology, by H. Kolb, H. Ripps, and S. Wu (Eds.), – 2001, ISBN 0-444-50677-2.
Volume 132: Glial Cell Function, by B. Castellano López and M. Nieto-Sampedro (Eds.) – 2001, ISBN 0-444-50508-3.
Volume 133: The Maternal Brain. Neurobiological and neuroendocrine adaptation and disorders in pregnancy and post partum, by J.A. Russell, A.J. Douglas, R.J. Windle and C.D. Ingram (Eds.) – 2001, ISBN 0-444-50548-2.
Volume 134: Vision: From Neurons to Cognition, by C. Casanova and M. Ptito (Eds.) – 2001, ISBN 0-444-50586-5.
Volume 135: Do Seizures Damage the Brain, by A. Pitkänen and T. Sutula (Eds.) – 2002, ISBN 0-444-50814-7.
Volume 136: Changing Views of Cajal's Neuron, by E.C. Azmitia, J. DeFelipe, E.G. Jones, P. Rakic and C.E. Ribak (Eds.) – 2002, ISBN 0-444-50815-5.
Volume 137: Spinal Cord Trauma: Regeneration, Neural Repair and Functional Recovery, by L. McKerracher, G. Doucet and S. Rossignol (Eds.) – 2002, ISBN 0-444-50817-1.
Volume 138: Plasticity in the Adult Brain: From Genes to Neurotherapy, by M.A. Hofman, G.J. Boer, A.J.G.D. Holtmaat, E.J.W. Van Someren, J. Verhaagen and D.F. Swaab (Eds.) – 2002, ISBN 0-444-50981-X.
Volume 139: Vasopressin and Oxytocin: From Genes to Clinical Applications, by D. Poulain, S. Oliet and D. Theodosis (Eds.) – 2002, ISBN 0-444-50982-8.

PROGRESS IN BRAIN RESEARCH

VOLUME 140

THE BRAIN'S EYE: NEUROBIOLOGICAL AND CLINICAL ASPECTS OF OCULOMOTOR RESEARCH

EDITED BY

J. HYÖNÄ
Department of Psychology, University of Turku, FIN-20014 Turku, Finland

D.P. MUNOZ
Centre for Neuroscience Studies, Department of Physiology, Queen's University, Kingston, ON K7L 3N6, Canada

W. HEIDE
Department of Neurology, University of Lübeck, Ratzeburger Allee 160, D-23538 Lübeck, Germany

R. RADACH
Technical University of Aachen, Institute of Psychology, Jaegerstrasse 17–19, 52056 Aachen, Germany

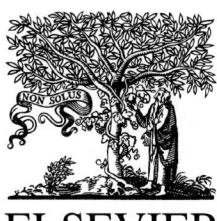

ELSEVIER

AMSTERDAM – BOSTON – LONDON – NEW YORK – OXFORD – PARIS
SAN DIEGO – SAN FRANCISCO – SINGAPORE – SYDNEY – TOKYO
2002

ELSEVIER SCIENCE B.V.
Sara Burgerhartstraat 25
P.O. Box 211, 1000 AE Amsterdam, The Netherlands

© 2002 Elsevier Science B.V. All rights reserved.

This work is protected under copyright by Elsevier Science, and the following terms and conditions apply to its use:

Photocopying
Single photocopies of single chapters may be made for personal use as allowed by national copyright laws. Permission of the Publisher and payment of a fee is required for all other photocopying, including multiple or systematic copying, copying for advertising or promotional purposes, resale, and all forms of document delivery. Special rates are available for educational institutions that wish to make photocopies for non-profit educational classroom use.

Permissions may be sought directly from Elsevier Science via their homepage (http://www.elsevier.com) by selecting 'Customer support' and then 'Permissions'. Alternatively you can send an e-mail to: permissions@elsevier.com, or fax to: (+44) 1865 853333.

In the USA, users may clear permissions and make payments through the Copyright Clearance Center, Inc., 222 Rosewood Drive, Danvers, MA 01923, USA; phone: (+1) 978 7508400, fax: (+1) 978 7504744, and in the UK through the Copyright Licensing Agency Rapid Clearance Service (CLARCS), 90 Tottenham Court Road, London W1P 0LP, UK; phone: (+44) 207 631 5555, fax: (+44) 207 631 5500. Other countries may have a local reprographic rights agency for payments.

Derivative Works
Tables of contents may be reproduced for internal circulation, but permission of Elsevier Science is required for resale or distribution of such material.
Permission of the Publisher is required for all other derivative works, including compilations and translations.

Electronic Storage or Usage
Permission of the Publisher is required to store or use electronically any material contained in this work, including any chapter or part of a chapter.

Except as outlined above, no part of this work may be reproduced, stored in a retrieval system or transmitted in any form or by any means, electronic, mechanical, photocopying, recording or otherwise, without prior written permission of the Publisher.
Address permissions requests to: Elsevier Science Global Rights Department, at the mail, fax and e-mail addresses noted above.

Notice
No responsibility is assumed by the Publisher for any injury and/or damage to persons or property as a matter of products liability, negligence or otherwise, or from any use or operation of any methods, products, instructions or ideas contained in the material herein. Because of rapid advances in the medical sciences, in particular, independent verification of diagnoses and drugs dosages should be made.

First edition 2002

Library of Congress Cataloging in Publication Data
A catalog record from the Library of Congress has been applied for.

British Library Cataloguing in Publication Data
A catalogue record from the British Library has been applied for.

ISBN: 0-444-51097-4 (volume)
ISBN: 0-444-80104-9 (series)
ISSN: 0079-6123

♾ The paper used in this publication meets the requirements of ANSI/NISO Z39.48-1992 (Permanence of Paper).
Printed in The Netherlands.

List of Contributors

R.V. Abadi, Department of Optometry and Neuroscience, UMIST, P.O. Box 88, Manchester, M60 1QD, UK

P. Aivar, Department of Neuroscience, Erasmus University, P.O. Box 1738, 3000 DR Rotterdam, The Netherlands

T.J. Anderson, Department of Neurology, Christchurch Hospital, Private Bag 4710, Christchurch, New Zealand

G.R. Barnes, Department of Optometry and Neuroscience, UMIST, P.O. Box 88, Manchester, M60 1QD, UK

H. Bekkering, Nijmegen Institute for Cognition and Information, P.O. Box 9104, 6500 HE Nijmegen, The Netherlands

T. Bekkour, Division of Orthoptics, University of Liverpool, Brownlow Hill, Thompson Yates Building, Liverpool, L69 3BX, UK

D. Bennett, Mental Health and Neural Systems Research Unit, Department of Psychology, Lancaster University, Lancaster LA1 4YF, UK

R.T. Born, Department of Neurobiology, Harvard Medical School, 220 Longwood Avenue, Boston, MA 02115-5701, USA

B. Bridgeman, Department of Psychology, University of California, Social Sciences 2, Santa Cruz, CA 95064, USA

D.S. Broomhead, Department of Mathematics, UMIST, P.O. Box 88, Manchester, M60 1QD, UK

D.P. Carey, Neuropsychology Research Group, Department of Psychology, University of Aberdeen, Old Aberdeen, AB24 2UB, UK

Y. Chen, Department of Psychiatry, Harvard Medical School, McLean Hospital, Belmont, MA 02478, USA

R.A. Clement, Visual Sciences Unit, Institute of Child Health, University College of London, 30 Guilford Street, London, WC1N 1EH, UK

J.D. Crawford, York University, Centre for Visual Research, Departments of Psychology and Biology, 4700 Keele Street, BSB, Room 291, Toronto, ON M3J 1P3, Canada

T.J. Crawford, Mental Health and Neural Systems Research Unit, Department of Psychology, Lancaster University, Lancaster LA1 4YF, UK

P. De Graef, Laboratory of Experimental Psychology, Department of Psychology, University of Leuven, Tiensestraat 102, B-3000 Leuven, Belgium

J.F.W. Deakin, Neurosciences and Psychiatry Unit, University of Manchester, G907, Stopford Building, Oxford Road, Manchester, M13 9PT, UK

S. Della Sala, Neuropsychology Research Group, Department of Psychology, University of Aberdeen, Old Aberdeen, AB24 2UB, UK

H. Deubel, Department of Psychology, Ludwig-Maximilians-Universität, Leopoldstrasse 13, 80802 Munich, Germany

S.M. Dornhoefer, Department of Psychology III, Dresden University of Technology, Mommsenstrasse 13, 01062 Dresden, Germany

A.S. Drew, Department of Exercise and Movement Science, Institute of Neuroscience, University of Oregon, Eugene, OR 97403-1240, USA

T. Eggert, Department of Neurology, Klinikum Grosshadern, Center for Sensorimotor Research, Marchioninistr. 23, D-81377 Munich, Germany

J.D. Enderle, Biomedical Engineering, University of Connecticut, 260 Glenbrook Road, Storrs, CT 06269-2157, USA

S. Everling, Departments of Physiology and Psychology, University of Western Ontario, Social Science Centre, London, ON N6A 5C2, Canada

J.H. Fecteau, Centre for Neuroscience Studies, CIHR Group in Sensory-Motor Systems, Department of Physiology, Queen's University, Kingston, ON K7L 3N6, Canada

D. Fernandez-Duque, Cognitive Neurology Unit A421 Sunnybrook, and Women's College Health Science Centre, Toronto, ON M4N 3M5, Canada

J.R. Flanagan, Department of Psychology, Centre for Neuroscience Studies, Queen's University, Kingston, ON K7L 3N6, Canada

M.S.H. Harris, Center for Cognitive Medicine, Department of Psychiatry, MC 913, The Neuropsychiatric Institute, University of Illinois at Chicago, 912 S. Wood Street, Chicago, IL 60612, USA

M. Hayhoe, Center for Visual Science, University of Rochester, Rochester, NY 14627, USA

W. Heide, Department of Neurology, Medical University, Ratzeburger Allee 160, D-23538 Lübeck, Germany

M.H. Heitger, Department of Medicine, Christchurch School of Medicine and Health Sciences, P.O.Box 4345, Christchurch, New Zealand

D. Heller, Technical University of Aachen, Institute of Psychology, Jaegerstrasse 17-19, 52056 Aachen, Germany

D.Y.P. Henriques, York University, Centre for Visual Research, Departments of Psychology and Biology, 4700 Keele Street, BSB, Room 291, Toronto, ON M3J 1P3, Canada

P.S. Holzman, Department of Psychiatry, Harvard Medical School, McLean Hospital, Belmont, MA 02478, USA

L. Huestegge, Technical University of Aachen, Institute of Psychology, Jaegerstrasse 17-19, 52056 Aachen, Germany

M. Ietswaart, Neuropsychology Research Group, Department of Psychology, University of Aberdeen, Old Aberdeen, AB24 2UB, UK

U.J. Ilg, Kognitive Neurologie, Neurologische Universitätsklinik, Hoppe-Seyler-Strasse 3, D-72076 Tübingen, Germany

C.B. Jarrett, Department of Optometry and Neuroscience, UMIST, P.O. Box 88, Manchester, M60 1QD, UK

R.D. Jones, Department of Medical Physics and Bioengineering, Christchurch Hospital, Private Bag 4710, Christchurch, New Zealand

A.Z. Khan, York University, Centre for Visual Research, Departments of Psychology and Biology, 4700 Keele Street, BSB, Room 291, Toronto, ON M3J 1P3, Canada

P.C. Knox, Division of Orthoptics, University of Liverpool, Thompson Yates Building, Brownlow Hill, Liverpool, L69 3BX, UK

D. Kömpf, Department of Neurology, Medical University, Ratzeburger Allee 160, D-23538 Lübeck, Germany

H.-J. Kunert, Technical University of Aachen, Clinic for Psychiatry and Psychotherapy, Pauwelstrasse 30, 52057 Aachen, Germany

A.L. Le Vasseur, Department of Physiology, Centre for Neuroscience Studies, Queen's University, Kingston, ON K7L 3N6, Canada

J.-H. Lee, Department of Exercise and Movement Science, Institute of Neuroscience, University of Oregon, Eugene, OR 97403-1240, USA

G. Lekwuwa, Lancashire Teaching Hospitals NHS Trust, Neuroscience Directorate, Departments of Neurology and Neurophysiology, Sharoe Green Lane, Preston, PR2 9HT, UK

D. Levy, Department of Psychiatry, Harvard University, Boston, MA, USA

M.R. MacAskill, Department of Medicine, Christchurch School of Medicine, P.O. Box 4345, Christchurch, New Zealand

W.P. Medendorp, York University, Centre for Visual Research, Departments of Psychology and Biology, 4700 Keele Street, BSB, Room 291, Toronto, ON M3J 1P3, Canada

R. Mruczek, Department of Neuroscience, Brown University, Providence, RI 02912, USA

D.P. Munoz, Centre for Neuroscience Studies, CIHR Group in Sensory-Motor Systems, Department of Physiology, Queen's University, Kingston, ON K7L 3N6, Canada

K. Nakayama, Department of Psychology, Harvard University, Cambridge, MA 02138, USA

D. Newsham, Division of Orthoptics, Department of Allied Health Professions, University of Liverpool, Thompson Yates Building, Brownlow Hill, Liverpool, L69 3GB, UK

C.C. Pack, Department of Neurobiology, Harvard Medical School, 220 Longwood Avenue, Boston, MA 02115-5701, USA

R. Radach, Technical University of Aachen, Institute of Psychology, Jaegerstrasse 17-19, 52056 Aachen, Germany

E. Reingold, Department of Psychology, University of Toronto, 100 St. George Street, Toronto, ON M5S 3G3, Canada

R.A. Rensink, Department of Psychology, University of British Columbia, 2136 West Mall, Vancouver, BC V6T 1Z4, Canada

J. Saiki, Graduate School of Informatics, Kyoto University, Yoshida-Honmachi, Sakyo-ku, Kyoto 606-8501, Japan

U. Sailer, Department of Neurology, Klinikum Grosshadern, Center for Sensorimotor Research, Marchioninistr. 23, D-81377 Munich, Germany

A.M. Schmid, NMR Center at the Massachusetts General Hospital, Charleston, MA 02129, USA

W.X. Schneider, Experimental Psychology, Ludwig-Maximilians-Universität, Leopoldstrasse 13, 80802 Munich, Germany

S. Shaunak, Lancashire Teaching Hospitals NHS Trust, Neuroscience Directorate, Departments of Neurology and Neurophysiology, Sharoe Green Lane, Preston, PR2 9HT, UK

A. Shrivastavah, Center for Visual Science, University of Rochester, Rochester, NY 14627, USA

A. Sprenger, Department of Neurology, Medical University, Ratzeburger Allee 160, D-23538 Lübeck, Germany

D.M. Stampe, Department of Psychology, University of Toronto, 100 St George Street, Toronto, ON M5S 3G3, Canada

A. Straube, Department of Neurology, Klinikum Grosshadern, Center for Sensorimotor Research, Marchioninistr. 23, D-81377 Munich, Germany

J.A. Sweeney, Center for Cognitive Medicine, Department of Psychiatry, MC 913, The Neuropsychiatric Institute, University of Illinois at Chicago, Chicago, IL 60612, USA

B.W. Tatler, Sussex Centre for Neuroscience, School of Biological Sciences, University of Sussex, Brighton, BN1 9QG, UK

I.M. Thornton, Max Planck Institute for Biological Cybernetics, Spemannstrasse 38, 72076 Tübingen, Germany

C.J. Tinsley, School of Psychology, The University of Nottingham, University Park, Nottingham, NG7 2RD, UK

P.J.A. Unema, Department of Experimental Psychology, Maastricht University, P.O. Box 616, 6200 MD Maastricht, The Netherlands

P. Van Donkelaar, Department of Exercise and Movement Science, Institute of Neuroscience, University of Oregon, Eugene, OR 97403-1240, USA

B.M. Velichkovsky, Department of Psychology III, Dresden University of Technology, Mommsenstrasse 13, 01062 Dresden, Germany

K. Verfaillie, Laboratory of Experimental Psychology, Department of Psychology, University of Leuven, Tiensestraat 102, B-3000 Leuven, Belgium

J.P. Whittle, The University of Sheffield, Department of Ophthalmology and Orthoptics, Royal Hallamshire Hospital, Glossop Road, Sheffield, S10 2JF, UK

D. Zambarbieri, Dipartimento di Informatica e Sistemistica, Università di Pavia, Via Ferrata 1, 27100 Pavia, Italy

R. Zhao, Department of Neurobiology, Harvard Medical School, 220 Longwood Avenue, Boston, MA 02115-5701, USA

Preface

The book comprises a selected collection of papers presented at the 11th European Conference on Eye Movements (August 22–25, 2001, Turku, Finland), supplemented by invited contributions and commentaries. The ECEM series of conferences was commenced in 1981 by Professor Rudolf Groner in Bern. It brings together researchers from various disciplines with an interest to study behavioral, cognitive, neurobiological and clinical aspects of eye movements. The book at hand consists of contributions that either directly deal with the neural basis of eye movements or make reference to neural mechanisms related to eye movement control. All chapters were reviewed by two referees, who typically were fellow contributors, but a number of outside referees were also recruited.

The book is divided into five sections: (I) Saccadic eye movements; (II) Change blindness and trans-saccadic integration; (III) Smooth pursuit eye movements; (IV) Eye-hand coordination; and (V) Clinical aspects of eye movement research. Each section ends with a commentary chapter written by a distinguished scholar. A sister book has also been published (Hyönä, Radach and Deubel (Eds.), *The Mind's Eye: Cognitive and Applied Aspects of Eye Movements*, Elsevier Science, Oxford), where the emphasis is on research that uses eye-tracking as a tool to study various cognitive functions.

Section I is comprised of a series of articles that address aspects of the saccadic system at various levels of control ranging from behavior to neurophysiological correlations with behavior to modeling. This multidisciplined approach has greatly enhanced our understanding of the system. Aspects of the control system that are addressed in this book include the control of reflexive visual or auditory saccades, voluntary saccades, and the ability to suppress unwanted saccades. Recent evidence has accumulated to suggest that control of these types of behaviors is distributed across a network of cortical and subcortical structures. The premotor circuitry comprising of the superior colliculus, brainstem reticular formation, and cerebellum is now understood at a level that is sufficient to allow for the design of sophisticated behavioral tasks to probe higher brain functions, using the eye movement system as the behavioral readout.

In Section II, two related topics are discussed that have recently received considerable interest in vision research, change blindness and trans-saccadic memory of visual information. Change blindness refers to human perceivers' poor ability to detect abrupt changes in the visual environment, when a change takes place at the same time when the stimulus is temporarily blanked or occluded. The detection may also be poor when the change is made during an eye blink or a saccadic movement. This brings the section to the question of what information is carried over from one eye fixation to the next to yield a stable and continuous percept of the visual world — a question that has interested students of visual perception since Helmholtz' days. In his commentary, Ronald Rensink concludes that the recent studies of change blindness have changed ideas about visual perception and have thus increased our understanding of how vision works.

Section III presents new aspects on the physiology of smooth pursuit eye movements in man and monkey, with a particular focus on low-level and high-level factors influencing their execution. Two of the contributions demonstrate that smooth pursuit is intimately linked to visual motion processing. They present new evidence how pursuit initiation is influenced by different visual motion parameters reflected in the neuronal activity of extrastriate areas MT and MST, with their specific timing and spatial frames of reference. However, pursuit initiation is also modulated by non-target influences such as distracters and disengagement from the fixation point, as well as by high-level vision features such as the cognitive load, the structure of the background, or the predictability of target trajectory. Three of the contributions summarize elaborate studies on the high-level influences of expectancy, learning, and attention. Thus the spotlight of attention is allocated ahead of the moving pursuit target. The commentary by Uwe Ilg integrates these different contributions and important data of his own group into a thorough state-of-the-art review, spanning from the processing of visual motion to cognitive aspects of smooth pursuit execution.

Contributions of Section IV on eye-hand co-ordination deal with the interfacing of the processes and mechanisms of oculomotor control with another very important sensorimotor system. Basic research in this area indicates that the eyes are usually ahead of the hand in moving to a target such that information for online corrections of hand movements can be acquired. However, it is also important to note that co-ordination is of a reciprocal nature: in complex situations, the eyes will also wait for the hands, if necessary. Discussions in this section are centered on such interesting issues as the question of whether both systems share common start signals and target representations and the question of the specific nature of these target representations. Special attention is given to the identification of brain areas that are involved in eye-hand co-ordination and to the clinical applicability of experimental results. One very important new feature of research in this area is that eye-hand co-ordination can now be studied in ecologically valid real life situations. In summary, as Harold Bekkering and Uta Sailer, the section commentators, put it, the research reported on this fascinating topic indicates that "... things are not as simple as they first seem, but secondly, this complexity also enables the enormous flexibility that allows us to effectively interact with our environment".

Section V provides a representative overview on different aspects of clinical eye movement research in neurology and psychiatry, illustrating how oculomotor paradigms can be used to learn about acute and chronic perturbations in brain function, deficits in brain development, disturbances in sensorimotor as well as cognitive systems, and the effects of therapeutic and illicit drugs on brain function. Whereas basic measures of saccadic or smooth pursuit eye movements may be preserved in cerebral hemispheric disease, specific deficits of cognitive, visuo-spatial or visuo-motor functions can nicely be detected by using more complex and natural eye movement tasks, like visual search, or by applying highly sophisticated paradigms for the analysis of specific cortical or cerebellar subfunctions, such as saccadic adaptation, the programming of saccadic sequences, and the inhibitory control of saccades. Finally, one chapter presents mathematical modeling of normal and abnormal eye movement behavior. The commentary by John Sweeney and colleagues discusses these contributions, provides an overview of broad methodological issues involved in applying eye movement studies to psychiatric populations and considers the potential of collaborations between eye movement and brain imaging researchers to advance understanding of clinical eye movement abnormalities and of what they reveal about the organization of the oculomotor system.

A note of thanks goes to all the contributors who made this book come to life and to all reviewers whose insights further improved the quality of submissions. During the course of this project, we felt sorry for the contributors and reviewers who had to perform under considerable time pressure imposed by us.

Jukka Hyönä
Douglas Munoz
Wolfgang Heide
Ralph Radach

May 2002

Contents

List of Contributors v

Preface ix

Section I. Saccadic eye movements
Section Editor: D.P. Munoz

1. Vying for dominance: dynamic interactions control visual fixation and saccadic initiation in the superior colliculus
   D.P. Munoz and J.H. Fecteau (Kingston, ON, Canada) 3

2. Neural control of saccades
   J.D. Enderle (Storrs, CT, USA) 21

3. The latency of saccades toward auditory targets in humans
   D. Zambarbieri (Pavia, Italy) 51

4. Contribution of the primate prefrontal cortex to the gap effect
   C.J. Tinsley and S. Everling (Oxford, UK) 61

5. Influence of stimulus characteristics on the latency of saccadic inhibition
   D.M. Stampe and E.M. Reingold (Toronto, ON, Canada) 73

6. Commentary: Saccadic eye movements: overview of neural circuitry
   D.P. Munoz (Kingston, ON, Canada) 89

Section II. Change blindness and transsaccadic integration
Section Editor: J. Hyönä

7. Converging evidence for the detection of change without awareness
   I.M. Thornton and D. Fernandez-Duque (Tübingen, Germany and Toronto, ON, Canada) 99

8. Blinks, blanks and saccades: how blind we really are for relevant visual events
   S.M. Dornhoefer, P.J.A. Unema and B.M. Velichkovsky (Dresden, Germany and Maastricht, The Netherlands) 119

9. Multiple-object permanence tracking: limitation in maintenance and transformation of perceptual objects
   J. Saiki (Kyoto, Japan) 133

10. What information survives saccades in the real world?
    B.W. Tatler (Sussex, UK) 149

11. Transsaccadic memory of position and form
    H. Deubel, W.X. Schneider and B. Bridgeman (Munich, Germany
    and Santa Cruz, CA, USA) 165

12. Transsaccadic memory for visual object detail
    P. De Graef and K. Verfaillie (Leuven, Belgium) 181

13. Commentary: Changes
    R.A. Rensink (Vancouver, BC, Canada) 197

Section III. Smooth pursuit eye movements
Section Editors: W. Heide and D.P. Munoz

14. Non-target influences on the initiation of smooth pursuit
    P.C. Knox and T. Bekkour (Liverpool, UK) 211

15. Integration of motion cues for the initiation of smooth pursuit eye movements
    R.T. Born, C.C. Pack and R. Zhao (Boston, MA, USA) 225

16. The role of expectancy and volition in smooth pursuit eye movements
    G.R. Barnes, A.M. Schmid and C.B. Jarrett (Manchester, UK and
    Charlestown, MA, USA) 239

17. Visual and cognitive control of attention in smooth pursuit
    Y. Chen, P.S. Holzman and K. Nakayama (Belmont, MA, USA and
    Cambridge, MA, USA) 255

18. The allocation of attention during smooth pursuit eye movements
    P. Van Donkelaar and A.S. Drew (Eugene, OR, USA)............... 267

19. Commentary: Smooth pursuit eye movements: from low-level to high-level vision
    U.J. Ilg (Tübingen, Germany) 279

Section IV. Eye-hand coordination
Section Editor: R. Radach

20. Cortical frames of reference for eye–hand coordination
    P. Van Donkelaar, J.-H. Lee and A.S. Drew (Eugene, OR, USA)..... 301

21. Neuropsychological perspectives on eye–hand coordination in visually-guided reaching
    D.P. Carey, S. Della Sala and M. Ietswaart (Old Aberdeen, UK) 311

22. Visuomotor transformations for eye–hand coordination
        D.Y.P. Henriques, W.P. Medendorp, A.Z. Khan and J.D. Crawford
        (Toronto, ON, Canada) 329

23. Implications of distracter effects for the organization of eye movements, hand
        movements, and perception
        U. Sailer, T. Eggert and A. Straube (Munich, Germany) 341

24. Visual short-term memory and motor planning
        M. Hayhoe, P. Aivar, A. Shrivastavah and R. Mruczek (Rochester,
        NY, USA, Rotterdam, The Netherlands and Providence, RI, USA) .. 349

25. Commentary: Coordination of eye and hand in time and space
        H. Bekkering and U. Sailer (Groningen, The Netherlands and Munich, Germany) 365

Section V. Clinical aspects of eye movement research
Section Editor: W. Heide

26. Visual search in long-term cannabis users with early age of onset
        L. Huestegge, R. Radach, H.-J. Kunert and D. Heller (Aachen,
        Germany) 377

27. Visual search in patients with left visual hemineglect
        A. Sprenger, D. Kömpf and W. Heide (Lübeck, Germany) 395

28. Saccadic adaptation in neurological disorders
        M.R. MacAskill, T.J. Anderson and R.D. Jones (Christchurch, New
        Zealand) 417

29. Saccade sequences as markers for cerebral dysfunction following mild closed
        head injury
        M.H. Heitger, T.J. Anderson and R.D. Jones (Christchurch, New
        Zealand) 433

30. Cognition and the inhibitory control of saccades in schizophrenia and Parkinson's disease
        T.J. Crawford, D. Bennett, G. Lekwuwa, S. Shaunak and J.F.W.
        Deakin (Lancaster, Preston and Manchester, UK) 449

31. Control of volitional and reflexive saccades in Tourette's syndrome
        D.P. Munoz, A.L. LeVasseur and J.R. Flanagan (Kingston, ON,
        Canada) 467

32. Oculomotor control in a group of very low birth weight (VLBW) children
        D. Newsham and P.C. Knox (Liverpool, UK) 483

33. A new framework for investigating both normal and abnormal eye movements
R.A. Clement, R.V. Abadi, D.S. Broomhead and J.P. Whittle (London, Manchester and Sheffield, UK) 499

34. Commentary: Eye movement research with clinical populations
J.A. Sweeney, D. Levy and M.S.H. Harris (Chicago, IL, USA and Boston, MA, USA) 507

Subject Index 523

SECTION I

Saccadic eye movements

Section Editor: D.P. Munoz

CHAPTER 1

Vying for dominance: dynamic interactions control visual fixation and saccadic initiation in the superior colliculus

Douglas P. Munoz* and Jillian H. Fecteau

Centre for Neuroscience Studies, CIHR Group in Sensory–Motor Systems, Department of Physiology, Queen's University, Kingston, ON K7L 3N6, Canada

Abstract: Visual fixation and saccadic initiation are the tools that we use to explore the visual environment. In the superior colliculi, these behaviors may be viewed as independent motor programs that compete for control. Here, we provide a model describing the superior colliculi's involvement in visual fixation and saccadic initiation, in which extrinsic signals (sensory, motor, and cognitive) are shaped into competing motor programs through its local circuitry. In addition to providing evidence in support of this model, we demonstrate that it can explain the differences in the timing of saccadic initiation that have been observed experimentally.

Introduction

By the time you finish reading this sentence, your eyes will have made a series of rapid movements, separated by short intervals in which they are still (e.g., McConkie and Rayner, 1975 and Yang and McConkie, 2001). This alternating pattern of saccadic initiation and visual fixation, respectively, is not limited to activities such as reading text, but occurs whenever the high acuity foveae of the eyes are directed to visual objects of interest (e.g., Yarbus, 1967), which occurs, on average, hundreds of thousands of times a day.

A complex collection of brain areas controls these behaviors including regions of the parietal and frontal cortices, basal ganglia, thalamus, superior colliculus, cerebellum, and brainstem reticular formation (Fig. 1; for recent reviews see: Moschovakis et al., 1996; Leigh and Zee, 1999; Schall and Thompson, 1999; Hikosaka et al., 2000; Munoz et al., 2000; Glimcher, 2001; Scudder et al., 2002). Considering the number of brain areas that are involved, fully understanding the physiological basis of visual fixation and saccadic initiation will not be a simple feat. Nonetheless, significant progress has been made in understanding the basis of these behaviors in the superior colliculi, wherein visual fixation and saccadic initiation can be viewed as independent motor plans that compete for expression. In this chapter, we describe the neurophysiological mechanisms responsible for shaping competing motor plans and how these processes evolve across time. In addition, we will show that differences in the timing of saccadic initiation may be explained through these mechanisms.

Dynamic reciprocal interactions shape visual fixation and saccadic initiation

At the most basic level, the relationship between visual fixation and saccadic initiation can be viewed as a game between two competing processes. Understanding the game requires careful consideration of the field upon which these competing processes hap-

---

* Correspondence to: D.P. Munoz, Centre for Neuroscience Studies, CIHR Group in Sensory–Motor Systems, Department of Physiology, Queen's University, Kingston, ON K7L 3N6, Canada. Tel.: +1-613-533-2111; Fax: +1-613-533-6840; E-mail: doug@eyeml.queensu.ca

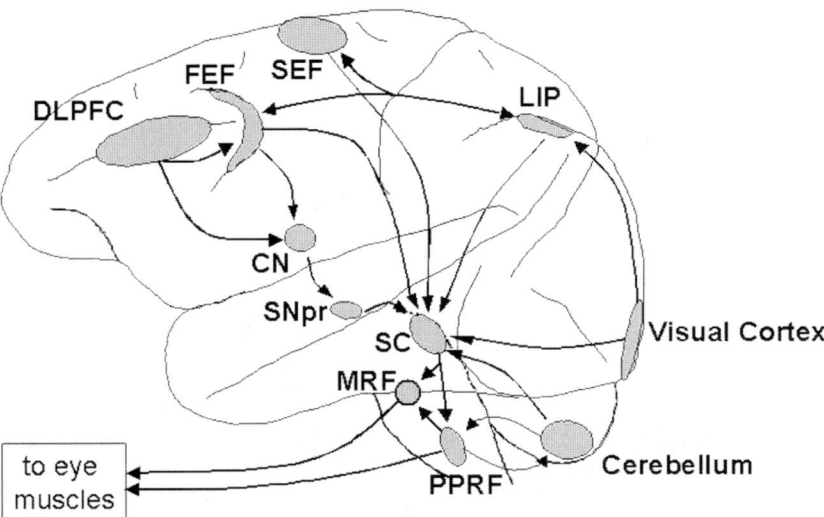

Fig. 1. Lateral view of monkey brain illustrating major areas that are involved in visual fixation and saccadic initiation. CN, caudate nucleus; DLPFC, dorsolateral prefrontal cortex; FEF, frontal eye fields; LIP, lateral intraparietal area; MRF, mesencephalic reticular formation; SC, superior colliculus; SEF, supplementary eye fields; SNpr, substantia nigra pars reticulata.

pen, the players involved, the mechanisms, or rules, governing these interactions, and watching the game unfold.

The intermediate layers of the superior colliculi are the fields upon which these interactions occur. At this depth, neurons are organized into a retinotopically coded motor map that specifies saccades into the contralateral visual field (e.g., Robinson, 1972). As illustrated in Fig. 2A, the amplitude of the saccade increases systematically along the rostral to caudal axis and the direction of the saccade shifts from upwards to downwards along the medial to lateral axis. Extrinsic input from sensory, motor, and cognitive areas modulates the activity of this map (Sparks and Hartwich-Young, 1989), which is shaped into independent motor plans, in part, through local inhibitory interneurons (Mize et al., 1991; Behan and Kime, 1996; Meredith and Ramoa, 1998; Munoz and Istvan, 1998; Olivier et al., 1999).

Broadly speaking, the competition is between two classes of neurons (Fig. 2B). Fixation neurons, located in the rostrolateral pole of the superior colliculus, produce tonic activity during visual fixation and pause during saccades (Munoz and Guitton, 1991; Munoz and Wurtz, 1993a). Saccadic neurons, located throughout the rest of the intermediate layers, produce bursts of action potentials prior to and during the execution of saccades made to their response field (Wurtz and Goldberg, 1972; Sparks et al., 1976; Munoz and Wurtz, 1995a). For ease of communication, the terms 'fixation' and 'saccadic' will be used throughout the rest of this chapter to describe neurons in and regions of the superior colliculus. It is important to realize, however, that this distinction is misleading for two reasons. First, rather than forming two distinct classes of neurons, fixation and saccadic neurons may consist of one class of neurons that encode actions (Munoz and Guitton, 1991; Munoz and Wurtz, 1995b; Krauzlis et al., 1997, 2000). The different characteristics expressed by these neurons arise from their position on the motor map. Fixation neurons respond to foveal and parafoveal input and encode actions specific to that location, maintaining gaze and initiating small (<2°) saccades. Saccadic neurons respond to more eccentric regions in the contralateral visual field and encode actions specific to that location, initiating saccades. Second, although the interactions between fixation and saccadic neurons will be focused upon in this review, it should be realized that competing motor plans can be formed anywhere across the motor map (Basso and Wurtz, 1997; Munoz and Istvan, 1998).

Two rules govern the interactions between the neurons in the intermediate layers. The first rule is that

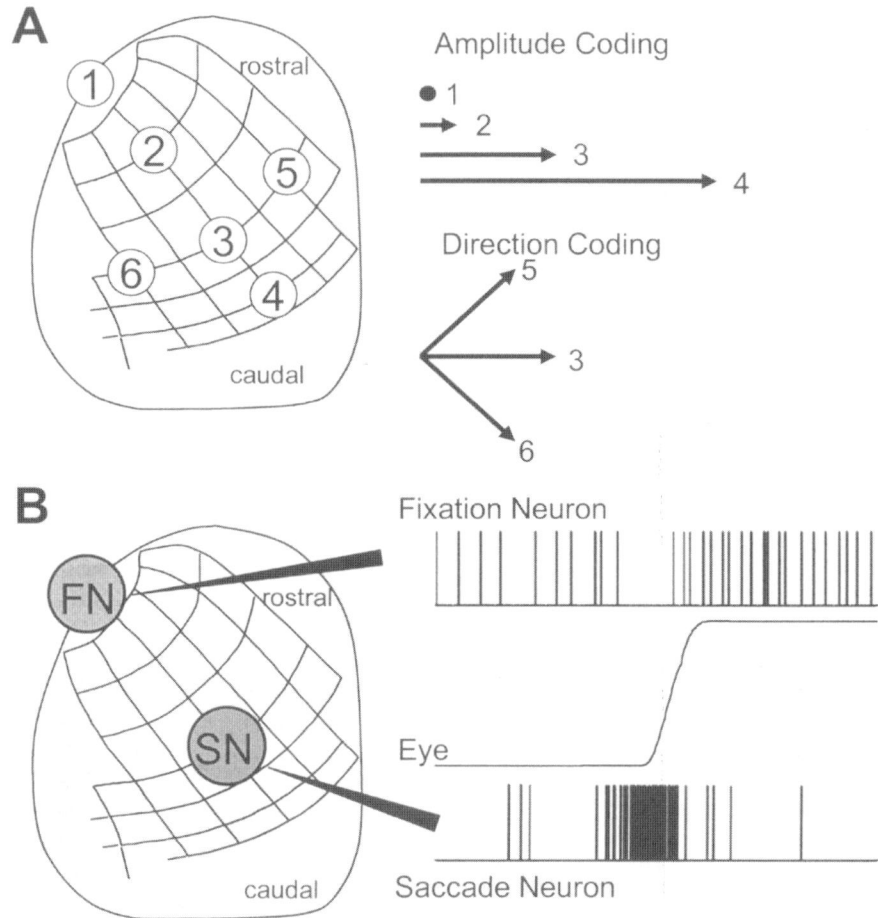

Fig. 2. Superior colliculus' retinotopic motor map. (A) Representation of amplitude (sites 1–4) and direction (sites 3, 5, 6) coding of rightward saccadic vectors in the left superior colliculus. (B) Typical discharge characteristics of a fixation neuron (FN) and a saccadic neuron (SN) in the left superior colliculus when monkey initiates a rightward saccade.

the activity of one region, or node, facilitates nodes that are nearby and inhibits nodes that are more distant, as illustrated in Fig. 3. The second rule is that the amount of activity expressed in the intermediate layers remains reasonably constant; with only the distribution of this activity changing. Therefore, if the activity of one node is strong, then the inhibition of distant nodes will be strong (solid line). If the activity of one node is weak, then the inhibition of distant nodes will be weak (dotted line).

'Watching' the game can be imagined with a simple example. The participant's job is to initiate saccades to visual targets that appear to the left side or to the right side of fixation. At the beginning of each trial, the participant maintains gaze at center and waits for the target to appear. Actively maintaining gaze constitutes a motor plan that is correlated with bilateral tonic activity in the fixation region in the rostral colliculi (Fig. 4A). Shortly after, a visual target appears to the right side. This sensory input enhances a point location in the left colliculus and changes the balance of activity across the intermediate layers: nearby nodes are facilitated and distant nodes are inhibited (Fig. 4B). Ultimately, the saccadic plan is initiated, which is correlated with a strong burst of action potentials in a caudal region of the left colliculus that shuts down the rest of the map in a winner-takes-all fashion (Fig. 4C).

If this dynamic interactions model is accurate, then altering the balance of activity in the interme-

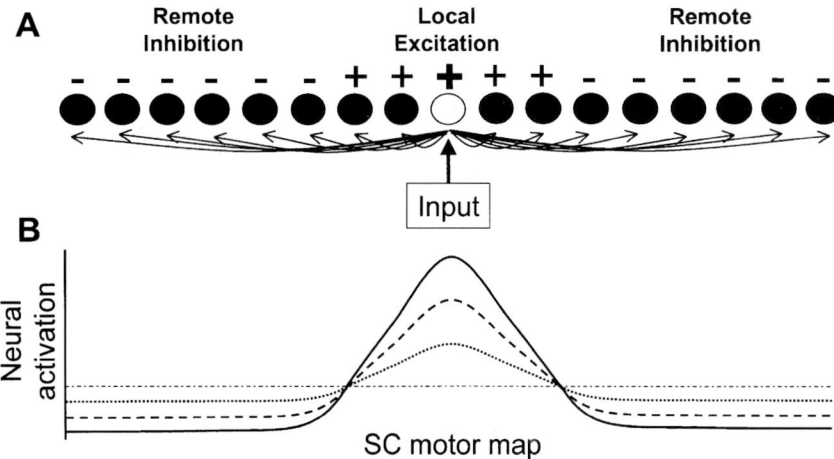

Fig. 3. Schematic representation of the dynamic interactions across the intermediate layers. (A) Local and distant interactions. Each circle represents an individual node. Extrinsic input to one node excites local nodes (plus signs) and inhibits distant nodes (minus signs). (B) Relative distribution of activity. The intensity of the extrinsic input alters the relative distribution of activity across the intermediate layers. See text for further details.

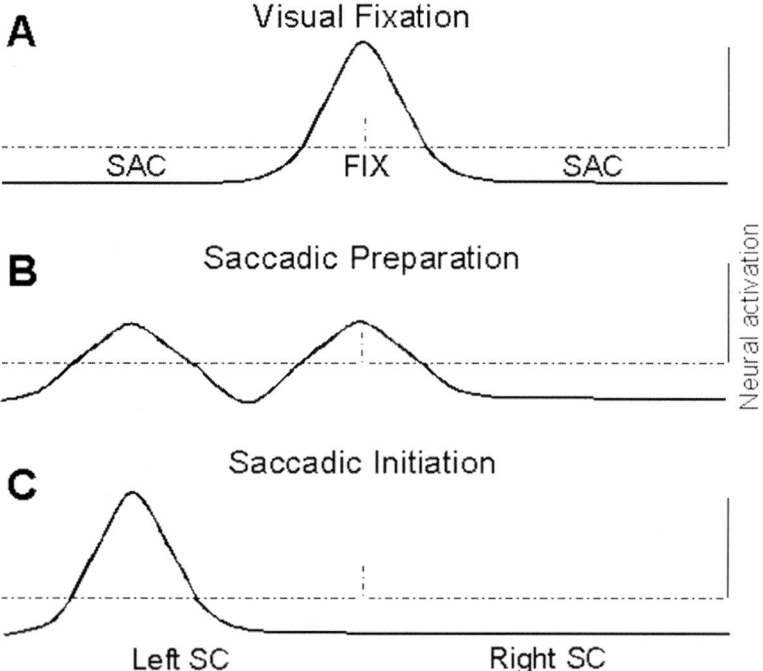

Fig. 4. Dynamic interactions unfold across time. Schematic representation of the distribution of activity across the intermediate layers of both colliculi during (A) visual fixation, (B) saccadic preparation, and (C) saccadic initiation.

diate layers, artificially, will have predictable consequences on neuronal excitability and behavior. This idea has been tested in two ways: (1) by facilitating confined regions of the intermediate layers with microstimulation and monitoring its influence on fixation and saccadic neurons located across the motor map (Munoz and Istvan, 1998), and (2) by facilitating and inhibiting regions of the intermediate layers with different chemical compounds and observing the consequences on behavior (Hikosaka and Wurtz, 1985; Munoz and Wurtz, 1993b).

Munoz and Istvan (1998) recorded the activity of fixation and saccadic neurons while monkeys initiated saccades to eccentric targets. On a selected proportion of trials, different regions of the intermediate layers were stimulated electrically and the ensuing effects on fixation and saccadic neurons were observed. The timing of microstimulation depended on the class of neurons that was being monitored. When fixation neurons were monitored, stimulation was applied when the monkey was actively fixating the central fixation marker (e.g., Fig. 4A). When saccadic neurons were monitored, stimulation was applied when a saccade was being initiated into the neuron's response field (e.g., Fig. 4C). Four regions of the superior colliculus were stimulated relative to the recording site; fixation regions or saccadic regions were stimulated on the same side as the recording electrode or on the opposite side as the recording electrode.

The findings from this study were consistent with the dynamic interactions model. Stimulating saccadic regions inhibited both fixation (Fig. 5A) and saccadic (not shown) neurons that were distant from the stimulation locus at very short latencies. Stimulating fixation regions inhibited saccadic neurons at very short latencies (Fig. 5B). In both instances, the inhibition was more potent and was evident earlier when the ipsilateral side was stimulated compared to the contralateral side. Importantly, stimulating one fixation region excited fixation neurons on the contralateral side (Munoz and Istvan, 1998). Based on these data and complementary studies in anaesthetized animals (McIlwain, 1982) and reduced preparations (Meredith and Ramoa, 1998), artificially enhancing specific regions of the intermediate layers with microstimulation, inhibits nodes that are distant and facilitates nodes that are, functionally, nearby.

Modifying the distribution of activity across the intermediate layers with pharmacological manipulations also has predictable consequences on behavior. Increasing the activity of one region should facilitate actions that are supported by that region and inhibit actions made elsewhere, whereas de-

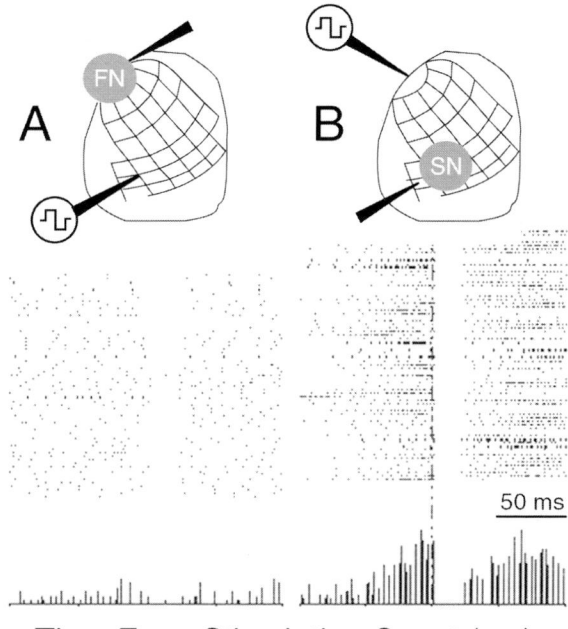

Fig. 5. Neurophysiological evidence supporting dynamic interactions model. (A) Stimulating saccadic regions produces potent, short-latency inhibition of fixation neurons (FN). (B). Stimulating fixation regions produces potent, short-latency inhibition of saccadic neurons (SN). Rasters and histograms are aligned on stimulation onset (dashed vertical line). Adapted from Munoz and Istvan (1998).

creasing the activity of one region should inhibit actions that are supported by that region and facilitate actions made elsewhere. These predictions have been confirmed. Facilitating the fixation region with bicuculline (black bars in Fig. 6A), a $GABA_A$ antagonist, increased the reaction time of saccades (Munoz and Wurtz, 1993b). Inhibiting the fixation region with a microinjection of muscimol (gray bars in Fig. 6A), a $GABA_A$ agonist, decreased saccadic reaction times (Munoz and Wurtz, 1993b). As illustrated in Fig. 6B, the opposite pattern was obtained when the excitability of saccadic neurons was altered. Microinjection of bicuculline into a saccadic region shortened saccadic reaction times, while injecting muscimol increased saccadic reaction times (Hikosaka and Wurtz, 1985). Thus, modifying the activity of specific regions of the motor map affects behavior in a manner that is consistent with the dynamic interactions model.

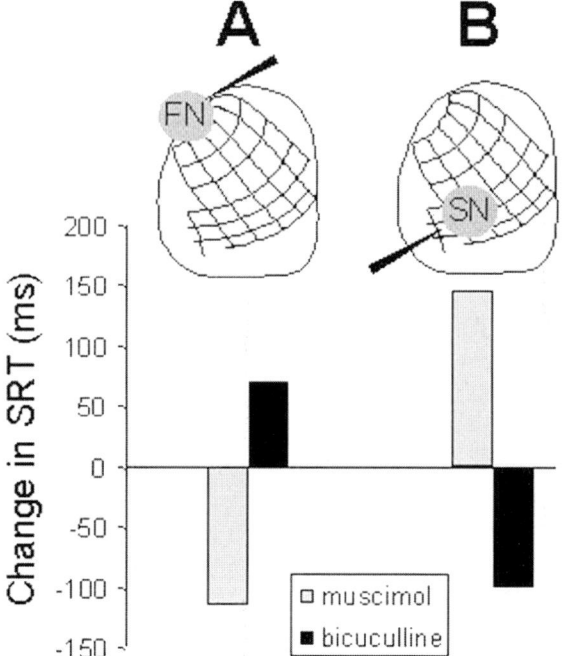

Fig. 6. Pharmacological manipulations support dynamic interactions model. (A) Modulating activity of fixation regions with muscimol (gray bars) decreases saccadic reaction times, whereas bicuculline (black bars) increases saccadic reaction times. (B) Modulating activity of saccadic regions with muscimol increases saccadic reaction times, whereas bicuculline decreases saccadic reaction times. Data adapted from Munoz and Wurtz (1993b) and Hikosaka and Wurtz (1985).

Up to this point, the evidence that we have described speaks to distant interactions across the intermediate layers, in most instances. Yet, the dynamic interactions model also makes specific predictions for local interactions. Using a different technique, we have probed both local and distant interactions across the intermediate layers. Behavioral evidence has demonstrated that presenting an irrelevant distractor influences responding to a target and its influence depends on the relative distance between target and distractor. If the distractor appears close to the target, then saccadic reaction time is reduced. If the distractor appears far from the target, then saccadic reaction time is increased (Walker et al., 1997; Olivier et al., 1999). These behavioral observations match the dynamic interactions model perfectly. Presenting a distractor will excite neighboring nodes in the intermediate layers, enhancing their responsiveness to a nearby target. Presenting a distractor will inhibit distant nodes, impairing their responsiveness to a remote target.

The activity of saccadic neurons was monitored as monkeys performed the distractor task that was described above (Olivier et al., 1999). As illustrated in Fig. 7, the results from this study provided compelling support for the dynamic interactions model. Compared to the control condition, in which no distractor was presented (Fig. 7A), presenting a distractor close to the target caused a saccade to be initiated immediately following presentation of the target (see arrow Fig. 7B), whereas presenting a distractor far from the target inhibited the low frequency activity of the neuron, making it more difficult for the neuron to reach threshold (see arrow Fig. 7C).

All told, a picture emerges in which the alternating pattern of visual fixation and saccadic initiation arises, at least in part, from dynamic interactions across the intermediate layers of the superior colliculi. Extrinsic input selectively enhances confined regions of the intermediate layers that changes the distribution of activity elsewhere in the map in a push–pull fashion: nearby nodes are facilitated and distant nodes are inhibited (see Fig. 3). These dynamic interactions shape competing motor plans across the intermediate layers. When one of these plans reaches threshold, it produces a strong burst of activity and inhibits other regions in a 'winner-take-all' fashion, allowing a saccade to be initiated (see Trappenberg et al., 2001 for implementation of the model). Enhancing or inhibiting specific regions of the intermediate layers has provided compelling support for this model.

Evidence supporting dynamic reciprocal interactions: behavioral anomalies explained

As a model of motor planning, saccadic eye movements are an ideal action to study because they are very stereotyped. However, this characteristic also makes it more difficult to push the boundaries of the dynamic interactions model to see if it can explain the exception to the rule, as well as the rule itself. In this section, we describe several instances in which the timing of saccadic initiation has been altered, allowing us to probe the predictions of the dynamic interactions model in these boundary conditions.

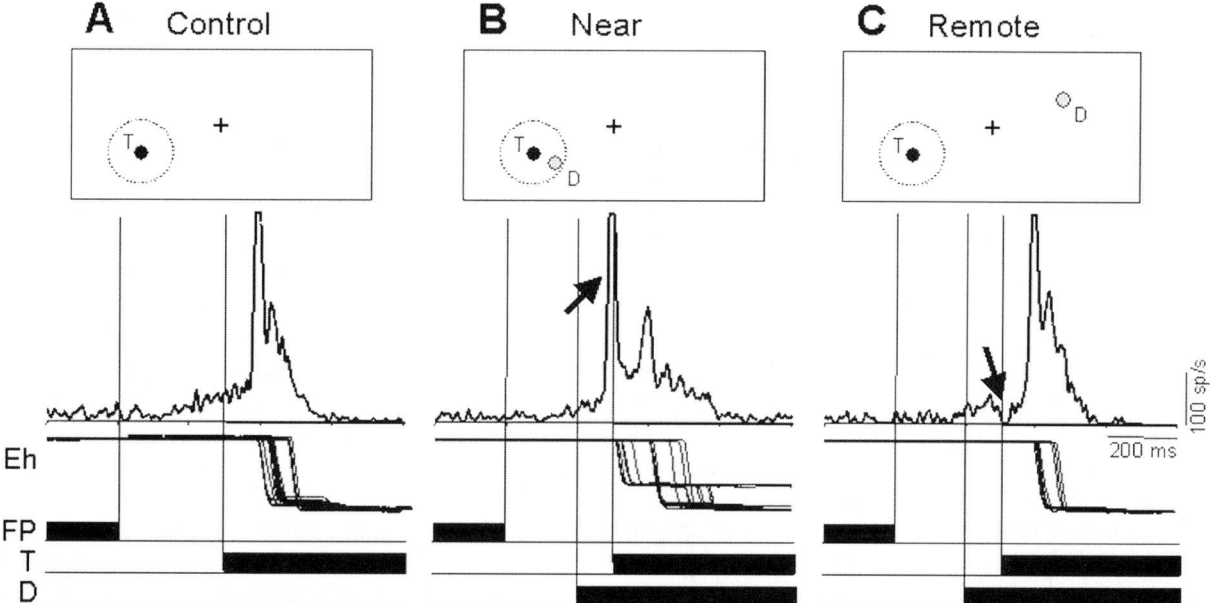

Fig. 7. Distractor effects on pretarget activity of saccadic neurons support dynamic interactions model. (A) Control trials reveal buildup of pretarget activity that precedes target- and saccade-related bursts after the target appears (black circle) in the neuron's response field (dotted circle). (B) Presentation of near distractor (gray circle) 100 ms before target appearance facilitates neuron (marked by black arrow) and often triggers express saccades to the distractor. (C) Remote distractor inhibits neurons (marked by black arrow) and delays the onset of the saccade. Illustrated from top to bottom in each panel are a schematic of target and distractor locations, the spike density waveform, horizontal eye position (Eh), and traces depicting the timing of fixation point (FP) disappearance, target (T) and distractor (D) appearance.

Before doing so, a brief reminder of the basic saccadic task will be provided because minor modifications to this task change the timing of saccadic initiation. In this task (Fig. 4), each trial begins with the monkey fixating a central marker. A target then appears to an eccentric position in the visual field to which the monkey initiates a saccade. In the following subsections, the modifications made to this paradigm, the corresponding behavioral and neurophysiological consequences, and the interpretation of these changes, with regard to the dynamic interactions model, are described.

The gap effect

The 'gap effect' refers to the observation that inserting a short temporal gap in between the disappearance of the fixation point and the appearance of a target reduces saccadic reaction times (Saslow, 1967). Two, not mutually exclusive, theories have been provided to explain this effect. First, the gap may act as a non-localized warning signal, increasing the observer's readiness to respond to the target (e.g., Kingstone and Klein, 1993; Paré and Munoz, 1996). Second, the gap may disengage attention, or oculomotor fixation, which reduces saccadic reaction times because one step involved in initiating the saccade has been eliminated (Mayfrank et al., 1986; Fischer and Weber, 1993).

Within the dynamic interactions framework, readiness and oculomotor disengagement have straightforward neurophysiological consequences. 'Readiness' may be evidenced as non-localized extrinsic input that modulates the excitability of the intermediate layers. 'Oculomotor disengagement' may be evidenced as decreased activity of fixation neurons.

Indeed, such neurophysiological correlates have been observed in the intermediate layers when monkeys perform the gap saccade task. Before we describe these effects fully, we will first provide additional detail about the characteristics of fixation and saccadic neurons because understanding these characteristics helps reveal the consequences of 'readiness' and 'oculomotor disengagement'.

Up to now, two 'classes' of neurons have been described in the intermediate layers, fixation neurons that represent foveal and parafoveal regions and saccadic neurons that represent more eccentric regions of the motor map. This simplistic representation is somewhat misleading because saccadic neurons have additional characteristics that can be used to divide them into different categories, including (1) the presence or absence of long-lead activity prior to saccadic initiation, (2) the shape of their movement fields, and (3) the depth below the dorsal surface of the superior colliculus (Munoz and Wurtz, 1995a,b)[1]. Burst neurons produce brief, high frequency discharges for saccades that fall within a small range of amplitudes and directions (i.e., closed movement field) and tend to reside more superficially in the intermediate layers. Buildup neurons often begin firing well before saccadic initiation, discharge for all saccades whose amplitudes are equal to or greater than their optimal (i.e., open-ended movement fields) and tend to reside deeper in the intermediate layers. Fixation neurons, like buildup neurons, are located in deeper parts of the intermediate layers and have open-ended movement fields.

The characteristic firing pattern of each neuron type is illustrated in Fig. 8 for the gap saccade task. Before the target appears, fixation neurons (Fig. 8B) are tonically active when the fixation marker is visible (left side of left vertical line) and this activity continues during the gap period, albeit at a reduced rate (right side of left vertical line); burst neurons (Fig. 8C) are silent during this interval, and buildup neurons (Fig. 8D) begin to discharge at a low frequency tonic rate during the gap period. After the target appears (right side of right vertical line), a saccade is initiated. At the time of saccadic initiation, fixation neurons pause and burst and buildup neurons produce a high frequency burst of action potentials. Owing to the shared characteristics of buildup and fixation neurons, we have proposed that these neurons participate in the dynamic interactions across the intermediate layers, whereas burst neurons amplify the saccade-related signals (Wurtz and Munoz, 1995; Trappenberg et al., 2001). We mention this difference because the neutal correlates of readiness and oculomotor disengagement are manifest in the low frequency, tonic activity of fixation and buildup neurons.

We explored the neurophysiological consequences of the gap effect on the dynamic interactions between fixation and buildup neurons (Dorris and Munoz, 1995; Dorris et al., 1997). If fixation and buildup neurons do interact in a reciprocal manner, then removing the fixation marker should decrease the activity of fixation neurons and increase the excitability of buildup neurons. As illustrated in Fig. 9A, this exact pattern was observed. From a relatively stable rate of discharge during visual fixation, the activity of fixation neurons began to decline about 100 ms after the fixation marker disappeared and reached a nadir 200–300 ms into the gap before rising toward a level slightly less than that observed during visual fixation. Correspondingly, the activity of buildup neurons increased during the gap starting ~100 ms after the fixation marker disappeared and reached a maximum rate about 250 ms into the gap period. As illustrated in Fig. 9B, the mean saccadic reaction times measured from trials with different gap durations followed the same pattern as the activity recorded from fixation and buildup neurons for long (≥ 600 ms) gap duration trials. That is, mean saccadic reaction times were lowest for gap durations of 200–300 ms, when the pretarget fixation activity was at its minimum and the buildup activity was at its maximum.

In summary, the gap effect can be interpreted easily within our model. The gap has two interactive influences; it decreases the tonic activity of fixation neurons and increases the low frequency, pretarget activity of buildup neurons. These reciprocal interactions in the intermediate layers produce the shorter saccadic reaction times that are observed in behavior.

Motor preparation

One shortcoming of the 'readiness' explanation is that the low frequency activity of buildup neurons can be localized in some circumstances (Glimcher and Sparks, 1992). Thus, rather than being an unlo-

---

[1] Like fixation and saccadic neurons, burst and buildup neurons may represent opposite ends of one continuum of neurons rather than two distinct classes of neurons.

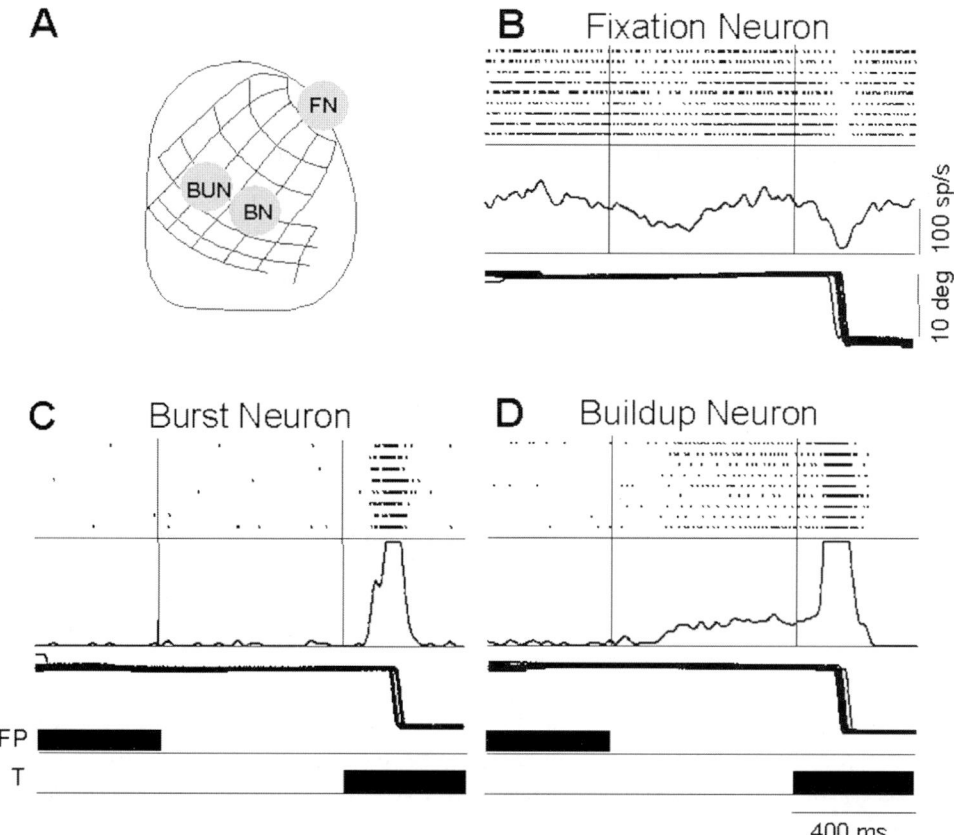

Fig. 8. Characteristic discharge patterns of a fixation neuron (B), a burst neuron (C), and a buildup neuron (D) during the gap saccade task. In this example, the fixation point (FP) disappears (left vertical line) 600 ms before the target (T) appears (right vertical line).

calized 'readiness' signal, this low frequency activity may signify 'motor preparation' that is specific to potential target locations. Considering that only two target locations were used in the gap saccade task (Dorris et al., 1997) and that multiple motor plans can be programmed concurrently (Basso and Wurtz, 1997; McPeek and Keller, 2002), this notion has substantial merit. We tested this question by manipulating the probable location of the target in the gap saccade task, which could appear in two locations equally often, or in one location 100% of the time (Dorris and Munoz, 1998). If the low frequency pretarget activity is a sign of 'readiness', then it should be similar in all three conditions. If, however, the low frequency activity is a sign of 'motor preparation', then the buildup activity should be greatest when the target appears in the neuron's response field 100% of the time, intermediate when the target appears in the neuron's response field 50% of the time, and virtually absent when the target never appears in the neuron's response field.

As illustrated in Fig. 10A, the findings from this study were entirely consistent with a motor preparation explanation. In addition, this finding supports the dynamic interactions model because the level of pretarget activity in the 100% in response field condition was approximately double of that observed in the 50% in response field condition, suggesting that the level of activity is being divided between two locations in the latter case (Fig. 10B).

Indeed, if the activity codes motor preparation, then greater pretarget activity should be correlated with shorter saccadic reaction times. This is precisely what was observed when pretarget activity of buildup neurons and saccadic reaction times were compared on a trial-by-trial basis (Dorris and Munoz, 1998).

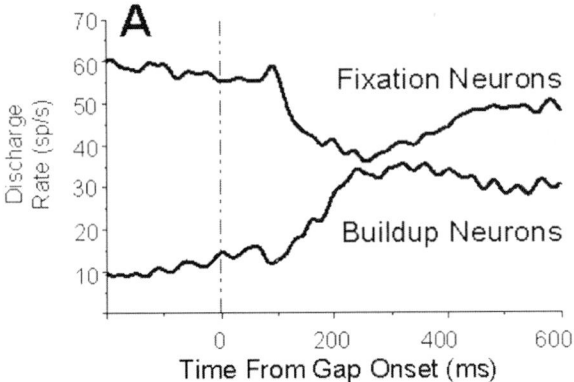

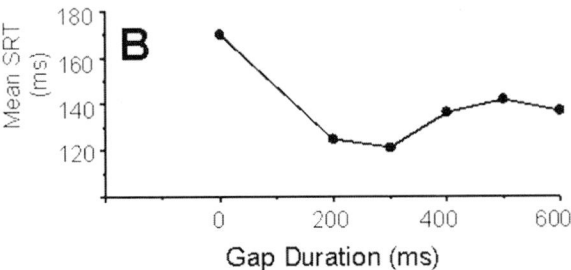

Fig. 9. Gap effect on pretarget activity and saccadic reaction times. (A) Population responses of fixation and buildup neurons in the gap saccade task with a gap period 600 ms. (B) Mean saccadic reaction times of trials with gap periods of 0, 200, 300, 400, 500, and 600 ms.

Thus, pretarget activity represents an early motor preparation signal that prepares the oculomotor system for an impending saccade.

Express saccades

Combining a gap period with a probability manipulation has the additional consequence of creating a bimodal distribution of saccadic reaction times, as illustrated in Fig. 11A. Regular latency saccades (>150 ms) exceed the minimum afferent and efferent conduction times that are needed for visual input to initiate a saccade (Carpenter, 1981). Express saccades (~100 ms), on the other hand, approach the minimal time required for sensory–motor transformation to occur (Fischer and Weber, 1993).

The gap effect describes the speeding up of regular saccades whenever a gap is introduced (Saslow, 1967). Express saccades, alternatively, require additional factors to be obtained, including a predictable target location and temporal regularity of its appearance (Fischer et al., 1984; Boch and Fischer, 1986; Rohrer and Sparks, 1993; Sommer, 1994; Paré and Munoz, 1996). Accordingly, we have hypothesized that express saccades require advanced motor preparation to be obtained (Paré and Munoz, 1996). Put into context of the dynamic interactions model, extrinsic preparatory input to a specific region of the motor map combined with increased excitability of saccadic regions (owing to decreased activity of fixation neurons) will produce express saccades when an abrupt visual transient appears at the location being prepared (Paré and Munoz, 1996).

Regular and express saccades have markedly different neurophysiological signatures (Edelman and Keller, 1996; Dorris et al., 1997). Regular saccades are associated with two bursts of action potentials, one in response to the target's appearance and one in response to the motor action (Fig. 11C). Express saccades, on the other hand, are associated with one burst of action potentials, a combined visuomotor burst (Fig. 11B).

We wondered if differences in pretarget activity might account for the differences between regular and express saccades. This appears to be the case (Dorris et al., 1997). Regular saccades were generated when pretarget activity was low. Express saccades were generated when pretarget activity was high. In all likelihood, pretarget activity may determine how close the system is to achieving threshold for saccadic initiation (Fig. 12). When pretarget activity is low, the target-related response does not exceed the saccadic threshold and a later signal is required to trigger a saccade. When pretarget activity is high, the target-related response exceeds saccadic threshold and triggers a saccade at express latency.

In summary, express saccades are a special instance of saccadic initiation, in which localized input to a particular region of the motor map elevates pretarget activity to a high level, allowing the appearance of a visual target to elicit a saccade immediately. Thus, express saccades depend on a unique combination of dynamic interactions that permit the immediate initiation of a saccade to a visual target.

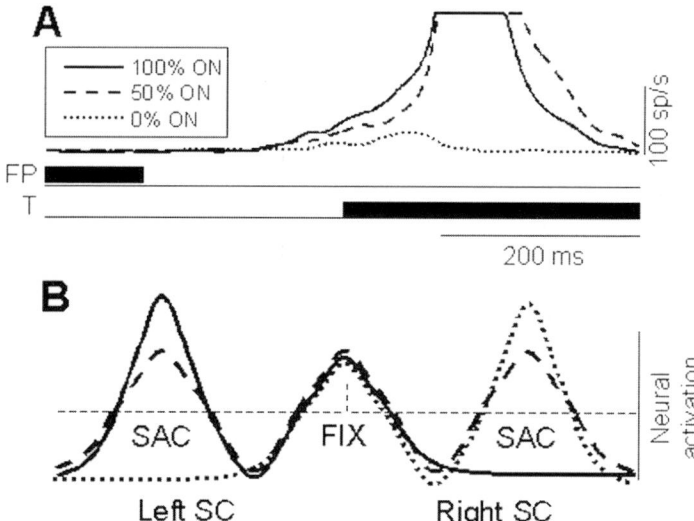

Fig. 10. Probability effects on pretarget activity of buildup neurons. (A) Spike density waveform of a buildup neuron when the target appeared in the neuron's response field 100% (solid line) 50% (dashed line) or 0% (dotted line) of the time. (B) Schematic representation of pretarget activity across intermediate layers when the probability of the target location is manipulated within a block of trials: 100% right (solid line), 100% left (dotted line), 50% right and 50% left (dashed line). Adapted from Dorris and Munoz (1998).

Antisaccades

Up to now, all of the tasks that have been described share one common feature, i.e., saccades were directed to a visual target. However, the relationship between visual targets and saccades can be more flexible than this. Indeed, a saccade may be initiated to any region of the visual field, even when a competing visual target is presented at the same time. The antisaccade task specifically assesses this ability. In this task, participants must (1) suppress the urge to initiate a saccade to a visual target, and (2) initiate a saccade to the target's mirror location (Hallett, 1978). Antisaccades provide a novel way of exploring the dynamic interactions across the intermediate layers because sensory and motor signals are dissociated and, therefore, are being represented in competing regions of the motor map in opposite colliculi.

We explored this possibility by monitoring fixation and saccadic neurons in the intermediate layers, while monkeys initiated prosaccades (saccade to target) and antisaccades (saccade away from target) in the same block of trials (Everling et al., 1998, 1999; Bell et al., 2000). The color of the fixation marker indicated the response that was required on each trial. In addition, a 200 ms gap was presented on half of the trials to further change the dynamics of the intermediate layers during this task.

Saccadic reaction times were longer and the number of errors was greater for antisaccades than for prosaccades, as illustrated in Fig. 13. Introducing a gap enhanced this difference, by increasing the number of direction errors that were made on antisaccade trials.

The neural correlates of prosaccades and antisaccades were compared in several different epochs (Everling et al., 1998, 1999). Understanding the purpose of each epoch requires breaking down a single trial into its basic components. The appearance of the fixation marker has two consequences: (1) it instructs the response (i.e., prosaccade or antisaccade) that is required on each trial and (2) it warns the participant that a target will appear soon. Thus, the fixation epoch induces a cognitive set for the upcoming trial. Then, the target appears or the fixation marker is removed for 200 ms before the target appears. As has been noted above, presenting or not presenting a gap modifies the excitability of saccadic regions in the intermediate layers. The target's position specifies the location to which a saccade must be initiated and then the saccadic plan is generated.

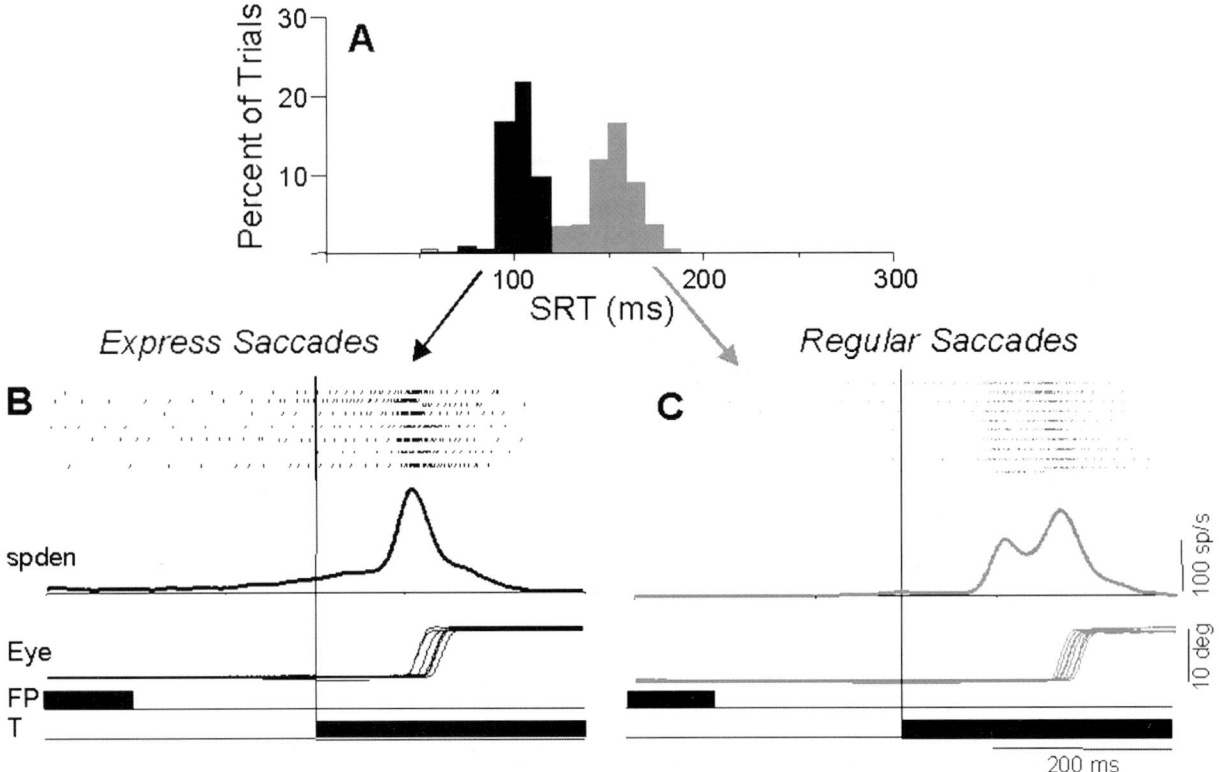

Fig. 11. Neurophysiological correlate of distribution of saccadic reaction times. (A) Bimodal distribution of saccadic reaction times in the gap saccade task. Neurophysiological signatures of (B) express saccades and (C) regular saccades recorded from a buildup neuron. Adapted from Dorris et al. (1997).

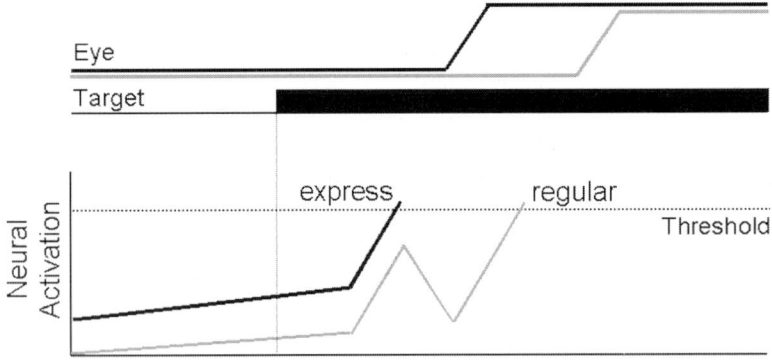

Fig. 12. Schematic representation of neural activity as it accumulates towards saccadic threshold. For express saccades, a high level of pretarget activity is combined with a target-related response and threshold for a saccade is met. For regular saccades, lower pretarget activity does not allow the target-related response to reach saccadic threshold; and a later saccade-related signal is required.

Fig. 14 illustrates the activity of a fixation neuron during prosaccade and antisaccade trials in the overlap (Fig. 14A) and in the gap (Fig. 14B) conditions. The activity of the fixation neuron changed depending on the trial that was being performed (Everling et al., 1999). Upon presentation of the fixation marker,

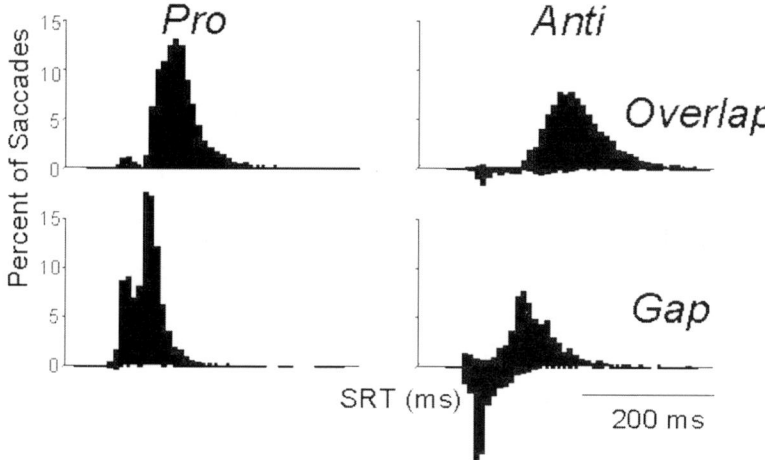

Fig. 13. Distribution of saccadic reaction times in the combined pro-/anti-saccade task. Values above *x*-axis represent correct responses, values below *x*-axis represent direction errors. Adapted from Bell et al. (2000).

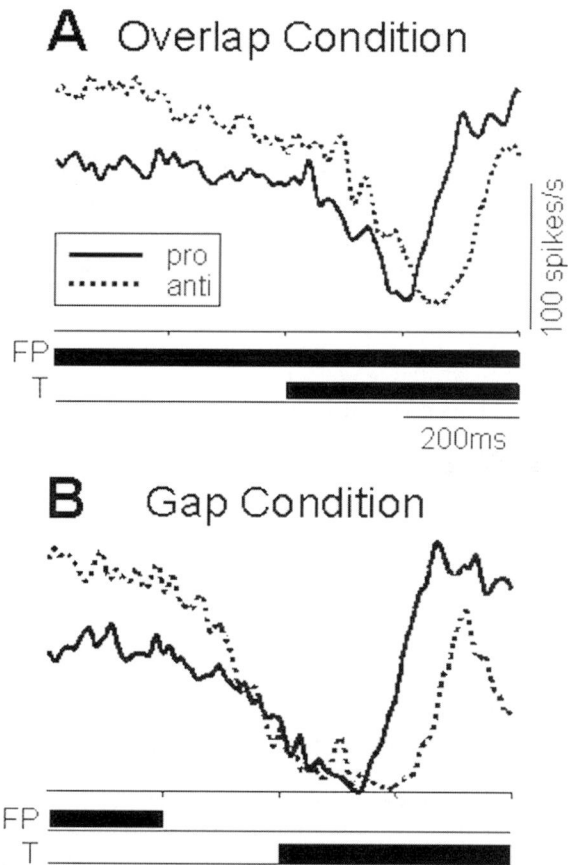

Fig. 14. Discharge of a fixation neuron in the combined pro-/anti-saccade task for overlap (A) and gap (B) conditions. Adapted from Everling et al. (1999).

the fixation neuron elicited more activity for antisaccade trials than for prosaccade trials. In the overlap condition (fixation marker illuminated throughout entire trial), this heightened level of tonic activity was maintained into the target epoch (Fig. 14A). In the gap condition, the tonic activity of the fixation neuron decreased during the gap period to the same rate in prosaccade and antisaccade trials (Fig. 14B). The fixation neuron then paused during the saccade in all conditions (Fig. 14).

Fig. 15 illustrates the activity of a buildup neuron during prosaccade and antisaccade trials in the gap condition when the target appeared in the neuron's response field (Fig. 15A) or the saccade was directed into the neuron's response field (Fig. 15B). The activity of the buildup neuron was greater for prosaccade trials than for antisaccade trials (Everling et al., 1999), which was particularly notable for target-related and saccade-related discharges. In addition, less pretarget activity was observed on antisaccade trials. A similar pattern of findings was obtained for the overlap condition (not shown).

These findings are consistent with the dynamic interactions model. For prosaccades, the target appeared in and the saccade was initiated to the same location. As a consequence, there was no disparity between the two signals and strong bursts of action potentials were elicited for both. For antisaccades, however, the target appeared in and the saccade was generated to opposite fields. As a consequence, the

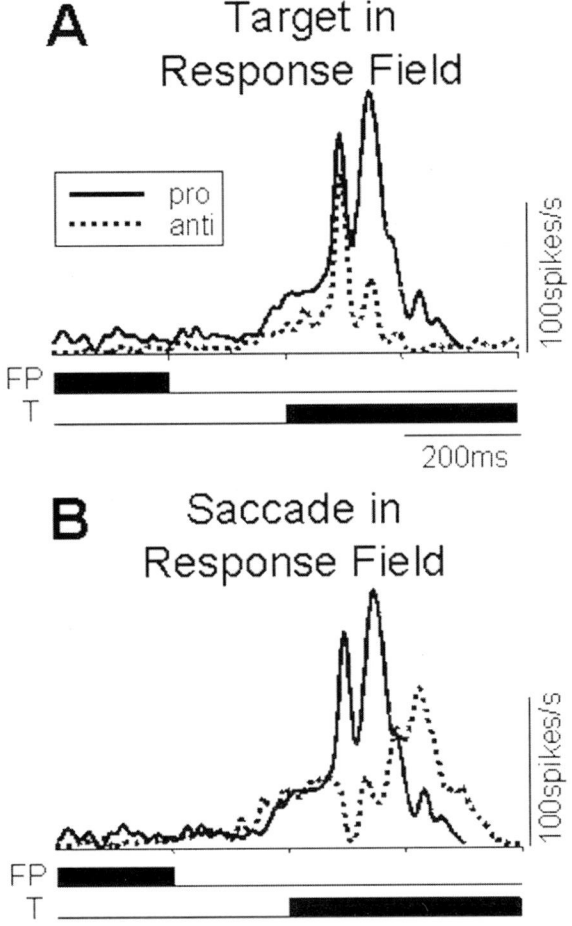

Fig. 15. Discharge of a buildup neuron in the combined pro-/anti-saccade task in the gap condition for trials in which the target (A) or the saccade (B) was directed into the neuron's response field. Adapted from Everling et al. (1999).

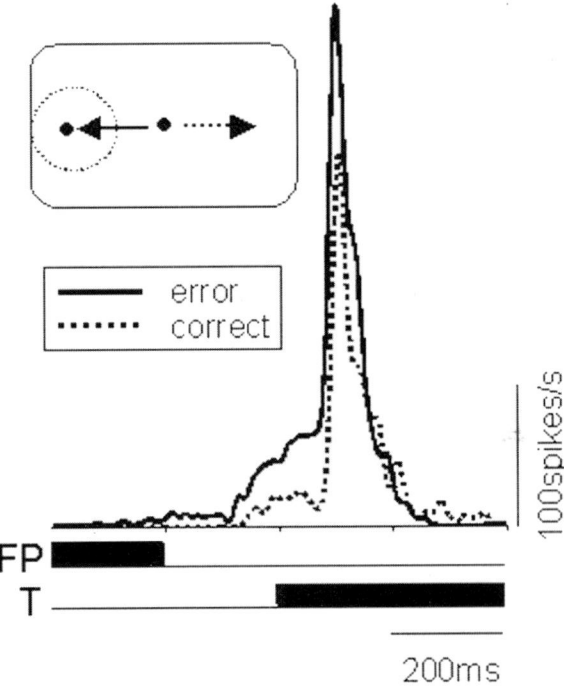

Fig. 16. Discharge of a buildup neuron for correct and error trials initiated in the anti-gap condition in which the target was located in the neuron's response field and the correct response was to look away. Adapted from Everling et al. (1998).

target-related and saccade-related signals were in competing regions of the motor map. These competitive interactions were responsible for the delay in saccadic reaction times for antisaccade trials (see Fig. 13). Also consider that pretarget activity may be detrimental for generation of correct antisaccade responses because, when the target-related response is added, this combined activity could exceed saccadic threshold (see Fig. 12) and a saccade would be generated to the target's location. For antisaccades initiating a saccade to the target is an error.

If this explanation is accurate, then comparing correctly executed and incorrectly executed responses should reveal greater pretarget activity when an error is made. As illustrated in Fig. 16, this expected pattern was obtained (Everling et al., 1998). More pretarget activity was observed for incorrectly executed trials. In many instances, the elevated pretarget activity was sufficient to initiate a saccade at express latency.

In summary, antisaccades have a special influence on the dynamic interactions across the intermediate layers because fixation neurons, saccadic neurons that encode the visual target, and saccadic neurons that encode the motor action act as competing motor plans. Fig. 17 depicts the dynamic interactions across the intermediate layers for prosaccade and antisaccade responses. During visual fixation (Fig. 17A), fixation neurons are more active on antisaccade trials, leading to greater inhibition of saccadic neurons. In this case, greater fixation-related activity is beneficial because it makes it harder for the visual target to trigger a saccade, allowing a saccade to be executed in the opposite direction. When the target appears to

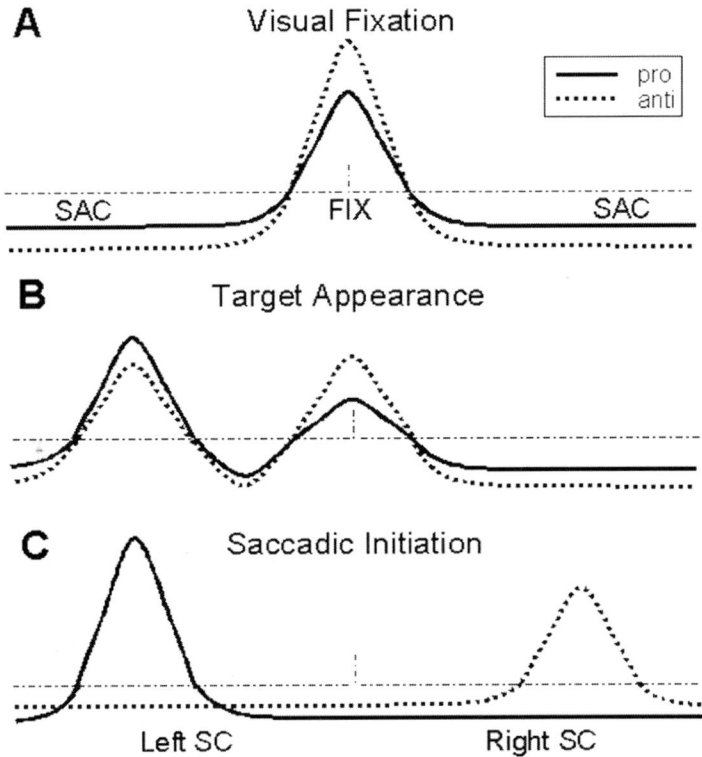

Fig. 17. Schematic representation contrasting activity on collicular motor map for prosaccade (solid lines) and antisaccade (dotted lines) trials.

the right side (Fig. 17B), it elicits a burst of action potentials in the left colliculus. This target-related activity is attenuated for antisaccade trials because the fixation-related activity is still exerting a strong influence on the interactions across the intermediate layers. Eventually a saccade is planned and this plan is initiated. For prosaccade trials, a large burst of action potentials is obtained (Fig. 17C). However, for antisaccade trials, a saccade is planned to the left side (right colliculus) that competes with the target-related activity in the left colliculus and the residual fixation-related activity at the fovea. These competing signals attenuate the saccade-related activity (Fig. 17C) and delay the development of the saccadic burst activity, leading to longer reaction times for antisaccades.

Summary

By the time you have reached this point, your daily count of alternating saccades and fixations will have increased considerably. So too will have your understanding of the dynamic interactions model.

In the superior colliculi, visual fixation and saccadic initiation may be viewed as independent motor plans that compete for dominance across the intermediate layers. Extrinsic input modifies a point location on the retinotopic motor map that is shaped into a motor plan through the intrinsic circuitry of the superior colliculi. Independent motor plans compete for selection in a push–pull fashion and when a saccadic plan ultimately reaches threshold, it produces a strong burst of action potentials that shuts down the remaining regions of the intermediate layers.

Modifying the activity of the intermediate layers changes these dynamic interactions in predictable ways. Enhancing the activity of one region facilitates nearby locations and inhibits distant locations. Diminishing the activity of one region inhibits nearby locations and facilitates distant locations. Such effects have been demonstrated in the neurophysiological activity of single cells (Munoz and Istvan, 1998;

Olivier et al., 1999) and in behavior (Hikosaka and Wurtz, 1985; Munoz and Wurtz, 1993b).

In addition to explaining visual fixation and saccadic initiation during basic saccadic tasks, the dynamic interactions model can explain changes in the timing of saccadic initiation that are observed when this task is modified. Namely, the gap effect, or decreased saccadic reaction times as a consequence of a gap period, occurs because removing fixation decreases the activity of fixation regions and, correspondingly, increases the excitability of saccadic regions. Express saccades, are a special instance of such dynamic interactions, in which decreased fixation activity and heightened motor preparation signals cause the target-related activity to be translated into a saccadic signal immediately. Finally, the slowing of saccadic initiation for antisaccades, can be interpreted as the consequence of multiple competing signals across the intermediate layers.

It should be emphasized that the dynamic interactions that we have described in this chapter are not limited to the superior colliculi. On the contrary, similar interactions take place at many levels of the neuraxis (Moschovakis et al., 1996; Leigh and Zee, 1999; Schall and Thompson, 1999; Hikosaka et al., 2000; Munoz et al., 2000; Glimcher, 2001; Scudder et al., 2002). At this juncture, however, the dynamic interactions involved in producing visual fixation and saccadic initiation are better understood in the superior colliculi because of its well-organized motor map and its well-characterized neuronal elements. Although we are a long way from understanding how the brain controls visual fixation and saccadic initiation, we have made substantial progress in understanding these behaviors in the superior colliculi.

Acknowledgements

We are indebted to Ann Lablans, Dave Hamburger, Sean Hickman, Kim Moore, and Chris Wellstood for outstanding technical assistance and Andrew Bell, Michael Dorris, Stefan Everling, Joanna Gore, Peter Istvan, and Martin Paré who participated in various aspects of this work. D.P. Munoz holds the Canada Research Chair in Neuroscience at Queen's University. J.H. Fecteau is supported by a postdoctoral fellowship from the National Sciences and Engineering Research Council of Canada. This work was supported by the Canadian Institutes for Health Research.

References

Basso, M.A. and Wurtz, R.H. (1997) Modulation of neuronal activity by target uncertainty. *Nature*, 389: 66–69.

Behan, M. and Kime, N.M. (1996) Intrinsic circuitry in the deep layers of the cat superior colliculus. *Vis. Neurosci.*, 13: 1031–1042.

Bell, A.H., Everling, S. and Munoz, D.P. (2000) Influence of stimulus eccentricity and direction on characteristics of pro- and antisaccades in non-human primates. *J. Neurophysiol.*, 84: 2595–2604.

Boch, R. and Fischer, B. (1986) Further observations on the occurrence of express-saccades in the monkey. *Exp. Brain Res.*, 63: 487–494.

Carpenter, R.H.S. (1981) Oculomotor procrastination. In: D.F. Fischer and R.A. Montey (Eds.), *Eye Movements: Cognition and Visual Perception*. Erlbaum, Hillsdale, NJ, pp. 237–246.

Dorris, M.C. and Munoz, D.P. (1995) A neural correlate for the gap effect on saccadic reaction times in monkey. *J. Neurophysiol.*, 95: 2558–2562.

Dorris, M.C. and Munoz, D.P. (1998) Saccadic probability influences motor preparation signals and time to saccadic initiation. *J. Neurosci.*, 18: 7015–7026.

Dorris, M.C., Pare, M. and Munoz, D.P. (1997) Neuronal activity in monkey superior colliculus related to the initiation of saccadic eye movements. *J. Neurosci.*, 17: 8566–8579.

Edelman, J.A. and Keller, E.L. (1996) Activity of visuomotor burst neurons in the superior colliculus accompanying express saccades. *J. Neurophysiol.*, 76: 1–19.

Everling, S., Dorris, M.C. and Munoz, D.P. (1998) Reflex suppression in the anti-saccade task is dependent on prestimulus neural processes. *J. Neurophysiol.*, 80: 1584–1589.

Everling, S., Dorris, M.C., Klein, R.M. and Munoz, D.P. (1999) Role of primate superior colliculus in preparation and execution of anti-saccades and pro-saccades. *J. Neurosci.*, 19: 2740–2754.

Fischer, B. and Weber, H. (1993) Express saccades and visual attention. *Behav. Brain Sci.*, 16: 533–610.

Fischer, B., Boch, R. and Ramsperger, E. (1984) Express-saccades of the monkey: effect of daily training on probability of occurrence and reaction time. *Exp. Brain Res.*, 55: 232–242.

Glimcher, P.W. (2001) Making choices: the neurophysiology of visual–saccadic decision making. *Trends Neurosci.*, 24: 654–659.

Glimcher, P.W. and Sparks, D.L. (1992) Movement selection in advance of action in the superior colliculus. *Nature*, 355: 542–545.

Hallett, P.E. (1978) Primary and secondary saccades to goals defined by instructions. *Vision Res.*, 18: 455–472.

Hikosaka, O. and Wurtz, R.H. (1985) Modification of saccadic eye movements by GABA-related substances. I. Effect of muscimol and bicuculline in monkey superior colliculus. *J. Neurophysiol.*, 53: 266–291.

Hikosaka, O., Takikawa, Y. and Kawagoe, R. (2000) Role of the basal ganglia in the control of purposive saccadic eye movements. *Physiol. Rev.*, 80: 953–978.

Kingstone, A. and Klein, R.M. (1993) Visual offsets facilitate saccadic latency: does predisengagement of visuospatial attention mediate this gap effect? *J. Exp. Psychol. Hum. Percept. Perform.*, 19: 1251–1265.

Krauzlis, R.J., Basso, M.A. and Wurtz, R.H. (1997) Shared motor error for multiple eye movements. *Science*, 276: 1693–1695.

Krauzlis, R.J., Basso, M.A. and Wurtz, R.H. (2000) Discharge properties of neurons in the rostral superior colliculus of the monkey during smooth-pursuit eye movements. *J. Neurophysiol.*, 84: 876–891.

Leigh, R.J. and Zee, D.S. (1999) *The Neurology of Eye Movements*. F.A. Davis Company, Philadelphia, PA.

Mayfrank, L., Mobashery, M., Kimmig, H. and Fischer, B. (1986) The role of fixation and visual attention in the occurrence of express saccades in man. *Eur. Arch. Psych. Neurol. Sci.*, 235: 269–275.

McConkie, G.W. and Rayner, K. (1975) The span of effective stimulus during a fixation in reading. *Perception and Psychophysics*, 17: 578–586.

McIlwain, J.T. (1982) Lateral spread of neural excitation during microstimulation in intermediate gray layer of cat's superior colliculus. *J. Neurophysiol.*, 47: 167–178.

McPeek, R.M. and Keller, E.L. (2002) Superior colliculus activity related to concurrent processing of saccade goals in a visual search task. *J. Neurophysiol.*, 87: 1805–1815.

Meredith, M.A. and Ramoa, A.S. (1998) Intrinsic circuitry of the superior colliculus: pharmacophysiological identification of horizontally oriented inhibitory interneurons. *J. Neurophysiol.*, 79: 1597–1602.

Mize, R.R., Jeon, C.J., Hamada, O.L. and Spencer, R.F. (1991) Organization of neurons labeled by antibodies to gamma-aminobutyric acid (GABA) in the superior colliculus of the Rhesus monkey. *Vis. Neurosci.*, 6: 75–92.

Moschovakis, A.K., Scudder, C.A. and Highstein, S.M. (1996) The microscopic anatomy and physiology of the mammalian saccadic system. *Prog. Neurobiol.*, 50: 133–254.

Munoz, D.P. and Guitton, D. (1991) Control of orienting gaze shifts by the tectoreticulospinal system in the head-free cat. II. Sustained discharges during motor preparation and fixation. *J. Neurophysiol.*, 66: 1624–1641.

Munoz, D.P. and Istvan, P.J. (1998) Lateral inhibitory interactions in the intermediate layers of the monkey superior colliculus. *J. Neurophysiol.*, 79: 1193–1209.

Munoz, D.P. and Wurtz, R.H. (1993a) Fixation cells in monkey superior colliculus, I. Characteristics of cell discharge. *J. Neurophysiol.*, 70: 559–575.

Munoz, D.P. and Wurtz, R.H. (1993b) Fixation cells in monkey superior colliculus, II. Reversible activation and deactivation. *J. Neurophysiol.*, 70: 576–589.

Munoz, D.P. and Wurtz, R.H. (1995a) Saccade-related activity in monkey superior colliculus, I. Characteristics of burst and buildup cells. *J. Neurophysiol.*, 73: 2313–2333.

Munoz, D.P. and Wurtz, R.H. (1995b) Saccade-related activity in monkey superior colliculus, II. Spread of activity during saccades. *J. Neurophysiol.*, 73: 2334–2348.

Munoz, D.P., Dorris, M.C., Pare, M. and Everling, S. (2000) On your mark, get set: brainstem circuitry underlying saccadic initiation. *Can. J. Physiol. Pharmacol.*, 78: 934–944.

Olivier, E., Dorris, M.C. and Munoz, D.P. (1999) Lateral interactions in the superior colliculus, not an extended fixation zone, can account for the remote distractor effect. *Behav. Brain Sci.*, 22: 694–695.

Paré, M. and Munoz, D.P. (1996) Saccadic reaction time in the monkey: advanced preparation of oculomotor programs is primarily responsible for express saccade occurrence. *J. Neurophysiol.*, 76: 3666–3681.

Robinson, D.A. (1972) Eye movements evoked by collicular stimulation in the alert monkey. *Vision Res.*, 12: 1795–1808.

Rohrer, W.H. and Sparks, D.L. (1993) Express saccades: the effects of spatial and temporal uncertainty. *Vision Res.*, 33: 2447–2460.

Saslow, M.G. (1967) Effects of components of displacement-step stimuli upon latency of saccadic eye movements. *J. Opt. Soc. Am.*, 57: 1024–1029.

Schall, J.D. and Thompson, K.G. (1999) Neural selection and control of visually guided eye movements. *Annu. Rev. Neurosci.*, 22: 241–259.

Scudder, C.A., Kaneko, C.R.S. and Fuchs, A.F. (2002) The brainstem burst generator for saccadic eye movements. *Exp. Brain Res.*, 142: 439–462.

Sommer, M.A. (1994) Express saccades elicited during visual scan in the monkey. *Vision Res.*, 34: 2023–2038.

Sparks, D.L. and Hartwich-Young, R. (1989) The deep layers of the superior colliculus. *Rev. Oculomot. Res.*, 89: 213–255.

Sparks, D.L., Holland, R. and Guthrie, B.L. (1976) Size and distribution of movement fields in the monkey superior colliculus. *Brain Res.*, 113: 21–34.

Trappenberg, T.P., Dorris, M.C., Munoz, D.P. and Klein, R.M. (2001) A model of saccade initiation based on the competitive integration of exogenous and endogenous signals in the superior colliculus. *J. Cogn. Neurosci.*, 15: 256–271.

Walker, R., Deubel, H., Schneider, W.X. and Findlay, J.M. (1997) Effect of remote distractors on saccade programming: evidence for an extended fixation zone. *J. Neurophysiol.*, 78: 1108–1119.

Wurtz, R.H. and Goldberg, M.E. (1972) Activity of superior colliculus in behaving monkey, III. Cells discharging before eye movements. *J. Neurophysiol.*, 35: 575–586.

Wurtz, R.H. and Munoz, D.P. (1995) Role of monkey superior colliculus in control of saccades and fixation. In: M.S. Gazzaniga (Ed.), *The Cognitive Neurosciences*. MIT Press, Cambridge, MA, pp. 533–548.

Yang, S.N. and McConkie, G.W. (2001) Eye movements during reading: A theory of saccade initiation times. *Vision Res.*, 41: 3567–3585.

Yarbus, A. (1967) *Eye Movements and Vision*. Plenum, New York.

CHAPTER 2

Neural control of saccades

John D. Enderle *

Biomedical Engineering, University of Connecticut, 260 Glenbrook Road, Storrs, CT 06269-2157, USA

Abstract: Quantitative models of the oculomotor plant and control of the saccadic eye movement system are presented in this chapter. Oculomotor plant models described here are linear, including a second-order model by Westheimer (1954), Bahill et al. (1980) and Enderle et al. (2000). The model of the saccade generator is initiated by the superior colliculus and terminated by the cerebellar fastigial nucleus that operates under a time optimal control strategy. A common mechanism for all types of saccades is described, including those with dynamic overshoot and glissadic behavior. Conflicting evidence exists regarding the operation of the excitatory burst neuron during saccades. The excitatory burst neuron operates within two states: complete inhibition, and without inhibition that is characterized by high firing at rates of up to 1000 Hz. While there is direct evidence of projections from the superior colliculus to the paramedian pontine reticular formation, there is conflictory evidence regarding the connections from the superior colliculus to the excitatory burst neuron, with the most recent experimental results supporting no direct connections. A model of the excitatory burst neuron is described using a Hodgkin–Huxley model of the neuron that fires at 1000 Hz automatically and without stimulation when released from inhibition. SIMULINK simulations using this neuron model have all of the characteristics of the excitatory burst neuron firing rate during a saccade. This model eliminates the need to introduce BIAS inputs that causes bursting in some models of the saccade generator. Such a model is also appropriate for modeling the Omnipause neurons.

Introduction

In this chapter a broad overview of the saccadic eye movement control system is presented. A saccade is a fast eye movement that involves quickly moving the fovea of the eye from one image to another image. This type of eye movement is very common and is observed most easily while reading when the end of a line is reached; the eyes are moved quickly to the beginning of the next line and begin to read the new line with the slow eye movement system. The final section provides a list of abbreviations used in this chapter. A qualitative description of the saccadic eye movement system is given first in the introduction, and then followed by a brief description of saccade characteristics. Next, the earliest quantitative saccade model is presented, and then followed by a more complex and physiologically accurate model. Finally, the saccade generator is then discussed on the basis of anatomical pathways and control theory. A special focus of this chapter is a neuron model of the EBN. The purpose of this review is focused on mathematical models of the saccadic eye movement system and neural control, rather than on how visual information is processed. The literature on the saccadic eye movement system is vast, and thus this review is not exhaustive, but rather a representative sample from the field.

The oculomotor system responds to visual, auditory and vestibular stimuli, which results in one of five types of eye movements: saccadic eye movements, smooth pursuit eye movements, vestibular ocular movements, vergence eye movements, and optokinetic eye movements. Each of these movements is controlled by a different neuronal system, and all of these controllers share the same final common

---

* Correspondence to: J.D. Enderle, Biomedical Engineering, University of Connecticut, 260 Glenbrook Road, Storrs, CT 06269-2157, USA. Tel.: +1-860-486-5521; Fax: +1-860-486-2500; E-mail: jenderle@bme.uconn.edu

pathway to the muscles of the eye. In addition to the five types of eye movements, these stimuli also cause head and body movements. Thus, the visual system is part of a multiple input–multiple output system.

Regardless of the input, the oculomotor system is responsible for movement of the eyes so that images are focused on the central one-half degree region of the retina, known as the fovea. Lining the retina are photoreceptive cells that translate images into neural impulses. These impulses are then transmitted along the optic nerve to the central nervous system via parallel pathways to the SC and the cerebral cortex. The fovea is more densely packed with photoreceptive cells than the retinal periphery; thus a higher resolution image (or higher visual acuity) is generated in the fovea than the retinal periphery. The purpose of the fovea is to allow us to *clearly* see an object, and the purpose of the retinal periphery is to allow us to *detect* a new object of interest. Once a new object of interest is detected in the periphery, the saccade system redirects the eyes to the new object. This type of saccade is typically called a goal-directed saccade.

During a saccade, the oculomotor system operates in an open-loop mode. The reason that the saccade system operates without feedback during a saccadic eye movement is simple, information from the retina and muscle proprioceptors is not transmitted quickly enough during the eye movement for use in altering the control signal. After the saccade is complete, the system operates in a closed-loop mode to ensure that the eyes reached the correct destination. Information from the retina and muscle proprioceptors is used to correct any error between the desired and current eye position. The saccade system operates in a closed-loop mode to reduce this error to zero with a corrective saccade. Later in this chapter, an internal closed-loop controller is described that operates to drive the eye to its destination based on an internal model.

The oculomotor plant and saccade generator are the basic elements of the saccadic system. The oculomotor plant consists of three muscle pairs and the eyeball. These three muscle pairs contract and lengthen to move the eye in horizontal, vertical and torsional directions. Each pair of muscles acts in an antagonistic fashion due to reciprocal innervation by the saccade generator. For simplicity, the models described here involve only horizontal eye movements and one pair of muscles, the lateral and medial rectus muscle.

Saccade characteristics

Saccadic eye movements, among the fastest voluntary muscle movements the human is capable of producing, are characterized by a rapid shift of gaze from one point of fixation to another. Saccadic eye movements are conjugate and ballistic, with a typical duration of 20–100 ms and a latency of 150–300 ms. The latent period is thought to be the time interval during which the CNS determines whether to make a saccade, and if so, calculates the distance the eyeball is to be moved, transforming retinal error into transient muscle activity.

Generally, saccades are extremely variable, with wide variations in the latent period, time to peak velocity, peak velocity, and saccade duration. Furthermore, variability is well coordinated for saccades of the same size; saccades with lower peak velocity are matched with longer saccade durations, and saccades with higher peak velocity are matched with shorter saccade durations. Thus, saccades driven to the same destination usually have different trajectories.

To appreciate differences in saccade dynamics, it is often helpful to describe them with saccade main sequence diagrams (Bahill et al., 1975; Enderle, 1988; Harwood et al., 1999). The main sequence diagrams plot saccade peak velocity–saccade magnitude, saccade duration–saccade magnitude, and saccade latent period–saccade magnitude. Peak velocity–saccade magnitude is basically a linear function until approximately 15°, after which it levels off to a constant for larger saccades. Many researchers have fit this relationship to an exponential function. A linear relationship between saccade duration and saccade magnitude exists in the main sequence diagram. The latent period–saccade magnitude data have been described with a latent period's value independent of saccade magnitude (Enderle, 1988), and with a linear relationship between the latent period and saccade magnitude (Bahill et al., 1975).

Westheimer saccadic eye movement model

The first quantitative saccadic eye movement model was published by Westheimer (1954). Based on visual inspection of a recorded 20° saccade, and the assumption of a step controller, Westheimer proposed the following second-order model:

$$J\ddot{\theta} + B\dot{\theta} + K\theta = \tau(t) \tag{1}$$

With Westheimer's parameter values, the duration is 37 ms for saccades of all sizes, which is independent of saccade magnitude and not in agreement with the experimental data that have a duration which increases as a function of saccade magnitude.

Peak velocity from this model is derived as $\dot{\theta}(t_{\mathrm{mv}}) = 55.02\Delta\theta$, that is, peak velocity is directly proportional to saccade magnitude. Evident from the main sequence diagram, experimental peak velocity data have an exponential form and not a linear function as predicted by the Westheimer model.

Westheimer noted the differences between saccade duration and saccade magnitude and between peak velocity and saccade magnitude in the model and the experimental data, and inferred that the saccade system was not linear because the peak vel-

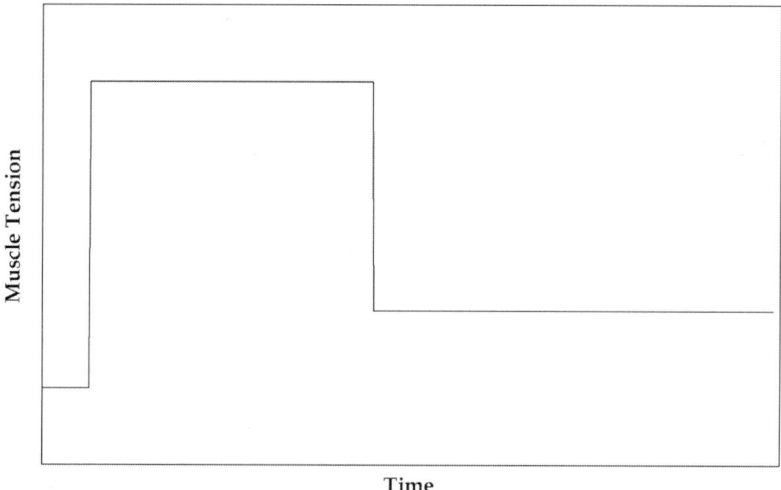

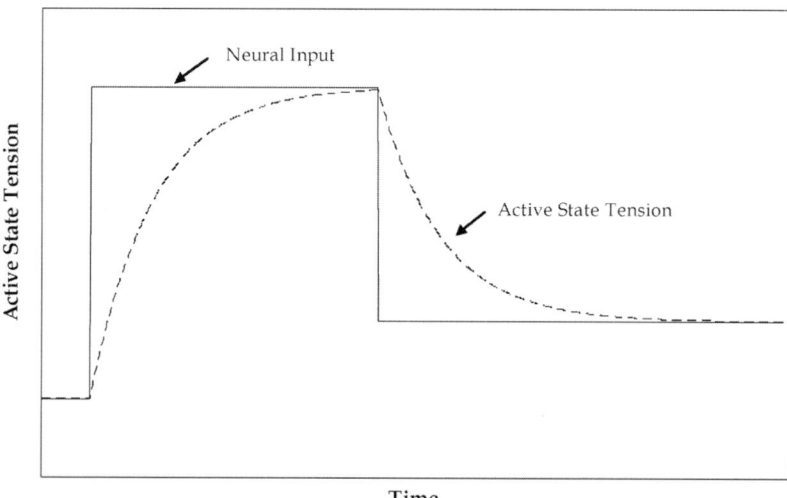

Fig. 1. Muscle tension and active state tension during a saccade. Note that the magnitude of the active state tension is typically larger than the muscle tension, and the pulse duration of the muscle tension is typically larger than the active state tension.

ocity–saccade magnitude plot was nonlinear, and the input was not an abrupt step function. Overall, this model provided a satisfactory fit to the eye position data for a saccade of 20°, but not for saccades of other magnitudes. Interestingly, Westheimer's second-order model proves to be an adequate model for saccades of all sizes, if one assumes a different input function as described in the next section. Due to its simplicity, the Westheimer model of the oculomotor plant is still popular today.

Robinson's model of the saccade controller

In 1964, Robinson performed an experiment to measure the input to the eyeballs during a saccade. To record the input, one eye was held fixed using a suction contact lens, while the other eye performed a saccade from target to target. Since the same innervation signal is sent to both eyes during a saccade, Robinson inferred that the input, recorded through the transducer attached to the fixed eyeball, was the same input driving the other eyeball. He estimated that the neural commands controlling the eyeballs during a saccade are a pulse–step input based on the recorded muscle tensions shown in Fig. 1.

It is important to distinguish between the muscle tension or force generated by a muscle, called muscle tension, and the force generator within the muscle, called the active state tension generator. The active state tension generator creates a force within the muscle that is transformed through the internal elements of the muscle into the muscle tension. Muscle tension is external and measurable, and the active state tension is internal and unmeasurable. Moreover, Robinson (1981) reports that the active state tensions are not identical to the neural controllers, but described by low-pass filtered pulse step waveforms as shown in Fig. 1. The agonist pulse input is required to quickly move the eye to the target, and the step is required to keep the eye at that location.

A linear homeomorphic saccadic eye movement model

In 1980, Bahill et al. presented a linear fourth-order model of the oculomotor plant, based on physiological evidence that provides a very good match between model predictions and eye movement data. This linear model of the oculomotor plant is derived from a nonlinear oculomotor plant model by Hsu et al. (1976), and based on a linearization of the force–velocity curve (Bahill et al., 1980). Muscle viscosity traditionally has been modeled with a hyperbolic force–velocity relationship. Using the linear model of muscle reported by Enderle et al. (1991), it is possible to avoid the linearization, and derive an updated linear homeomorphic saccadic eye movement model that has superior characteristics compared with the Bahill model as described next (Enderle et al., 2000).

The linear muscle model has the static and dynamic properties of rectus eye muscle, a model without any nonlinear elements. The model has a nonlinear force–velocity relationship that matches muscle data using linear viscous elements, and the length tension characteristics are also in good agreement with muscle data within the operating range of the muscle (Enderle et al., 1991). Fig. 2 illustrates the mechanical components of the updated oculomotor plant for horizontal eye movements, the lateral and medial rectus muscle, and the eyeball.

The differential equation describing the oculomotor plant model shown in Fig. 2 is derived by summing the forces acting at junctions 2 (variable x_2) and 3 (variable x_3), and the torques acting on the eyeball and junction 5 (variable θ_5), and using Laplace variable analysis about the operating point, and given by:

$$\delta \Big(K_{SE} K_{12} (F_{AG} - F_{ANT}) \\ + (K_{SE} B_{34} + B_2 K_{12})(\dot{F}_{AG} - \dot{F}_{ANT}) \\ + B_2 B_{34} (\ddot{F}_{AG} - \ddot{F}_{ANT}) \Big) \\ = \ddddot{\theta} + P_3 \dddot{\theta} + P_2 \ddot{\theta} + P_1 \dot{\theta} + P_0 \theta \quad (2)$$

where
$$J = \frac{57.296 J_p}{r^2}, \quad B_3 = \frac{57.296 B_{p1}}{r^2}, \quad B_4 = \frac{57.296 B_{p2}}{r^2}$$

$$K_1 = \frac{57.296 K_{p1}}{r^2}, \quad K_2 = \frac{57.296 K_{p2}}{r^2},$$

$$B_{12} = B_1 + B_2, \quad B_{34} = B_3 + B_4, \quad K_{12} = K_1 + K_2,$$

$$\delta = \frac{57.296}{r J B_{12} B_4},$$

$$C_3 = \frac{B_{12}(JK_2 + B_3 B_4) + JB_4 K_{ST} + 2B_1 B_2 B_{34}}{J B_{12} B_4}$$

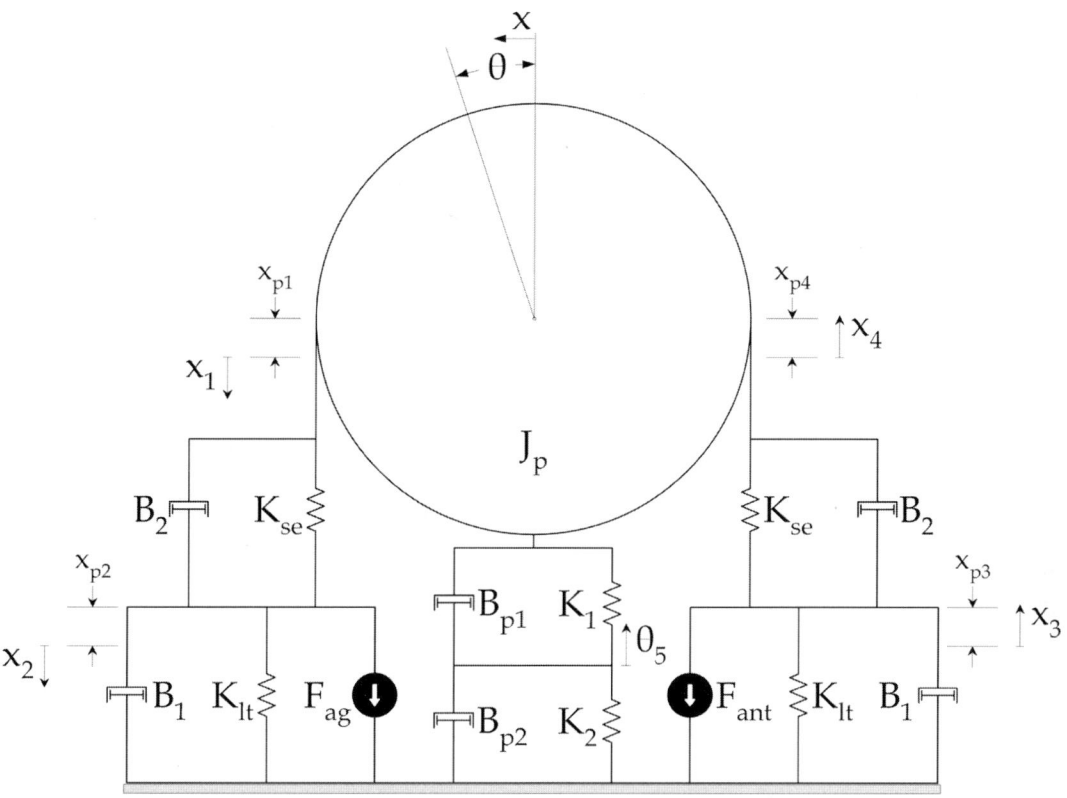

Fig. 2. This diagram illustrates the mechanical components of the updated oculomotor plant. The muscles are shown to be extended from equilibrium, a position of rest, at the primary position (looking straight ahead), consistent with physiological evidence. The radius of the eyeball is r. The agonist muscle is drawn in the lower left with active state tension generator F_{ag} and other viscoelastic elements connected to the eyeball at point x_1. The antagonist muscle is drawn in the right with active state tension generator F_{ant} and other viscoelastic elements connected to the eyeball at point x_4. The eyeball is connected to a pair of viscoelastic elements.

$$C_2 = \frac{JK_{ST}K_2 + B_3B_4K_{ST} + B_{12}B_3K_2 + 2K_{SE}B_{34}B_1}{JB_{12}B_4}$$
$$+ \frac{K_1B_{12}B_4 + 2B_2K_{LT}B_{34} + 2B_1K_{12}B_2}{JB_{12}B_4}$$

$$C_1 = \frac{K_{ST}(B_3K_2 + K_1B_4) + K_1K_2B_{12}}{JB_{12}B_4}$$
$$+ \frac{2K_{LT}K_{SE}B_{34} + 2B_1K_{12}K_{SE} + 2B_2K_{LT}K_{12}}{JB_{12}B_4}$$

$$C_0 = \frac{2K_{LT}K_{SE}K_{12} + K_1K_{ST}K_2}{JB_{12}B_4}$$

Based on an analysis of experimental data, suitable parameter estimates for the oculomotor plant are: $K_{SE} = 125$ N m^{-1}, $K_{LT} = 60.7$ N m^{-1}, $B_1 = 4.6$ N s m^{-1}, $B_2 = 0.5$ N s m^{-1}, $J = 2.2 \times 10^{-3}$ N s^2 m^{-1}, $B_3 = 0.538$ N s m^{-1}, $B_4 = 41.54$ N s m^{-1}, $K_1 = 26.9$ N m^{-1}, and $K_2 = 41.54$ N m^{-1}. With the updated model of muscle (Enderle et al., 1991) and length tension data (Collins, 1975), steady state active state tensions are determined as:

$$F = \begin{cases} 0.4 + 0.0175\theta & \text{N} \quad \text{for} \quad \theta \geq 0° \\ 0.4 - 0.0125\theta & \text{N} \quad \text{for} \quad \theta < 0° \end{cases} \quad (3)$$

Saccadic eye movements simulated with this model have characteristics which are in good agreement with the data, including position, velocity and acceleration, and the main sequence diagrams.

Saccade generator

Studies of the saccadic control mechanism have been based on the system identification technique and control systems, single-unit microelectrode recordings, muscle tension measurements, and general observations from the main sequence diagram. In comparison with other systems, the oculomotor system is the best understood of all human control systems. However, significant and important differences still exist regarding the control mechanism during saccadic eye movements. Physiological evidence indicates that saccades are controlled through a parallel-distributed network involving the cortex, cerebellum, and brain stem. The saccadic neural activity of the SC and cerebellum, in particular have been identified as the saccade initiator and terminator, respectively, although neither is required for a saccade.

To execute a saccade, a sequence of complex activities takes place within the brain, beginning from the detection of an error on the retina, to the actual movement of the eyes. A saccade is directly caused by a burst discharge (pulse) from motoneurons stimulating the agonist muscle and a pause in firing from motoneurons stimulating the antagonist muscle. During periods of fixation, the motoneurons fire at a rate necessary to keep the eye stable (step). The pulse discharge in the motoneurons is caused by the EBN and the step discharge is caused by the TN in the PPRF.

Consider the saccade network programmed to move the eyes 20° illustrated in Fig. 3. Qualitatively, a saccade occurs according to the following sequence of events according to the model presented here. First, the ipsilateral LLBN is stimulated by the contralateral SC. The LLBN then inhibits the tonic firing of the OPN. When the OPN ceases firing, the MLBN is released from inhibition and begins firing. The ipsilateral IBNs are stimulated by the ipsilateral LLBNs and the contralateral FNs of the cerebellum. When released from inhibition, the ipsilateral EBNs fire spontaneously. The EBNs are also stimulated by the contralateral FNs of the cerebellum; however, FN stimulation is not required for a saccade to be generated. The burst firing in the ipsilateral IBN inhibits the contralateral EBN and abducens nucleus, and the ipsilateral oculomotor nucleus. The burst firing in the ipsilateral EBN causes the burst in the ipsilateral abducens nucleus, which stimulates the ipsilateral lateral rectus muscle and the contralateral oculomotor nucleus. With the stimulation of the ipsilateral lateral rectus muscle by the ipsilateral abducens nucleus and the inhibition of the ipsilateral medial rectus muscle via the oculomotor nucleus, a saccade occurs in the right eye.

Simultaneously, the contralateral medial rectus muscle is stimulated by the contralateral oculomotor nucleus, and with the inhibition of the contralateral lateral rectus muscle via the abducens nucleus, a saccade occurs in the left eye. Thus the eyes move conjugately under the control of a single drive center.

The end of the saccade is normally terminated by the cerebellum. At the termination time, the cerebellar vermis through the Purkinje cells inhibits the contralateral FN and stimulates the ipsilateral FN. The ipsilateral FN then stimulates the contralateral IBN and EBN. The contralateral IBN then inhibits the ipsilateral EBN, TN and abducens nucleus, and contralateral oculomotor nucleus. With this inhibition, the stimulus to the agonist muscles ceases. The antagonist muscles receive stimulation from the contralateral EBN through the contralateral abducens nucleus and ipsilateral oculomotor nucleus, causing a dynamic break.

The cerebellum is included in the saccade generator as a gating element, using three active sites during a saccade: the oculomotor vermis, FN and flocculus. The vermis is concerned with the absolute starting position of a saccade in the movement field, and corrects control signals for initial eye position. Using proprioceptors in the oculomotor muscles and an internal eye position reference, the vermis is aware of the current position of the eye. The vermis is also aware of the DME used to generate the saccade via the connection with the NRTP and the SC. The oculomotor vermis and FN are important in the control of saccade amplitude, and the flocculus, perihypoglossal nuclei of the rostral medulla, and possibly the pontine and mesencephalic reticular formation are thought to form the integrator within the cerebellum. One important function of the flocculus may be to increase the time constant of the neural integrator for saccades starting at locations different from primary position. The output of the FN is excitatory and projects ipsilaterally and contralaterally as shown in Fig. 3. During fixation, the FN fires tonically at low rates. Twenty milliseconds prior to a saccade, the contralateral FN bursts, and the ipsilateral FN pauses and then discharges with a burst. The pause in ipsilateral firing is due to Purkinje

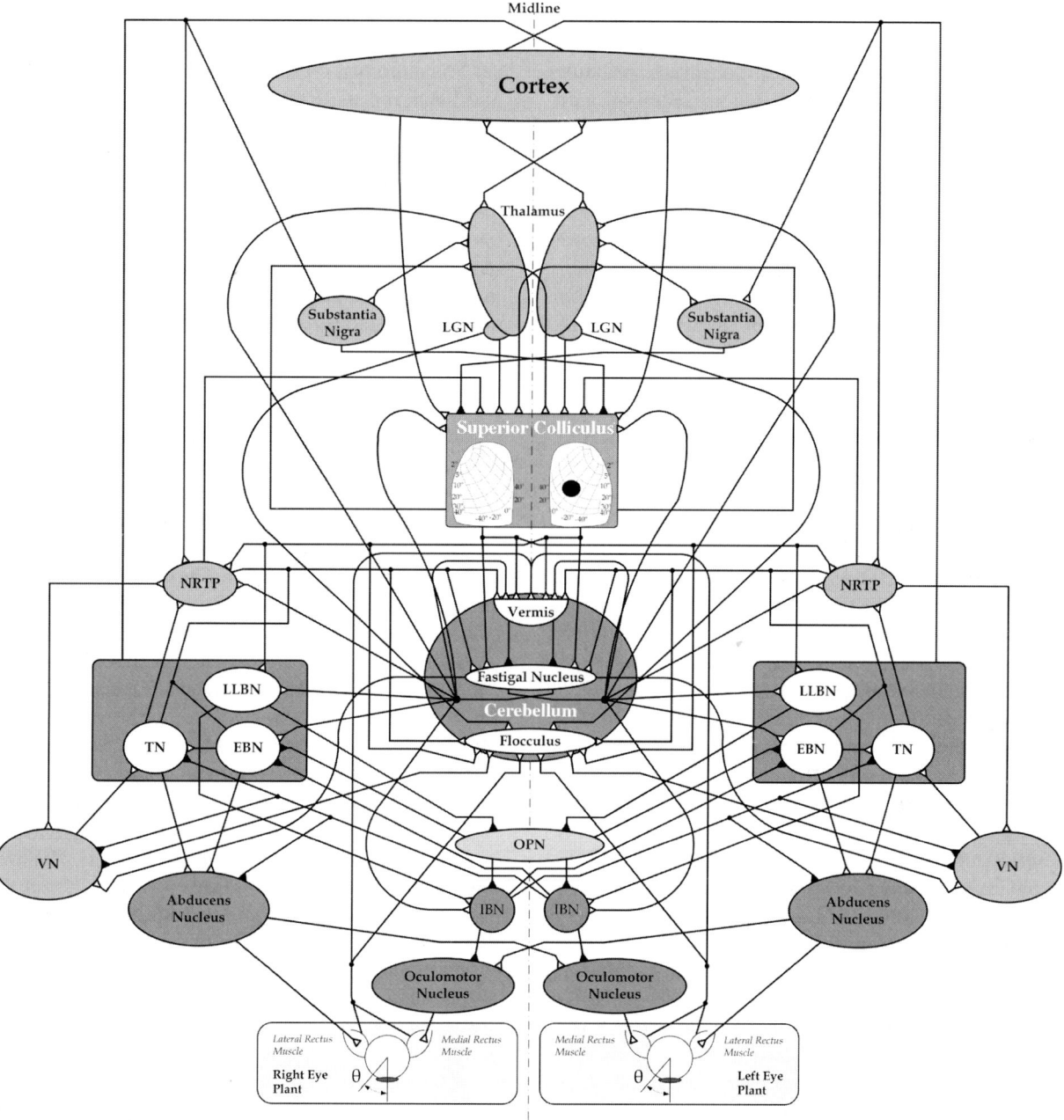

Fig. 3. Shown is a diagram illustrating important sites for the generation of a conjugate horizontal saccade in both eyes. Excitatory inputs are shown with △, inhibitory inputs are shown with a ▲. Consistent with current knowledge, the left and right structures of the neural circuit model are maintained. Since interest is in goal directed visual saccades, the cortex has not been partitioned into the frontal eye field and posterior eye field (striate, prestriate, and inferior parietal cortices).

cell input to the FN. The sequential organization of Purkinje cells along beams of parallel fibers suggests that the cerebellar cortex might function as a delay, producing a set of timed pulses which could be used to program the duration of the saccade. If one considers non-primary position saccades, different temporal and spatial schemes, via cerebellar control, are necessary to produce the same size saccade. It is postulated here that the cerebellum acts as a gating device that precisely terminates a saccade based on the initial position of the eye in the orbit.

The deep layers of the SC initiate a saccade based on the distance between the current position of the eye and the desired target (vector model). The neural activity in the SC is organized into movement fields that are associated with the direction and saccade amplitude, and does not involve the initial position of the eyeball whatsoever. The movement field is shown in Fig. 3 for a 20° saccade. Neurons active during a particular saccade are shown as the dark circle, representing a desired 20° eye movement. Active neurons in the deep layers of the SC generate a high frequency burst of activity beginning 18–20 ms before a saccade and ending sometime toward the end of the saccade; the exact timing for the end of the burst firing is quite random and can occur slightly before or slightly after the saccade ends. Neurons discharging for small saccades have smaller movement fields, and those for larger saccades have larger movement fields. All of the movement fields are connected to the same set of LLBNs. It should be noted that the contralateral SC and ipsilateral LLBN often continue firing after the saccade has ended. The saccade is actually terminated by the cerebellum as previously described. With the cessation of firing in the ipsilateral LLBN, the OPN is no longer inhibited and resumes firing at approximately 200 Hz, providing inhibition of the MLBN.

Paramedian pontine reticular formation

The PPRF has neurons responsible for the pulse and step discharges that drive the eyeball during a saccade. Neurons that fire at steady rates during fixation are called TNs and are responsible for holding the eye steady. The TN firing rate depends on the position of the eye (presumably through a local integrator type network involving the EBN). The TN is thought to provide the step component to the motoneuron. There are two types of burst neurons in the PPRF called the LLBN and the MLBN; during periods of fixation, these neurons are silent. The LLBNs burst at least 12 ms before a saccade and the MLBNs burst less than 12 ms (typically 6–8 ms) before the saccade. The MLBNs are connected monosynaptically with the abducens nucleus.

There are two types of neurons within the MLBN, the EBN and the IBN. The EBN and IBN label describes the synaptic activity upon the other neurons; the EBN excites and is responsible for the burst firing, and the IBN inhibits and is responsible for the pause. A mirror image of these neurons exists on both sides of the midline as shown in Fig. 3. As shown, the IBN inhibits the EBN on the contralateral side. EBNs are located ipsilaterally just rostral to the abducens nucleus. EBNs exhibit a burst of spikes for lateral saccades, and some produce monosynaptic excitation in the ipsilateral abducens motoneurons. IBNs are located in the dorso-medial medullary reticular formation just caudal to the abducens nucleus. They discharge a burst of spikes for lateral saccades and produce monosynaptic IPSP in contralateral abducens motoneurons.

Also within the brainstem is another type of saccade neuron called the OPN. The OPN fires tonically at approximately 200 Hz during periods of fixation, and is silent during saccades. The OPN stops firing approximately 10–12 ms before a saccade and resumes tonic firing approximately 10 ms before the end of the saccade. The OPNs are known to inhibit the MLBNs, and are inhibited by the LLBNs. The OPN activity is responsible for the precise timing between groups of neurons that causes a saccade. The existence of each of these PPRF neuron groups is uniformly accepted. The manner in which these neurons are connected, however, is not uniformly accepted. Many models of the OPN use a bias input for its firing rate during periods of fixation.

Direct projections from the SC to the PPRF have been demonstrated anatomically. Previous electrophysiological experiments in the monkey have demonstrated that direct projections from the SC to LLBNs exist, but have failed to find evidence for monosynaptic connections from the SC to EBN (Keller et al., 2000). In other experiments in the cat, direct connections to EBNs were found (Chimoto et al., 1996). Keller conducted experiments to determine whether direct connections from the SC to EBNs exist in the monkey. The experiment consisted of single-pulse stimuli delivered at sites in the SC at current levels well above those required to evoke saccades with pulse train stimuli shortly after the onset of ipsilateral or contralateral saccades and also slightly after the end of saccades. Twenty-one EBNs were recorded and none were activated by postsaccadic stimulation or during contralateral saccades. No evidence for direct connections to EBNs was found in this study. The variance in results obtained for cat and monkey may be due to a species difference that reflects the more complex signal processing required in the monkey's saccadic system, or even inhibitory projections from other neurons.

In contrast with the study of Keller et al., existence of direct connections to the region of the EBN from both the SC and the FEF has been shown by anatomic means (Harting, 1977; Stanton et al., 1988; Olivier et al., 1993; Moschovakis et al., 1996). Nevertheless, stimulation of the deeper layers of the SC in the alert monkey by Raybourn and Keller (1977) were unable to activate EBNs with single-pulse stimuli, although they did produce activation of EBNs following triple-pulse stimuli with resultant latencies in the poly-synaptic range. Moreover, they described LLBNs that were also found in the PPRF in close proximity to EBNs, which were readily activated from the SC, many in the range of latencies suggesting monosynaptic connections. LLBN characteristics are not as clearly related to saccadic parameters such as duration and velocity as are those of EBNs (Fuchs et al., 1985; Keller, 1991). Keller et al. (2000) noted that EBNs in the monkey do not generally receive direct input from the SC, but fall short of proving that no such connections exist, because of difficulties in interpretation when stimuli are delivered during ipsilateral saccades. There is no clear direct evidence that LLBNs project directly to the EBNs (Moschovakis et al., 1996).

Postinhibitory rebound burst firing

Electrophysiological evidence for postinhibitory rebound burst firing activity during saccadic eye movements is prevalent in the literature (for example, see fig. 4 in Robinson, 1981). This behavior is described by high neural firing rates without any regard for the size of the eye movement or apparent stimulation at the start of EBN activity during the first 10 ms of firing. Here it is proposed that postinhibitory rebound burst firing begins with a rapid rise to a peak occurring within a few ms, and then decaying to a lower steady state firing rate at approximately 10 ms. It is proposed here that the decay may be attributable to a reduction in ions or energy necessary to maintain the peak firing rate. Further, postinhibitory rebound burst firing activity after marked hyperpolarization is postulated to occur in the EBN due to a low membrane threshold voltage within the axon hillock of the neuron. With this biophysical property, a single neuron is capable of firing at high rates automatically without stimulation when released from inhibition. According to this hypothesis, when released from inhibition, the EBNs maximally fire automatically and without stimulation.

Hodgkin–Huxley model of an EBN

To investigate the effect of threshold voltage on the firing characteristics of a neuron, simulations are presented using the nonlinear Hodgkin–Huxley model (Hodgkin et al., 1952) of neuron described by the circuit diagram Fig. 4. This model describes the membrane potential at the axon hillock due to conductance changes. The following equation is the node equation for the circuit, and is parameterized for the squid giant axon defining the membrane potential V_m as a function of stimulus current I_m and active gate conductance for sodium and potassium.

$$I_m = \bar{g}_K n^4 (V_m - E_K) + \bar{g}_{Na} m^3 h (V_m - E_{Na}) + \frac{(V_m - E_l)}{R_l} + C_m \frac{dV_m}{dt} \quad (4)$$

where

$$\frac{dn}{dt} = \alpha_n (1-n) - \beta_n n$$

$$\frac{dm}{dt} = \alpha_m (1-m) - \beta_m m$$

$$\frac{dh}{dt} = \alpha_h (1-h) - \beta_h h$$

$$\alpha_n = 0.01 \times \frac{V+10}{e^{\frac{V+10}{10}} - 1} \text{ ms}^{-1}$$

$$\beta_n = 0.125 e^{\frac{V}{18}} \text{ ms}^{-1}$$

$$\alpha_m = 0.1 \times \frac{V+25}{e^{\frac{V+25}{10}} - 1} \text{ ms}^{-1}$$

$$\beta_m = 4 e^{\frac{V}{18}} \text{ ms}^{-1}$$

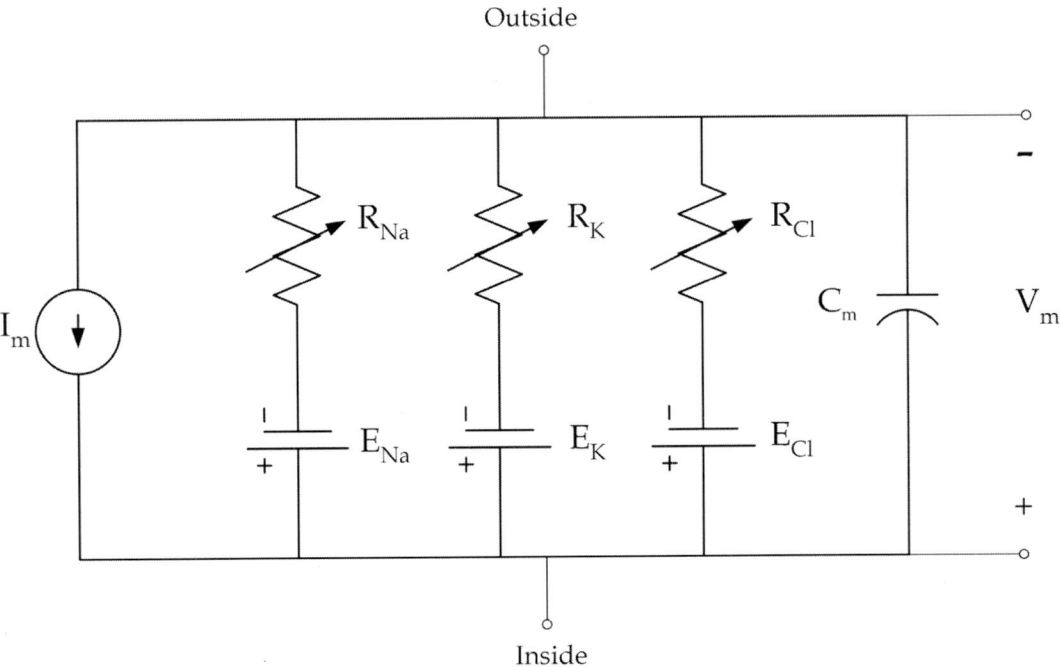

Fig. 4. Circuit model of an unmyelinated section of squid giant axon. The channels for K$^+$ and Na$^+$ are represented using variable voltage–time conductances given by $R_K = 1/(\bar{g}_K n^4)$ and $R_{Na} = 1/(\bar{g}_{Na} m^3 h)$. The passive gates for Na$^+$, K$^+$, and Cl$^-$ are given by a leakage channel with resistance, $R_l = 1/(0.3 \times 10^{-3})\Omega$. The batteries are given by the Nernst potential for each ion, $E_l = 49.4 \times 10^{-3}$ V, $E_{Na} = 55 \times 10^{-3}$ V and $E_K = -72 \times 10^{-3}$ V.

$$\alpha_h = 0.07 e^{\frac{V}{20}} \text{ ms}^{-1}$$

$$\beta_h = \frac{1}{e^{\frac{V+30}{10}} + 1} \text{ ms}^{-1}$$

$$V = V_{rp} - V_m \text{ mV}$$

$$\bar{g}_K = 36 \times 10^{-3} \text{ S}$$

$$\bar{g}_{Na} = 120 \times 10^{-3} \text{ S}$$

To investigate the effects of low threshold voltage, simulations using the Hodgkin–Huxley model of a neuron are presented using SIMULINK, a continuous time simulator. Threshold voltage is defined as when the sodium current, I_{Na}, characterized by the m and h differential equations, is greater than the potassium current, I_K, characterized by the n differential equation, and leakage current. Since sodium current changes more rapidly than the potassium current at the beginning of the action potential, changes in threshold voltage are accomplished by changing a parameter value in the sodium equation. Since sodium current has a rising component (the m differential equation) and a falling component (the h differential equation), threshold is modified here using the m differential equation. Thus changes to threshold are carried out by changing the value of 25 to 10 in the algebraic equation for α_m, yielding

$$\alpha_m = 0.1 \times \frac{V+10}{e^{\frac{V+10}{10}} - 1} \text{ ms}^{-1} \quad (5)$$

The value of 10 is selected since threshold is approximately $V_m = -45$ mV, resting potential $V_{rp} = -60$ mV, and the variable $V = V_{rp} - V_m = -60 + 45 = -15$ mV. Thus to change threshold to -60 mV, 15 is subtracted from the quantity $(V + 25)$ leaving $(V + 10)$ in the m differential equation. To change the firing rate of the Hodgkin–Huxley neuron model so that it bursts at 1000 Hz, the right-hand side of the n, m and h equations are multiplied by 35,000, effectively reducing the apparent time constant for these differential equations to model data.

To illustrate how changing threshold voltage affects the firing rates of the neuron, three simulations are presented in the following figures. Fig. 5 illustrates a normal action potential stimulated by a

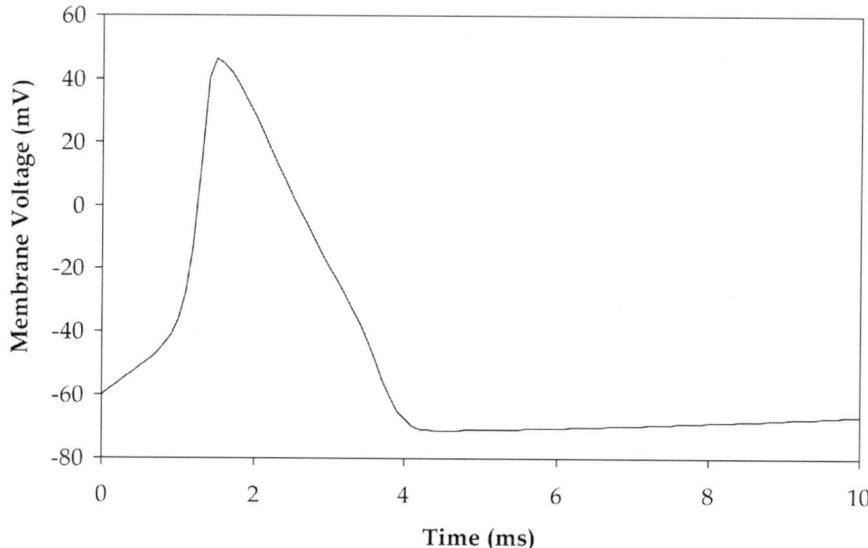

Fig. 5. An action potential simulated with the Hodgkin–Huxley model of Eq. 4. The current pulse starts at time zero with a magnitude of 20 μA and then turns off at 6 ms.

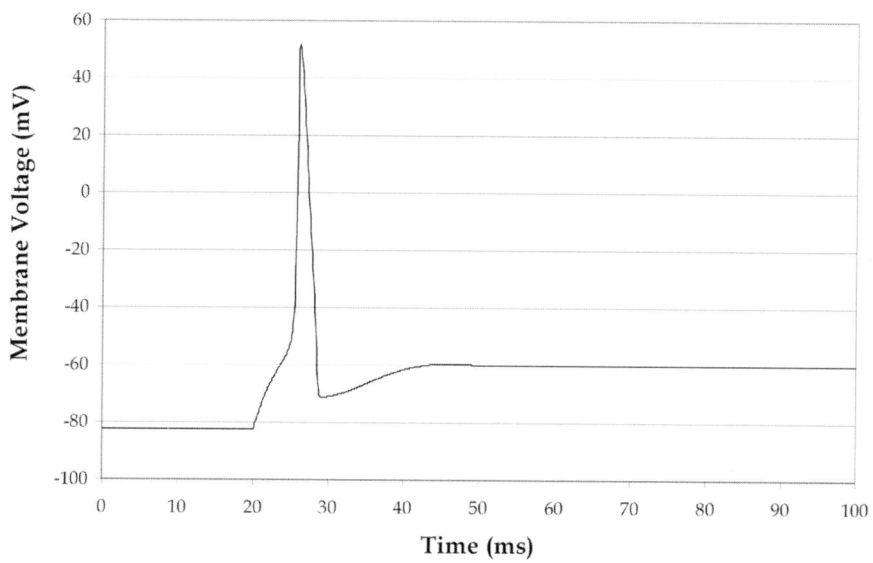

Fig. 6. With the Hodgkin–Huxley model of Equation 4, a −10 μA current pulse is used to hyperpolarize the cell membrane to approximately −80 mv for a very long time, and then turns off at 20 ms. After release from hyperpolarization at 20 ms, a single action potential occurs, without any stimulation.

current pulse of 20 μA for 6 ms with no initial hyperpolarization. Fig. 6 illustrates a single burst firing for a neuron after coming out of marked hyperpolarization with the normal Hodgkin–Huxley model, and without stimulation. Unique in this simulation is that no excitatory stimulus is used to cause the action potential; an action potential is caused by the hyperpolarization.

Fig. 7 illustrates spontaneous burst firing without stimulation in a neuron after coming out of

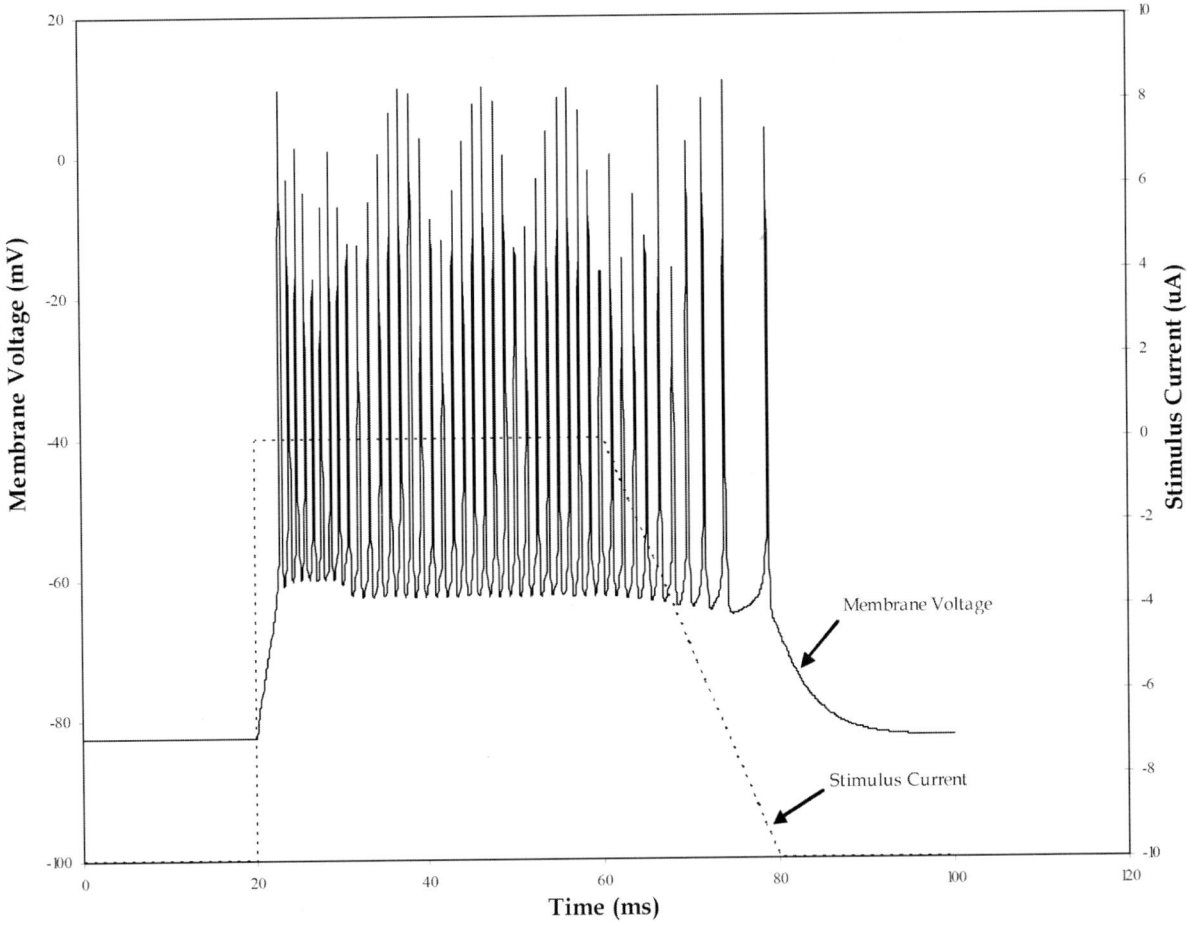

Fig. 7. The Hodgkin–Huxley model of Eq. 4, with the equation for α_m replaced by Equation 5 and the time constant for the n, m and h differential equations scaled appropriately is used in this simulation. A -10 μA current pulse is used to hyperpolarize the cell membrane to -80 mv for a very long time, and then is turned off at 20 ms, and reapplied at 60 ms. After release from hyperpolarization at 20 ms, the neuron fires spontaneously at approximately 1000 Hz without any stimulation until it is hyperpolarized again at 60 ms.

marked hyperpolarization at 20 ms using the modified Hodgkin–Huxley Eq. 5 in Eq. 4, an action potential occurring each time V_m reaches -60 mV. This continues without pause until the membrane is hyperpolarized at 80 ms when the membrane returns to a constant voltage of approximately -80 mV. To match EBN firing rate as in fig. 4 of Robinson (1981), the right-hand side of the n, m and h equations are multiplied by 35,000 from 20 to 30 ms to achieve a 1000 Hz firing rate, and then by 30,000 from 30 to 80 ms to achieve an approximate 800 Hz firing rate. Further, the current pulse is reapplied over a 20 ms interval from 60 to 80 ms to match the decay from steady state firing observed in the data.

After release from hyperpolarization, the simulation shown in Fig. 7 has a firing rate of approximately 1000 Hz initially, drops to 800 Hz, and then returns to zero after the neuron is hyperpolarized again. Notice that instead of having a plateau firing rate of 800 Hz in Fig. 7, a slow decay in the interval 30–80 ms could have been modeled by lowering the constant from 30,000 linearly over the interval. Fig. 8 summarizes the firing frequency in Fig. 7, with the EBN firing rate calculated from the inverse of the time interval between each action potential. A duration of 60 ms EBN burst usually results in a 10° saccade. The results in Fig. 7 summarized in Fig. 8 match the characteristics of EBN data shown in fig. 4 of

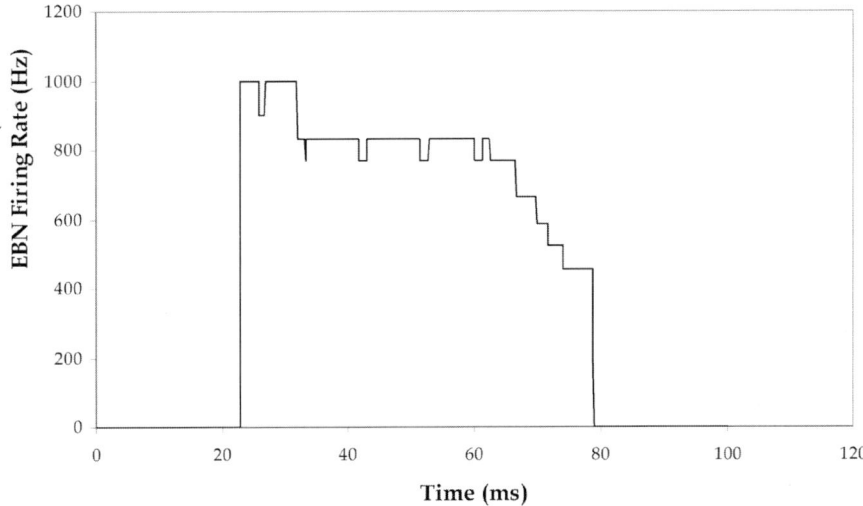

Fig. 8. EBN firing rate calculated from Fig. 7. The firing rate is calculated from the inverse of the time interval between each action potential.

Robinson (1981) very closely (see figure for the 11° saccade).

Direct projections from the SC to the PPRF have been demonstrated anatomically in numerous studies. Previous electrophysiological experiments in monkey have demonstrated that direct projections from the SC to LLBN exist, but recently have failed to find evidence for monosynaptic connections from the SC to EBN. Other investigators support direct connections between the SC and EBN. Perhaps some of the trouble in accepting that the EBN is not directly stimulated by the SC or other neurons is the difficulty in discerning how the EBN firing rate characteristics are so closely tied to the saccade without direct stimulation by a neural controller. Since a direct cause and effect relationship is normally expected in such a system, just releasing a group of neurons from inhibition that causes 'spontaneous' firing does not at first appear reasonable. Another difficulty is the relationship between the firing rate of the EBN and saccade accuracy as the two are tightly coupled. Here, a model of the EBN is described using a Hodgkin–Huxley model of the neuron in which the threshold and time constant have been adjusted to yield a spontaneously firing neuron that has EBN characteristics. With this updated biophysical property in the Hodgkin–Huxley model, the EBN is capable of firing at 1000 Hz automatically and without stimulation when released from inhibition, and has tightly linked characteristics to the saccade based solely on the duration of the burst firing under time optimal control (Enderle and Wolfe, 1987). It should be noted that the EBNs have been reported to receive projections from the vestibular fibers and burster-driving neurons in the vestibular nuclei, sites that are not active during goal directed saccades considered (Markham, 1981; Ohki et al., 1988; Galiana, 1991). It is not clear how these inputs would impact the EBN, but further study is certainly warranted.

The role of the LLBN is not exactly clear based on experimental evidence, with some supporting an LLBN to EBN projection, and some not supporting the LLBN to EBN projection (Scudder, 1988a,b; Moschovakis et al., 1996; Gancarz and Grossberg, 1998). It is clear that the LLBN receives projections from the SC, and the LLBN may be involving in an integrating mechanism, but the integrative mechanism is not uniformly accepted (Gancarz and Grossberg, 1998). The firing characteristics of the LLBN follow those of the SC rather closely, but do not follow the EBN after the OPNs have been inhibited. It is clear that the firing characteristics of the LLBN are not tightly related to the characteristics of the saccade (main sequence), even during the time interval when the OPN is inhibited. The EBN has been described with (1) a resettable leaky integrator in models of the EBN to match the characteristics of experimental data in some studies (Moschovakis et al., 1996; Gancarz and Grossberg, 1998); (2) a BIAS input in order to match the characteristics of experimental data for small saccades (for example, see Scudder, 1988b; Gancarz and Grossberg, 1998).

Neither (1) or (2) above are required with the EBN model proposed here. There is no memory associated with the spontaneously firing EBN, and the neuron fires at high rates for all saccades, which matches the experimental data.

The focus of this work has been the EBN, but it can also be applied to the OPN, which does not seem to have any inputs as well. Some have proposed that the OPNs are stimulated by a thalamic circuit, while others seem to suggest an unknown BIAS circuit. In fact the neuron model presented here can be easily parameterized to match the OPN firing rates of 100–200 Hz.

Components of the burst

Shown in Fig. 9 are sketches of the EBN firing rate drawn to generally match the data in fig. 4 of Robinson (1981) with (A), and the data in fig. 6a of Gancarz and Grossberg (1998) with (B). The interval 0 to T_1 is the minimum duration for EBN burst firing as supported by physiological evidence for saccades of all sizes. For example, a 1° saccade would have a burst of T_1 s, as would a 4° saccade. This interval represents the time it takes to switch off and on the OPN due to the inherent time delays in signal transmission. The interval T_1 to T_2 is the time which the EBN drives the eyes to their destination. The interval T_2 until the EBN ceases firing is when the OPN resumes its inhibition of the EBN; this part of the waveform is the same for saccades of all sizes.

The EBN model presented here is designed to have a constant plateau of firing during the interval 30 to 60 ms to model the firing rate of fig. 4 of Robinson (1981). It can also be modified to have a small reduction in firing rate during this interval to match experimental data shown in fig. 6a of Gancarz and Grossberg (1998). The decay can be implemented as previously described with a linear reduction in firing rate of this interval, and might be attributable to a reduction in ions or energy necessary to maintain the firing rate. It should be noted that the firing rate of the EBN is quite random from saccade to saccade. Gancarz and Grossberg indicate that the decreasing firing rate in the interval T_1 to T_2 for the EBN is due to IBN inhibition of the LLBN. Since the LLBNs in their model drive the EBN, a reduction the LLBN firing rate causes a reduction in the EBN firing rate. Such a strategy implies that the EBN reflects an error signal. Such results are not consistently observed in the data published in the literature.

Regardless of the firing rate of the EBN during the interval T_1 to T_2, the motoneurons and muscles experience a saturation effect above a certain firing rate, which is approximately 400 Hz. Therefore, whether the firing rate in the interval T_1 to T_2 is a constant or decaying slowly is of little importance due to the muscle saturation affecting the signals driving the eyeballs to their destination.

A minimum duration for an EBN once released from inhibition is T_1 as shown in Fig. 9. T_1 is the smallest possible interval in which the EBN can be switched on and off. This phenomenon is observed in the data, even for microsaccades. To account for minimum burst duration, fewer neurons in the SC fire for small saccades as shown Fig. 10. This figure shows a detailed view of the SC for a 20° movement and a 2° movement. Notice the locus of points for the 2° movement is smaller than that for the 20° movement implying that fewer neurons are firing for the smaller movement. Above 7°, the size of the movement field remains constant in the SC. Below 7°, the size of the movement field decreases as 0 is approached. Since fewer cells firing in the SC means fewer cells in the LLBN, this implies that fewer EBNs are released from inhibition via OPN release, and fewer cells are driving the eyes to their destination. This also explains why small saccades all have approximately the same duration up to about 7°.

Superior colliculus and the moving hill hypothesis

Very few saccade generator models incorporate a functional model of the SC and the influence of the cerebellum on the SC. Recent work on the intracollicular activities within the SC during a saccade described a moving hill of neural activity (Munoz et al., 1991, 1996; Munoz and Wurtz, 1992, 1993a,b,

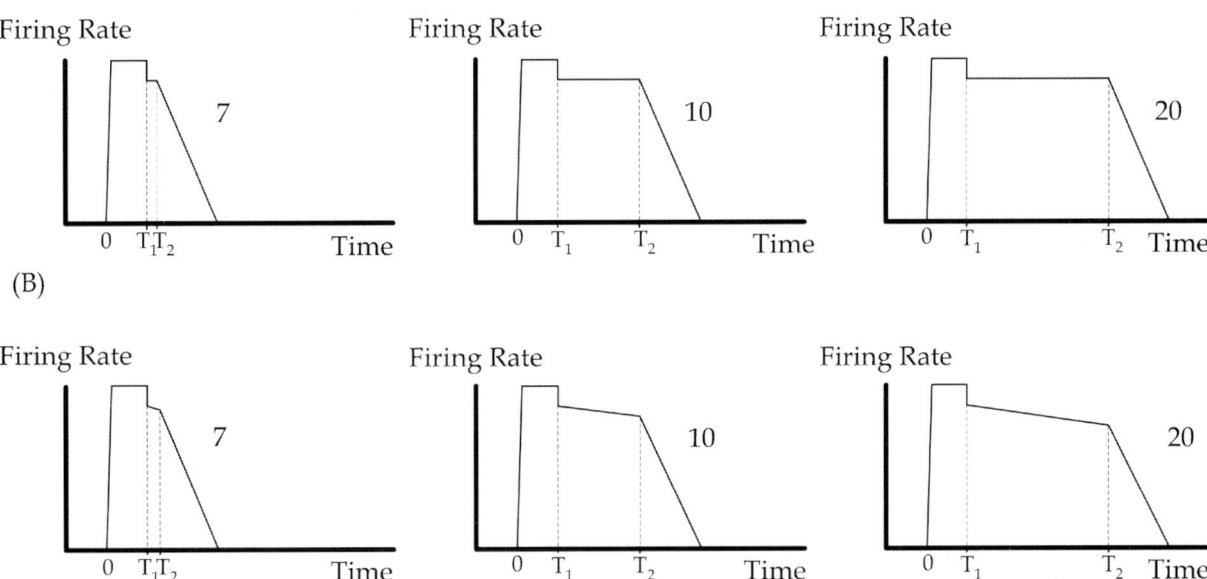

Fig. 9. Block sketch of EBN firing rates for 5°, 10°, and 20° saccades drawn to match the data in Robinson (1981) shown in A, and in Gancarz and Grossberg (1998) in B. Notice that the functions are identical from 0 to T_1 for all cases, where this represents the minimum time for an EBN burst.

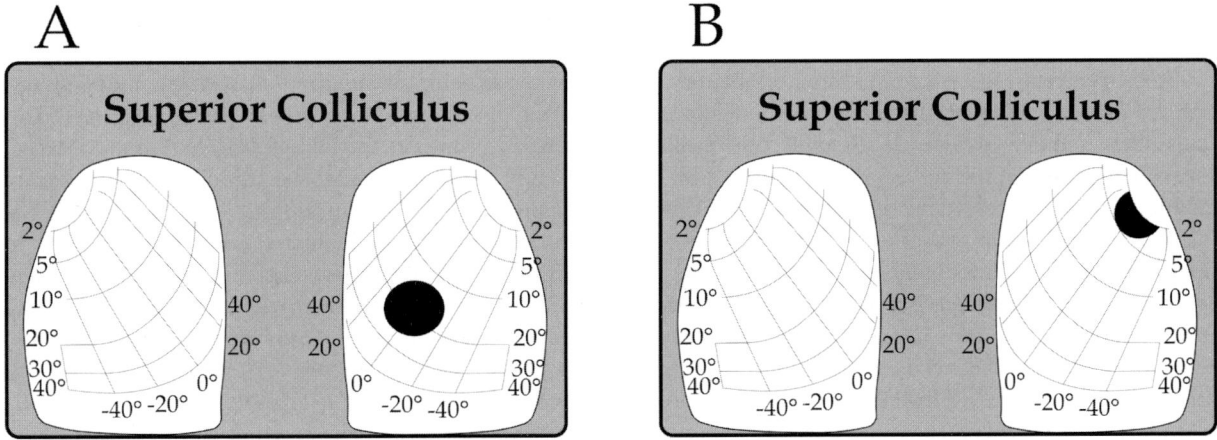

Fig. 10. A detailed view of the superior colliculus for a 20° movement (A), and a 2° movement (B). Notice that the locus of points for the 2° movement is smaller than that for the 20° movement implying that fewer neurons are firing for the smaller movement. The movement field within the superior colliculus also reflects that the number of neurons firing for saccades less than 7° are fewer than those firing for saccades greater than 7°. For saccades above 7°, the movement field is approximately constant.

1995a,b; Munoz and Istvan, 1998). However, Anderson et al. (1998) observed very little movement of activity within the SC and therefore questioned the existence of a moving hill of activity. Further work by Port et al. (2000) demonstrated a moving hill within the SC. A model of the SC is presented here based on the hypothesis of Munoz et al. that explains all the observations found by Munoz et al. (Short and Enderle, 2001). This model generates only horizontal movements and focuses on the series of events within the SC using SIMULINK to simulate saccades, but could easily be expanded to horizontal and vertical saccades.

The SC is modeled as three separate subsystems, the superficial, intermediate, and deep layers. The superficial layer acts as a relay of visual information from the retina to the LGN and NRTP. The intermediate layer models the burst layer of the SC and as such receives both excitatory and inhibitory afferent signals, and projects to the PPRF. The deep layer receives signals relating desired eye movement and converts the polar position coordinate to rectangular collicular coordinates. The location on the collicular map is related to the burst layer to define the future active site within that layer. Activity within the deep layer begins 100 ms prior to saccade initiation at the site of desired motor error. Once the eye movement begins, the deep layer uses a feedback system to model the moving hill. As the moving hill approaches the rostral pole, activity within the population of fixation neurons increases. This increases activation of inhibitory interneurons that then begin to inhibit the activity of the more caudal burst neurons. The intermediate burst layer creates an active region centered at the point of optimal saccade amplitude.

Activity occurs in up to three-quarters of the SC map in the buildup layer, the actual amount activated dependent on size of saccade. Several studies have been done to examine the population activity both spatially and temporally. Both Munoz and Wurtz (1995a,b), and Anderson et al. (1998) support that activity in the buildup layer encompasses a larger portion of the whole map for any size saccade than activity for the same saccade in the burst layer. Moreover, the size of the active zone changes with the amplitude of the saccade. However, Munoz and Wurtz demonstrated a movement of the locus of activity within the buildup layer as a saccade develops so that the active region in the buildup layer moves rostrally across the retinotopic map and excites the fixation neurons, ending the saccade. Anderson et al. observed some movement in the buildup layer, but that the movement failed to reach the rostral pole. Anderson et al. also examined clipped saccade metrics via stimulation of the rostral pole versus saccades clipped via OPN stimulation. These results indicate that there were some differences in the outcomes of the two experiments, most notably revealing that fixation neurons are not the primary controller for the OPN. These seemingly contradictory pieces of information are easily explained if the fixation pole of the SC is considered an inhibitory unit for the SC only, and not the rest of the saccadic system.

While information is shared between the OPN and the fixation pole, this connection operates as a supporting connection only. If the burst from the SC is silenced by the fixation neurons, then the signal to the LLBN is clipped and the OPNs are released from inhibition. The OPNs then inhibit the EBNs which ends the saccade. Signals sent from the fixation cells to the OPN may serve to reduce the latency between the end of LLBN activity and the resumption of tonic activity. Both Anderson et al. and Munoz et al. performed experiments to determine the spatial profile of population activity in the buildup layer. Results indicate a buildup layer with very irregular activity profiles that vary from one measurement to the next.

Within the model by Short and Enderle (2001), feedback is introduced to force the moving hill across the motor map. This feedback comes from the NPH projection to the SC. As the buildup layer receives the current gaze error, the Gaussian peak of the buildup population shifts to the updated gaze error. The buildup layer uses lateral inhibition to control fixation and movement cell activity. As movement cell activity increases, the fixation neurons are inhibited. The location on the collicular surface that correlates with the center of population activity defines the saccade amplitude and direction. The cell that receives this input then activates neighboring cells. Current motor error is sent back to the buildup layer, moving the hill of activity toward the rostral pole.

This SC model is intended to simulate afferent and efferent connections of the SC with respect to the generation of horizontal saccadic eye movements as well as demonstrate intracollicular interactions. Here, the focus is simulated activity within SC as the saccade is generated. The series of diagrams in Fig. 11 depict the change in activation within the buildup layer of the SC as the saccade proceeds. Clearly demonstrated is the initial activation of the fixation pole, the simultaneous rise of the movement neuron activity and fall of the fixation neuron activ-

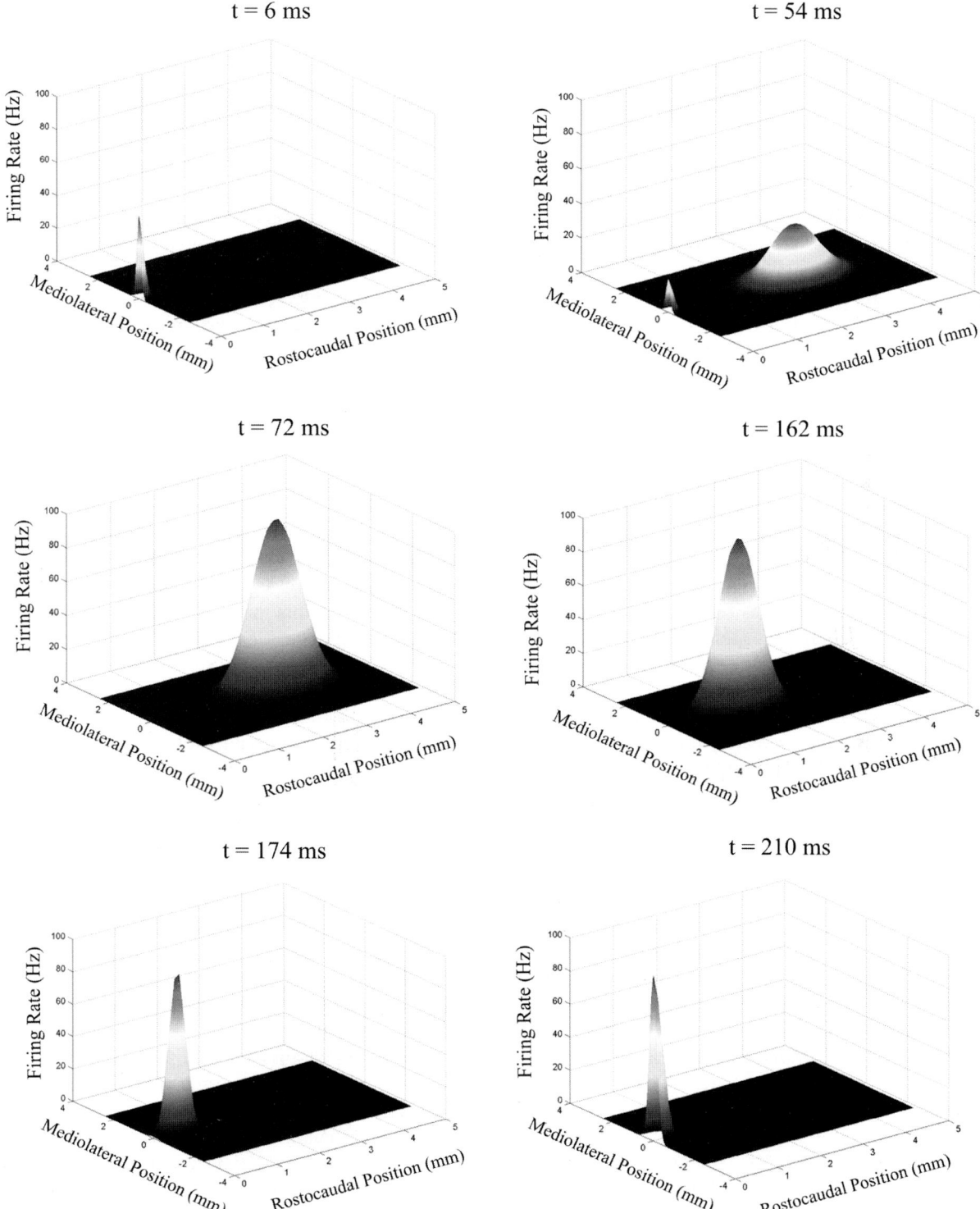

Fig. 11. Sequence of population activity within the intermediate layer of the superior colliculus.

ity, and the resumption of tonic fixation pole firing after saccade termination. Note also the change in active population as the remaining error decreases below 10°.

The operation of the moving hill in the SC provides a rudimentary control system consisting of a simple feedback circuit. If the FN is lesioned, the SC does terminate the saccade, but the saccade overshoots its destination. The SC termination is due to the influence of the substantia nigra and the fixation pole of the buildup layer. With cerebellar control in place, the hill of activity within the buildup layer does not always reach the rostral pole. Indeed, Anderson et al. (1998) determined that there was no strong evidence to support the moving hill hypothesis, statistical analysis did not show activation of these cells serially ordered from caudal as opposed to in random order. Activity of individual neurons does not correlate well with the resulting saccadic eye movement as individual burst neurons do not always reflect their positions within the retinotopic motor map. However, the response of the entire active population does correlate well with the desired motor error. Therefore, it is not surprising that individual buildup neurons would demonstrate optimal movement fields that seem contrary to the expected activity defined by their location.

Anderson et al. (1998) noted that oculomotor neurons cease firing approximately 6 ms before the saccade ends which would mean that collicular events would need to lead eye movements by approximately 8 ms. Since the experimental data collected failed to demonstrate this timing sequence, the robustness of the moving hill is challenged unless the operation of the total saccade network is considered. The original moving hill hypothesis proposed that the rostral spread of activity served as a terminator of the saccade. While this mechanism functions in this capacity, the SC provides a less accurate control system that is superseded by the precise control of the cerebellum. The rostral spread of activity in the SC can serve to terminate a saccade, with less accuracy, if the FN does not terminate the saccade first.

Cerebellum

The cerebellum is responsible for the coordination of movement and identified as the saccade terminator. It is composed of a cortex of gray matter, internal white matter and three pairs of deep nuclei: FN, the interposed and globose nucleus, and dentate nucleus. The deep cerebellar nuclei and the vestibular nuclei transmit the entire output of the cerebellum. Output of the cerebellar cortex is carried through Purkinje cells. Purkinje cells send their axons to the deep cerebellar nuclei and have an inhibitory effect on these nuclei. The cerebellum is involved with both eye and head movements, and both tonic and phasic activity are reported in the cerebellum. The cerebellum is not directly responsible for the initiation or execution of a saccade, but contributes to saccade precision. Consistent with the operation of the cerebellum for other movement activities, the cerebellum is postulated here to act as the coordinator for a saccade, and act as a precise gating mechanism.

The cerebellum is included in the saccade generator as a time-optimal gating element, using three active sites during a saccade: the vermis, FN and flocculus. The vermis is concerned with the absolute starting position of a saccade in the movement field, and corrects control signals for initial eye position. Using proprioceptors in the oculomotor muscles and an internal eye position reference, the vermis is aware of the current position of the eye. The vermis is also aware of the DME used to generate the saccade via the connection with the NRTP and the SC.

With regard to the oculomotor system, the cerebellum has inputs from SC, lateral geniculate nucleus (LGN), oculomotor muscle proprioceptors, and striate cortex via NRTP. The cerebellum sends inputs to the NRTP, LLBN, EBN, VN, thalamus, and SC as shown in Fig. 3. The oculomotor vermis and FN are important in the control of saccade amplitude, and the flocculus, perihypoglossal nuclei of the rostral medulla, and possibly the pontine and mesencephalic reticular formation are thought to form the integrator with the cerebellum. One important function of the flocculus may be to increase the time constant of the neural integrator for saccades starting at locations different from primary position.

Purkinje cells exert an inhibitory action on the output of the cerebellum (deep nuclei axons) as shown in Fig. 3. As a result, an initial burst of excitation in the deep cerebellar nuclei is followed by inhibition delivered by the Purkinje cells. This mechanism enables the cerebellum to serve as a precise timing device. By means of its output projections to the thalamus and motor cortex and to the red nucleus, the cerebellum regulates the timing necessary to generate the complex patters of muscle activation. Of these nuclei, FN plays an important role in saccadic eye movement system (Dean, 1995; Hashimoto and Ohtsuka, 1995; Ohtsuka and Noda, 1995; Enderle and Engelken, 1996; Leichnetz et al., 1984; Leichnetz and Gonzalo-Ruiz, 1996; Schweighofer et al., 1996; Versino et al., 1996; Goffart and Pelisson, 1997; Krauzlis and Miles, 1998; Takagi et al., 1998). Cells in the FN exit the cerebellum taking two paths. Crossing axons from the FN pass to the vestibular nuclei and reticular formation of the pons and medulla. Uncrossed fibers pass via the inferior cerebellar peduncle to reach the vestibular nuclei and reticular formation.

The oculomotor vermis is connected with the absolute starting position of a saccade (Vilis et al., 1983; Krauzlis and Miles, 1998; Takagi et al., 1998). The vermis is topographically organized as determined through stimulation studies. It is known that non-primary position saccades have different characteristics than saccades initiated from primary position. For instance, a saccade starting from 30° and moving to primary position has higher peak velocity and shorter duration than a saccade moving from primary position to 30° (this is due to the oculomotor plant elastic elements, etc.). In lesion studies, a saccade is still executed after the cerebellum is removed. However, the accuracy of saccade execution is greatly diminished with marked postsaccadic drift (Optican and Miles, 1980). Here the saccade is terminated with the less accurate SC termination circuit as discussed previously without cerebellar termination. In addition to the cerebellum's role as a coordinator for saccadic eye movements, it is also involved in long term adaptive control (Optican and Miles, 1980, 1985).

The FN receives input from the SC, as well as other sites. The output of the FN is excitatory and projects ipsilaterally and contralaterally as shown in Fig. 3. During fixation, the FN fires tonically at low rates. Twenty milliseconds prior to a saccade, the contralateral FN bursts, and the ipsilateral FN pauses and then discharges with a burst. The pause in ipsilateral firing is due to Purkinje cell input to the FN. The sequential organization of Purkinje cells along beams of parallel fibers suggests that the cerebellar cortex might function as a delay, producing a set of timed pulses which could be used to program the duration of the saccade. If one considers non-primary position saccades, different temporal and spatial schemes, via cerebellar control, are necessary to produce the same size saccade.

Fastigial cells exhibit unique responses depending on the direction of saccades and are involved in terminating the saccade. Purkinje cells in the oculomotor vermis (lobules VIc and VII) are thought to modulate these discharges of fastigial cells (Sato and Kawasaki, 1990; Sato and Noda, 1992; Dean, 1995; Goffart and Pelisson, 1997). The cerebellar vermis and its associated deep cerebellar nucleus, the caudal fastigial, is directly implicated in every aspect of the on-line control of saccades: initiation (latency), accuracy (amplitude and direction) and dynamics (velocity and acceleration), and also in the acquisition of adaptive oculomotor behavior. The FNs receive topographically organized projections from the anterior and posterior lobe vermis and project bilaterally to the brain stem reticular formation and to the lateral vestibular nuclei. The FNs also have crossed ascending projections that reach the motor cortex after relaying in the ventrolateral nucleus.

Interestingly, experimental data relating the cerebellar vermis and FN to the precise execution of a saccade have resulted in very few mathematical models (Schweighofer et al., 1996; Lefèvre et al., 1998; Enderle, 2000). A first-order time optimal neural control model for horizontal saccadic eye movement mechanism was proposed by Enderle and Wolfe (1987), Enderle (1994), Enderle et al. (2000). In this model, the control mechanism is initiated by the SC and terminated by the cerebellar FN. Agonist burst cell activity is initiated with maximal firing due to an error between the target and eye position, and continues until the internal eye position in the cerebellar vermis reaches the desired position, then decays to zero. After the agonist burst, antagonist neural activity rises with a stochastic rebound burst and from input from the FN, then falls to a tonic firing level necessary to keep the eye at its destination. Each of the neural sites in the model fires similarly to experimental data, and simulate saccadic eye movements.

Saccade controller

Qualitatively, all studies support the crude pulse–step, or more refined pulse–slide–step for the neural control of saccades, the sum of EBN and TN firing rates. Additionally, some support a stochastic antagonist neural brake operating at the end of the saccade (Robinson, 1981; Van Gisbergen et al., 1981; Van Opstal et al., 1985). Quantitatively, two general patterns of neural activity have evolved. One supports a firing rate–saccade amplitude independent saccadic control mechanism during the pulse or burst phase. The other supports a firing rate–saccade amplitude dependent saccadic control mechanism during the pulse phase.

In 1964, Robinson first suggested the notion of a time optimal controller based on force measurements with a suction contact lens. In 1970, Fuchs and Luschei presented microelectrode results that indicate firing frequency during the pulse phase of saccadic eye movements is independent of saccade amplitude, and that the duration of the pulse alone determines the size of the saccade for saccades greater than 10° (Fuchs and Luschei, 1970). Schiller (1970) also used microelectrode results to demonstrate that firing frequency during the pulse phase of saccadic eye movements is independent of saccade amplitude for saccades of all sizes, and that the size of the saccade is determined by the duration of the burst. Firing rate–saccade amplitude independent results are also seen in Robinson, 1981 (fig. 4), and in Van Gisbergen et al., 1981 (figs. 2 and 4) for saccades as low as 7° (but were not interpreted as such by these investigators). Theoretical and experimental results by Enderle and Wolfe (1987) further support firing rate–saccade amplitude independence to saccades of all sizes by proposing a first-order time optimal control of horizontal saccadic eye movements. Currently, most oculomotor researchers support a firing rate–saccade amplitude dependent saccadic control mechanism during the pulse phase. Robinson first reported a firing rate–saccade amplitude dependent saccadic control (Robinson, 1970) based on microelectrode results. In 1975, Collins reported that the amplitude and duration of the pulse phase determines the magnitude of a saccade based on muscle tension recordings; specifically, he determined a logarithmic relationship between innervation amplitude and saccade magnitude.

Microelectrode investigators previously identified as supporting a firing rate–saccade amplitude independent saccadic control mechanism, now support a firing rate–saccade amplitude dependent saccade controller. Interestingly, Van Gisbergen et al. (1981) and Robinson (1981) described a firing rate–saccade amplitude dependent saccade controller, yet, as Scudder (1988b), and Enderle and Wolfe (1987) point out, their microelectrode results clearly support a firing rate–saccade amplitude independent controller.

Today, an increasing number of investigators are describing the saccade controller via a local feedback loop that continuously drives the eye to its destination. This hypothesis, first presented by Vossius (1960), did not start to gain acceptance until Robinson (1975) re-examined it. Subsequently, a number of other investigators have modified the local feedback mechanism proposed by Robinson to better describe the neural connections and firing patterns of brainstem neurons during saccades. Several models of the saccade generator have evolved with a few listed here: the Robinson model (as modified by Van Gisbergen et al., 1981), the Scudder model (1988b), the Schweighofer model (1996), the Gancarz and Grossberg model (1998), the Lefèvre model (1998), and the Enderle time optimal control model (1987, 1994, 2000). The Robinson's saccade generator model is a firing rate–saccade amplitude dependent controller. The Scudder saccade generator model is structured to provide a control signal that is firing rate–saccade amplitude dependent, and is based on microelectrode results. The Schweighofer model is a firing rate–saccade amplitude dependent controller that incorporates the cerebellum as an adaptive controller of the saccade gain. The Gancarz and Grossberg model also uses a firing rate–saccade amplitude dependent controller. The Lefèvre model is a firing rate–saccade amplitude dependent controller with the cerebellum involved with residual motor error. The time optimal saccade generator model discussed here uses a firing rate–saccade amplitude independent controller initiated by the SC, and terminated by the FN of the cerebellum. Except for the time optimal saccade generator model, all of the other models use an inaccurate model of the oculomotor plant.

Significant differences exist among interpretation of microelectrode recordings, especially for small saccades. For large saccades (those greater than 10°), most investigators support 'an identical high level of rather steady discharge' in the ipsilateral EBN. The saccade size is determined by the duration of the burst. Under a time optimal controller discussed here, small saccades of size less than 7° have a constant burst duration T_1; the size of the saccade is determined by the number of EBN firing due to a smaller movement field in the SC. The time optimal saccade generator during small saccades has the appearance of a controller which depends on the size of the saccade, but is actually due to a firing rate–saccade amplitude independent controller given the constraint that the neuron burst has minimum burst duration.

Based on an inverse method, Van Opstal et al. (1985) calculated the firing rate (more properly viewed as active state tension because of low-pass filtering and saturation effects within the muscle) during saccades, and then postulated a firing rate–saccade amplitude dependent controller. The conclusion by Van Opstal et al. gives the appearance of a firing rate–saccade amplitude dependent controller, but these characteristics can be due to the low-pass filtering and muscle saturation effects on a firing rate–saccade amplitude independent controller. The calculated firing rate results reported fit a firing rate–saccade amplitude independent controller as previously described, that is, for small saccades, fewer cells firing results in a smaller active state tension. Cullen et al. (1996) used a system identification technique and found a firing rate–saccade amplitude dependent controller, but used a first-order oculomotor plant, which may have impacted their results.

Time optimal control of saccades

The saccade generator described here is based on work by Enderle (1994), Enderle and Wolfe (1987), Enderle et al. (2000). The model is first-order time optimal, initiated by the intermediate layers of the SC and terminated by the FN of the cerebellum. Under a time optimal saccade controller, the agonist muscle is stimulated by a pulse (the ipsilateral EBN burst) that fires maximally regardless of the size of the saccade, and only the duration of the pulse affects the size of the saccade. In general, whenever a retinal error exists, the contralateral SC fires driving the DME to zero as described previously with the moving hill, initiating burst activity through the network described in Fig. 3. Agonist burst cell activity is initiated with maximal firing due to an error between the target and eye position, and continues until the internal eye position in the cerebellar vermis reaches the desired position, then decays to zero. The cerebellar vermis is responsible for adapting the duration of maximal firing based on the initial position of the eye. After the agonist burst, antagonist neural activity rises with a stochastic rebound burst from FN input, and then falls to a tonic firing level necessary to keep the eye at its destination. The onset of the antagonist tonic firing is stochastic, weakly coordinated with the end of the agonist burst, and under cerebellar control.

Both the agonist and antagonist controllers exhibit random behavior from saccade to saccade. This controller is different than others presented in the literature that are either based on a position model or a vector model. The EBN model presented here supports a time optimal controller in which the firing frequency does not depend on the saccade size and can vary from saccade to saccade of the same size. The saccade size is determined solely by the length of time that the ipsilateral EBN is bursting in the interval 0 to T_2, and the number of neurons firing. Lefèvre et al. (1998) describe two different types of saccade controllers: (1) temporal coding of the DME by the activity of SC based on the dependence of SC burst neuron firing as a function of DME; (2) spatial coding of DME is reflected via a moving hill in the SC.

Both controllers produce accurate saccades and are based on a local area feedback. The model by Lefèvre and the time optimal model also produce accurate saccades, but are different than (1) and (2) because of the use of the cerebellum as the terminator of the saccade. A problem with both controllers of type 1 and 2 identified by Lefèvre involves lesion studies and the incorrect output of the models, with only the Lefèvre and time optimal models providing a correct output. The Lefèvre model operates by having the SC project to the MLBN directly with excitatory signals dependent on the DME. Further, the Lefèvre model uses the concept of increasing SC projection weights to the MLBN as saccade amplitude increases (a firing rate–saccade amplitude dependent controller), a second-order oculomotor

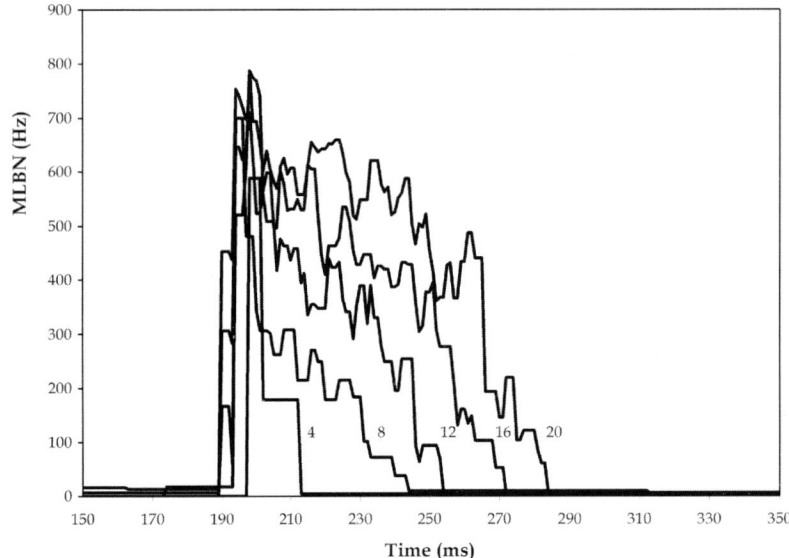
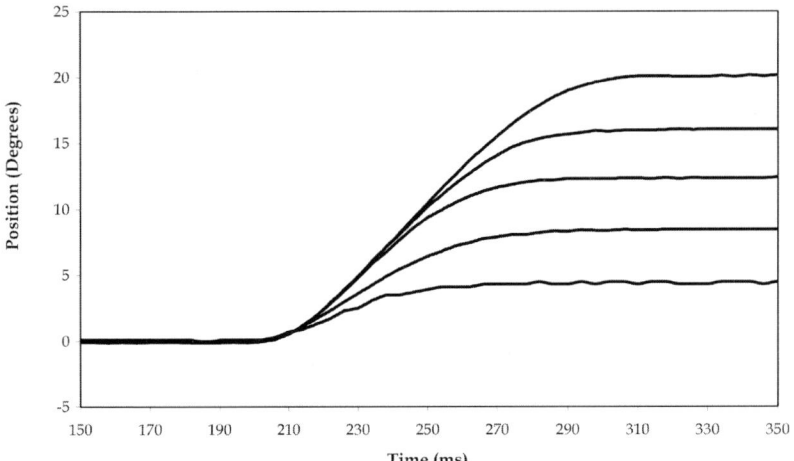
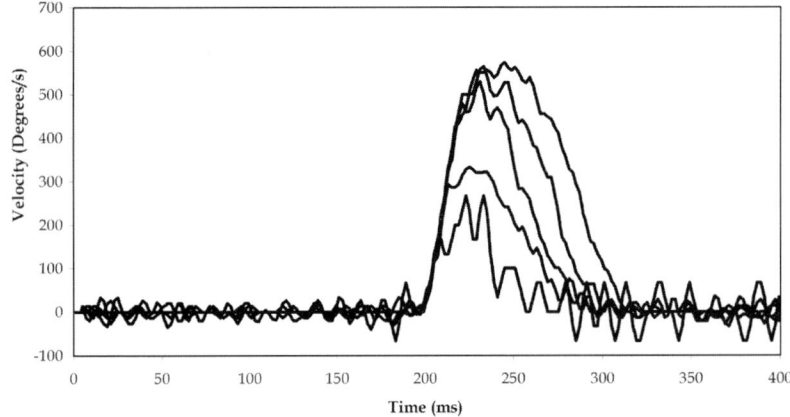

plant, and an OPN with a bias similar to the Scudder model. All of the models except for the time optimal model provide an EBN firing rate proportional to the DME. The concept of EBN firing in proportion to the DME is supported indirectly by even new studies (Van Opstal and Kappen, 1993; Cullen et al., 1996); however, EBN data reported in the literature do not consistently support this type of controller and even data that are highlighted as supportive do not have a one-to-one relationship between DME and EBN firing rate, nor do they take into account the number of neurons firing.

Generally, saccades recorded for any size amplitude are extremely variable, with wide variations in the latent period, time to peak velocity, peak velocity (indicative of variations in pulse magnitude), and saccade duration. Furthermore, variability is well coordinated for saccades of the same size. Saccades with lower peak velocity are matched with longer saccade durations and saccades with higher peak velocity are matched with shorter saccade durations. Thus, saccades driven to the same destination usually have different trajectories. It is known that saccade dynamics are determined by the number of motoneurons firing in synchrony and their firing rate. Some investigators incorrectly identify the cause of the peak velocity–saccade amplitude profile in the main sequence diagram as due to a nonlinear oculomotor plant driven by a nonlinear saccade amplitude dependent controller. Van Opstal et al. (1985) note "as saccades become larger, their duration increases and peak velocity shows a less-than-linear increase. For a linear system, instead, duration would be the same for all amplitudes and peak velocity would have a linear relation with amplitude".

Shown in Fig. 12 are five saccades elicited from target movements of 4, 8, 12, 16 and 20°. Notice that the 8, 12, 16 and 20° eye movements follow the same trajectory before separating toward the end of the eye movement, consistent with a firing rate-independent controller. The 4° eye movement follows a different trajectory and is due to a smaller population of neurons firing maximally, and is time optimal according to the hypothesis presented here. It is envisioned that the reduced number of neurons is based on the 'time constant of the burster', that is, once firing is initiated in the EBN, it takes approximately 10 ms to turn off. Thus, small saccades could never occur with all neurons firing maximally as observed in the microelectrode recordings, if the system did not compensate by reducing the number of active neurons.

Using the system identification technique, Enderle and Wolfe (1988) demonstrated that the oculomotor plant is essentially linear, and does not significantly affect the main sequence diagram. It should be noted that the main sequence diagram profile is due to the characteristics of the input. Enderle et al. (1991, 2000), Enderle (1994) also described a linear muscle model and oculomotor plant that matches the data very closely. Under a time optimal control of saccades, saccade amplitude is determined by the duration of the pulse (interval 0 to T_2), whereby the pulse magnitude remains constant for saccades of all sizes. Given a time optimal input, peak velocity increases in a quasi-linear manner with saccade amplitude up to approximately 15°, after which it reaches a soft saturation level, consistent with the main sequence diagram. For saccades less than 15°, overall maximal peak velocity is not reached because the EBN burst is turned off before this can happen. Note that if the input were a step waveform, then peak velocity would be the same as the point of soft saturation for the pulse–step input at approximately 15°. Because of muscle saturation, these results are unchanged whether the input in Fig. 9A or B is used.

A firing rate–saccade amplitude dependent controller yields saccades which almost immediately separate into separate trajectories. A firing rate–saccade amplitude independent (time optimal) controller yields saccades which follow the same trajectory during the pulse phase for saccades over 7°, and

Fig. 12. Extracellular single-unit recordings from within the abducens nucleus (MLBN), eye position and velocity obtained from rhesus monkeys during saccadic eye movements. Eye position data were recorded using magnetic coils, neural activity were recorded using tungsten microelectrodes. No filtering of the data was carried out, but the firing frequency was placed in the usual format of frequency of firing over 1 ms intervals, rather than the electrical activity itself. Details of the experiment and training are reported elsewhere (Sparks et al., 1976; data provided by Dr. David Sparks).

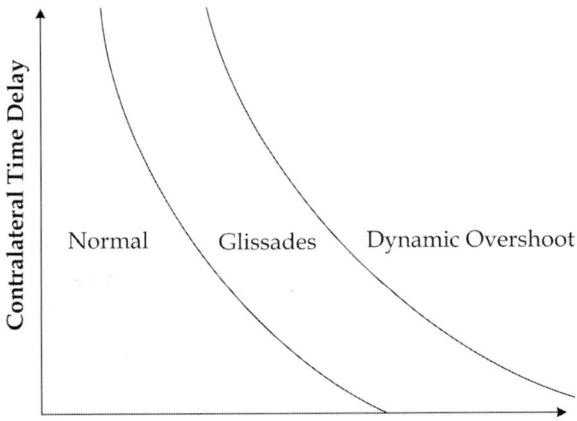

Fig. 13. Diagram illustrating a common mechanism of action for postsaccade phenomena involving normal saccades, dynamic overshoot and glissadic behavior.

then separate. This is usually difficult to appreciate given the large variability in saccades of the same size. A firing rate–saccade amplitude independent (time optimal) controller yields saccades which almost immediately separate into separate trajectories during the pulse phase for saccades under 7° because fewer EBNs are firing as described here. Similar statements can be made for saccade velocity. Note that in Fig. 12, the data for position and velocity support a firing rate–saccade amplitude independent (time optimal) controller. In general, families of recorded saccades are not frequently reported in the literature. Of those saccade families reported, Van Opstal et al. (1985) in fig. 2a and Robinson (1964) support saccades with the characteristics like those in Fig. 12.

Dynamic overshoot and glissades

Using a Hodgkin–Huxley model of an EBN, it is possible to explain many postsaccade phenomena, such as dynamic overshoot and glissades. Undershoot is the phenomenon whereby the final eye position falls short of the target position. Dynamic overshoot is an eye position overshoot, followed by a quick saccade-like return to a lower steady state eye position. Glissadic overshoot is similar to dynamic overshoot, but with a return to steady state that is more gradual. Glissadic undershoot is an initial eye position undershoot, followed by a gradual rise to a higher steady eye position.

Marked inhibition of neurons within the PPRF often results in postinhibitory rebound burst firing activity at the beginning and end of a saccade. Ipsilateral IBN inhibition of the contralateral EBN may cause the postinhibitory rebound burst firing activity within these cells, shortly after the DME returns to zero as observed in the cerebellar vermis. This burst might be responsible for the small burst identified in some data before being inhibited by the OPN. The occurrence of postinhibitory rebound bursts are a random and unplanned portion of the firing rate. However, the average effects of the rebound burst are adaptively compensated through cerebellar interaction.

One consequence of the termination of the saccade by the cerebellar circuit is that it offers a common mechanism for saccades of all types, including those with dynamic overshoot, glissadic behavior and undershoot. Depending on the timing of the termination signal by the cerebellum and any rebound burst observed in the antagonist muscle by the contralateral EBN, one of three types of behavior can occur as shown in Fig. 13. The occurrence of dynamic overshoot during saccadic eye movements is quite varied and reported from 5% to 70% depending on the subject (Bahill et al., 1975; Lehman and Stark, 1983; Kapoula et al., 1986). Furthermore, the incidence of dynamic overshoot decreases as saccade size increases. Here, it is suggested that dynamic overshoot is primarily caused by unplanned postinhibitory rebound burst firing as the DME as monitored in the cerebellar vermis returns to zero, and the time gap in inhibition of the contralateral EBN by the ipsilateral IBN and the OPN. The timing of the postinhibitory rebound burst is critical for dynamic overshoot; it is surmised here that the rebound burst must be delayed approximately 15 ms (or more) after the initiation of the DME return to zero. Moreover, the amplitude of the rebound burst must be of sufficiently high amplitude for dynamic overshoot to occur with a sufficient number of neurons firing. With muscle saturation effects, these cells do not need to fire at 1000 Hz to cause a dynamic break, but fire at the 100–200 Hz rate observed in the data of Robinson (1981) and Van Gisbergen et al. (1981).

One reported mechanism of action for glissadic overshoot describes a central nervous system (CNS) dependent error in computing the duration of the agonist EBN burst and not the level of EBN firing (Bahill et al., 1975, 1978). Support for this hypothesis is derived from reported lower peak velocities of glissades, as compared to other types of saccades. Experimental results, however, indicate that glissades have the same distribution of peak velocities as other types of saccades. Another mechanism of action for glissadic overshoot uses an adaptive mechanism for suppression of postsaccadic drift (Optican and Miles, 1985). This mechanism supports a CNS error in the gain of the step and the time constant of the slide for glissade generation. Glissades are quite common, with a frequency of occurrence of approximately 35%. This is a rather high CNS error rate for the pulse width glissadic error mechanism and an adaptive mechanism.

Here it is suggested that glissadic overshoot and undershoot are primarily caused by postinhibitory rebound burst firing. As with dynamic overshoot, both the amplitude and timing of the rebound burst is important in generating a glissade. An inherent coordination error exists between the return to tonic firing levels in the abducens and oculomotor nucleus during the completion of a saccade. Ipsilateral abducens nucleus fires (although dynamically changing) during an abducting saccade. Oculomotor nucleus firing activity is inhibited during the pulse phase during an abducting saccade. Because of the ipsilateral IBN inhibition of the contralateral EBN and TN, and ipsilateral oculomotor nucleus, resumption of tonic firing and rebound burst activity in the oculomotor nucleus does not begin until shortly before the ipsilateral IBNs cease firing, a delay of approximately 10 ms after the DME initiates the return to zero. This same delay exists in the abducens nucleus for adducting saccades.

There are significantly more internuclear neurons between the contralateral EBNs and TNs, and the ipsilateral oculomotor nucleus (antagonist neurons during an abducting saccade), than the ipsilateral EBNs and TNs, and ipsilateral abducens nucleus (antagonist neurons during an adducting saccade) (Zee and Leigh, 1983). Due to the greater number of internuclear neurons operating during an abducting saccade, a longer time delay exists before the resumption of activity in the oculomotor nucleus after the pulse phase for abducting than adducting saccades. The abducting time delay is in addition to the time delay present because of IBN activity during the pulse phase as previously discussed.

Since the time delay before the resumption of activity in the oculomotor nucleus after the pulse phase of a saccade is greater for abducting saccades than with adducting saccades, the incidence of saccades with dynamic overshoot should be greater for abducting saccades than adducting saccades. This is precisely what is observed in saccadic eye movement recordings. Nearly all saccades with dynamic overshoot occur in the abducting direction. Additionally, because the contralateral TN firing rate decreases as ipsilateral saccade amplitude increases, the rate of dynamic overshoot decreases since fewer saccades have sufficiently high postinhibitory rebound burst amplitudes. This is also what is observed in saccadic eye movement recordings.

Essentially nothing is known about the distribution of the onset and amplitude of the postinhibitory rebound burst firing. Based on the variability observed in saccadic eye movement response, these variables are stochastic. It appears that the mean onset time of the rebound burst (after the DME return to zero is initiated) is approximately 12 ms for abducting saccades and 10 ms for adducting saccades, both with a standard deviation of 2 ms. Moreover, the mean peak amplitude of the rebound burst is approximately 100 Hz, with a standard deviation of 33 Hz for both abducting and adducting saccades. Certainly, appropriate microelectrode studies are needed to more completely describe these distributions.

Future directions

Future work on the saccadic system may focus on the creation of a three-dimensional homeomorphic oculomotor plant with a saccade generator. Work on the creation of a three-dimensional eye movement model has been carried out by a number of researchers. Korentis (2001) and Korentis and Enderle (2001) have focused on using homeomorphic muscle model with *Pro/Engineer 2000* and *Pro/Mechanica 2000* to construct a 3-D oculomotor plant. They identified central variables associated with modeling 3-D ocular movements with the axes of rotation and the muscle forces that produce them. A major issue related to this work was that the 3-D model must describe the orientation of the eye within its orbit, a far more complex situation than a model involving a horizontal eye movement system. The paths of action in which the muscles act during the entire movement are of paramount importance in modeling the proper dynamic behavior of 3-D eye movements. To accommodate the 3-D oculomotor plant, the saccade generator for horizontal eye movements described in Fig. 3 needs to be expanded for 3-D saccades.

Work by Miller and Demer (1999) has focused on soft rectus muscle pulleys in the oculomotor system in which the muscle telescopes within mid-orbital. Pulleys have important implications for ocular plant dynamics in that pulley models have different mechanics and produce different axes of rotation than those without. Tweed (1997) developed a neural control model based on noncommutative, rotational quaternions relating the orientation of the eye in the head to the integral of the eye velocity command generated by the CNS. A major thrust in this effort is that both Donder's law and Listing's law are neurally satisfied. Raphan (1998) proposed that the oculomotor plant appears commutative to the neural controller as a result of muscle pulleys reported by Miller.

Conclusion

This chapter has focused on quantitative models of the oculomotor plant and control of the saccadic eye movement system. Saccades are extremely variable with wide variations in trajectories, but highly coordinated such that they accurately reach their destination. Each of the oculomotor plant models described here are linear, including the second-order model by Westheimer (1954), one by Bahill et al. (1980) and one by Enderle et al. (2000). The control of saccades is initiated by the SC and terminated by the cerebellar FN. Based on electrophysiological evidence, system identification techniques and main sequence characteristics, a time optimal controller of saccades is presented that provides a common mechanism for all types of saccades including those with dynamic overshoot and glissadic behavior.

To execute a saccade, the ipsilateral LLBN is stimulated by the contralateral SC. Once stimulated, the LLBN then inhibits the tonic firing of the OPN, which allows the MLBN to begin firing. The ipsilateral IBN is stimulated by the ipsilateral LLBN and the contralateral FN of the cerebellum. When released from inhibition, the ipsilateral EBN fires spontaneously. The EBN is also stimulated by the contralateral FN of the cerebellum; however, FN stimulation is not required for a saccade to be generated. The burst firing in the ipsilateral IBN inhibits the contralateral EBN and abducens nucleus, and the ipsilateral oculomotor nucleus. The burst firing in the ipsilateral EBN causes the burst in the ipsilateral abducens nucleus, which stimulates the ipsilateral lateral rectus muscle and the contralateral oculomotor nucleus. With the stimulation of the ipsilateral lateral rectus muscle by the ipsilateral abducens nucleus and the inhibition of the ipsilateral medial rectus muscle via the oculomotor nucleus, a saccade occurs in the right eye. Simultaneously, the contralateral medial rectus muscle is stimulated by the contralateral oculomotor nucleus, and with the inhibition of the contralateral lateral rectus muscle via the abducens nucleus, a saccade occurs in the left eye. Thus the eyes move conjugately under the control of a single drive center.

The end of the saccade is normally terminated by the cerebellum. At the termination time, the cerebellar vermis through the Purkinje cells inhibits the contralateral FN and stimulates the ipsilateral FN. The ipsilateral FN then stimulates the contralateral IBN and EBN. The contralateral IBN then inhibits the ipsilateral EBN, TN and abducens nucleus, and contralateral oculomotor nucleus. With this inhibition, the stimulus to the agonist muscles ceases. The antagonist muscles receive stimulation from the contralateral EBN through the contralateral abducens nucleus and ipsilateral oculomotor nucleus, causing a dynamic break.

Conflicting evidence exists regarding the operation of the EBN during saccades. The EBN operates within two states: complete inhibition, and without inhibition that is characterized by high firing at rates of up to 1000 Hz. While there is direct evidence of projections from the SC to the PPRF, there is conflictory evidence regarding the connections from the SC to the EBN, with the most recent experimental results supporting no direct connections from the SC to the EBN. The only excitatory projection to the EBN active during visually elicited saccades is from the FN. The input from the FN has been shown not to cause the high firing rates in the EBN when the EBN is released from inhibition. Thus there are no known excitatory inputs that cause the 800 to 1000 Hz discharge rate in the EBN. Here, a model of the EBN is described using a Hodgkin–Huxley model of the neuron in which the threshold and time constant has been adjusted. With this updated biophysical property, the EBN is capable of firing at 1000 Hz automatically and without stimulation when released from inhibition. SIMULINK simulations using this neuron model have all of the characteristics of the EBN firing rate during a saccade. This model eliminates the need to introduce BIAS inputs that causes bursting in some models of the saccade generator. Such a model is also appropriate for modeling the omnipause neurons.

Abbreviations

DME	dynamic motor error
EBN	excitatory burst neuron
FN	fastigial nucleus
IBN	inhibitory burst neuron
LLBN	long lead burst neuron
MLBN	medium lead burst neuron
NRTP	nucleus reticularis tegmenti pontis
PPRF	paramedian pontine reticular formation
OPN	omnipause neuron
SN	substantia nigra
SC	superior colliculus
TN	tonic neuron
VN	vestibular nucleus

References

Anderson, R.W., Keller, E.L., Gandhi, N.J. and Das, S. (1998) Two-dimensional saccade-related population activity in superior colliculus in monkey. *J. Neurophys.*, 80(2): 798–817.

Bahill, A.T., Clark, M.R. and Stark, L. (1975) The main sequence, a tool for studying human eye movements. *Math. Biosci.*, 24: 194–204.

Bahill, A.T., Hsu, F.K. and Stark, L. (1978) Glissadic overshoots are due to pulse width errors. *Arch. Neurol.*, 35: 138–142.

Bahill, A.T., Latimer, J.R. and Troost, B.T. (1980) Linear homeomorphic model for human movement. *IEEE Trans. Biomed. Eng.*, 27: 631–639.

Chimoto, S., Iwamoto, Y., Shimazu, H. and Yoshida, K. (1996) Functional connectivity of the superior colliculus with saccade-related brain stem neurons in the cat. *Prog. Brain Res.*, 112: 157–165.

Collins, C.C. (1975) The human oculomotor control system. In: G. Lennerstrand and P. Bach-y-Rita (Eds.), *Basic Mechanisms of Ocular Motility and Their Clinical Implications*. Pergamon, Oxford, pp. 145–180.

Cullen, K.E., Rey, C.G., Guitton, D. and Galiana, H.L. (1996) The use of system identification techniques in the analysis of oculomotor burst neuron spike train dynamics. *J. Comput. Neurosci.*, 3: 347–368.

Dean, P. (1995) Modelling the role of the cerebellar fastigial nuclei in producing accurate saccades: the importance of burst timing. *Neuroscience*, 68(4): 1059–1077.

Enderle, J.D. (1988) Observations on pilot neurosensory control performance during saccadic eye movements. *Aviat. Space Environ. Med.*, 59: 309–313.

Enderle, J.D. (1994) A physiological neural network for saccadic eye movement control. *Armstrong Laboratory/AO-TR-1994-0023*. Air Force Material Command, Brooks Air Force Base, TX.

Enderle, J.D. (2000) The fast eye movement control system. In: J. Bronzino (Ed.), *The Biomedical Engineering Handbook*. CRC Press, Boca Raton, FL, Vol. 2, 2nd ed., Ch. 166, pp. 166-1–166-21.

Enderle, J.D. and Engelken, E.J. (1996) Effects of Cerebellar Lesions on Saccade Simulations. *Biomed. Sci. Instrum.*, 32: 13–22.

Enderle, J.D. and Wolfe, J.W. (1987) Time-optimal control of saccadic eye movements. *IEEE Trans. Biomed. Eng.*, 34(1): 43–55.

Enderle, J.D. and Wolfe, J.W. (1988) Frequency response analysis of human saccadic eye movements. *Comput. Biol. Med.*, 18(3): 195–219.

Enderle, J.D., Engelken, E.J. and Stiles, R.N. (1991) A comparison of static and dynamic characteristics between rectus eye muscle and linear muscle model predictions. *IEEE Trans. Biomed. Eng.*, 38: 1235–1245.

Enderle, J.D., Blanchard, S.M. and Bronzino, J.D. (2000) Physiological modeling. In: *Introduction to Biomedical Engineering*. Academic Press, San Diego, CA, pp. 279–368.

Fuchs, A.F. and Luschei, E.S. (1970) Firing patterns of abducens neurons of alert monkeys in relationship to horizontal eye movement. *J. Neurophys.*, 33: 382–392.

Fuchs, A.F., Kaneko, C.R.S. and Scudder, C.A. (1985) Brainstem control of saccadic eye movements. *Annu. Rev. Neurosci.*, 8: 307–337.

Galiana, H.L. (1991) A Nystagmus strategy to linearize the vestibulo-ocular reflex. *IEEE Trans. Biomed. Eng.*, 38: 532–543.

Gancarz, G. and Grossberg, S. (1998) A neural model of the saccade generator in reticular formation. *Neural Netw.*, 11: 1159–1174.

Goffart, L. and Pelisson, D. (1997) Changes in initiation of orienting gaze shifts after muscimol inactivation of the caudal fastigial nucleus in the cat. *J. Physiol.*, 503(3): 657–671.

Harting, J.K. (1977) Descending pathways from the superior colliculus: an autoradiographic analysis in the rhesus monkey (*Macaca mulatta*). *J. Comp. Neurol.*, 173: 583–612.

Harwood, M.R., Mezey, L.E. and Harris, C.M. (1999) The spectral main sequence of human saccades. *J. Neurosci.*, 19(20): 9098–9106.

Hashimoto, M. and Ohtsuka, K. (1995) Transcranial magnetic stimulation over the posterior cerebellum during visually guided saccades in man. *Brain*, 118(5): 1185–1193.

Hodgkin, A.L., Huxley, A.F. and Katz, B. (1952) Measurement of current–voltage relations in the membrane of the giant axon of *Loligo*. *J. Physiol.*, 116: 424–448.

Hsu, F.K., Bahill, A.T. and Stark, L. (1976) Parametric sensitivity of a homeomorphic model for saccadic and vergence eye movements. *Comp. Progr. Biomed.*, 6: 108–116.

Kapoula, Z.A., Robinson, D.A. and Hain, T.C. (1986) Motion of the eye immediately after a saccade. *Exp. Brain Res.*, 61: 386–394.

Keller, E.L. (1991) The brainstem. In: R.H.S. Carpenter (Ed.), *Eye Movements*. Macmillan, London, pp. 200–223.

Keller, E.L., McPeek, R.M. and Salz, T. (2000) Evidence against direct connections to PPRF EBNs from SC in the monkey. *J. Neurophys.*, 84(3): 1303–1313.

Korentis, G.A. (2001) *Feature Based, Parametric Modeling of the 3-D Oculomotor Plant*. Master Thesis, University of Connecticut, Storrs.

Korentis, G.A. and Enderle, J.D. (2001) Dynamic system modeling of the 3-D oculomotor plant: the 1st step in discerning ocular motor control. *Biomed. Sci. Instrum.*, 37: 355–360.

Krauzlis, R.J. and Miles, F.A. (1998) Role of the oculomotor vermis in generating pursuit and saccades: effects of microstimulation. *J. Neurophys.*, 80(4): 2046–2062.

Lefèvre, P., Quaia, C. and Optican, L.M. (1998) Distributed model of control of saccades by superior colliculus and cerebellum. *Neural Netw.*, 11: 1175–1190.

Lehman, S. and Stark, L. (1983) Multipulse controller signals. *Biol. Cybern.*, 48: 1–10.

Leichnetz, G.R. and Gonzalo-Ruiz, A. (1996) Prearcuate cortex in the Cebus monkey has cortical and subcortical connections like the macaque frontal eye field and projects to fastigial-recipient oculomotor-related brainstem nuclei [published erratum appears in Brain Res. Bull. 1997; 42(1): following III]. *Brain Res. Bull.*, 41(1): 1–29.

Leichnetz, G.R., Smith, D.J. and Spencer, R.F. (1984) Cortical projections to paramedian tegmental and basilar pons in the monkey. *J. Comp. Neurol.*, 228: 388–408.

Markham, C.H. (1981) Cat medial pontine neurons in vestibular nystagmus. *Ann. N.Y. Acad. Sci.*, 374: 189–209.

Miller, J.M. and Demer, J.L. (1999) Clinical applications of computer models for strabismus. In: A. Rosenbaum and A.P. Santiago (Eds.), *Clinical Strabismus Management*. Saunders, Philadelphia, PA.

Moschovakis, A.K., Scudder, C.A. and Highstein, S.M. (1996) The microscopic anatomy and physiology of the mammalian saccadic system. *Prog. Neurobiol.*, 50(2–3): 133–254.

Munoz, D.P. and Istvan, P.J. (1998) Lateral inhibitory interactions in the intermediate layers of the monkey superior colliculus. *J. Neurophys.*, 79(3): 1193–1209.

Munoz, D.P. and Wurtz, R.H. (1992) Role of the rostral superior colliculus in active visual fixation and execution of express saccades. *J. Neurophys.*, 67(4): 1000–1002.

Munoz, D.P. and Wurtz, R.H. (1993a) Fixation cells in the monkey superior colliculus. I. Characteristics of cell discharge. *J. Neurophys.*, 70(2): 559–575.

Munoz, D.P. and Wurtz, R.H. (1993b) Fixation cells in the monkey superior colliculus. II. Reversible activation and deactivation. *J. Neurophys.*, 70(2): 576–589.

Munoz, D.P. and Wurtz, R.H. (1995a) Saccade related activity in monkey superior colliculus. II. Spread of activity during saccades. *J. Neurophys.*, 73(6): 2334–2348.

Munoz, D.P. and Wurtz, R.H. (1995b) Saccade related activity in monkey superior colliculus. I. Characteristics of burst and buildup cells. *J. Neurophys.*, 73(6): 2313–2333.

Munoz, D.P., Pelisson, D. and Guitton, D. (1991) Movement of neural activity on the superior colliculus motor map during gaze shifts. *Science*, 251(4999): 1358–1360.

Munoz, D.P., Waitzman, D.M. and Wurtz, R.H. (1996) Activity of neurons in monkey superior colliculus during interrupted saccades. *J. Neurophys.*, 75(6): 2562–2580.

Ohki, Y., Shimazu, H. and Suzuki, I. (1988) Excitatory input to burst neurons from the labyrinth and its mediating pathway in the cat: location and functional characteristics of burster-driving neurons. *Exp. Brain Res.*, 72: 457–472.

Ohtsuka, K. and Noda, H. (1995) Discharge properties of Purkinje cells in the oculomotor vermis during visually guided saccades in the macaque monkey. *J. Neurophys.*, 74(5): 1828–1840.

Olivier, E., Grantyn, A., Chat, M. and Berthoz, A. (1993) The control of slow orienting eye movements by tectoreticulospinal neurons in the cat behavior, discharge patterns and underlying connections. *Exp. Brain Res.*, 93: 435–449.

Optican, L.M. and Miles, F.A. (1980) Cerebellar-dependent adaptive control of primate saccadic system. *J. Neurophys.*, 44(6): 1058–1076.

Optican, L.M. and Miles, F.A. (1985) Visually induced adaptive changes in primate saccadic oculomotor control signals. *J. Neurophys.*, 54: 940–958.

Port, N.L., Sommer, M.A. and Wurtz, R.H. (2000) Multielectrode evidence for spreading activity across the superior colliculus movement map. *J. Neurophys.*, 84(1): 344–357.

Raphan, T. (1998) Modeling control of eye orientation in three dimensions. I. Role of muscle pulleys in determining saccadic trajectory. *J. Neurophys.*, 79(5): 2653–2667.

Raybourn, M.S. and Keller, E.L. (1977) Colliculoreticular organization in primate oculomotor system. *J. Neurophys.*, 40: 861–878.

Robinson, D.A. (1964) The mechanics of human saccadic eye movement. *J. Physiol. (Lond.)*, 174: 245–264.

Robinson, D.A. (1970) Oculomotor unit behavior in the monkey. *J. Physiol.*, 33: 393–404.

Robinson, D.A. (1975) Oculomotor control signals. In: G. Lennerstrand and P. Bach-y-Rita (Eds.), *Basic Mechanisms of Ocular Motility and their Clinical Implication*. Pergamon Press, Oxford, pp. 337–374.

Robinson, D.A. (1981) Models of mechanics of eye movements. In: B.L. Zuber (Ed.), *Models of Oculomotor Behavior and Control*. CRC Press, Boca Raton, FL, pp. 21–41.

Sato, Y. and Kawasaki, T. (1990) Operational unit responsible for plane-specific control of eye movement by cerebellar flocculus in cat. *J. Neurophys.*, 64(2): 551–564.

Sato, H. and Noda, H. (1992) Saccadic dysmetria induced by transient functional decoration of the cerebellar vermis. *Brain Res. Rev.*, 8(2): 455–458.

Schiller, P.H. (1970) The discharge characteristics of single units in the oculomotor and abducens nuclei of the unanesthetized monkey. *Exp. Brain Res.*, 10: 347–362.

Schweighofer, N., Arbib, M.A. and Dominey, P.F. (1996) A model of the cerebellum in adaptive control of saccadic gain. II. Simulation results. *Biol. Cybern.*, 75(1): 29–36.

Scudder, C.A. (1988a) Characteristics and functional identification of saccadic inhibitory burst neurons in the alert monkey. *J. Neurophys.*, 59(4): 1430–1454.

Scudder, C.A. (1988b) A new local feedback model of the saccadic burst generator. *J. Neurophysiol.*, 59(4): 1454–1475.

Short, S.J. and Enderle, J.D. (2001) A model of the internal control system within the superior colliculus. *Biomed. Sci. Instrument.*, 37: 349–354.

Sparks, D.L., Holland, R. and Guthrie, B.L. (1976) Size and distribution of movement fields in the monkey superior colliculus. *Brain Res.*, 113: 21–34.

Stanton, G.B., Goldberg, M.E. and Bruce, C. (1988) Frontal eye field efferents in the macaque monkey. I. Subcortical pathways and topography of striatal and thalamic terminal fields. *J. Comp. Neurol.*, 271: 473–492.

Takagi, M., Zee, D.S. and Tamargo, R.J. (1998) Effects of lesions of the oculomotor vermis on eye movements in primate: saccades. *J. Neurophysiol.*, 80(4): 1911–1931.

Tweed, D. (1997) Three-dimensional model of human eye–head saccadic system. *J. Neurophys.*, 77(2): 654–666.

Van Gisbergen, J.A.M., Robinson, D.A. and Gielen, S. (1981) A quantitative analysis of generation of saccadic eye movements by burst neurons. *J. Neurophys.*, 45(3): 417–442.

Van Opstal, J. and Kappen, H. (1993) A two-dimensional ensemble coding model for spatial–temporal transformation of saccades in monkey superior colliculus. *Network*, 4: 19–38.

Van Opstal, A.J., Van Gisbergen, J.A.M. and Eggermont, J.J. (1985) Reconstruction of neural control signals for saccades based on an inverse method. *Vision Res.*, 25(6): 789–801.

Versino, M., Hurko, O. and Zee, D.S. (1996) Disorders of binocular control of eye movements in patients with cerebellar dysfunction. *Brain*, 119(Pt 6): 1933–1950.

Vilis, T., Snow, R. and Hore, J. (1983) Cerebellar saccadic dysmetria is not equal in the two eyes. *Exp. Brain Res.*, 51: 343–350.

Vossius, G. (1960) The system of eye movement. *Z. Biol.*, 112: 27–57.

Westheimer, G. (1954) Mechanism of saccadic eye movements. *A.M.A. Arch. Ophthalmol.*, 52: 710–724.

Zee, D.S. and Leigh, R.J. (1983) *The Neurology of Eye Movement*. F.A. Davis, Philadelphia, PA.

CHAPTER 3

The latency of saccades toward auditory targets in humans

Daniela Zambarbieri *

Dipartimento di Informatica e Sistemistica, Università di Pavia, Via Ferrata 1, 27100 Pavia, Italy

Abstract: Auditory targets can be used to evoke saccadic eye movements since they provide a position reference signal in space. Comparison of the characteristics of saccades evoked by both visual and auditory stimuli can give further information on the oculomotor control system.

In particular, the latency of auditory saccades evoked in different experimental situations, such as the step, gap and overlap protocols, and with different starting positions of the eyes in the orbit can provide useful insight into the central processing underlying saccade generation.

The aim of this chapter is to provide a review of auditory saccade characteristics and to present latency data obtained in human subjects in different experimental conditions.

Introduction

Eye movement characteristics are normally investigated by using visual stimulation. Nevertheless other sensory information could be used in order to further investigate the behavior of the oculomotor control system. In particular, auditory targets are able to provide position reference in space and therefore elicit saccadic eye movements.

A different situation is created when auditory targets are used with respect to visual targets. The position of an auditory target in space is localized based on the difference in time and intensity of the sound at the two ears. Therefore the incoming sensory information is organized in a craniotopic map which is different from the reference frame in which eye movements are controlled and executed (retinotopic). Moreover, eye movements are executed in open loop conditions since no retinal error neither retinal slip velocity are available. Thus, eye movements evoked by auditory target presentation can provide further information on the characteristics of the oculomotor control system.

A review will be provided in the following sections on the characteristics of horizontal saccades in humans toward auditory targets in different experimental protocols. In particular, attention will be focused on the latency of auditory saccades.

The latency of a saccadic response represents the time required by the central nervous system to perform a number of different processes such as acquisition of sensory information, central reconstruction of target position and execution of eye movement. Due to the difference previously described between visual and auditory targets, the investigation of auditory saccade latency can give further insights into the behavior of the saccadic mechanisms.

Methods

The results reported in the literature on auditory saccades in humans are sometimes different, due mainly to experimental differences that can be attributed to the type of sound used as auditory target (tones, buzzers, clicks, bursts, white noise, etc.) and its duration, the instruction given to the subject (to be quick, or accurate, or both), the range of target positions

---

* Correspondence to: D. Zambarbieri, Dipartimento di Informatica e Sistemistica, Università di Pavia, Via Ferrata 1, 27100 Pavia, Italy. Tel.: +39-0382-505353; Fax: +39-0382-505353; E-mail: dani@unipv.it

considered in the experiments. Therefore in order to make a reliable comparison on auditory saccade latency in different experimental protocols, the results obtained with the same experimental set-up and in the same population of subjects will be considered in the following sections.

Thirteen subjects (6 male and 7 female, aged between 25 and 28 years) with normal visual, auditory and oculomotor functions were examined. Subjects were seated, in total darkness with their head restrained, at a center of a circular frame, 2.2 m in diameter, supporting visual and auditory targets placed every 5° from 90° to the right to 90° to the left. Auditory targets were 5 cm diameter loudspeakers continuously fed with a 15 Hz square-wave signal so as to produce a 60 dB noise burst. Visual targets were red-light emitting diodes (LED) placed above each loudspeaker.

Eye movements were recorded using conventional electro-oculography (EOG). The EOG signal was low-pass filtered with a cut-off frequency of 40 Hz and sampled at a frequency of 250 Hz. The EOG signal was calibrated at the beginning of each test.

A visual target was first presented to the subject in order to keep his eyes in a specific position in the orbit. The position of this visual fixation target could be either 0°, 20° or −20°. After a random interval, varying between 2 and 4 s, a lateral target, either visual or auditory, was presented to the subject for 2 s. The lateral target position was randomly selected among the 14 available positions in the range ±35°. Each target position was presented three times within a random sequence. In the case of an auditory target presentation, the LED placed in the same position of the loudspeaker was then switched on for a further 2 s in order to elicit visual corrective saccades in the case of an error in the estimation of auditory target position. Subjects were asked to orient their eyes toward the target as accurately as possible.

Different timing of visual fixation target disappearance with respect to the presentation of the lateral target have been considered in the experiments. The visual fixation target disappears simultaneously with lateral target presentation (*step paradigm*), or before lateral target presentation (*gap paradigm*), or after lateral target presentation (*overlap paradigm*). Subjects' instructions in gap and overlap paradigms was to move at target appearance. All 13 subjects were tested in the step and gap experimental protocols and by using both visual and auditory targets. Six among the 13 subjects were also tested in the overlap protocol.

Saccade parameters (latency, duration, amplitude and peak velocity) were computed off-line by using an interactive program which used a velocity threshold of 25°/s for saccade identification. Only responses with primary saccade latency ranging between 100 and 900 ms have been considered, since outside this range responses could have been affected by either anticipation or lack of attention.

For the sake of simplicity, in the following sections, saccadic eye movements following the presentation of visual and auditory targets will be referred to as 'visual saccades' and 'auditory saccades', respectively. Moreover, 'target position' will be used to indicate the absolute position of the target in space, that is with respect to the head. Both 'target eccentricity' and 'target displacement' will be used to indicate the position of the target with respect to the initial eye position in the orbit determined by the position of the visual fixation target.

Dynamics of auditory saccades

Before entering into the details of the latency of auditory saccades a summary of the results reported in the literature on saccade dynamics will be presented.

Auditory saccades are slower with respect to visual saccades (Zahn et al., 1978; Zambarbieri et al., 1982; Jay and Sparks, 1990; Lueck et al., 1990). For the same saccade amplitude they have a longer duration and a lower peak velocity. A 20° amplitude saccade has a duration of about 92 ms in auditory responses and 77 ms in visual responses. The same amplitude saccade reaches peak velocity of about 330°/s in auditory responses and about 400°/s in visual responses (Zambarbieri et al., 1982).

For what concerns the precision of auditory saccades a distinction is needed between primary saccade amplitude and total amplitude of the response. In fact a great percentage, about 50%, of responses is composed by a primary saccade followed by one or more corrective saccades (Zambarbieri et al., 1982; Traccis et al., 1984). Only about 14% of primary saccades is correct, whereas 75% is hypometric and 11% is hypermetric.

When the precision of auditory responses is examined in terms of the total eye displacement at the end of target presentation, an average final error of less then 3° was found for all target positions. No significant difference in the precision of single and multiple saccade responses was noted (Zambarbieri et al., 1982). A similar error was found by Jay and Sparks (1990), whereas Yao and Peck (1997), considering only single saccade responses, found that for target eccentricity of ±10°, the accuracy of visual and auditory saccades were not significantly different.

Latency of auditory saccades

Simple reaction time

By measuring the simple reaction time of subjects asked to press a button at the appearance of both visual and auditory targets in space, it has been found that simple reaction time is independent from target position in space. The processing time of sound detection in space is less than the time required for visual target detection. The mean value of simple reaction time is 221 ms for auditory targets and 262 ms for visual targets (Zambarbieri et al., 1982).

Step paradigm

When a subject is asked to orient his eyes as accurately as possible toward an auditory target randomly presented in space, and starting from a visual fixation target at 0°, the latency of auditory saccades was proved to decrease with target position as shown in Fig. 1. The results obtained from the same population of subjects by using visual targets are presented in the same figure for comparison. The latency of visual saccades only slightly increases with target position.

For target position up to 15–20° to the right and to the left, auditory saccade latency is significantly greater than that of visual saccades. For 5° target position, auditory saccade latency reaches values greater than 400 ms. The difference between saccades to the right and to the left in Fig. 1 is not a constant behavior. In other experimental studies (Zambarbieri et al., 1995) the difference is reversed demonstrating therefore not to be significant. At the largest target positions auditory and visual saccades

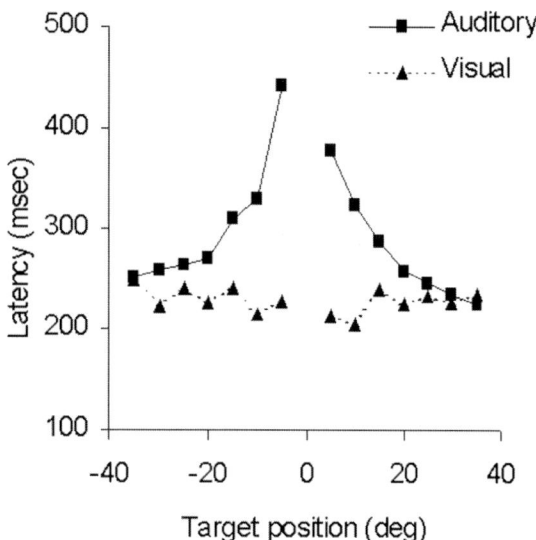

Fig. 1. Mean latency of auditory and visual saccades versus target position in space in the step paradigm with visual fixation target at 0°.

latencies are very similar. For the same target position the latency of primary saccades was found to be unrelated to saccade amplitude.

A similar relationship between latency and target position has been obtained by Zahn et al. (1978), Engelken and Stevens (1989), Lueck et al. (1990), Yao and Peck (1997), even if the range of latency values varies among studies. Only Jay and Sparks (1990) found that the auditory saccade latency is greater than visual saccade latency only for target positions of ±10°. For largest target positions, auditory saccade latency is smaller than visual latency. Nevertheless, also in this study auditory saccade latency was found to decrease with target position.

In the case of a central visual fixation target, the craniotopic representation of the auditory space and the retinotopic map of eye movements are coincident, and therefore target position and target eccentricity are the same. Nevertheless, a difference can be easily created between the two maps by simply considering a visual fixation target different from the central position with respect to the orbit.

When a difference is created between the craniotopic and the retinotopic position of the target the latency of auditory saccades presents the longest values for the smallest target eccentricities with respect to the eyes (Fig. 2). That means that, given an au-

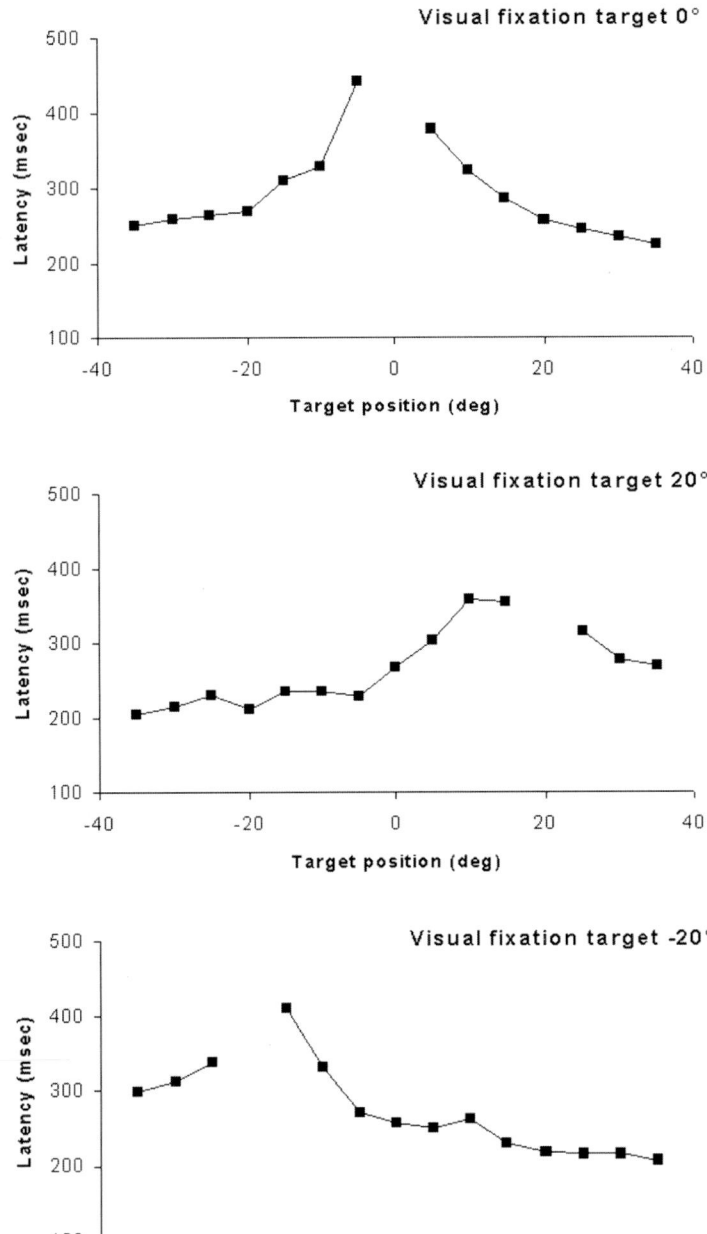

Fig. 2. Mean latency of auditory saccades versus target position in space for three different positions of the visual fixation target in the step paradigm.

ditory target placed at 25° to the right in space, the latency of the saccade oriented towards this target is 250 ms if the starting eye position is 0°, 315 ms if the starting eye position is 20° to the right, and 215 ms if the starting eye position is 20° to the left. These results have led to the conclusion that the latency of auditory saccades depends on the relative position of the sound with respect to the eyes (Zambarbieri et al., 1995). Similar results have been obtained by Zahn et al. (1979), Lueck et al. (1990), and Yao and Peck (1997).

Gap and overlap paradigms

In order to further investigate the latency of auditory saccades, experiments were performed in the gap and overlap paradigms, in which the timing of disappearance of the fixation target and the appearance of the peripheral target are not coincident. Also in the case of gap and overlap paradigms three different positions of the visual fixation target have been considered.

Since the pioneering study of Saslow (1967) it is known from the literature that in the case of visual target presentation a gap (dark period) between the disappearance of the fixation target and the appearance of the lateral target induces a reduction of saccade latency. When the lateral target is switched on before the disappearance of the fixation target (overlap, period during which both targets are present), the latency of saccades is increased.

In some studies dealing with the interpretation of the gap effect, auditory targets have been considered but only two target positions in space have been used. Fendrich et al. (1991) found a difference between the gap and overlap paradigms of about 31 ms with auditory targets, compared with a difference of 43 ms with visual targets. Shafiq et al. (1998) observed a gap effect with respect to the step paradigm of 17 ms with auditory targets and 32 ms with visual targets. Taylor et al. (1999) used auditory targets to investigate the presence and disappearance of the fixation target in the gap effect.

The results obtained by considering the whole range of target positions in space, as in the previous experiments, show that when auditory targets are presented to the subjects in the gap paradigm, with a gap period of 300 ms, a mean reduction of saccade latency can be observed of about 80 ms. But, as shown in Fig. 3, the relationship between saccade latency and target position with respect to the eyes still remains unchanged. In the same population of subjects the mean gap effect in the visual case was of about 60 ms.

An analogous behavior has been observed in the overlap paradigm, with overlap duration of 300 ms. Saccade latency is increased with respect to the step paradigm, even if not in an homogeneous way for all target positions. Nevertheless, the relationship between target eccentricities and latency remains unchanged. Fig. 4 shows the results obtained in the overlap and step paradigms in a population of six subjects. In the lower part of the figure the latency values of the gap and step paradigms from the same population of subjects are presented for comparison. Data obtained with different positions of the visual fixation target have been pooled by considering the latency as a function of target displacement, that is the position of the target with respect to the eyes. The difference with respect to the step paradigm varied between 10 and 120 ms. Also in the visual case the overlap effect on latency varies among target positions and ranges between 10 and 60 ms.

Discussion

Auditory targets can be used to evoke saccadic eye movements in order to further investigate the behavior of the saccadic mechanism. Auditory targets can provide a real position reference signal but, if compared with visual targets, the absence of retinal error and retinal slip velocity makes the system to operate in open loop conditions. Moreover the craniotopic reference frame of the incoming sensory signal is different from the retinotopic reference frame of eye movement execution. Therefore the comparison of saccade characteristics toward auditory targets with those of visually triggered saccades can provide further information on the saccadic mechanism.

Some interesting results that give an insight in the central processing underlying the generation of saccadic responses are those related to the latency. In spite of a detection time which is shorter in the case of auditory target presentation and is independent from target position in space, the latency of auditory saccades has been found to be related to target position with respect to the eyes. The latency decreases as target eccentricity increases and for small target eccentricities the latency is much greater than the latency toward visual targets at the same eccentricity. Gap and overlap in target presentation induce a

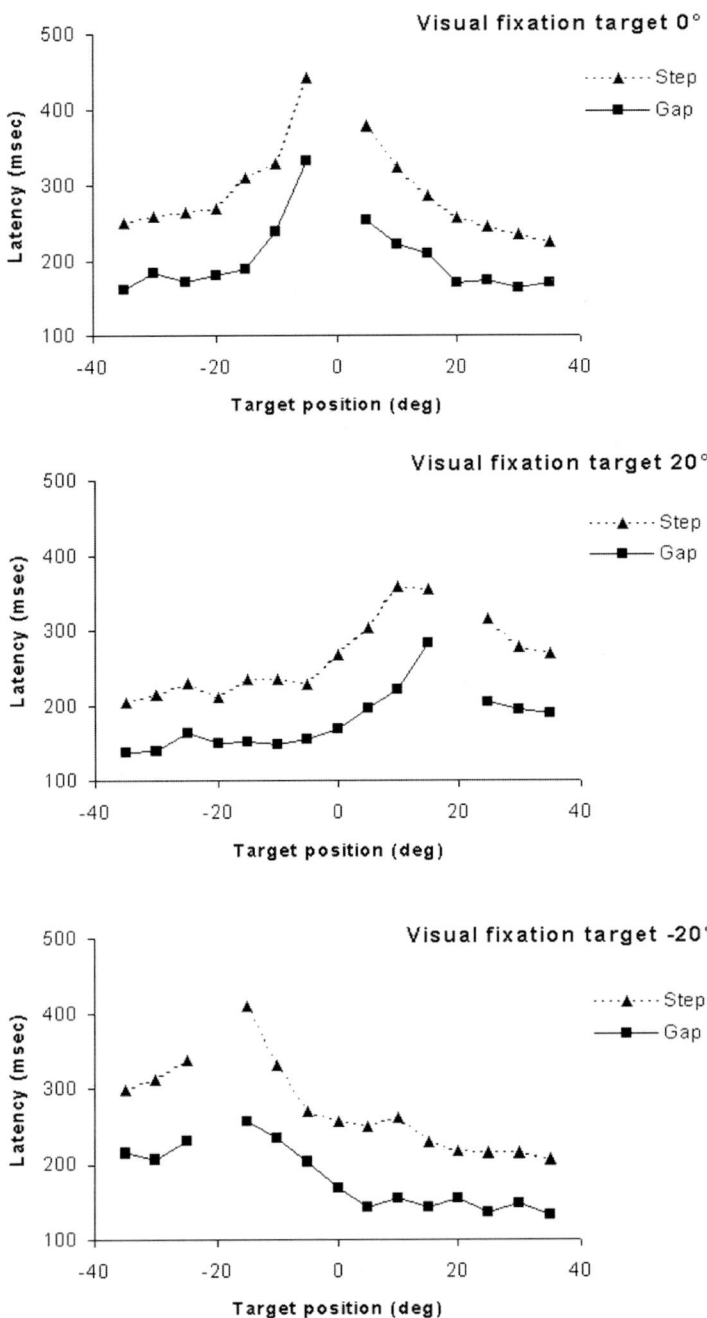

Fig. 3. Mean latency of auditory saccades versus target position in the step and gap paradigms with three different positions of the visual fixation target.

reduction and an increase, respectively, in saccade latency without modifying the relationship existing between latency and target eccentricity.

The latency of saccades reflects the time required to perform a number of processes inside the central nervous system. These processes, underlying

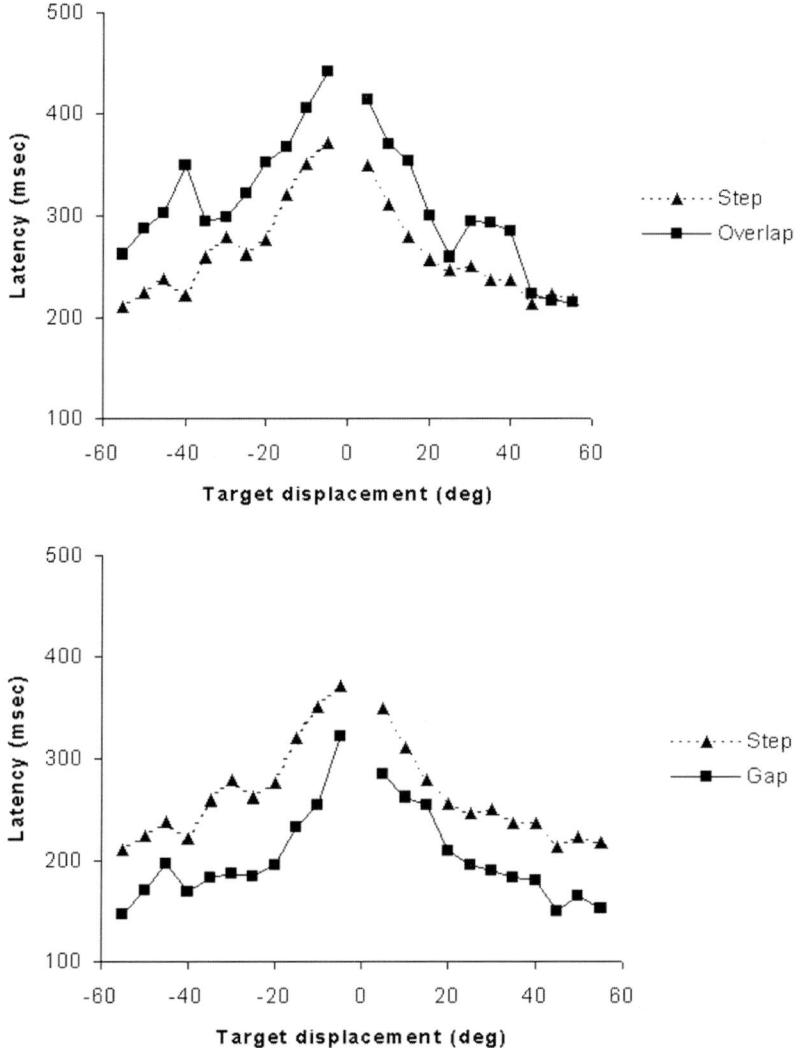

Fig. 4. Comparison of the mean latency of auditory saccades in different experimental paradigms. Upper diagram: step versus overlap paradigm; lower diagram: step versus gap paradigm. Latency values obtained with three different positions of the visual fixation target have been pooled and reported versus target displacement, that means versus the position of the target with respect to eye position in the orbit.

the generation of a saccadic response toward a real target, can be identified in three successive steps (Fig. 5). Step I represents the process of target localization which is based on the incoming sensory signals. Step II corresponds to the central processing at the level of the superior colliculus (SC) where target position information, coded in the reference frame of the relevant sensory system, is further elaborated. Finally, Step III represents the generation of the motor command to the saccadic mechanism.

Let us make the assumption that the input signal entering each one of these steps is affected by uncertainty. Thus, the time required to produce the output depends on the level of this uncertainty. The uncertainty can be imagined as a noise affecting the signal. The greater the noise, the longer the time required to reach a threshold level in the estimation process. A variation in the signal-to-noise ratio reflects the time required to execute any one of these steps and will therefore induce a variation in saccade latency.

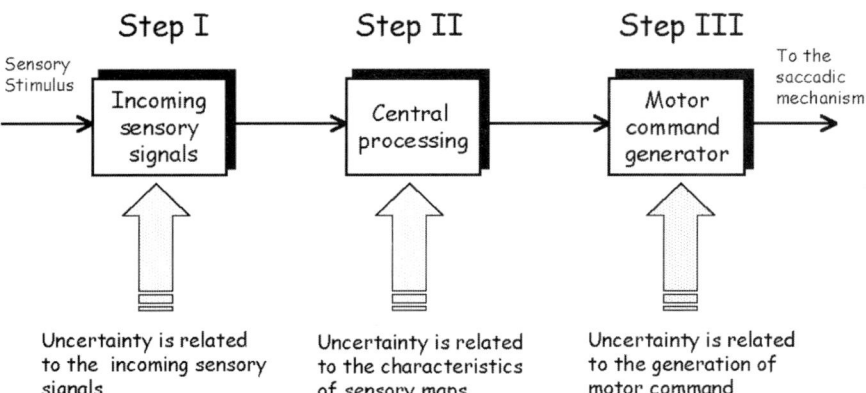

Fig. 5. Schematic representation of the central processing underlying saccade generation and the uncertainty that can affect each step of the processing (redrawn from Zambarbieri et al., 1995).

A model of saccade generation in which the acquisition of target position and the central processing were stochastic processes has been proposed (Schmid et al., 1982) and simulation results were able to predict the variation of auditory saccade latency with target position. The model was based on the assumption that any incoming sensory information is more or less affected by noise. Target localization can therefore be viewed as a running estimate through a procedure that progressively reduces the effect of noise.

In the model, the origin of this noise was supposed to be related to the uncertainty affecting the incoming sensory signal as in the case of an auditory target placed near the midline, where the intra-aural difference in time and intensity is small, or in the case of a low light intensity of a visual target. That means that following this hypothesis the origin of latency behavior is due to the Step I in Fig. 5.

But the experiments in which the visual fixation target was different from 0° have indicated that the latency depends on target position with respect to the eyes rather than on target position in space (Zambarbieri et al., 1995). Therefore, the hypothesis attributing to Step I the origin of latency variation cannot be considered the only source of uncertainty. Nevertheless, the same stochastic process for the reduction of noise to reach an estimate could be related to the excitation of the receptive field at the level of SC. Larger receptive fields are less selective and can induce a longer time to reach the threshold level.

As a matter of fact, some experiments in animals have indicated that the auditory map shifts according to eye position. A shift of 54% of eye position was found in monkeys (Jay and Sparks, 1984, 1987) and of 61% in cats (Hartline et al., 1995; Peck et al., 1995). In this way any feature of the auditory map also shifts and influences saccade latency depending on target eccentricity rather than on target position. If the receptive fields in the auditory map have different levels of selectivity and need longer latency to generate small saccades, this behavior will be related to the amplitude of the required saccade independently from target position in space. Therefore, Step II could be considered as the origin of the latency behavior of auditory saccades.

Also the frontal eye field (FEF) that strongly projects to the SC can be involved in this central processing. Russo and Bruce (1994) have demonstrated not only that, in monkeys, FEF activity appears to have a role in auditory as well as visually guided saccades, but also that the movement fields associated with auditory saccades were a function of the location of the target relative to gaze direction.

Nevertheless, a further hypothesis cannot been excluded that involves the third step of motor command generation. At this level of processing, target position has to be compared with the actual eye position in the orbit in order to generate a motor error that drives the burst units. The smaller the difference between these two signals, the greater the effect of uncertainty on motor command evaluation. Moreover, at this stage of the processing also attention effect and visual fixation disengagement could influence saccade latency as it has been demonstrated by gap and overlap effects in visual saccades.

But gap and overlap paradigms in auditory saccades have indicated that, in spite of a general reduction or increase of the latency values, no modifications can be observed in the relationship between latency and target position with respect to the eyes.

In conclusion, by considering all together the results of auditory saccade latency in different experimental conditions, the most reasonable hypothesis seems the one that involves the step of central processing at the level of SC and FEF where the auditory map is in register with eye position.

References

Engelken, E.J. and Stevens, K.W. (1989) Saccadic eye movements in response to visual, auditory, and bisensory stimuli. *Aviat. Space Environ. Med.*, 60: 762–768.

Fendrich, R., Hughes, H.C. and Reuter-Lorenz, P.A. (1991) Fixation-point offsets reduce the latency of saccades to acoustic targets. *Percept. Psychophys.*, 50: 383–387.

Hartline, P.H., Pandey Vimal, R.L., King, A.J., Kurylo, D.D. and Northmore, D.P.M. (1995) Effects of eye position on auditory localization and neural representation of space in superior colliculus of cats. *Exp. Brain Res.*, 104: 402–408.

Jay, M.F. and Sparks, D.L. (1984) Auditory receptive fields in the primate superior colliculus that shifts with changes in eye positions. *Nature*, 309: 345–347.

Jay, M.F. and Sparks, D.L. (1987) Sensorimotor integration in the primate superior colliculus, II. Coordinates of auditory signals. *J. Neurophysiol.*, 57: 35–55.

Jay, M.F. and Sparks, D.L. (1990) Localization of auditory and visual targets for the initiation of saccadic eye movements. In: M.A. Berkley and W.C. Stebbin (Eds.), *Comparative Perception, Vol. I. Basic Mechanisms*. Wiley, New York, NY, pp. 351–374.

Lueck, C.J., Crawford, T.J., Savage, C.J. and Kennard, C. (1990) Auditory–visual interaction in the generation of saccades in man. *Exp. Brain Res.*, 82: 149–157.

Peck, C.K., Baro, J.A. and Warder, S.M. (1995) Effects of eye position on saccadic eye movements and on the neuronal responses to auditory and visual stimuli in cat superior colliculus. *Exp. Brain Res.*, 103: 227–242.

Russo, G.S. and Bruce, C.J. (1994) Frontal eye field activity preceding aurally guided saccades. *J. Neurophysiol.*, 71: 1250–1253.

Saslow, M.G. (1967) Effects of components of displacement-step stimuli upon the latency for saccadic eye movements. *J. Opt. Soc. Am.*, 57: 1024–1029.

Schmid, R., Magenes, G. and Zambarbieri, D. (1982). A stochastic model of central processing in the generation of fixation saccades. In: A. Roucoux and M. Crommelink (Eds.), *Physiological and Pathological Aspects of Eye Movements*. Junk, The Hague, pp. 301–311.

Shafiq, R., Stuart, G.W., Sandbach, J., Maruff, P. and Currie, J. (1998) The gap effect and express saccades in the auditory modality. *Exp. Brain Res.*, 118: 221–229.

Taylor, T.L., Klein, R.M. and Munoz, D.P. (1999) Saccadic performance as a function of the presence and disappearance of auditory and visual fixation stimuli. *J. Cogn. Neurosci.*, 11: 206–213.

Traccis, S., Abel, L.A. and Dell'Osso, L.F. (1984) Audio-ocular responses: saccade programming. *Aviat. Space Environ. Med.*, 55: 735–739.

Yao, L. and Peck, C.K. (1997) Saccadic eye movements to visual and auditory targets. *Exp. Brain Res.*, 115: 25–34.

Zahn, J.R., Abel, L.A. and Dell'Osso, L.F. (1978) Audio-ocular response characteristics. *Sensory Process*, 2: 32–37.

Zahn, J.R., Abel, L.A., Dell'Osso, L.F. and Daroff, R.B. (1979) The audio-ocular response: intersensory delay. *Sensory Process*, 3: 60–65.

Zambarbieri, D., Schmid, R., Magenes, G. and Prablanc, C. (1982) Saccadic responses evoked by presentation of visual and auditory targets. *Exp. Brain Res.*, 47: 417–427.

Zambarbieri, D., Beltrami, G. and Versino, M. (1995) Saccade latency toward auditory targets depends on the relative position of the sound with respect to the eyes. *Vision Res.*, 35: 3305–3312.

CHAPTER 4

Contribution of the primate prefrontal cortex to the gap effect

Christopher J. Tinsley [1] and Stefan Everling *

Department of Experimental Psychology, University of Oxford, South Parks Road, Oxford OX1 3UD, UK

Abstract: The introduction of a brief temporal gap between the disappearance of the initial fixation point and the presentation of a peripheral target leads to a general reduction in saccadic reaction times (SRTs), known as the gap effect. Moreover, extremely short latency express saccades frequently occur in this paradigm. Disorders of the prefrontal cortex (PFC) are often associated with increased numbers of express saccades and an inability to suppress reflexive saccades. To investigate the role of the PFC in the gap effect and in express saccade generation, we trained two rhesus monkeys on a gap saccade task in which the initial fixation point (FP) disappeared 200 ms or 600 ms before a peripheral stimulus appeared either 8° to its left or right side. We recorded from the lateral PFC (areas 8 Ar and 46) in both monkeys the activity of 214 neurons, 84 (39%) of which exhibited task-related activity. These neurons could be further categorized into separate groups based on their discharge behaviour: fixation neurons with a decrease in activity during the gap (27%), FP offset neurons (12%), preparatory neurons with an increase in activity during the gap (30%), visual neurons (6%), post-saccadic neurons (8%), and reward-related neurons (12%). There were no obvious differences in the topography of these groups. Significant differences between express and regular saccade trials were found for fixation-related neurons. These neurons had a lower activity during the gap prior to the generation of contralateral express saccades. We hypothesize that a reduction in the activity of fixation-related neurons in the PFC may contribute to the elevated rate of express saccades in prefrontal disorders.

Introduction

Saccadic eye movements towards visual targets display a large trial-to-trial variability in their reaction times. A behavioral paradigm that is widely used to investigate the neural basis of this variability is the gap saccade task in which the initial fixation point disappears before the peripheral stimulus appears (Saslow, 1967). The introduction of this temporal gap leads to a general reduction in saccadic reaction times (SRTs), known as the *gap effect*. Moreover, the gap saccade task often results in a bimodal SRT distribution with a first mode (~80 ms in monkeys; ~100 ms in humans) of express saccades and a second mode (~140 ms) of regular saccades (Fischer and Boch, 1983; Pare and Munoz, 1996).

Neurophysiological studies have demonstrated that an increased motor preparation in the primate superior colliculus (SC) is associated with express saccade generation (for review see Munoz et al., 2000). Although fixation-related neurons in the SC also modulate their activity during the gap period, they do not show different activities before express and regular saccades (Dorris et al., 1997; Everling et al., 1998a). In contrast, a subset of SC saccade-related neurons shows a discharge behaviour that

---

[1] Present address: School of Psychology, The University of Nottingham, University Park, Nottingham NG7 2RD, UK. Tel.: +44-115-951-5328; Fax: +44-115-951-5324; E-mail: cjt@psychology.nottingham.ac.uk

* Correspondence to: S. Everling, Departments of Physiology and Psychology, University of Western Ontario, Social Science Centre, London, ON N6A 5C2, Canada. Tel.: +1-519-661-2111 Ext. 84637; Fax: +1-519-661-3961; E-mail: severlin@uwo.ca

can account for the generation of express saccades. First, these neurons show a higher level of pretarget activity in the gap period prior to an express saccade compared with a regular saccade (Dorris et al., 1997). Second, these cells display two bursts of action potentials for regular saccades, a small stimulus-related burst and a larger saccade-related burst. Prior to an express saccade, these cells discharge only one large burst, which seems to be both stimulus-related and saccade-related (Edelman and Keller, 1996; Dorris et al., 1997). Therefore, it has been hypothesized that if the pretarget excitation of SC saccade cells is high enough then the stimulus-related burst can drive the system over the threshold and directly trigger an express saccade. Recently, it has been demonstrated that saccade-related neurons in the frontal eye field (FEF) that project to the SC display almost identical discharge properties (Everling and Munoz, 2000).

Why do saccade-related neurons in the SC and FEF have a higher level of pretarget activity on express saccade trials? A variety of studies indicate that the prefrontal cortex (PFC) may have an inhibitory effect on the saccade circuit. Patients with lesions of the PFC and psychiatric disorders that affect the PFC show an increased frequency of express saccades and an inability to suppress unwanted saccades (Guitton et al., 1985; Pierrot-Deseilligny et al., 1991; Braun et al., 1992; Matsue et al., 1994; Clementz, 1996; Gaymard et al., 1998). Further, brief inactivation of the PFC with transcranial magnetic stimulation increases the frequency of express saccades (Muri et al., 1999). Indeed, the PFC has strong anatomical links to both the SC and FEF (Goldman and Nauta, 1976; Leichnetz et al., 1981; Fries, 1984) and therefore would be in an ideal position to modulate the activity of both areas.

The objective of the present study is to investigate the role of the lateral PFC in express saccade generation. Further, the gap saccade task has been used in previous studies to compare the discharges of neurons in the brainstem saccade generator (Everling et al., 1998a), SC (Dorris et al., 1997; Sparks et al., 2000), FEF (Dias and Bruce, 1994; Everling and Munoz, 2000), and lateral intraparietal area (Ben Hamed et al., 1999). It is therefore of interest to investigate the activity of PFC neurons in the same task to reach a better understanding of the neural basis of fixation and saccade initiation.

Methods

The subjects in this study were two male rhesus monkeys (*Macaca mulatta*). Their weights were 5 and 10 kg. All procedures undertaken were in accordance with UK home office regulations. Both animals were prepared for chronic experiments by undergoing surgical procedures in order to place an implant upon their skull. The implant contained both a recording chamber and a head bolt. Anaesthesia was induced with ketamine hydrochloride (10 mg/kg i.m.) and maintained with thiopentone sodium solution (5%) administered through an intravenous cannula throughout the surgery. Heart rate, respiratory rate, and body temperature were monitored closely for the duration of the surgery. For a 10-day period starting just prior to the surgery, animals received a daily dose of antibiotic (penicillin, i.m.) to prevent infection. Animals were also given the analgesic buprenorphine hydrochloride (0.01 mg/kg) postoperatively to alleviate any discomfort.

In a first surgery, a head implant was constructed from dental acrylic and anchored to the skull with stainless steel screws. A stainless steel head bolt to restrain the head was anchored into the acrylic implant. After training on the gap saccade task and another paradigm that is not part of this report (Everling et al., 2000), animals underwent a second surgery for preparation of eye movement recordings using the magnetic search coil technique (Fuchs and Robinson, 1966) and for preparation of chronic neuron recordings. A preformed eye coil (three turns of stainless steel wire, Cooner Wire) was implanted into one eye behind the conjunctiva (Judge et al., 1980). The coil lead was passed subcutaneously to the acrylic implant that anchored the connector. A craniotomy (19 mm diameter) was performed over the PF cortex (A-P 31 mm, M-L 18 mm; left hemisphere in monkey A and right hemisphere in monkey B). Stainless steel recording chambers were placed over the trephination and dental acrylic was applied so that the entire implant was attached firmly to the skull.

Behavioral control and presentation of visual stimuli

Two Pentium PCs running CORTEX, a program developed in the laboratory of Dr. Robert Desimone (NIMH) for conducting neurophysiological and behavioural experiments, were used to present the stimuli, to control the behavioural paradigm, to deliver the rewards, and to store the behavioural data. Monkeys were seated comfortably in a primate chair within a sound-attenuating isolation chamber with their heads restrained and a juice-spout placed at their mouth for computer-controlled reward delivery (Crist Instruments). The stimuli were presented on a 21 inch colour computer screen 42 cm in front of the animals. During the training after the first surgery, horizontal and vertical eye movements were monitored at 60 Hz using a video eye tracker (IS-CAN). During the recording sessions after the second surgery, horizontal and vertical eye movements were sampled at 1000 Hz using a magnetic search coil system (David Northmore Instruments).

Gap saccade task paradigm

The monkeys were trained to perform the gap saccade task (Fig. 1A). The background was black throughout the entire experiment. Once the fixation point (FP; white filled circle, 0.2° diameter) appeared at the centre of the screen, the animal had 2000 ms to look at it and maintain steady fixation. After a random period of 700–900 ms, the FP was extinguished, and there was a period of no visual stimuli (gap period) before a peripheral target stimulus (white filled circle, 0.2° diameter) was presented. The gap period was set to a constant duration of 200 ms or 600 ms. The target was presented at one of two possible horizontal locations pseudorandomly interleaved and with equal probability, either 8° to the left or 8° to the right of the FP. The monkey received a juice reward if it started fixation, maintained steady fixation during the visual fixation and the gap periods and made a saccade to the target within 400 ms after its appearance. No rewards were given on trials where the monkey did not start or did not maintain fixation, and a 2-s time-out period was imposed.

The order of tasks within a recording session was usually (1) an attention paradigm that is not part of this report (Everling et al., 2000), and (2) the gap saccade task with at least 50 trials of each direction. A recording session was ended if the isolation of one or more neurons was lost or if the monkeys stopped performing the paradigms. Monkeys received liquid until satiation after performing the paradigms and were returned to their home cages. Records were kept of the weight and health status of the monkeys, and additional water and fruit was provided as needed.

Recordings

We recorded from all neurons that we were able to isolate; this was done to ensure an unbiased sampling of PFC activity. We used dura piercing tungsten electrodes (FHC Inc., #UEWLGDSMNNIE) and advanced arrays of between two and six electrodes using custom-built screw microdrives. The microdrives were attached to a 1-mm delgrin grid (Crist et al., 1988) placed inside the recording chamber. Neural activity was amplified using the Plexon MAP system (Plexon, Dallas, TX) and associated software was also used to sort the signals off-line using cluster separation techniques.

Confirmation of recording sites

After the electrophysiological experiments were completed we confirmed the location of the recording sites using a surgical procedure. The conditions of anaesthesia were the same as those described above. The precise position of the centre of the recording chamber and craniotomy was determined using a stereotaxic pointer. After this the implant was removed and the dura mater was cut in order to reveal the position of the arcuate and principal sulcus with respect to the recording chamber. Several stereotaxic readings were taken along the line of these sulci in order to obtain their shape and location. The readings confirmed that the recording locations were anterior to the arcuate sulcus in and around the principal sulcus with a bias towards dorsal recording sites. The dura was then sewn and the wound closed. Again monkeys received antibiotic treatment in order to prevent infection.

Data analysis

Data analysis was performed using Matlab (Mathworks) and the Spike Tool Box (developed by Wael Assad in the laboratory of Dr. Earl Miller, MIT). Saccade onset was defined as the time when the radial velocity exceeded 30°/s and the end of the saccade was defined as the time when the radial velocity fell below 30°/s. The times for each saccade

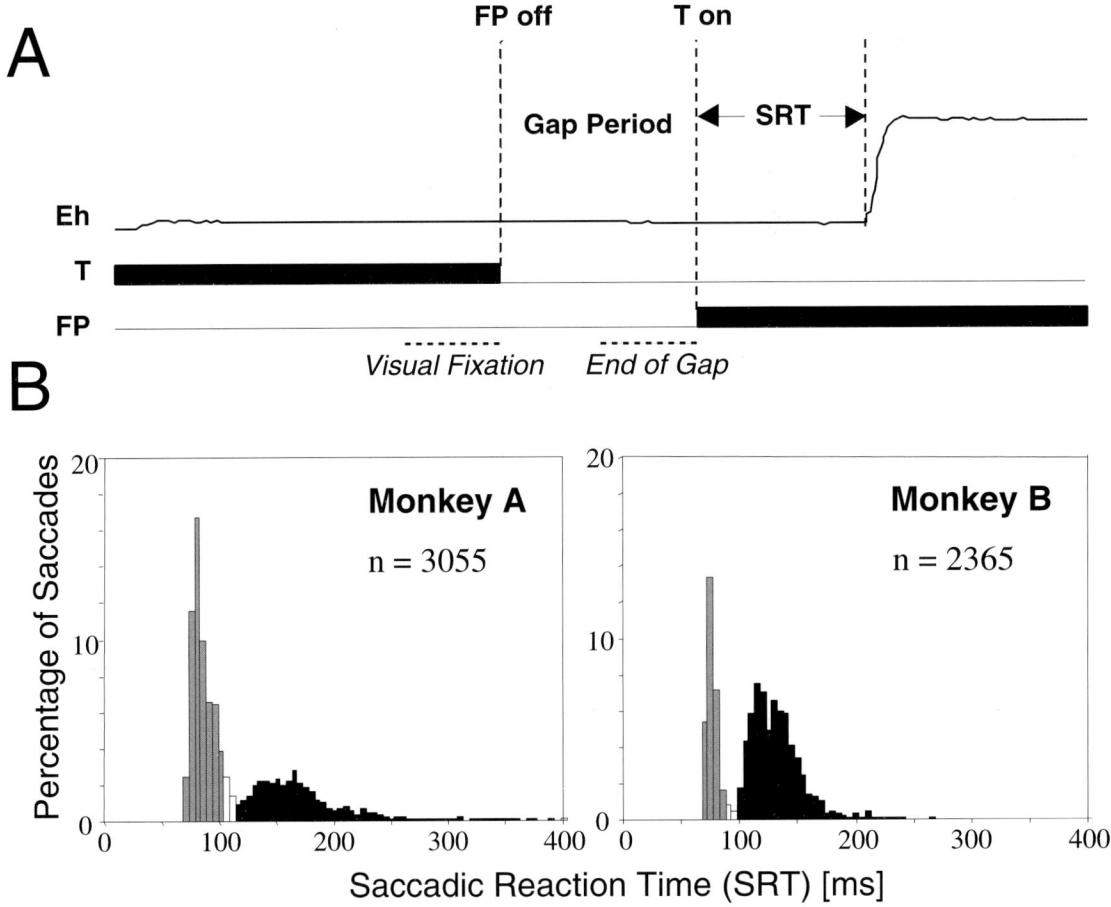

Fig. 1. Gap saccade task and behaviour. (A) Schematic representation of the gap saccade task. Time is represented on the horizontal axis, and presentations of the visual stimuli (FP, central fixation point; T, peripheral target) are indicated by the horizontal bars. Monkeys had to fixate the FP that was turned off 200 ms before the T appeared. Saccadic reaction time (SRT) was defined as the time from target appearance to the onset of the saccadic eye movement (Eh). The activity of neurons in this task was calculated during the final 100 ms of FP presentation (visual fixation) and the final 100 ms of the gap period (end of gap). (B) Distribution of SRTs of all saccades for each monkey obtained while recording from neurons in the PFC. The grey bars represent express saccades (70–100 ms in monkey A; 70–90 ms in monkey B) and the black bars represent regular latency saccades (110–400 ms in monkey A; 100–400 ms in monkey B).

onset were checked and corrected by an experimenter if necessary (this was performed with the aid of a custom-written program). Saccades with an SRT below 70 ms had a 50% chance of being in the correct direction and were excluded as anticipations. Saccades with SRTs above 400 ms were excluded as no response trials.

We were interested in comparing the neural activity associated with express and regular saccades. To do this we first produced a plot displaying the distribution of SRTs for each monkey (see Fig. 1B). For monkey A, express saccade trials were defined as those trials with SRTs between 70 and 110 ms; regular saccades were defined as trials of SRTs between 110 and 400 ms. The SRTs of monkey B were faster than the SRTs of monkey A. Therefore, for this monkey express saccades were classified as those saccades between 70 and 90 ms; regular saccades for this monkey were trials with SRTs between 100 and 400 ms. In order for us to analyze neural activity during the time course of the trials we constructed raster plots of discharge rate against time for individual neurons and neuronal populations. Raster plots using continuous activation waveforms were constructed for the whole length of the trial. To produce the activation waveform each spike was convolved with an asymmetric function that resembled a postsynaptic potential $A(t) = \left[1 - \exp(-t/\tau_\mathrm{g})\right]\left[\exp(-t/\tau_\mathrm{d})\right]$. The time constant for the growth time is τ_g and the time constant for the delay time is τ_d (see Thompson et al., 1996). For our analysis the growth time constant was set to 1 ms and the delay time constant was set to 20 ms.

Results

Prefrontal cortex activity during the gap saccade task

Two hundred and fourteen neurons were recorded from areas 8 Ar and 46 of the PFC of two monkeys (Fig. 2). There were 84 neurons (39%) which displayed task-related activity. These neurons could be further divided into three main groups: (1) neurons with foveal-on or fixation-related activity, (2) neurons with preparatory activity prior to saccade generation, and (3) foveal-off neurons.

Fixation neurons (27/84, or 32%) were tonically active during visual fixation and decreased their discharge rate during the gap period (Fig. 3A). Some of the fixation neurons displayed a transient burst in discharge just after the presentation of the peripheral target; however, the majority of these fixation neurons gave a pause in discharge both prior and during the saccade.

Foveal-off neurons (10/84, or 12%) displayed a rapid burst of action potentials soon after the disappearance of the FP (Fig. 3B). The onset of this burst occurred at approximately 70 ms after the removal of the FP from the screen.

Preparatory neurons (25/84, or 30%) displayed an increasing level of activity during the gap period (Fig. 3C). The increase in discharge rate of these neurons began abruptly at approximately 100 ms after the disappearance of the FP.

There were small groups of neurons, which responded to the task in differing ways to those detailed above. A small group of neurons (5/84, or 6%) had a transient phasic increase in discharge after target appearance 8° right or left in the gap saccade task (Fig. 3D). These neurons did not show any other modulation in discharge during the task. We did not attempt to determine the response field of a particular neuron, therefore it is likely that the actual number of neurons in this category is higher in the PFC (see Boch and Goldberg, 1989).

Another group of neurons displayed post-saccadic activity (7/84, or 8%). These neurons showed a discrete burst of action potentials after the saccade (Fig. 3E). A further neuronal population (10/84, or 12%) displayed an increase in discharge rate at approximately 300 ms after the appearance of the target stimulus (Fig. 3F). We termed the latter group here reward neurons, but the gap saccade task did not allow us to dissociate reward-related responses from activity related to the sound of the acoustic reward signal, the licking movements, or the taste of the fruit juice. Unmodulated or inactive neurons (132/216, or

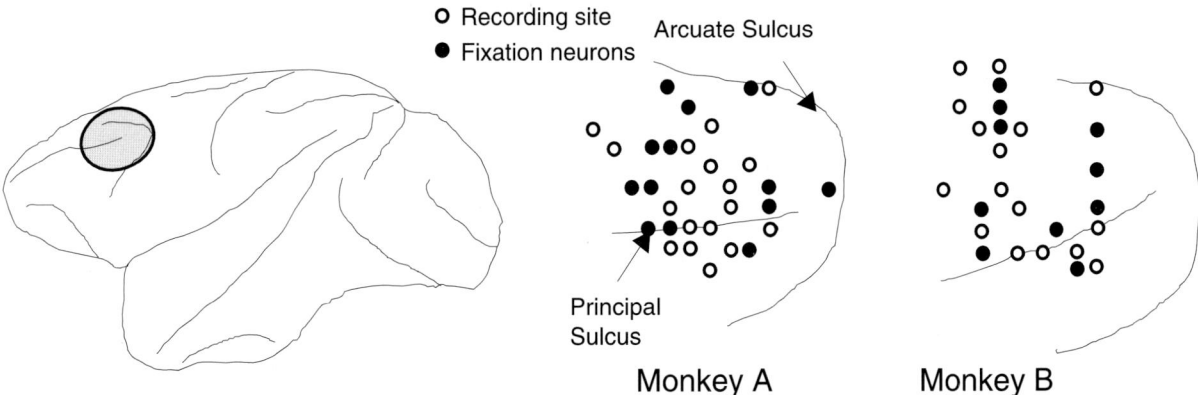

Fig. 2. Recording locations in both monkeys. Unfilled circles indicate recording locations and filled circles indicate recording sites where fixation-related neurons were found. There was no obvious topography of fixation-related neurons.

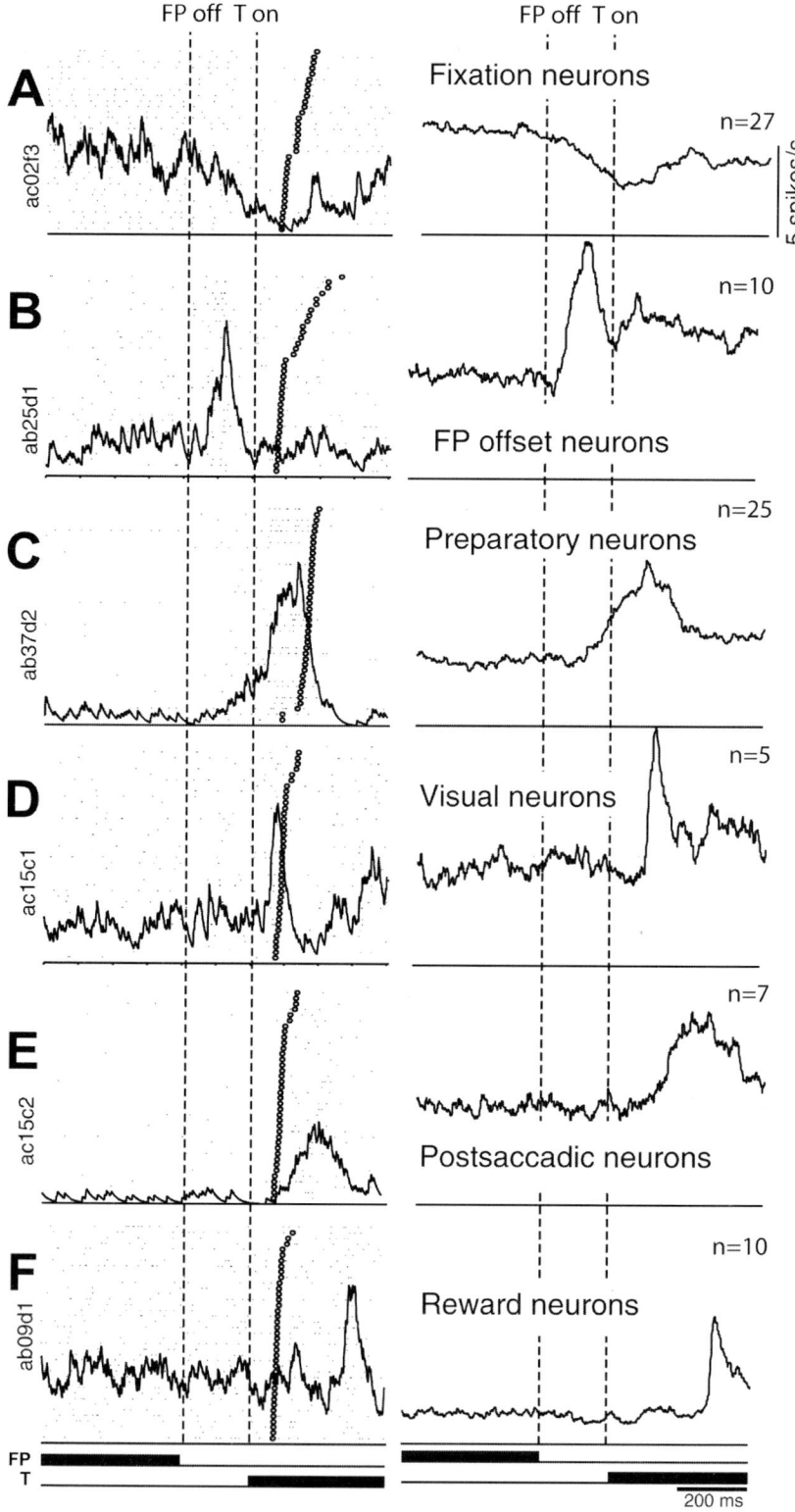

61%) did not discharge or did not modulate their activity during the trial.

Neural activity and express and regular saccades

To assess if the neural activity associated with express and regular saccades was different, we compared trial activity for express saccades with that of regular saccades. This analysis was limited to fixation and preparatory neurons due to the low number of neurons within the other groups. For a comparison of express versus regular saccades, data sets were required to have a minimum of five express saccade trials and five regular saccade trials. We measured the average discharge rate of neurons in the last 100 ms of the visual fixation period for express and regular saccades. We also obtained the average neural discharge for neurons in the last 100 ms of the gap period for both types of saccade.

During the fixation period, preparatory neurons ($n = 24$) did not show significant differences in their discharge rates for express and regular saccades (Fig. 4A,B). The mean discharge rate for preparatory neurons for contralateral targets was 5.2 ± 1.6 spikes/s before express saccades and 5.5 ± 1.3 spikes/s before regular saccades (Wilcoxon signed rank test, $p = 0.49$). For ipsilateral targets, the mean discharge rate prior to express saccades 6.4 ± 1.8 spikes/s and was 5.8 ± 1.3 spikes/s prior to regular saccades (Wilcoxon signed rank test, $p = 0.27$). By definition the mean discharge rate of preparatory neurons was increased towards the end of the gap period. However, these neurons showed no difference in discharge rate for express and regular saccades. The mean discharge rate of these neurons for contralateral targets was 8.5 ± 2.2 spikes/s before express saccades and 8.4 ± 1.8 spikes/s before regular saccades (Wilcoxon signed rank test, $p = 0.57$). For ipsilateral targets the mean discharge rate was 10.3 ± 3.3 spikes/s prior to express saccades and 9.5 ± 3.2 spikes/s before regular saccades (Wilcoxon signed rank test, $p = 0.33$). Therefore, preparatory neurons showed no difference in discharge rate for express and regular saccades either at the end of the fixation period or at the end of the gap period.

The activity of fixation neurons during the gap task prior to express and regular saccades is depicted in parts C and D of Fig. 4. For fixation neurons at the end of the fixation period the mean discharge rate for contralateral targets was 6.3 ± 1.1 spikes/s before express saccades and 8.7 ± 1.8 spikes/s before regular saccades. There was no significant difference between these groups (Wilcoxon signed rank test, $p = 0.60$). The result was similar for ipsilateral targets, the average discharge rate prior to express saccades was 7.2 ± 1.7 spikes/s, the rate before regular saccades was 6.3 ± 1.5 spikes/s (Wilcoxon signed rank test, $p = 0.28$). At the end of the gap period, before contralateral targets the mean activity of fixation neurons was 3.5 ± 0.9 spikes/s before express saccades and 5.0 ± 1.0 spikes/s before regular saccades. Fig. 5A shows the mean discharge rate of 24 fixation neurons at the end of the gap period prior to express saccades compared to the mean discharge rate prior to regular saccades. Most neurons in our sample (19/24, or 79%) showed a higher discharge rate prior to regular saccades (Fig. 5B). This difference was significant (Wilcoxon signed rank test, $p = 0.01$). For ipsilateral targets, the mean discharge rate was 4.5 ± 1.0 spikes/s prior to express saccades and 3.6 ± 0.9 spikes/s before regular saccades (Fig. 5C,D). These differences were not significant (Wilcoxon signed rank test, $p = 0.13$). These data show that express saccade generation is associated with a low level of pretarget activity in fixation-related PFC neurons in the hemisphere contralateral to where the target is due to appear.

Discussion

The results from our experiments show that neuronal activity in the primate PFC change over the course

---

Fig. 3. Neuron types recorded in the PFC. (Left panel) Activity of single task-related PFC neurons for target presentations contralateral to the recording hemisphere. Activity is aligned on the disappearance of the fixation point (FP off) and the appearance of the target (T on). Each dot indicates the time of an action potential, and each row represents one trial. The trials are sorted according to saccadic reaction times (indicated by open circles). Superimposed is the mean spike density function for all trials. (Right panel) Mean spike density of the sample of neurons in the various groups.

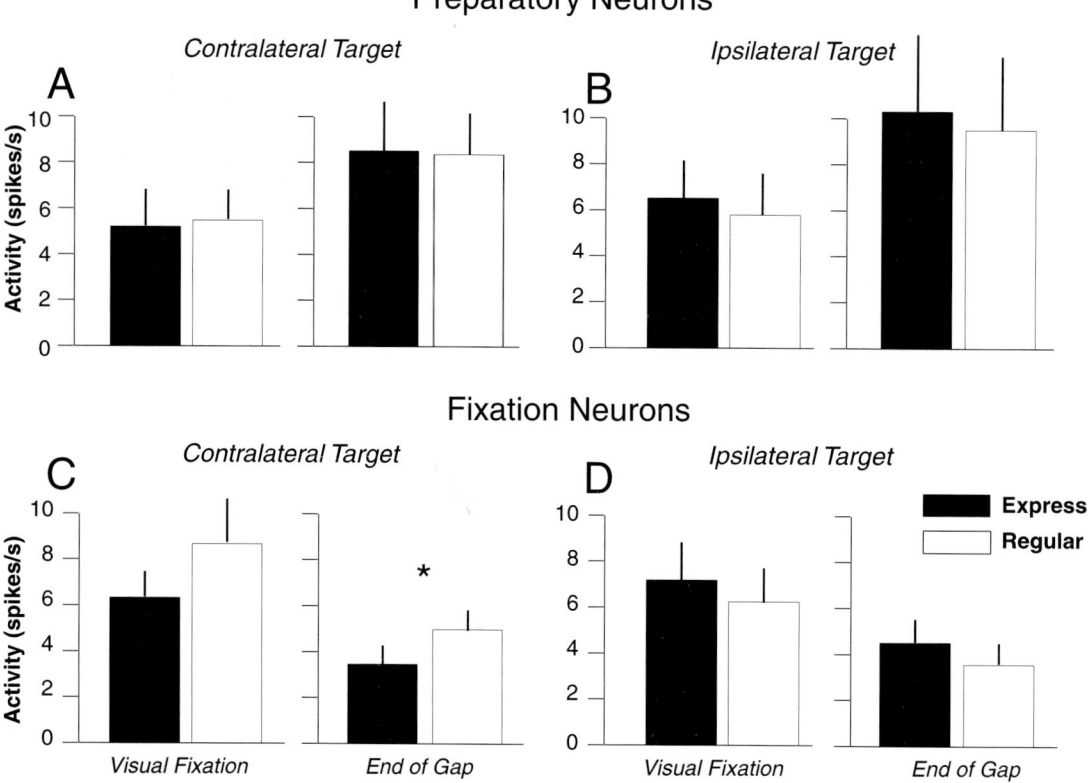

Fig. 4. Mean discharge rate prior to express and regular saccades for the population of preparatory (A,B) and fixation (C,D) neurons during visual fixation (left panels) and the end of the gap epochs (right panels) for contralateral (A,C) and ipsilateral targets (B,D). * Significant difference ($p < 0.05$) between express and regular saccades within sample period.

of the trial during the gap saccade task. We found preparatory neurons and fixation neurons within this part of the PFC. We also found evidence for a possible role of these fixation neurons in the generation of express saccades. These neurons have an activity profile which is the inverse of the activity profile of saccade-related neurons in the SC (Dorris et al., 1997) and FEF (Everling and Munoz, 2000).

PFC neurons have been described previously (Suzuki and Azuma, 1977; Barone and Joseph, 1989; Boch and Goldberg, 1989; Miller et al., 1996); however, this is the first study to report that the pretarget activity of these neurons differs between express and regular saccades. We found that low levels of contralateral pretarget activity were associated with a subsequent express saccade.

The lower activity of PFC fixation neurons prior to contralateral express saccades may be due to random variations in their activity. In fact, our paradigm did not allow the monkeys to predict the direction of the next saccade target. However, it has been shown that even in paradigms with randomly interleaved left and right target locations, monkeys have slightly shorter SRTs if the target appears at the same location as the previous target (Dorris et al., 2000). These faster SRTs are accompanied by a higher pretarget activity of saccade-related neurons in the SC. The increased discharge of SC neurons for the previous target location may reflect the monkey's bias to program a saccade to the location that had been rewarded before. Indeed, several experimental manipulations have demonstrated that the low level pretarget activity of SC neurons is not merely the result of the removal of the initial fixation stimulus, but is influenced by cognitive programs that include attentional shifts (Kustov and Robinson, 1996), tar-

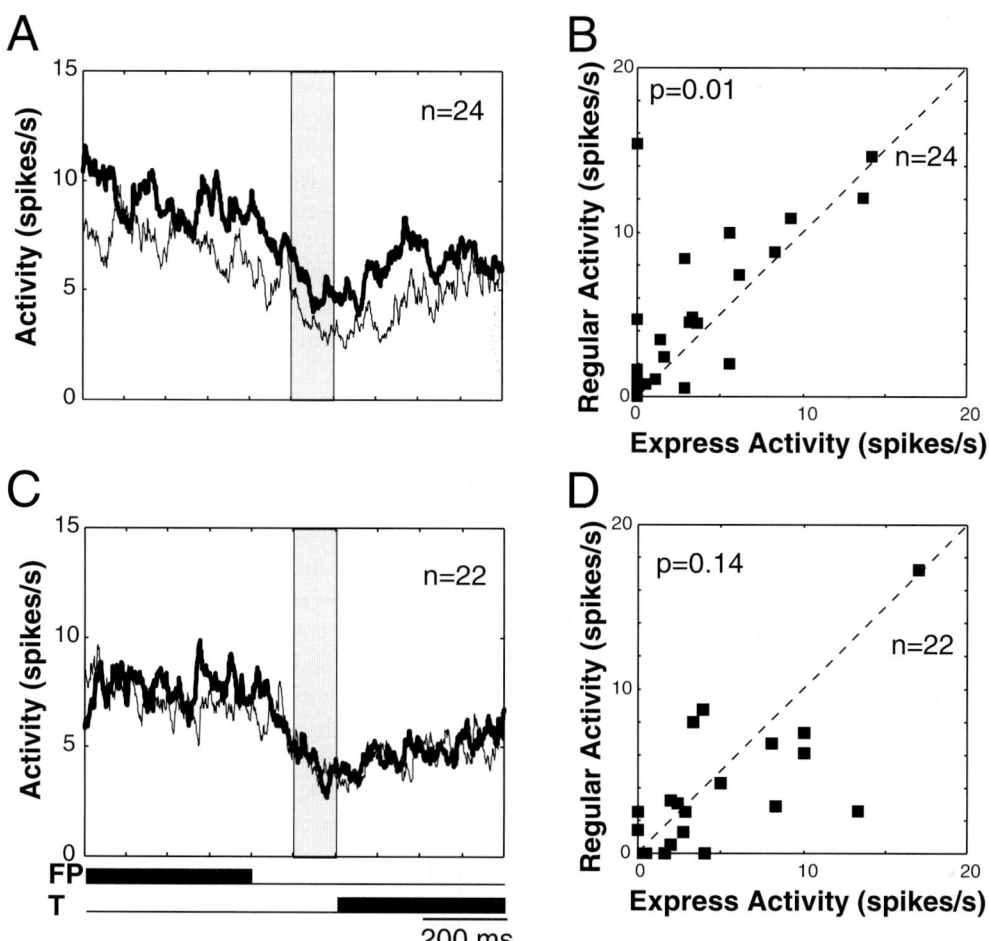

Fig. 5. Average activity of the sample of fixation-related PFC neurons on express and regular saccade trials. (A) Spike density function of express (thin) and regular (thick) saccade trials for target presentations contralateral to the recording hemisphere. (B) The mean activity in the interval 100 ms before stimulus presentation (shaded region in A) of individual neurons (squares) is plotted before express saccades (abscissa) and regular saccades (ordinate). The oblique dashed line represents the unity line (slope is 1). (C,D) Same as in A,B but for target presentations ipsilateral to the recording hemisphere.

get probability (Basso and Wurtz, 1998; Dorris and Munoz, 1998), and movement preparation (Glimcher and Sparks, 1992). Further experiments are necessary to determine whether the activity of PFC fixation neurons is also systematically modulated by such cognitive programs.

Besides in the PFC, neurons with fixation-related activity have been found in the paramedian pontine reticular formation (Luschei and Fuchs, 1972; Keller, 1974; Everling et al., 1998a), SC (Munoz and Wurtz, 1993a,b), zona incerta (Ma, 1996), subthalamic nucleus (Matsumura et al., 1992), thalamus (Schlag and Schlag-Rey, 1984), substantia nigra pars reticulata (Katsanis et al., 2000), FEF (Bruce and Goldberg, 1985; Burman and Bruce, 1997; Hanes et al., 1998), supplementary eye field (Schall, 1991; Bon and Lucchetti, 1992; Schlag et al., 1992), and posterior parietal cortex (Lynch et al., 1977; Sakata et al., 1980).

The neural control of visual fixation is still poorly understood. In particular, it is unclear whether neurons with a fixation-related activity form a global fixation network within the brain or whether they act as local fixation systems that only indirectly influence each other. Previous studies that examined fixation neurons in the SC (Dorris et al., 1997) and omnipause neurons in the paramedian pontine reticular formation (Everling et al., 1998a) did not find differences in the activity pattern of these neurons between express and regular saccades. Therefore, it is unlikely that the PFC fixation neurons that we described in this study influence express saccade generation by projections to fixation neurons in the SC or brainstem. Alternatively, fixation-related PFC neurons may provide a tonic inhibitory input to saccade-related neurons in the SC and FEF in the same hemisphere. A reduction in the activity of PFC fixation-related neurons would release SC and FEF neurons from this inhibition and would result in an increase in pretarget activity of these neurons. In the case of an express saccade, the reduced inhibition from PFC neurons may be sufficient to allow the incoming visual signal to pass the saccade threshold and directly trigger an express saccade (Sommer, 1994; Edelman and Keller, 1996; Dorris et al., 1997).

Our findings may provide a neural correlate for the well-known finding that patients with prefrontal lesions or psychiatric disorders with a suspected prefrontal pathology show an increased frequency of express saccades and unwanted reflexive saccades (for review see Everling and Fischer, 1998). Moreover, children have great difficulty suppressing short-latency reflexive saccades until age 10–15 (Fischer et al., 1997; Munoz et al., 1998). This corresponds with the time of prefrontal cortical maturation (for review see Fuster, 1991). Furthermore, functional brain imaging has demonstrated an involvement of the PFC in the maintenance of active fixation (Anderson et al., 1994). Scalp recordings in humans also showed lower levels of pretarget activations prior to express saccades and unwanted reflexive saccades at frontal electrodes (Everling et al., 1996, 1998b; Klein et al., 2000).

It is, however, unlikely that the cortical modulation of express saccade occurrence depends on the PFC alone. The differences between express and regular saccades are more prominent in saccade-related neurons in the SC (Dorris et al., 1997) and the FEF (Everling and Munoz, 2000) than in fixation neurons in the PFC. Ben Hamed et al. (1999) recently described three classes of foveal neurons in the dorsal LIP in a gap saccade task which share many similarities with the fixation, preparatory, and foveal off neurons that we found in the PFC. Further, some supplementary eye field neurons have a lower pretarget activity prior to errors in an anti-saccade task, of which many were express saccades (Schlag-Rey et al., 1997). It remains to be determined whether PFC fixation neurons are also involved in the suppression of unwanted reflexive saccades. In conclusion, a large proportion of PFC neurons change their activity in a gap saccade task and the activity of a subpopulation of these neurons may be involved in the timing of saccades in this task.

Acknowledgements

The authors wish to thank Earl K. Miller and Trina Norden-Krichmar for help in setting up CORTEX, Wael Assad for supplying the SpikeToolbox, Susan Mygdal and Martin Brown for excellent surgical assistance, and David Gaffan for help in the confirmation of recording locations. Paul Gribble provided helpful comments on an earlier version of the manuscript. This research was supported by the National Alliance for Research on Schizophrenia and Depression to S. Everling and the Medical Research Council of the United Kingdom. S. Everling is currently a Canadian Institutes of Health Research New Investigator.

References

Anderson, T.J., Jenkins, I.H., Brooks, D.J., Hawken, M.B., Frackowiak, R.S. and Kennard, C. (1994) Cortical control of saccades and fixation in man. A PET study. *Brain*, 117: 1073–1084.

Barone, P. and Joseph, J.P. (1989) Prefrontal cortex and spatial sequencing in macaque monkey. *Exp. Brain Res.*, 78: 447–464.

Basso, M.A. and Wurtz, R.H. (1998) Modulation of neuronal activity in superior colliculus by changes in target probability. *J. Neurosci.*, 18: 7519–7534.

Ben Hamed, S., Bihouee, A., Deneve, S. and Duhamel, J.R. (1999) Neural correlates of visual fixation in the dorsal lateral intraparietal area of the macaque (LIPd). *Soc. Neurosci. Abstr.*, 25: 471.5.

Boch, R.A. and Goldberg, M.E. (1989) Participation of prefrontal neurons in the preparation of visually guided eye movements in the rhesus monkey. *J. Neurophysiol.*, 61: 1064–1084.

Bon, L. and Lucchetti, C. (1992) The dorsomedial frontal cortex of the macaca monkey: fixation and saccade-related activity. *Exp. Brain Res.*, 89: 571–580.

Braun, D., Weber, H., Mergner, T. and Schulte-Monting, J. (1992)

Saccadic reaction times in patients with frontal and parietal lesions. *Brain*, 115: 1359–1386.

Bruce, C.J. and Goldberg, M.E. (1985) Primate frontal eye fields. I. Single neurons discharging before saccades. *J. Neurophysiol.*, 53: 603–635.

Burman, D.D. and Bruce, C.J. (1997) Suppression of task-related saccades by electrical stimulation in the primate's frontal eye field. *J. Neurophysiol.*, 77: 2252–2267.

Clementz, B.A. (1996) The ability to produce express saccades as a function of gap interval among schizophrenia patients. *Exp. Brain Res.*, 111: 121–130.

Crist, C.F., Yamasaki, D.S., Komatsu, H. and Wurtz, R.H. (1988) A grid system and a microsyringe for single cell recording. *J. Neurosci. Methods*, 26: 117–122.

Dias, E.C. and Bruce, C.J. (1994) Physiological correlate of fixation disengagement in the primate's frontal eye field. *J. Neurophysiol.*, 72: 2532–2537.

Dorris, M.C. and Munoz, D.P. (1998) Saccadic probability influences motor preparation signals and time to saccadic initiation. *J. Neurosci.*, 18: 7015–7026.

Dorris, M.C., Pare, M. and Munoz, D.P. (1997) Neuronal activity in monkey superior colliculus related to the initiation of saccadic eye movements. *J. Neurosci.*, 17: 8566–8579.

Dorris, M.C., Pare, M. and Munoz, D.P. (2000) Immediate neural plasticity shapes motor performance. *J. Neurosci.*, 20: RC52.

Edelman, J.A. and Keller, E.L. (1996) Activity of visuomotor burst neurons in the superior colliculus accompanying express saccades. *J. Neurophysiol.*, 76: 908–926.

Everling, S. and Fischer, B. (1998) The antisaccade: a review of basic research and clinical studies. *Neuropsychologia*, 36: 885–899.

Everling, S. and Munoz, D.P. (2000) Neuronal correlates for preparatory set associated with pro-saccades and anti-saccades in the primate frontal eye field. *J. Neurosci.*, 20: 387–400.

Everling, S., Krappmann, P., Spantekow, A. and Flohr, H. (1996) Cortical potentials during the gap prior to express saccades and fast regular saccades. *Exp. Brain Res.*, 111: 139–143.

Everling, S., Pare, M., Dorris, M.C. and Munoz, D.P. (1998a) Comparison of the discharge characteristics of brain stem omnipause neurons and superior colliculus fixation neurons in monkey: implications for control of fixation and saccade behavior. *J. Neurophysiol.*, 79: 511–528.

Everling, S., Spantekow, A., Krappmann, P. and Flohr, H. (1998b) Event-related potentials associated with correct and incorrect responses in a cued antisaccade task. *Exp. Brain Res.*, 118: 27–34.

Everling, S., Tinsley, C.J., Gaffan, D. and Duncan, J. (2000) Neural activity in primate prefrontal cortex in a focused attention task. *Soc. Neurosci. Abstr.*, 30: 837.19.

Fischer, B. and Boch, R. (1983) Saccadic eye movements after extremely short reaction times in the monkey. *Brain Res.*, 260: 21–26.

Fischer, B., Biscaldi, M. and Gezeck, S. (1997) On the development of voluntary and reflexive components in human saccade generation. *Brain Res.*, 754: 285–297.

Fries, W. (1984) Cortical projections to the superior colliculus in the macaque monkey: a retrograde study using horseradish peroxidase. *J. Comp. Neurol.*, 230: 55–76.

Fuchs, A.F. and Robinson, D.A. (1966) A method for measuring horizontal and vertical eye movement chronically in the monkey. *J. Appl. Physiol.*, 21: 1068–1070.

Fuster, J.M. (1991) The prefrontal cortex: anatomy, physiology, and neuropsychology of the frontal lobe. Raven, New York.

Gaymard, B., Ploner, C.J., Rivaud, S., Vermersch, A.I. and Pierrot-Deseilligny, C. (1998) Cortical control of saccades. *Exp. Brain Res.*, 123: 159–163.

Glimcher, P.W. and Sparks, D.L. (1992) Movement selection in advance of action in the superior colliculus. *Nature*, 355: 542–545.

Goldman, P.S. and Nauta, W.J. (1976) Autoradiographic demonstration of a projection from prefrontal association cortex to the superior colliculus in the rhesus monkey. *Brain Res.*, 116: 145–149.

Guitton, D., Buchtel, H.A. and Douglas, R.M. (1985) Frontal lobe lesions in man cause difficulties in suppressing reflexive glances and in generating goal-directed saccades. *Exp. Brain Res.*, 58: 455–472.

Hanes, D.P., Patterson, W.F. and Schall, J.D. (1998) Role of frontal eye fields in countermanding saccades: visual, movement, and fixation activity. *J. Neurophysiol.*, 79: 817–834.

Judge, S.J., Richmond, B.J. and Chu, F.C. (1980) Implantation of magnetic search coils for measurement of eye position: an improved method. *Vision Res.*, 20: 535–538.

Katsanis, J., Taylor, J., Iacono, W.G. and Hammer, M.A. (2000) Heritability of different measures of smooth pursuit eye tracking dysfunction: a study of normal twins. *Psychophysiology*, 37: 724–730.

Keller, E.L. (1974) Participation of medial pontine reticular formation in eye movement generation in monkey. *J. Neurophysiol.*, 37: 316–332.

Klein, C., Heinks, T., Andresen, B., Berg, P. and Moritz, S. (2000) Impaired modulation of the saccadic contingent negative variation preceding antisaccades in schizophrenia. *Biol. Psychiatry*, 47: 978–990.

Kustov, A.A. and Robinson, D.L. (1996) Shared neural control of attentional shifts and eye movements. *Nature*, 384: 74–77.

Leichnetz, G.R., Spencer, R.F., Hardy, S.G. and Astruc, J. (1981) The prefrontal corticotectal projection in the monkey; an anterograde and retrograde horseradish peroxidase study. *Neuroscience*, 6: 1023–1041.

Luschei, E.S. and Fuchs, A.F. (1972) Activity of brain stem neurons during eye movements of alert monkeys. *J. Neurophysiol.*, 35: 445–461.

Lynch, J.C., Mountcastle, V.B., Talbot, W.H. and Yin, T.C. (1977) Parietal lobe mechanisms for directed visual attention. *J. Neurophysiol.*, 40: 362–389.

Ma, T.P. (1996) Saccade-related omnivectoral pause neurons in the primate zona incerta. *Neuroreport*, 7: 2713–2716.

Matsue, Y., Osakabe, K., Saito, H., Goto, Y., Ueno, T., Matsuoka, H., Chiba, H., Fuse, Y. and Sato, M. (1994) Smooth pursuit eye movements and express saccades in schizophrenic patients. *Schizophr. Res.*, 12: 121–130.

Matsumura, M., Kojima, J., Gardiner, T.W. and Hikosaka, O.

(1992) Visual and oculomotor functions of monkey subthalamic nucleus. *J. Neurophysiol.*, 67: 1615–1632.

Miller, E.K., Erickson, C.A. and Desimone, R. (1996) Neural mechanisms of visual working memory in prefrontal cortex of the macaque. *J. Neurosci.*, 16: 5154–5167.

Munoz, D.P. and Wurtz, R.H. (1993a) Fixation cells in monkey superior colliculus. I. Characteristics of cell discharge. *J. Neurophysiol.*, 70: 559–575.

Munoz, D.P. and Wurtz, R.H. (1993b) Fixation cells in monkey superior colliculus. II. Reversible activation and deactivation. *J. Neurophysiol.*, 70: 576–589.

Munoz, D.P., Broughton, J.R., Goldring, J.E. and Armstrong, I.T. (1998) Age-related performance of human subjects on saccadic eye movement tasks. *Exp. Brain Res.*, 121: 391–400.

Munoz, D.P., Dorris, M.C., Pare, M. and Everling, S. (2000) On your mark, get set: brainstem circuitry underlying saccadic initiation. *Can. J. Physiol. Pharmacol.*, 78: 934–944.

Muri, R.M., Rivaud, S., Gaymard, B., Ploner, C.J., Vermersch, A.I., Hess, C.W. and Pierrot-Deseilligny, C. (1999) Role of the prefrontal cortex in the control of express saccades: a transcranial magnetic stimulation study. *Neuropsychologia*, 37: 199–206.

Pare, M. and Munoz, D.P. (1996) Saccadic reaction time in the monkey: advanced preparation of oculomotor programs is primarily responsible for express saccade occurrence. *J. Neurophysiol.*, 76: 3666–3681.

Pierrot-Deseilligny, C., Rivaud, S., Gaymard, B. and Agid, Y. (1991) Cortical control of reflexive visually guided saccades. *Brain*, 114: 1473–1485.

Sakata, H., Shibutani, H. and Kawano, K. (1980) Spatial properties of visual fixation neurons in posterior parietal association cortex of the monkey. *J. Neurophysiol.*, 43: 1654–1672.

Saslow, M.G. (1967) Effects of components of displacement-step stimuli upon latency of saccadic eye movements. *J. Opt. Soc. Am.*, 57: 1024–1029.

Schall, J.D. (1991) Neuronal activity related to visually guided saccadic eye movements in the supplementary motor area of rhesus monkeys. *J. Neurophysiol.*, 66: 530–558.

Schlag, J. and Schlag-Rey, M. (1984) Visuomotor functions of central thalamus in monkey. II. Unit activity related to visual events, targeting, and fixation. *J. Neurophysiol.*, 51: 1175–1195.

Schlag, J., Schlag-Rey, M. and Pigarev, I. (1992) Supplementary eye field: influence of eye position on neural signals of fixation. *Exp. Brain Res.*, 90: 302–306.

Schlag-Rey, M., Amador, N., Sanchez, H. and Schlag, J. (1997) Antisaccade performance predicted by neuronal activity in the supplementary eye field. *Nature*, 390: 398–401.

Sommer, M.A. (1994) Express saccades elicited during visual scan in the monkey. *Vision Res.*, 34: 2023–2038.

Sparks, D., Rohrer, W.H. and Zhang, Y. (2000) The role of the superior colliculus in saccade initiation: a study of express saccades and the gap effect. *Vision Res.*, 40: 2763–2777.

Suzuki, H. and Azuma, M. (1977) Prefrontal neuronal activity during gazing at a light spot in the monkey. *Brain Res.*, 126: 497–508.

Thompson, K.G., Hanes, D.P., Bichot, N.P. and Schall, J.D. (1996) Perceptual and motor processing stages identified in the activity of macaque frontal eye field neurons during visual search. *J. Neurophysiol.*, 76: 4040–4055.

CHAPTER 5

Influence of stimulus characteristics on the latency of saccadic inhibition

Dave M. Stampe and Eyal M. Reingold *

Department of Psychology, University of Toronto, 100 St. George Street, Toronto, ON M5S 3G3, Canada

Abstract: Participants read or performed visual search while the normal task display was replaced for 33 ms by a transient image at random intervals. This produced a sharp reduction in saccadic frequency (saccadic inhibition) beginning as early as 70 ms following the display change. It was found that the latency of inhibition onset was determined by the difference between the normal and transient images, with changes in high spatial frequency content of the display resulting in longer latencies than changes in low spatial frequencies. Luminance changes evoked the fastest inhibition onset regardless of the spatial frequency content of the display change.

Introduction

Recently, Reingold and Stampe (1997, 2000, 2002a,b, 2002c) introduced a new paradigm for measuring the effect of changes in visual input on saccade production. In one version of this paradigm, participants perform a task such as reading or visual search, which produced saccades at the rate of 3 to 4 per second. At random intervals, the task display (henceforth the normal image) is replaced with another image (henceforth the transient image) for 33 ms. For example, in a reading task the normal display of text on a white background might be replaced by a black screen. The result is an irregular flickering, which the participants are instructed to ignore. Employing this paradigm Reingold and Stampe (1997, 2000, 2002b,c) documented a decrease in saccadic frequency time-locked to the presentation of the transient image and occurring as early as 60 to 70 ms following its onset. It was argued that the fast latency of this effect, which approaches the limits imposed by delays in the visual and saccadic systems, strongly suggests a low-level, reflex-like, oculomotor effect, which was referred to as saccadic inhibition.

A typical histogram of saccadic frequency is shown in Fig. 1, which illustrates the saccadic inhibition profile. Specifically, for the first 50 ms following the display change, the proportion of saccades remained constant. Approximately 60 to 70 ms following the onset of the flicker, the proportion of saccades decreased below this initial level forming a dip that reflects saccadic inhibition. Following the dip, an increase above the initial level of saccadic frequency occurred, forming a peak, which likely reflects the recovery from inhibition. Finally, following the peak, the proportion of saccades returned to initial levels.

Reingold and Stampe (1997, 2000, 2002b,c) demonstrated robust saccadic inhibition of scanning saccades produced during complex visual tasks such as reading and visual search. In addition, in order to investigate the saccadic inhibition phenomenon under conditions that are more similar to the experimental paradigms typically used in behavioral and neurophysiological studies of the saccadic system,

---

* Correspondence to: E. Reingold, Department of Psychology, University of Toronto, 100 St. George Street, Toronto, ON M5S 3G3, Canada. Tel.: +1-416-978-3990; Fax: +1-905-625-0337; E-mail: reingold@psych.utoronto.ca

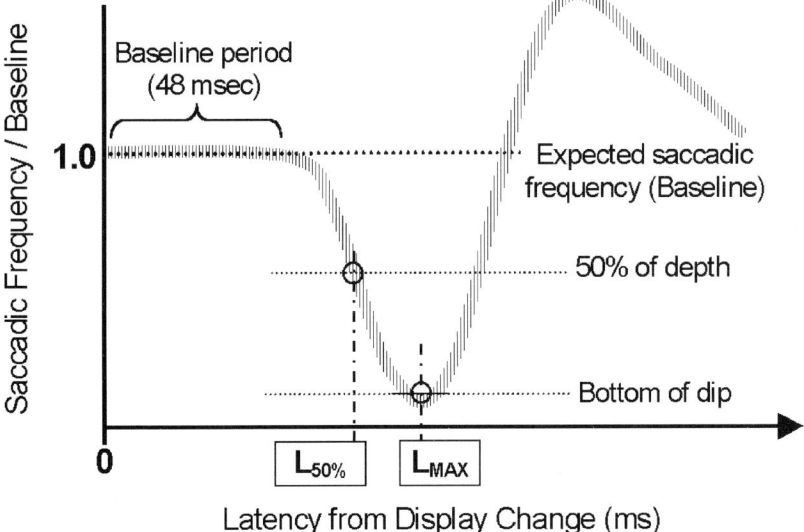

Fig. 1. A typical histogram of saccadic frequency elicited by randomly scheduled display changes, showing the dip and peak due to saccadic inhibition. The latencies of the onset of saccadic inhibition ($L_{50\%}$) and the latency of the maximum strength of inhibition (L_{MAX}) are illustrated.

Reingold and Stampe (2002a) developed a discrete trial version of the saccadic inhibition paradigm. Employing the discrete trial version of the paradigm, Reingold and Stampe (2002a) documented saccadic inhibition of stimulus elicited saccades in the gap paradigm, and saccadic inhibition of voluntary saccades in the antisaccade paradigm.

Thus, consistent with the hypothesis that saccadic inhibition is a low level oculomotor effect, this effect was demonstrated across a wide range of saccadic tasks. In this paper, we will investigate how saccadic inhibition is affected by the low level characteristics of the display change. Specifically, we will examine the effects of changes in spatial frequency content and luminance on the latency of the inhibition. As illustrated in Fig. 1, two latency measures were employed: $L_{50\%}$ and L_{MAX}, which represent the latency from the onset of the display change at which inhibition achieved 50% and 100% of its magnitude, respectively (see Reingold and Stampe, 2002a,b).

While the neurological structures and pathways underlying saccadic inhibition are not yet known (but see Reingold and Stampe, 2002a for a proposal of a neurophysiological model), its short latency suggests that it is evoked by input from the early stages of the visual system. If this is the case, then the effects of stimulus characteristics on visually evoked saccadic inhibition may be similar to those observed for visually evoked potentials (VEP). These potentials arise directly from the activity of neurons in the cerebral cortex in response to changes in visual input, and therefore, the latency of early components of the VEP closely reflect delays in the early visual system. Accordingly, we will contrast previous findings in the VEP literature with the effects produced using similar manipulations of luminance and spatial frequency on saccadic inhibition.

In Experiment 1, we will investigate the effects of changes limited to the luminance or detail of text in a reading task. Experiment 2 will compare the effect of the spatial frequency content of the transient image on the latency of saccadic inhibition to similar effects reported from VEP studies. Experiment 3 investigates the interaction of luminance changes and the spatial frequency content of the task display (normal image). Finally, Experiment 4 will investigate the effects of spatial frequency on saccadic inhibition in a visual search task using natural scenes.

General method

Participants, apparatus and display

A group of 10 participants participated in each experiment. All experiments were performed with the understanding and written consent of each participant. All participants had normal or corrected-to-normal vision, and were paid $10.00 for each one hour session. Eye movements were monitored using an SR Research Ltd. EyeLink eye tracking system. The high spatial resolution (0.005°) and sampling rate (250 Hz or 4 ms temporal resolution) of this tracker allowed the onset of saccades to be accurately determined. The on-line saccade detector of the eye tracker was set to detect saccades with an amplitude of 0.5° or greater, using an acceleration threshold of $9500°/s^2$ and a velocity threshold of 30°/s. The three cameras on the EyeLink headband permitted simultaneous tracking of both eyes and of head position, which was used to compute true gaze position with unrestrained head motion. By default, only the participant's dominant eye was tracked in our studies. An Ethernet link between the eye tracker and display computer supplied real-time gaze position data for the generation of the gaze-contingent window.

Participants viewed the stimuli on a 17″ ViewSonic 17PS monitor from a distance of 60 cm, at which the display subtended a visual angle of 30° horizontally and 22.5° vertically. Displays were generated using an S3 VGA card and special software which supported 120 Hz frame rates, fast switching between several images, and gaze-contingent windows. The average delay between an eye movement and the update of the gaze-contingent window on the monitor was 14 ms.

Reading task

Participants read a short story for comprehension, which was presented in black text on a white background. The luminance of the background was determined by the stimulus requirements of each experiment, but was held constant for all trials within each experiment. An anti-aliased, proportionally spaced text font was used, which had an average of 2.2 characters per degree of visual angle and 10 lines of text per page. One page of text in the story was presented in each trial. After reading each page, participants pressed a button to end the trial and proceed to the next page of the story. The pages were presented in the same order to all participants, but the experimental condition for each page was determined randomly for each participant, with no more than three contiguous trials of the same condition.

Visual search task

During the trial, one of 64 gray-scale scenes of residential interiors were displayed as normal images. Participants searched the scenes for four small targets whose positions were randomly changed for each participant and trial. The targets were 0.5° checkerboards with 0.083° squares, with contrasts of 35%. The average luminance of the targets was matched to the surrounding area of the image in order to make the search difficult and to produce many saccades per trial. Participants were allowed up to 30 s for the search and could terminate the trial with a button press if all the targets were found before the deadline. Each of the 64 original images were presented once in each condition, with random ordering of the scenes and experimental conditions such that no more than three contiguous trials of the same condition occurred.

Procedure

A 9-point calibration was performed at the start of the experiment followed by a 9-point calibration accuracy test. Calibration was repeated if the error at any point was more than 1°, or if the average error for all points was greater than 0.5°. Before each screen of text, a black fixation target was presented at the top left corner of the display for the reading task, and at the center of the display for the visual search task. The participant fixated this target, and the gaze position measured during this fixation was used to correct any post-calibration drift errors. Throughout the reading of each screen, the experimenter was able to view on a separate monitor the text the participant was reading, overlaid with a cursor corresponding to real-time gaze position. If the experimenter judged that gaze-tracking accuracy had declined, the experimenter initiated a full calibration before the next screen. This occurred very infrequently.

During each experimental trial, one page of text or one picture was presented as the normal image. This was replaced by the transient image for 33 ms, after which the normal image was restored. This display change occurred at random intervals of 300 ms to 400 ms during the reading task, and 250 ms to 350 ms during the visual search task. The time of the onset of the transient image was recorded along with eye-movement data for later analysis. The transient image for each trial was determined by the experimental condition. In Experiment 4, the transient image filled the entire display. In all other experiments the transient image was displayed only within a 6° square gaze-contingent window centered on the participant's point of gaze, and the normal image remained visible outside the gaze-contingent window.

Data analysis

Eye tracker data files were processed to produce histograms of saccade frequency by latency from each change from the normal to the transient image. Saccades that occurred during display of the transient image or with amplitudes of less than 0.5° were discarded. A separate histogram was compiled for each participant and condition, and analyzed to produce measures of the evoked saccadic inhibition. Composite histograms were also generated for each condition using saccades from all participants, and are reproduced in this paper to illustrate the results of each experiment. The histogram bin width was 4 ms, determined by the maximum temporal resolution of the eye tracker. These narrow bins provide high temporal resolution but resulted in noisy histograms, which required that individual participant histograms be smoothed by a 7-bin box average filter before analysis. Composite histograms were not filtered, as the large numbers of saccades resulted in much less noise. All bins of the histogram were divided by the baseline saccadic frequency (average saccadic frequency during the first 48 ms following the display change) to compute the normalized saccadic frequency, which is defined as the ratio of expected (baseline) to measured saccadic frequency for each bin. The strength of saccadic inhibition for any histogram bin, defined as the proportion of saccades that were inhibited, could then be estimated by subtracting the normalized saccadic frequency in that bin from 1.0.

Quantitative measures of the latency (L_{MAX} and $L_{50\%}$) of the saccadic inhibition were computed from the sharp reduction in saccadic frequency in the histograms (the 'dip') caused by the saccadic inhibition. The dip was first located by finding the histogram bin with the minimum normalized saccadic frequency at latencies between 55 and 175 ms. The latency of the maximum strength of inhibition (L_{MAX}), defined as the latency of the bottom of the dip, was computed from the average latency of all bins that had a normalized saccadic frequency within 0.1 of the minimum in the dip. The latency of the onset of saccadic inhibition ($L_{50\%}$) was defined as the latency from the display change at which inhibition first reached 50% of its greatest strength. This criterion was chosen to reduce bias caused by the slope of the sides of the dip, which might have been reduced by the filtering of the histogram. The effects of noise were reduced by computing $L_{50\%}$ as the average latency of all bins to the left of L_{MAX} in which inhibition was between 33% and 67% of its greatest strength.

Experiment 1

In previous studies (Reingold and Stampe, 2000, 2002b,c), saccadic inhibition was evoked by replacing black text on a white background with a black transient image. This stimulus resulted in the disappearance of the text and at the same time caused a large change in the luminance of the image, either of which could have been responsible for the observed inhibition. In this experiment, we wished to study the saccadic inhibition evoked by each component of the display change in isolation, and therefore contrasted a pure luminance change to blanking the text with no change to the average luminance of the display.

Method

During each trial, a normal image of black text on a white background with an average luminance of 33 cd/m^2 was displayed. A different transient image was used in each of the two conditions. In the luminance condition, a pure luminance change was produced by displaying as the transient image a brightened version of the normal image, with the

TABLE 1

Results of experiments (mean ± 95% CI)

Experiment	Condition	$L_{50\%}$ (ms)	L_{MAX} (ms)
1	Luminance	71.9 ± 2.2	95.4 ± 4.3
	Blanked	83.5 ± 2.5	107.2 ± 4.6
2	0.5 c/deg grating	76.6 ± 2.3	95.0 ± 3.6
	6.0 c/deg grating	88.6 ± 5.0	109.8 ± 4.4
	Black	74.0 ± 2.4	95.2 ± 4.3
	Blanked	85.6 ± 3.2	103.2 ± 3.5
3	LF text, black	72.8 ± 4.6	93.2 ± 5.7
	HF text, black	72.4 ± 4.3	95.2 ± 6.1
	LF text, blanked	82.0 ± 4.7	102.8 ± 4.3
	HF text, blanked	101.1 ± 3.7	125.6 ± 5.9
4	Black	72.8 ± 3.2	93.6 ± 4.0
	Blanked	76.0 ± 2.0	97.6 ± 4.3
	Sharpened	96.4 ± 7.9	120.8 ± 4.5

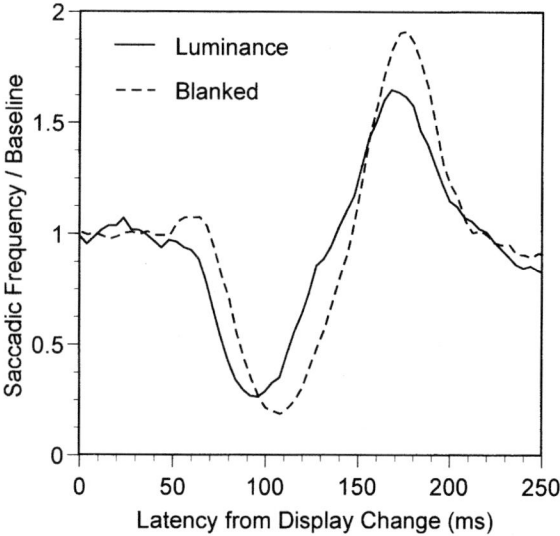

Fig. 2. Saccade frequency histograms showing the time course of the saccadic inhibition evoked by stimuli in Experiment 1. The pure luminance change in the luminance condition evoked the most rapid inhibition, while removal of the text without a luminance change in the blanked condition resulted in inhibition of substantially longer latency.

luminance of both the text and background increased by 33 cd/m². In the blanked condition, the text was removed without changing the average luminance of the display by displaying a blanked transient image matched to the average luminance of the normal image. As it was expected that the lower spatial acuity of the peripheral visual field would cause the blanking of the text to be reduced in saliency compared to the luminance change, the display changes were limited to the center of the visual field by a 6° square gaze-contingent window centered on the participant's point of gaze. A total of 90 pages of text were presented, with 45 pages randomly assigned to each condition.

Results and discussion

An average of 2523 saccades were collected from each participant in each condition. These were used to create individual histograms for each participant and condition, from which the latency measures in Table 1 were computed. Saccades from all participants were combined to create the histograms of saccadic frequency in Fig. 2, which show the time course of the saccadic inhibition produced in each experimental condition. Both the luminance change and the blanking of the text clearly evoked strong saccadic inhibition. Therefore, production of saccadic inhibition does not require the disappearance of the text, but instead, appears to be a response of the oculomotor system to changes in low level characteristics of the visual input such as luminance.

Blanking the text without a luminance change evoked saccadic inhibition of a significantly longer latency than that evoked by changing the luminance of the display. The difference in latencies between the two conditions was 11.8 ms ($t(9) = 6.38$, $p < 0.001$), as measured by L_{MAX}, and 11.6 ms ($t(9) = 13.71$, $p < 0.001$), as measured by $L_{50\%}$. While it is possible that this difference is due to fundamental differences in the mechanism by which saccadic inhibition is evoked in the two conditions, a more parsimonious explanation is that the latency of saccadic inhibition may be sensitive to the low level visual characteristics of the display changes in each condition. In addition, the rapid time course of saccadic inhibition, indicative of a reflexive oculomotor mechanism, is also compatible with this hypothesis. Similar latency effects caused by low level stimulus characteristics have been observed in studies of visual evoked potentials (VEP) in which the fastest components of the response have latencies similar to that of saccadic inhibition. In several such studies, it has been reported that response latencies are longer for stimuli containing high spatial frequencies (such as text), when compared to stimuli containing low spatial frequencies or luminance changes. The hypothesis that the frequency content of the display change stimulus was responsible for the observed differences in latency in this experiment will be explored in detail throughout the remainder of this paper.

Experiment 2

A consistent finding from VEP studies is that presentation of high frequency gratings resulted in increased response latency when compared to low frequency gratings (Parker and Salzen, 1977, 1982; Parker et al., 1982; Vassilev et al., 1983; Musselwhite and Jeffreys, 1985; Vassilev and Stomonyakov, 1987). This effect has been observed (1) for the onset, offset, and reversal of sinusoidal gratings (Parker and Salzen, 1977, 1982), (2) over a wide range of contrasts (Vassilev et al., 1983), and (3) for both sinusoidal and square wave gratings (Musselwhite and Jeffreys, 1985). The effect of spatial frequency on latency may arise in the retina and optic nerve, as both Y cells (magnocellular) and X cells (parvocellular) in the cat have been observed to show a clear correlation between the spatial frequency of the stimulus and the latency of the neural response at the lateral geniculate nucleus (LGN) (Sestokas and Lehmkuhle, 1986). This subcortical frequency-dependent delay should influence the latency of all cortical and subcortical responses, including the unknown pathways involved in saccadic inhibition. The contributions of subcortical visual pathways to the frequency-dependent latency effect are best measured from the C1 peak of the VEP response, which has a latency of 50–100 ms (Clark and Hillyard, 1996), and which is thought to be the earliest cortical component of VEP and thus should be least contaminated by cortical processing effects. In a study by Musselwhite and Jeffreys (1985), the latency of C1 was found to be relatively constant for spatial frequencies below 2 cycles per degree (c/deg), and was increased by 15 to 30 ms at 10 c/deg, which corresponds to about 5 to 10 ms per octave of frequency. A similar latency shift was observed by Vassilev and Stomonyakov (1987) using sinusoidal gratings at 4 and 6 times the

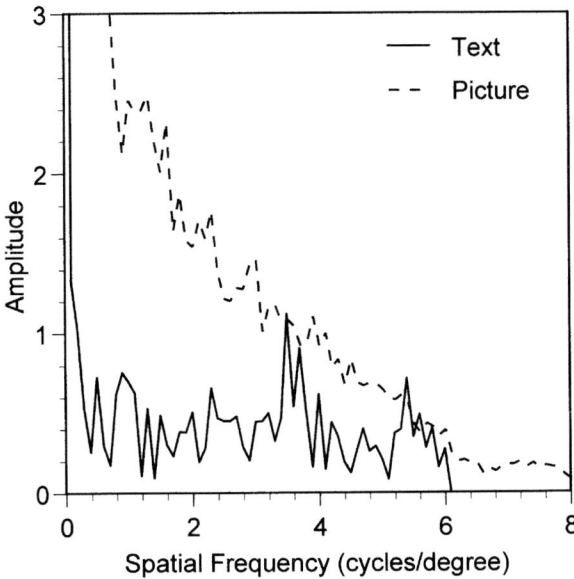

Fig. 3. Spatial frequency content of text, compared to frequency content of a typical photograph used in Experiment 4. Most of the energy in the text is above 2 c/deg, while the energy of the photograph is concentrated at low spatial frequencies. This plot was generated by summing the square of the frequency components (spectral energy) of a two-dimensional Fourier transform of sample images from the studies into 0.1 c/deg bins. Amplitude is computed as the square root of the total energy in each bin.

psychophysical contrast threshold, with C1 latency increasing by 30 ms between 2 and 16 c/deg, or about 10 ms per octave of frequency.

The increased latency of neural responses to stimuli consisting of high spatial frequencies may explain the delayed saccadic inhibition evoked by the blanking of the text that was observed in Experiment 1. Blanking the text would have caused a change in the frequency content of the display equal to the frequency content of the normal text image that is plotted in Fig. 3. Most of the spectral energy in the text is at frequencies above 2 c/deg, which is also the frequency above which the latency of VEP responses has been observed to increase for grating stimuli. Therefore, the largely high frequency stimulus, generated by the disappearance of the text, would be expected to evoke delayed VEP responses, and perhaps delayed saccadic inhibition as well.

To show that the observed latency differences in Experiment 1 were caused by the spatial frequency content of the stimuli, we must first demonstrate that the latency of saccadic inhibition evoked by the display change is in fact influenced by the frequency content of the stimulus in the same fashion as the C1 peak was observed to be in VEP studies. Specifically, we must show that the inhibition evoked by a low frequency sinusoidal grating is of shorter latency than the inhibition produced by a high frequency grating. In the VEP studies, the grating was flashed on a blank background or was counterphased in order to create a pure frequency stimulus. However, displaying the gratings as a transient image will not produce a pure frequency stimulus in this paradigm, as the disappearance of the text during display of the grating adds extraneous high- and low frequency components to the display change. To evaluate the effects of these extraneous components, we included a blanked transient image condition similar to that in Experiment 1. This condition removed the text without displaying a grating, and will be used as a control for the grating conditions. A black transient image condition was also included, which added a luminance change to the disappearance of the text. Based on the frequency and luminance content of the display change in each condition, it was predicted that the lowest latency saccadic inhibition should be evoked by the black and low frequency grating transient images, and the highest latency inhibition should be evoked by the blanked and high frequency grating transient images.

Method

In all conditions, the normal images consisted of black text on a white background as in Experiment 1. Low frequency (0.5 c/deg) and high frequency (6.0 c/deg) sinusoidal gratings were used as transient images, with the average luminance of the gratings adjusted to be equal to that of the normal text image (34 cd/m^2). The contrast of each grating was 50%, computed as (max − min)/(max + min) where max and min are the maximum and minimum luminance of the gratings respectively. A luminance-matched blanked transient image was used to remove the text without displaying a grating, and a black transient image (4 cd/m^2) both removed the text and changed the luminance of the display. Transient images were displayed for 33 ms within a 6° gaze-contingent window centered on the participant's point of gaze. A total of 112 pages of text were presented, with 28 pages randomly assigned to each of the four conditions.

Results and discussion

An average of 2386 saccades were collected from each participant in each condition. These were used to compute the latency measures reported in Table 1, and saccades from all participants were combined to create the histograms of saccadic frequency shown in Fig. 4. The fastest saccadic inhibition was evoked by the black transient image, which caused a large change in the luminance of the display. The inhibition evoked by the low frequency grating was of slightly longer latency than produced by the black transient image as measured by $L_{50\%}$ ($t(9) = 2.75$, $p < 0.05$), but no difference was seen for L_{MAX} ($t(9) = 0.15$, $p = 0.89$). As predicted, the inhibition evoked by the high frequency grating was of significantly longer latency than that evoked by the low frequency grating, with the latency of the onset of inhibition ($L_{50\%}$) delayed by 12.0 ms ($t(9) = 5.28$, $p < 0.01$) for the 6.0 c/deg grating transient image compared to the 0.5 c/deg grating. A similar effect was observed for L_{MAX}, with a difference of 14.8 ms between the gratings ($t(9) = 8.14$, $p < 0.001$). This confirmed that the spatial frequency content of the stimulus affected the latency of visually evoked saccadic inhibition in the same fashion as had been reported for visually evoked potentials. The difference observed in L_{MAX} between the 0.5 c/deg and 6.0 c/deg grating conditions was 14.8 ms, which corresponds to a change of 4 ms per octave. This is somewhat lower than the latency effect observed in VEP studies, computed from the change in the C1 latency for gratings of similar frequencies (5–10 ms/octave, Musselwhite and Jeffreys, 1985; 10 ms/octave, Vassilev and Stomonyakov, 1987). The smaller effect of frequency on latency observed in this experiment may be due to the presence of the extraneous frequency components added by the disappearance of the text.

All of the display changes in this experiment contained extraneous frequency components caused by the disappearance of the text, in addition to the desired luminance or frequency components from the transient images. These extraneous components were also present in isolation in the blanked tran-

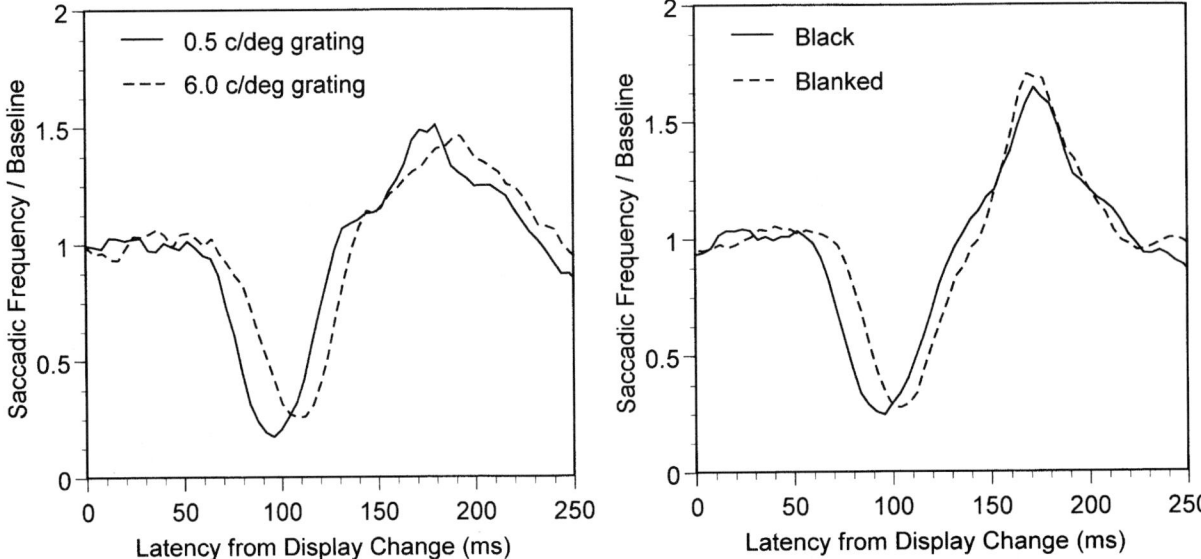

Fig. 4. Saccade frequency histograms showing the time course of the saccadic inhibition evoked by stimuli in Experiment 2. (Left panel) Inhibition evoked by low and high frequency gratings, showing the difference in latency caused by grating frequency. (Right) Comparison of inhibition evoked by black and blanked transient images, showing a latency difference caused by the presence of the luminance change.

sient image condition, which may be utilized as a control condition. By comparing the blanked transient image condition to each of the others, we may evaluate the effect that the desired component of the display change had when added to the disappearance of the text. The black transient image condition added a luminance component to the display change, which resulted in faster inhibition than in the blanked condition, by 11.6 ms as measured by $L_{50\%}$ ($t(9) = 8.77$, $p < 0.001$), and 8.0 ms for L_{MAX} ($t(9) = 12.00$, $p < 0.001$). The low frequency grating condition added a low frequency component, which also produced significantly shorter latencies than did the blanked condition, by 9.0 ms for $L_{50\%}$ ($t(9) = 8.63$, $p < 0.001$), and 8.2 ms for L_{MAX} ($t(9) = 8.94$, $p < 0.001$). In contrast, the high frequency grating produced inhibition with a non-significant difference in latency compared to that evoked by the blanked image as measured by the onset of inhibition (3.0 ms for $L_{50\%}$) ($t(9) = 1.31$, $p = 0.224$), but showed a 6.6 ms longer latency to peak inhibition as measured by L_{MAX} ($t(9) = 4.11$, $p < 0.01$).

This pattern of comparisons shows that the blanked transient image and high frequency grating evoked inhibition of comparable onset latencies due to the largely high frequency content of both display changes. The results of this experiment clearly demonstrated that the low level stimulus characteristics of the display change determined the latency of the inhibition observed in each condition. Specifically, changes in the luminance of the display evoked the fastest saccadic inhibition, changes in the low frequency content of the display resulted in slightly longer latencies, and changes in the high frequency content resulted in significantly delayed saccadic inhibition.

Experiment 3

In Experiment 2, saccadic inhibition of relatively long latency was produced when the normal text image, containing mostly high spatial frequency content, was momentarily replaced by a luminance-matched blanked image. The latency of the evoked inhibition appeared to be determined by the difference in spatial frequency content between the normal and transient images, rather than the contents of either image individually. If this is indeed the case, then manipulating the frequency content of the text in the normal image should change the latency of saccadic inhibition evoked by the blanked transient image. Specifically, replacing a text image containing mainly low frequency components with a blanked transient image should cause a change in low frequency content and evoke low latency inhibition, while the same blanked transient image when paired with a text image containing mostly high frequency components should cause a change in high frequency content and evoke saccadic inhibition of significantly longer latency.

It was also observed in the previous experiment that the luminance change caused by the black transient image evoked low latency inhibition, despite the presence of a change in high spatial frequency content caused by the removal of the text. This suggests that the presence of a sufficiently strong luminance component may override other frequency components of the display change in determining the latency of the evoked saccadic inhibition. If this is the case, then presenting a black instead of a blanked transient image should reduce or eliminate any latency effects caused by the frequency content of the normal image. This experiment will test all of these hypothesized interactions of the frequency content of the normal image and luminance changes, by presenting filtered text in combination with both black and blanked transient images.

Method

The frequency content of images of text similar to those used in the previous experiments was manipulated by high-pass or low-pass filtering. A Gaussian low-pass filter with a standard deviation of 2.0 c/deg in the frequency domain was applied to create low frequency text (LF text) images. High frequency text (HF text) images were created by subtracting the LF text images from the original text images, and adding a constant value to each pixel to equalize the average luminance of the HF and LF text images. The text was only slightly degraded in readability by the filtering, which caused mild blurring of the LF text and added white borders to the characters in the HF text. The frequency content of the filtered text is plotted in Fig. 5. Each type of text was presented as a normal image in combination with both a black transient image (4 cd/m^2) and a blanked image matched

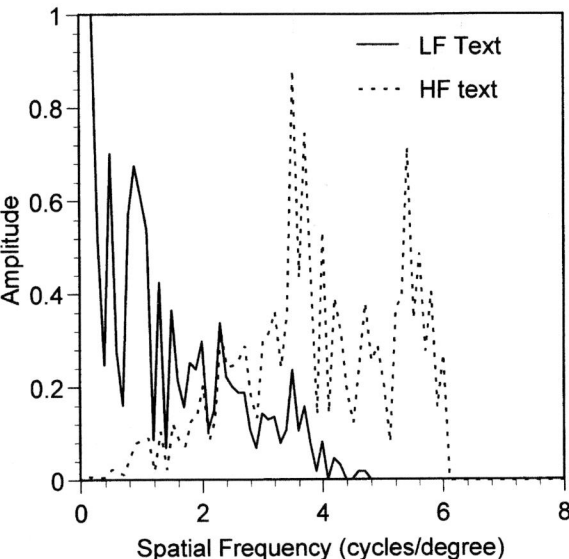

Fig. 5. Spatial frequency content of filtered text. A Gaussian low-pass filter with a standard deviation of 2.0 c/deg was used to create the LF text. The HF text was high-pass filtered by subtracting the LF text image from the original text image.

in luminance to the filtered text images (40 cd/m^2). The transient images were presented for 33 ms in a 6° gaze-contingent window centered on the participant's point of gaze, as in previous experiments. A total of 120 pages of text were presented, randomly assigned with 30 pages in each of the 4 conditions.

Results and discussion

An average of 1752 saccades were collected from each participant in each condition, and used to compute the measures of latency reported in Table 1. Saccadic frequency histograms showing the time course of the inhibition evoked by the black and blanked transient images when paired with the LF and HF filtered text are shown in Fig. 6. The saccadic inhibition evoked by the blanked transient image differed in latency when paired with the LF text compared to the HF text normal images, confirming that it is not the transient image alone that is the stimulus for saccadic inhibition, but the difference between the normal and transient images. As predicted, the latency of inhibition was longer for the HF text, by 18.7 ms for $L_{50\%}$ ($t(9) = 6.11$, $p < 0.001$) and 22.8 ms for L_{MAX} ($t(9) = 10.01$, $p < 0.001$). These

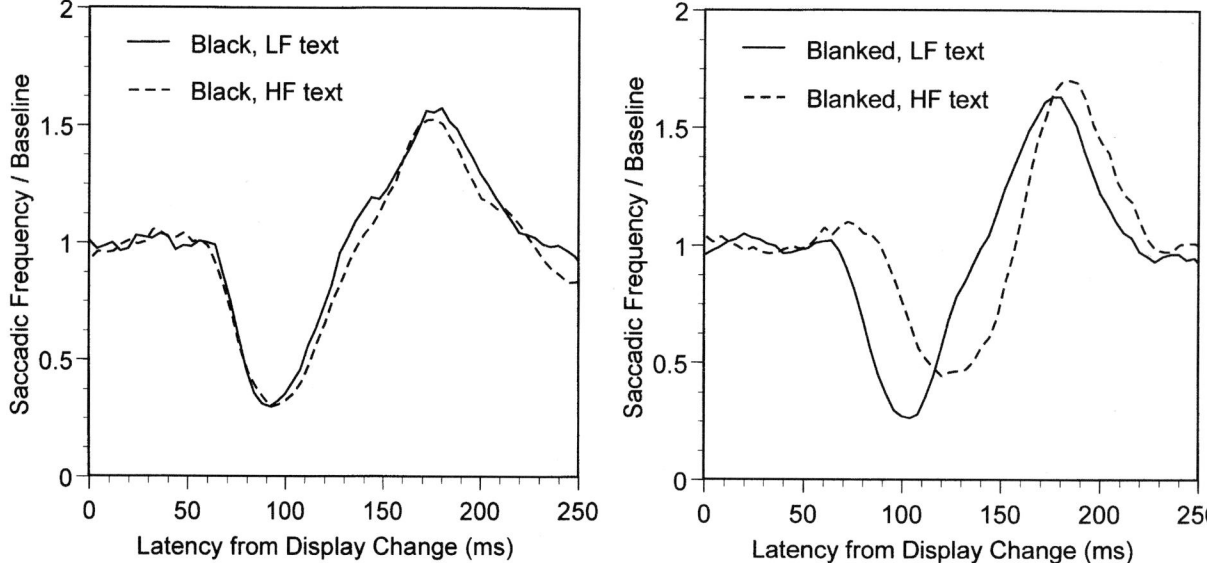

Fig. 6. Saccade frequency histograms showing the time course of saccadic inhibition evoked in Experiment 3. (Left) Comparison of inhibition evoked by the black transient image replacing LF and HF text. No differences were seen in the time course of inhibition. (Right) Comparison of inhibition evoked by the blanked transient image. A very large latency difference is observed between LF and HF text conditions.

differences in latency are almost twice as large as those observed between the sinusoidal grating conditions in Experiment 2, where extraneous frequency components added by the disappearance of the text prevented a pure manipulation of frequency content. The present experiment achieved a purer manipulation of high and low frequency content by using filtered text, which appears to have resulted in a larger latency effect.

In contrast, no differences in the time course of the saccadic inhibition evoked by black transient image were observed between the LF or HF text normal images. The saccadic frequency histograms in Fig. 6 for these conditions appear to be almost identical, and no significant differences were found for either measure of latency ($t(9) < 1$ for all comparisons). The interaction between the two transient images and the two types of normal text were highly significant, both for $L_{50\%}$ ($F(1,9) = 27.8$, $p < 0.01$) and L_{MAX} ($F(1,9) = 51.7$, $p < 0.001$). The black transient image also consistently evoked faster inhibition than the blanked transient image when paired with either LF and HF text, as measured by both $L_{50\%}$ (LF text, $t(9) = 3.76$, $p < 0.01$; HF text $t(9) = 13.70$, $p < 0.001$) and L_{MAX} (LF text, $t(9) = 6.47$, $p < 9.001$; HF text $t(9) = 10.01$, $p < 0.001$). These findings show that the time course of the inhibition was completely determined by the luminance change caused by the black transient image, despite the presence of other frequency components in the display change. Conversely, the blanked transient image produced no luminance change and the time course of the saccadic inhibition was determined by the frequency components present in the normal image.

Experiment 4

In the preceding experiments, it was demonstrated that the latency of saccadic inhibition during reading was dependent on the luminance and frequency content of the display change stimulus. We will now demonstrate that this latency effect is also present in a visual search task, which is similar to that used in a previous study of saccadic inhibition (Reingold and Stampe, 2000). This was done in order to illustrate the generality of the saccadic inhibition effect. More specifically, we attempted to demonstrate that the effects that the low level characteristics of display changes have on saccadic inhibition are similar for both the visual search task and the reading task. For the visual search task, participants searched gray-scale photographs of residential interiors for several small targets that were made difficult to find in order to produce many saccades per trial. As in the reading task, display changes were generated by momentarily replacing the normal images (the photographs) with a transient image. However, the pictures used in this task were very different in their spatial frequency content when compared to the text used in previous experiments. As shown in Fig. 3, most of the energy in the text was at frequencies above 2.0 c/deg, while the photographs contained largely low frequency energy. Because of this, replacing the pictures with a blanked luminance-matched transient image should cause a change in the low frequency content of the display, and thus evoke low latency saccadic inhibition. By comparison, when text was replaced by the blanked transient image in Experiments 1 and 2, longer latency inhibition resulted because of the largely high frequency content of the display change.

In this experiment, the inhibition evoked by the blanked transient image was contrasted with the inhibition evoked by a change in the luminance or in the high frequency content of the display. The luminance change was produced by replacing the normal images with a black transient image as used in previous experiments. The change in high frequency content was achieved by replacing the normal images with a transient image in which the high spatial frequency energy has been increased by a sharpening filter. If the effect of the low level characteristics of these display changes are the same for the visual search task as for the reading task, it is predicted that the luminance change caused by the black transient image should evoke the fastest inhibition, the change in low frequency content caused by the blanked transient image should evoke inhibition of slightly longer latency, and the high frequency change produced by the sharpened transient image should result in inhibition of significantly longer latency than in any other condition.

Method

During each trial, one of 64 gray-scale photographs of residential interiors was displayed as a normal im-

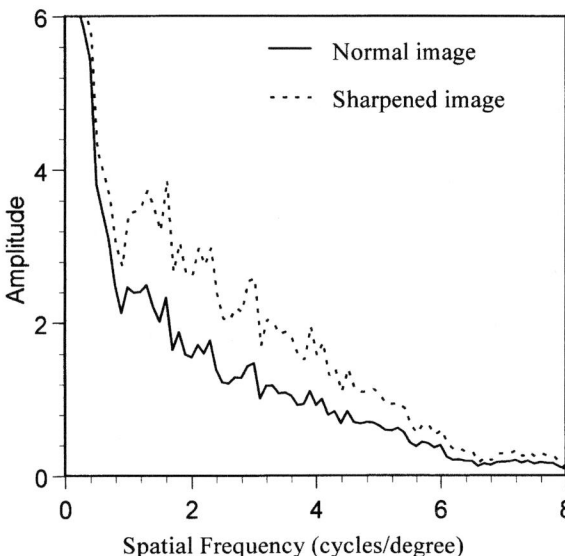

Fig. 7. Spatial frequency content of a sample photograph used in Experiment 4. Sharpened images were generated by subtracting a Gaussian low-pass filtered image (standard deviation of 1.0 c/deg) from the original image to create a high-pass filtered version, then adding this to the original image to double its high frequency content.

age. Participants searched each image for four small targets (low-contrast checkerboards matched in luminance to the part of the photograph under them). The transient image for each trial was black (4 cd/m^2), blanked with the same average luminance as the normal image (18 cd/m^2 to 50 cd/m^2), or a sharpened version of the normal image. The sharpening filter multiplied each pixel in the image by 2, then subtracted a Gaussian low-pass filtered (1.0 c/deg standard deviation) version of the original image. This resulted in the accentuation of contours in the image, and doubled the amplitude of all frequency components above 1.0 c/deg. The frequency content of the original and sharpened images are shown in Fig. 7. Unlike previous experiments, the entire display was replaced by the transient image for 33 ms. Each of the 64 original images were presented once in each of the 3 conditions, for a total of 192 trials.

Results and discussion

An average of 2285 saccades were collected from each participant in each condition, and were used

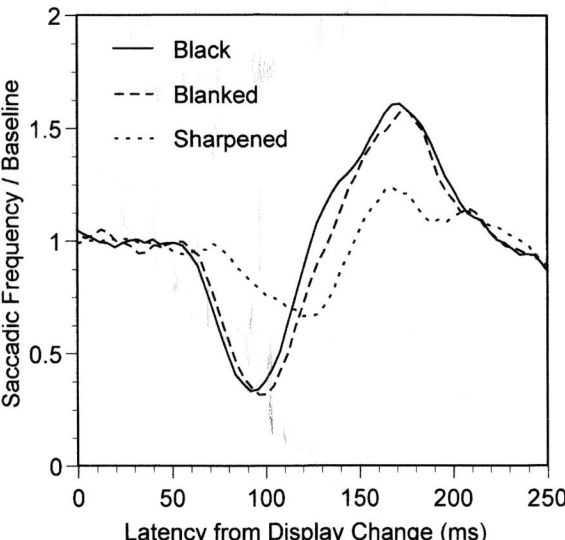

Fig. 8. Saccade frequency histograms showing the time course of saccadic inhibition observed in Experiment 4. The change from the picture to the black transient image produced inhibition of only slightly lower latency than did the luminance-matched blanked transient image. The boost in high spatial frequencies caused by the sharpened transient image produced saccadic inhibition with significantly longer latency.

to compute the measures of latency reported in Table 1. The saccadic frequency histograms and time course of the inhibition in each condition are shown in Fig. 8. As predicted, both the black and blanked transient images evoked a short latency saccadic inhibition, when compared to that produced by the sharpened transient image. The inhibition evoked by the black transient image was of slightly shorter latency than that produced by the blanked image, by 3.2 ms for $L_{50\%}$ ($t(9) = 4.00$, $p < 0.01$) and 4.0 ms for L_{MAX} ($t(9) = 4.47$, $p < 0.01$). The inhibition evoked by the sharpened transient image had a much longer latency than that produced by the blanked transient image, by 20.4 ms for $L_{50\%}$ ($t(9) = 5.46$, $p < 0.001$) and 23.2 ms for L_{MAX} ($t(9) = 8.97$, $p < 0.001$). This large difference in latency reflects the nearly pure high or low frequency composition of the display changes in these two conditions. In addition, the inhibition evoked by the sharpened transient image appeared to be rather weak, which may reflect the low saliency of the display change in this condition and the limited high frequency content of the pictures. This pattern of results clearly demonstrates that the luminance and frequency content of the display change had a similar effect on the latency of saccadic inhibition in both the reading task and the visual search task, despite the very different nature of the tasks and stimuli in each of these paradigms.

General discussion

The results of the present experiments establish that the latency of visually evoked saccadic inhibition is influenced by the spatial frequency content of the display change. Specifically, changes in the high frequency content of the display evoke inhibition with longer latency than do changes in low frequency content or the luminance of the display. These findings are qualitatively similar to findings for visually evoked potentials (Parker and Salzen, 1977, 1982; Parker et al., 1982; Vassilev et al., 1983; Musselwhite and Jeffreys, 1985; Vassilev and Stomonyakov, 1987). In the experiments presented here, saccadic inhibition was evoked by momentarily replacing the text being read with a transient image. As shown in Experiment 3, it is the difference between the normal image and the transient image, and not the transient image alone that is the stimulus for saccadic inhibition. For example, changing the frequency content of the text by filtering also changed the latency of the inhibition evoked by the presentation of the blanked transient image. In this case, the stimulus was the disappearance of the normal text image, and the frequency content of the display change was that of the text. Similarly, early VEP responses appear to be evoked by changes in the visual stimulus, such as the onset, offset, or reversal of sinusoidal gratings (e.g. Parker and Salzen, 1977, 1982).

The present experiments also demonstrated that adding a luminance component to the display change by using a black, rather than a blanked but luminance-matched, transient image resulted in low latency saccadic inhibition, and the frequency content of the normal image then had no effect on the evoked inhibition. These findings may be explained by a simple race model, where saccadic inhibition is always initiated by the first component of the display change to arrive at the neural substrate of inhibition. Since the luminance change produced saccadic inhibition of lower latency than any other frequency component, luminance information should arrive at the locus of saccadic inhibition before any other component of the display change and thus determine the latency of the resulting saccadic inhibition. This model also explains why inhibition of low latency was produced by the onset of the low frequency grating in Experiment 2, despite the presence of high frequency components from the simultaneous disappearance of the text. In this case, the low frequency components caused by the onset of the low frequency grating arrived first and triggered the saccadic inhibition.

The paradigm used to study visually evoked saccadic inhibition in this paper enabled the calculation of the latency of the strongest point of saccadic inhibition (L_{MAX}), as well as the latency of the onset of inhibition ($L_{50\%}$) (see Reingold and Stampe, 2002a,b). The results shown in Table 1 demonstrate that these measures of saccadic inhibition gave highly reproducible results for all 10 participants, with 95% confidence intervals of 4.6 ms (4.5% of the mean) for L_{MAX}, and 3.7 ms (4.6% of the mean) for $L_{50\%}$, averaged across all experiments and conditions. The patterns of results were similar for both measures of latency, with an average difference computed across all experiments and conditions of 20.9 ms between $L_{50\%}$ and L_{MAX}. The L_{MAX} measure is similar to the measures of latencies of peaks typically reported in VEP studies. However, the equivalence of the $L_{50\%}$ measure is rarely seen in VEP studies, as the latency of the onset of peaks is difficult to determine due to the complex nature of the VEP response, which consists of several overlaid positive and negative peaks. The much simpler shape of the saccadic frequency histogram produced by the random display change paradigm used in this study, which shows only a single dip followed by a recovery peak, allowed the reliable measurement of the timing of both the onset and the maximum strength of the inhibition.

Luminance changes evoked saccadic inhibition with an exceptionally short onset latency for an oculomotor response. Reingold and Stampe (2000, 2002a,b, 2002c) estimated onset latencies in the range of 60–70 ms for a black transient image. The $L_{50\%}$ measure used in this study produced comparable latencies: for example, the pure luminance change condition of Experiment 1 produced significant inhibition 71.9 ms after the brightening of the display. This very fast response was observed for all participants, with individual values of $L_{50\%}$ ranging from 66 to 76 ms. This is, to our knowledge, the fastest known visuomotor response of the human saccadic system. By comparison, the fastest (express) saccades produced in response to the onset of a visual target have latencies of approximately 90 ms (see Fischer et al., 1993; Kingstone and Klein, 1993). Based on the available neurophysiological evidence, Reingold and Stampe (2000, 2002a,b) suggested that the superior colliculus is the primary candidate for mediating the fast saccadic inhibition onset latencies, and that this effect may be related to inhibitory processes in the superior colliculus that were documented by Munoz and colleagues (e.g. Munoz and Wurtz, 1992, 1993a,b, 1995a,b; Dorris et al., 1997; Dorris and Munoz, 1998; Munoz and Istvan, 1998; see Munoz et al., 2000 for a review). The superior colliculus is ideally suited to mediate fast visuomotor responses, as it receives direct input from fast, transient M ganglion cells in the retina (Schiller and Malpeli, 1977). Collicular visual neurons (pandirectional cells) respond nonspecifically to visual input in as little as 35 ms (Rizzolatti et al., 1980), and collicular output directly activates the saccade generator in the brainstem (for reviews see Sparks and Hartwich-Young, 1989; Wurtz and Goldberg, 1989; Moschovakis et al., 1996). Furthermore, lesions of the superior colliculus abolish short latency (express) saccades in monkeys (Schiller et al., 1987).

The role of saccadic inhibition in normal vision is unclear, but we may speculate on its possible advantages. Saccades are required for the acquisition of visual information, but their performance also has perceptual costs. During saccades, the availability of visual information is reduced by motion blur and saccadic suppression (e.g. Burr et al., 1994; Deubel et al., 1996). It may also be impossible to stop or redirect the saccade in response to new visual information that becomes available at a late stage in the preparation of the saccade (e.g. Becker and Jurgens, 1979). It is therefore advantageous for the human visual and saccadic systems to minimize the costs associated with saccadic production by temporarily delaying the generation of saccades when new visual information is detected.

Acknowledgements

Preparation of this paper was supported by a grant to Eyal Reingold from the Natural Science and Engineering Research Council of Canada. The authors thank Colleen Ray and Elizabeth Bosman for their helpful comments on an earlier draft of the manuscript.

References

Becker, W. and Jurgens, R. (1979) An analysis of the saccadic system by means of double step stimuli. *Vision Res.*, 19: 967–983.

Burr, D.C., Morrone, M.C. and Ross, J. (1994) Selective suppression of the magnocellular visual pathway during saccadic eye movements. *Nature*, 371: 511–513.

Clark, V.P. and Hillyard, S.A. (1996) Spatial selective attention affects early extrastriate but not striate components of the visual evoked potential. *J. Cogn. Neurosci.*, 8: 387–402.

Deubel, H., Schneider, W.X. and Bridgeman, B. (1996) Postsaccadic target blanking prevents saccadic suppression of image displacement. *Vision Res.*, 36: 985–996.

Dorris, M.C. and Munoz, D.P. (1998) Saccadic probability influences motor preparation signals and time to saccadic initiation. *J. Neurosci.*, 18: 7015–7026.

Dorris, M.C., Paré, M. and Munoz, D.P. (1997) Neuronal activity in monkey superior colliculus related to the initiation of saccadic eye movements. *J. Neurosci.*, 17: 8566–8579.

Fischer, B., Weber, H., Biscaldi, M., Aiple, F., Otto, P. and Stuhr, V. (1993) Separate populations of visually guided saccades in humans: reaction times and amplitudes. *Exp. Brain Res.*, 92: 528–541.

Kingstone, A. and Klein, R.M. (1993) What are human express saccades? *Percept. Psychophys.*, 54: 260–273.

Moschovakis, A.K., Scudder, C.A. and Highstein, S.M. (1996) The microscopic anatomy and physiology of the mammalian saccadic system. *Prog. Neurobiol.*, 50: 133–254.

Munoz, D.P. and Istvan, P.J. (1998) Lateral inhibitory interactions in the intermediate layers of the monkey superior colliculus. *J. Neurophysiol.*, 79: 1193–1209.

Munoz, D.P. and Wurtz, R.H. (1992) Role of the rostral superior colliculus in active visual fixation and execution of express saccades. *J. Neurophysiol.*, 67: 1000–1002.

Munoz, D.P. and Wurtz, R.H. (1993a) Fixation cells in monkey superior colliculus. I. Characteristics of cell discharge. *J. Neurophysiol.*, 70: 559–575.

Munoz, D.P. and Wurtz, R.H. (1993b) Fixation cells in monkey superior colliculus. II. Reversible activation and deactivation. *J. Neurophysiol.*, 70: 576–589.

Munoz, D.P. and Wurtz, R.H. (1995a) Saccade-related activity in monkey superior colliculus. I. Characteristics of burst and buildup cells. *J. Neurophysiol.*, 73: 2313–2333.

Munoz, D.P. and Wurtz, R.H. (1995b) Saccade-related activity in monkey superior colliculus. II. Spread of activity during saccades. *J. Neurophysiol.*, 73: 2334–2348.

Munoz, D.P., Dorris, M.C., Pare, M. and Everling, S. (2000) On your mark, get set: brainstem circuitry underlying saccadic initiation. *Can. J. Physiol. Pharmacol.*, 78: 934–944.

Musselwhite, M.J. and Jeffreys, D.A. (1985) The influence of spatial frequency on the reaction times and evoked potentials recorded to grating pattern stimuli. *Vision Res.*, 25: 1545–1555.

Parker, D.M. and Salzen, E.A. (1977) Latency changes in the human visual evoked response to sinusoidal gratings. *Vision Res.*, 17: 1201–1204.

Parker, D.M. and Salzen, E.A. (1982) Evoked potentials and reaction times to the offset and contrast reversal of sinusoidal gratings. *Vision Res.*, 22: 205–207.

Parker, D.M., Salzen, E.A. and Lishman, J.R. (1982) The early wave of the visual evoked potential to sinusoidal gratings: responses to quadrant stimulation as a function of spatial frequency. *Electroencephalogr. Clin. Neurophysiol.*, 53: 427–435.

Reingold, E.M. and Stampe, D.M. (1997) Transient saccadic inhibition in reading. Paper presented at the 9th European Conference on Eye Movements, Ulm.

Reingold, E.M. and Stampe, D.M. (2000) Saccadic inhibition and gaze contingent research paradigms. In: A. Kennedy, R. Radach, D. Heller and J. Pynte (Eds.), *Reading as a Perceptual Process*. Elsevier, Amsterdam, pp. 119–145.

Reingold, E.M. and Stampe, D.M. (2002a) Saccadic inhibition in voluntary and reflexive saccades. *J. Cogn. Neurosci.*, 14: 371–388.

Reingold, E.M. and Stampe, D.M. (2002b) Saccadic inhibition in reading. *J. Exp. Psychol. Hum. Percept. Perform.*, in press.

Reingold, E.M. and Stampe, D.M. (2002c) Saccadic inhibition in reading: Implications for models of saccadic control in reading. In: J. Hyönä, R. Radach and H. Deubel (Eds.), *The Mind's Eyes: Cognitive and Applied Aspects of Eye Movements*. Elsevier, Amsterdam, in press.

Rizzolatti, G., Buchtel, H.A., Camarda, R. and Scandolara, C. (1980) Neurons with complex visual properties in the superior colliculus of the macaque monkey. *Exp. Brain Res.*, 38: 37–42.

Schiller, P.H. and Malpeli, J.G. (1977) Properties and tectal projections of monkey retinal ganglion cells. *J. Neurophysiol.*, 40: 428–445.

Schiller, P.H., Sandell, J.H. and Maunsell, J.H. (1987) The effect of frontal eye field and superior colliculus lesions on saccadic latencies in the rhesus monkey. *J. Neurophysiol.*, 57: 1033–1049.

Sestokas, A.K. and Lehmkuhle, S. (1986) Visual response latency of X and Y cells in the dorsal lateral geniculate nucleus of the cat. *Vision Res.*, 26: 1041–1054.

Sparks, D.L. and Hartwich-Young, R. (1989) The deep layers of the superior colliculus. In: R.H. Wurtz and M.E. Goldberg (Eds.), *The Neurobiology of Saccadic Eye Movements*. Elsevier, Amsterdam, pp. 213–256.

Vassilev, A. and Stomonyakov, V. (1987) The effect of grating spatial frequency on the early VEP-component CI. *Vision Res.*, 27: 727–729.

Vassilev, A., Manahilov, V. and Mitov, D. (1983) Spatial frequency and the pattern onset–offset response. *Vision Res.*, 23: 1417–1422.

Wurtz, R.H. and Goldberg, M.E. (Eds.) (1989) *The Neurobiology of Saccadic Eye Movements*. Elsevier, Amsterdam.

CHAPTER 6

Commentary: Saccadic eye movements: overview of neural circuitry

Douglas P. Munoz *

Centre for Neuroscience Studies, Department of Physiology, Queen's University, Kingston, ON K7L 3N6, Canada

Abstract: Recent neuroanatomical, neurophysiological, clinical, and brain imaging studies have generated a wealth of data describing the neural control of saccadic eye movements and visual fixation. These studies have identified many of the cortical and subcortical structures involved in controlling the behavior. Critical nodes in the network include regions of the parietal and frontal cortices, basal ganglia, thalamus, superior colliculus, cerebellum, and brainstem reticular formation. Specific functions are likely not localized to only one brain area, but rather, they may be distributed across multiple areas. This commentary is used to review briefly the neural circuitry controlling saccadic eye movements and visual fixation.

Introduction

One of the most important functions of the central nervous system is the generation of movement in response to sensory stimulation. The visual guidance of saccadic eye movements represents one form of sensory-to-motor transformation that has provided significant insight into our understanding of motor control and sensorimotor processing. The eyes have a simple and well defined repertoire of movements and the neural circuitry regulating the production of saccadic eye movements is now understood at a level that is sufficient to link cortical and subcortical areas together. The contributions to this section of the book by Munoz and Fecteau, Enderle, Zambarbieri, Tinsley and Everling, and Stampe and Reingold address aspects of saccadic processing at various stages of the neuraxis from the brainstem reticular formation, the superior colliculus, the cerebellum, to the cerebral cortex. This commentary will therefore be used to review briefly the neural circuitry controlling saccadic eye movements.

Before reviewing the details of the neural circuitry it is first important to recognize why saccadic eye movements have evolved and what they are used for. The primate retina has a specialized region in its center, called the fovea, which serves the central 1° of the visual field and provides the greatest visual acuity (Perry and Cowey, 1985). In most cortical and subcortical visual areas, the fovea has the greatest representation, emphasizing the importance of foveal vision in most aspects of visual processing and visually guided behavior (Dow et al., 1981; Van Essen et al., 1984). In order to maximize the efficiency of foveal vision, we must have the ability to align the fovea rapidly upon novel targets that may appear unexpectedly in the visual world and then keep the fovea aligned upon these targets for a sufficient period of time for the visual system to perform a comprehensive analysis of the image. Thus, we have the ability to both move the eyes from one target of interest to another and we also have the ability to suppress eye movements to irrelevant stimuli or locations and maintain foveal vision at a specific location

---

* Correspondence to: D.P. Munoz, Department of Physiology, Queen's University, Kingston, ON K7L 3N6, Canada. Tel.: +1-613-533-2111; Fax: +1-613-533-6840; E-mail: doug@eyeml.queenu.ca

as demanded by the task. Thus, saccades are used to redirect the fovea from one target of interest to another and a fixation mechanism is used to keep the fovea aligned on the target during subsequent image analysis. This alternating behavior of saccade–fixate is repeated several hundred thousand times a day and is critical for complex acts such as visual search, reading, or driving an automobile.

Overview of brain areas

Experiments in both humans and animals have contributed extensively to our understanding of the neural circuitry controlling visual fixation and saccade generation. Human experiments typically involve either studying patient groups with discrete lesions to a specific part of the brain that is involved in controlling some aspect of the behavior, or more recently, employing various functional imaging techniques to correlate changes in blood flow or oxygen metabolism in specific brain areas to aspects of the behavior. Additional techniques can be employed in animal experiments such as single cell recording, artificial activation via electrical microstimulation, reversible activation or deactivation of neurons with microinjection of transmitter substance, or irreversible lesions.

These different techniques have provided a wealth of data describing the role of various brain areas in the control of visual fixation and saccade generation. Fig. 1 highlights some of the areas that have been identified in non-human primates and analogous areas that have been identified in the human brain. Critical nodes in the network include regions of the parietal and frontal cortices, basal ganglia, thalamus, superior colliculus, cerebellum, and brainstem reticular formation (see Wurtz and Goldberg, 1989; Leigh and Zee, 1991; Moschovakis et al., 1996; Schall and Thompson, 1999; Hikosaka et al., 2000; Munoz et al., 2000; Scudder et al., 2002 for detailed review of aspects of the circuitry). Because these brain areas span almost the entire neuraxis, neurological immaturity, degeneration or malfunction may influence the ability of a subject to maintain visual fixation and generate accurate saccades. Indeed, many neurological and psychiatric disorders are accompanied by disturbances in eye movements and visual fixation, which have become important cues in the identification of the affected brain regions.

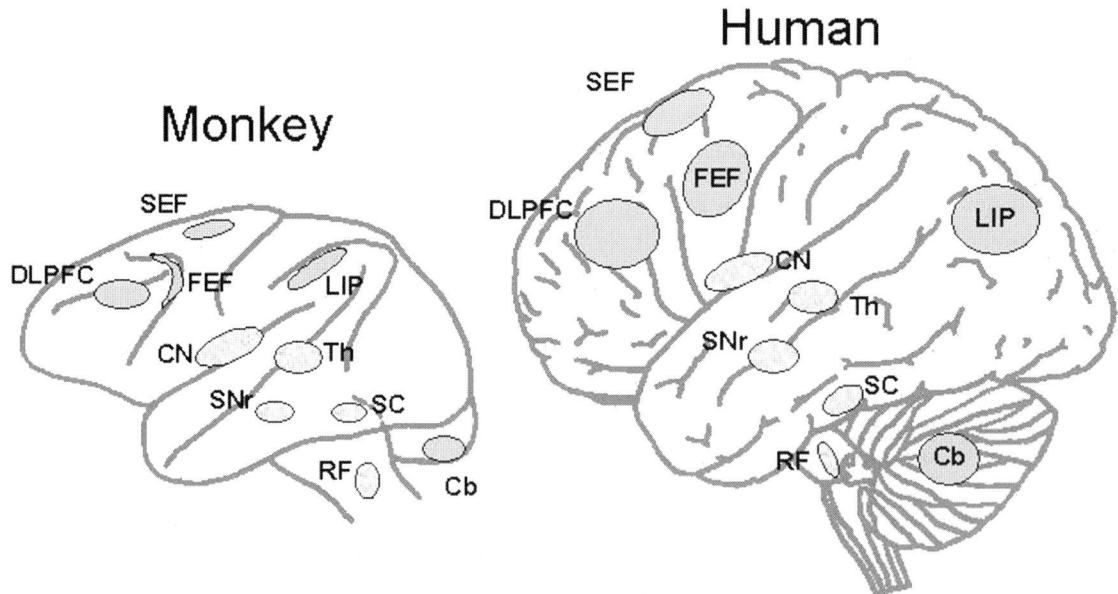

Fig. 1. Brain areas contributing to the control of saccadic eye movements in human and non-human primates. Abbreviations: Cb, cerebellum; CN, caudate nucleus; DLPFC, dorsolateral prefrontal; FEF, frontal eye field; LIP, lateral intraparietal area; RF, reticular formation; SC, superior colliculus; SEF, supplementary eye field; SNr, substantia nigra pars reticulata; Th, thalamus.

Brainstem saccadic burst generator

Many studies involving neuronal recording in awake animals and pathway tracing between areas have provided detailed information regarding the premotor circuitry for the control of saccadic eye movements (Fig. 2). Eye movements are controlled by the synergistic action of six extraocular muscles that are organized into three orthogonal pairs (lateral and medial rectus; inferior rectus and superior oblique; superior rectus and inferior oblique). The motoneurons (MN) that innervate the extraocular muscles are located in cranial nerve nuclei III, IV, and VI in the brainstem (for details see Leigh and Zee, 1991). The MN have a pulse–step discharge during saccadic eye movements. The MN discharge a burst of action potentials (the pulse) for saccades in the on-direction and have pause in their discharge for saccades in the off-direction. The frequency of this burst is correlated to eye velocity and the number of spikes in the burst scales with amplitude. In addition, there is a tonic component of the discharge of MN (the step) that is correlated to eye position and is present following a saccade to maintain the eye at an eccentric position in the orbit.

The reciprocal pattern of discharge (on-direction burst, off-direction pause) among the MN to create the saccade is generated by premotor neurons located in the mesencephalic, pontine and medullary regions of the reticular formation. The burst component of the MN discharge is generated by the saccadic burst generator circuit in the brainstem reticular formation (see Moschovakis et al., 1996; Scudder et al., 2002 for detailed review). Excitatory and inhibitory

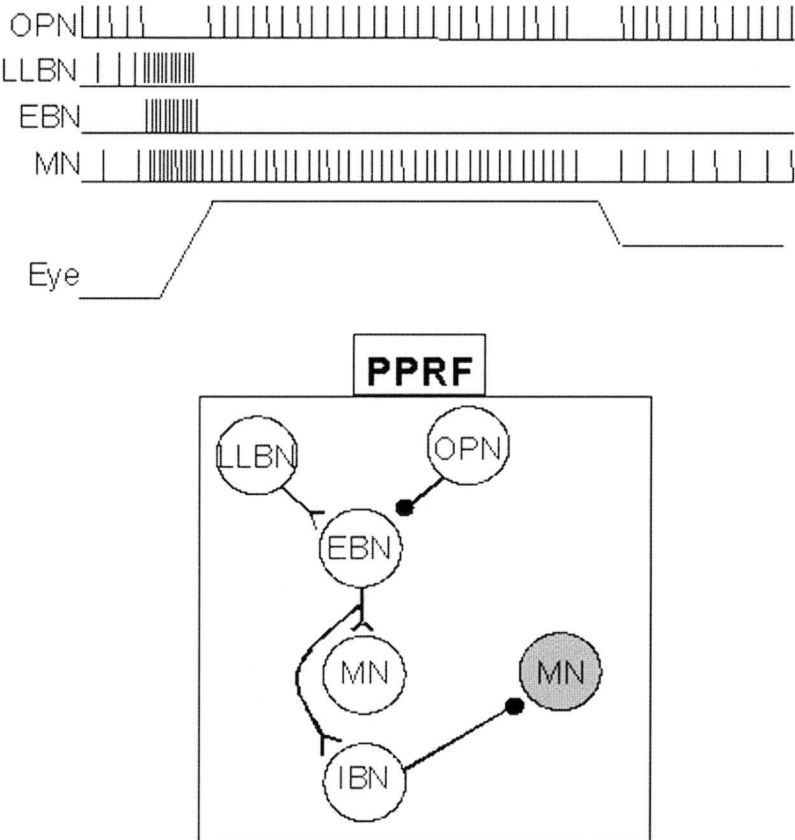

Fig. 2. Identification of elements in the brainstem premotor circuit controlling saccade generation. Agonist motoneuron is white and antagonist motoneuron is shaded gray. Abbreviations: EBN, excitatory burst neuron; IBN, inhibitory burst neuron; LLBN, long-lead burst neuron; MN, motoneuron; OPN, omnipause neuron.

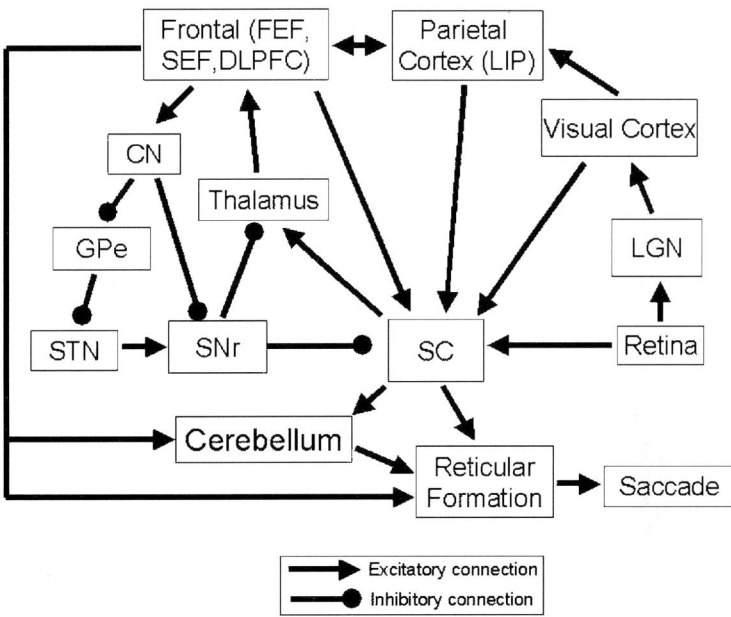

Fig. 3. Circuitry connecting brain areas involved in controlling saccadic eye movements. Abbreviations: CN, caudate nucleus; DLPFC, dorsolateral prefrontal; FEF, frontal eye field; GPe, globus pallidus external; LGN, lateral geniculate nucleus; LIP, lateral intraparietal area; SC, superior colliculus; SEF, supplementary eye field; SNr, substantia nigra pars reticulata; STN, subthalamic nucleus.

burst neurons (EBN and IBN) are silent during fixation and discharge bursts of action potentials for saccades in the on-direction. The EBN excite the on-direction MN monosynaptically and also excite the IBN, which in turn inhibit the antagonist MN. The EBN and IBN for horizontal saccades are located in the paramedian pontine reticular formation (PPRF); the EBN and IBN for vertical saccades are located in the rostral interstitial nucleus of the medial longitudinal fasciculus in the mesencephalon.

Other neurons in the PPRF are believed to control the discharge of EBN and IBN (see Moschovakis et al., 1996; Scudder et al., 2002 for review). Long-lead burst neurons (LLBN), also located in the brainstem reticular formation, discharge a high frequency burst for saccades into the contralateral hemifield. In addition to the burst, these cells also have a low frequency buildup of activity before the burst. It is believed that LLBN project to the EBN and IBN to provide the burst input. The EBN and IBN for horizontal and vertical systems are subject to potent inhibition from omnipause neurons (OPN), also located in the PPRF, which discharge tonically during all fixations and pause for saccades in all directions. Thus,

in order to generate a saccade, OPN must be silenced and the LLBN then activate the appropriate pools of EBN and IBN to produce the saccade command that is sent to the MN. Following completion of the saccade, OPN are reactivated to inhibit the EBN and IBN. The tonic activity of OPN ensures that any early, presaccadic activity among other premotor elements cannot lead to spurious activity among EBN and IBN, which would disrupt fixation.

It has been hypothesized that the step response that is carried by the MN is produced by integration of the pulse (Robinson, 1975). This eye position signal arises from different populations of brainstem neurons (see Scudder et al., 2002 for detailed review). A major source of the horizontal eye position signal to the MN is provided by neurons in the nucleus prepositus hypoglossi, located caudal to abducens nucleus. Neurons in the interstitial nucleus of Cajal in the mesencephalon produce the tonic, step response for the vertical saccadic system. Many neurons in these nuclei have combined burst–tonic discharges: they burst for on-direction saccades and produce tonic discharges that are correlated to eye position. Neural integration of the burst is believed to be achieved via a distributed network that includes these nuclei and elements in the vestibular nuclei.

Inputs to the brainstem premotor circuitry arise from several structures including the frontal cortex, superior colliculus and cerebellum (Fig. 3). Although our understanding of how these inputs are coordinated to control the actions of the burst generator circuit are incomplete, significant progress has been made in recent years (see Scudder et al., 2002 for detailed review).

Superior colliculus inputs to the saccadic burst generator

The superior colliculus (SC) plays a critical role in the control of visual fixation and saccadic eye movements. The superficial layers of the SC contain neurons that receive direct retinal inputs as well as inputs from other visual areas (Robinson and McClurkin, 1989). These visual neurons are organized into a visual map of the contralateral visual hemifield.

The intermediate layers of the SC contain neurons whose discharges are modulated by saccadic eye movements and visual fixation (see Munoz et al., 2000; Scudder et al., 2002 for review). These neurons are organized into a retinotopically coded motor map specifying saccades into the contralateral visual field. Neurons that increase their discharge before and during saccades, referred to as saccadic neurons, are distributed throughout the intermediate layers of the SC. Neurons that are tonically active during visual fixation and pause during saccades, referred to as fixation neurons, are located in the rostrolateral pole of the SC where the fovea is represented. These saccadic and fixation neurons in the SC project to the premotor circuitry in the brainstem reticular formation to influence behavior.

Munoz and Fecteau (2002, this volume) describe characteristics of a dynamic interactions model in which signals related to visual fixation and saccadic initiation interact across the motor map within the superior colliculus. Local interconnections are used as the substrate for motor programs to compete. The outputs from these interactions are then passed to the brainstem premotor circuitry to help guide behavior. Thus, the superior colliculus provides signals to the brainstem premotor circuitry that specify where and when a saccade will occur.

The superior colliculus is a site of multisensory convergence. That is, visual, auditory, and somatosensory information converges onto single neurons in the intermediate layers where it is integrated to guide behavior (see Stein and Meredith, 1993 for review). Such integration is critical for dealing with real world situations in which targets or objects of interest to the saccadic system may not be only visual. This multisensory convergence however leads to a fundamental problem because each of the sensory systems (visual, auditory, and somatosensory) uses very different coordinate systems. Visual inputs are coded retinotopically, auditory inputs are coded craniotopically, and tactile inputs are coded somatotopically. Despite the very different coding systems on the sensory side, the same motor system is used to localize a target. Zambarbieri (2002, this volume) addresses this issue. She provides a review of auditory saccade characteristics that provide novel insight into the behavior of saccadic mechanisms.

Cerebellar inputs to the saccadic burst generator

There are also important inputs to the brainstem saccadic burst generator that arise from the cerebellum (see Scudder et al., 2002 for review). The superior colliculus and oculomotor areas in the frontal cortex project to the nucleus reticularis tegmenti pontis and other pontine nuclei. Neurons in these nuclei then project to the cerebellar vermis. Neurons in the oculomotor vermis discharge in relation to saccades and microstimulation in this region of the cerebellum can elicit saccades. Purkinje cells in the oculomotor vermis project to the caudal fastigial nucleus. Neurons in the oculomotor region of the caudal fastigial nucleus then project back to the brainstem burst generator circuit to terminate directly on the EBN and IBN. It has been hypothesized that these cerebellar inputs to the premotor circuitry are critical for maintaining saccadic accuracy.

Early models of the saccadic generating system focused only upon the neural elements in the PPRF (Robinson, 1975; Scudder, 1988). In these models, the superior colliculus was believed to provide the input to the burst generator circuit. However, more recently, models have included the superior colliculus, cerebellum, and elements within the PPRF (e.g., Quaia et al., 1999). Enderle (2002, this volume) describes in considerable detail aspects of a new model of saccade generation that includes inputs to the burst generator from the superior colliculus and cerebellum. In this model, saccades are initiated by inputs to the burst generator circuitry from the superior colliculus and the saccades are then terminated by inputs from the caudal fastigial nucleus. In addition, he provides a novel mechanism for the control of the EBN which provides a large component of the excitatory drive to the MN during saccade execution. Specifically, Enderle uses a Hodgkin–Huxley model of an EBN and proposes that EBN are driven at least initially by a post-inhibitory rebound. In other words, he proposes that when EBN are released from the OPN inhibition, they will discharge at a high frequency automatically without stimulation.

Higher centers involved in presaccadic processing

Inputs to the superior colliculus, cerebellum, and brainstem reticular formation from posterior parietal and frontal cortices and basal ganglia (see Fig. 3) play a critical role in selection of potential saccadic targets to ultimately influence behavior. Visual inputs that are important for maintaining visual fixation or generating saccades are sent initially via the retina and lateral geniculate nucleus to the visual cortex. Projections via the dorsal stream of extrastriate cortex proceed to regions of posterior parietal cortex involved in sensory–motor transformations and attentional processing (see Andersen et al., 1997; Colby and Goldberg, 1999; Glimcher, 2001 for detailed review). One area in particular that lies at the sensory–motor interface and may play an important role in decision making is the lateral intraparietal area (LIP). Visual inputs important for fixation and saccade control can be directed from visual cortex and LIP directly to the superior colliculus to influence premotor processing and ultimately influence behavior.

Frontal cortical oculomotor areas include the frontal eye fields (FEF), the supplementary eye fields (SEF), and the dorsolateral prefrontal cortex (DLPFC). Area LIP projects directly to the FEF and SEF (see Schall, 1997; Schall and Thompson, 1999 for review). The FEF, SEF, and DLPFC all project to the superior colliculus, the cerebellum, and brainstem reticular formation. In addition, these frontal oculomotor areas are also interconnected. Tinsley and Everling (2002, this volume) describe a role for neurons in the DLPFC in fixation control. In their chapter, they demonstrate that many neurons in DLPFC have discharges that are modulated by the gap period of a gap saccade task. Such modulations are similar to those described previously in the FEF and superior colliculus.

There are several pathways from the frontal cortex through the basal ganglia (see Fig. 3) that participate in presaccadic processing (for detailed review see Hikosaka et al., 2000). These pathways through the basal ganglia allow for the integration of motivation and reward information with saccade planning. There is a *direct pathway* in which the frontal areas project to the caudate nucleus to excite GABAergic neurons which in turn project directly to the substantia nigra pars reticulata. The neurons in the substantia nigra pars reticulata form the major output of the basal ganglia. They are GABAergic and they project to the intermediate layers of the superior colliculus and the thalamus. The thalamus then projects back to frontal and parietal cortices. Via this direct pathway through the basal ganglia, activation of cortical inputs will lead to disinhibition of the superior colliculus and thalamus because the signals pass through two inhibitory synapses.

There is also an *indirect pathway* through the basal ganglia in which a separate set of GABAergic neurons in the caudate nucleus project to the external segment of the globus pallidus. Neurons in external segment of the globus pallidus are GABAergic and project to the subthalamic nucleus. Neurons in the subthalamic nucleus then send excitatory projections to the substantia nigra pars reticulata, which in turn projects to the superior colliculus and thalamus. Thus, the indirect pathway travels through three inhibitory synapses and activation of cortical input will serve to inhibit the superior colliculus and thalamus.

Reflexive versus voluntary saccade control

Saccades can be generated reflexively, to stimuli that appear suddenly in the periphery, or voluntarily, in the absence of any overt sensory stimuli. In addition, the brain has evolved mechanisms to suppress unwanted or reflexive saccades during periods of visual fixation. There are many cortical areas that participate in the control of saccadic eye movements (Fig. 3). Evidence suggests that different classes of saccades are mediated by different cortical areas (Pierrot-Deseilligny et al., 1991; Gaymard et al., 1998). Pathways from visual and posterior parietal cortices may provide the dominant input to the superior colliculus for the execution of visually triggered saccades. Lesions of posterior parietal cortex increase reaction time of visually guided saccades (Heide and Kompf, 1998).

Regions of frontal cortex that project directly, and indirectly via the basal ganglia, to the superior colliculus play a more critical role in suppressing reflexive saccades and generating voluntary saccades. Lesions of the frontal eye fields (FEF) have only a modest effect on visually guided saccades, but they produce significant impairment in the generation of voluntary or memory-guided saccades (Gaymard et al., 1998, 1999). These movements have increased reaction times and reduced saccadic velocities. Lesions of the DLPFC reduce the ability of subjects to suppress reflexive pro-saccades in the anti-saccade task (Guitton et al., 1985; Pierrot-Deseilligny et al., 1991). Thus, a critical function of the DLPFC may be the voluntary suppression of unwanted or reflexive saccades.

Indeed saccadic inhibition is a very important concept and the neural mechanisms of this phenomenon are only beginning to be understood. In addition to voluntary saccadic suppression, evidence is emerging that there may be a bottom-up mechanism for saccadic suppression in which sudden changes in the visual environment may transiently inhibit the generation of saccadic eye movements. Stampe and Reingold (2002, this volume) describe such mechanisms in their chapter. They show that when subjects perform a visual search task, a sudden change in the visual display will produce a sharp reduction in saccadic frequency within 70 ms. They speculate that such a mechanism may be important to suppress saccades when new visual information is available that may be important to guide behavior.

Conclusions

Fixation and saccadic signals are distributed across a network of brain areas that extends from the parietal and frontal cortices, through the basal ganglia and thalamus, to the superior colliculus, cerebellum, and brainstem reticular formation. Evidence is accumulating to show that these competing signals may interact at multiple levels of the neuraxis. Thus, it is likely that specific functions are not localized to only one brain area. Rather, they may be distributed across multiple areas. The chapters in this section provide compelling evidence for the distributed nature of the neural mechanisms that control saccadic eye movements.

References

Andersen, R.A., Snyder, L.H., Bradley, D.C. and Xing, J. (1997) Multimodal representation of space in the posterior parietal cortex and its use in planning movements. *Annu. Rev. Neurosci.*, 20: 303–330.

Colby, C.L. and Goldberg, M.E. (1999) Space and attention in parietal cortex. *Annu. Rev. Neurosci.*, 22: 319–349.

Dow, B.M., Snyder, A.Z., Vautin, R.G. and Bauer, R. (1981) Magnification factor and receptive field size in foveal striate cortex of the monkey. *Exp. Brain Res.*, 44: 213–228.

Enderle, J.D. (2002) Neural control of saccades. In: J. Hyönä, D.P. Munoz, W. Heide and R. Radach (Eds.), *The Brain's Eye: Neurobiological and Clinical Aspects of Oculomotor Research*. Progress in Brain Research, Vol. 140, Elsevier, Amsterdam, pp. 21–49.

Gaymard, B., Ploner, C.J., Rivaud, S., Vermersch, A.I. and Pierrot-Deseilligny, C. (1998) Cortical control of saccades. *Exp. Brain Res.*, 123: 159–163.

Gaymard, B., Ploner, C.J., Rivaud-Pechoux, S. and Pierrot-Deseilligny, C. (1999) The frontal eye field is involved in spatial short-term memory but not in reflexive saccade inhibition. *Exp. Brain Res.*, 129: 288–301.

Glimcher, P.W. (2001) Making choices: the neurophysiology of visual–saccadic decision making. *Trends Neurosci.*, 24: 654–659.

Guitton, D., Buchtel, H.A. and Douglas, R.M. (1985) Frontal lobe lesions in man cause difficulties in suppressing reflexive glances and in generating goal-directed saccades. *Exp. Brain Res.*, 58: 455–472.

Heide, W. and Kompf, D. (1998) Combined deficits of saccades and visuo-spatial orientation after cortical lesions. *Exp. Brain Res.*, 123: 164–171.

Hikosaka, O., Takikawa, Y. and Kawagoe, R. (2000) Role of the basal ganglia in the control of purposive saccadic eye movements. *Physiol. Rev.*, 80: 953–978.

Leigh, R.J. and Zee, D.S. (1991) *The Neurology of Eye Movements*. F.A. Davis, Philadelphia, PA.

Moschovakis, A.K., Scudder, C.A. and Highstein, S.M. (1996) The microscopic anatomy and physiology of the mammalian saccadic system. *Prog. Neurobiol.*, 50: 133–254.

Munoz, D.P. and Fecteau, J.H. (2002) Vying for dominance: Dynamic interactions control visual fixation and saccadic initiation in the superior colliculus. In: J. Hyönä, D.P. Munoz, W. Heide and R. Radach (Eds.), *The Brain's Eye: Neurobiological and Clinical Aspects of Oculomotor Research*. Progress in Brain Research, Vol. 140, Elsevier, Amsterdam, pp. 3–20.

Munoz, D.P., Dorris, M.C., Pare, M. and Everling, S. (2000) On your mark, get set: brainstem circuitry underlying saccadic initiation. *Can. J. Physiol. Pharmacol.*, 78: 934–944.

Perry, V.H. and Cowey, A. (1985) The ganglion cell and cone distributions in the monkey's retina: implications for central magnification factors. *Vis. Res.*, 25: 1795–1810.

Pierrot-Deseilligny, C., Rivaud, S., Gaymard, B. and Agid, Y. (1991) Cortical control of reflexive visually guided saccades. *Brain*, 114: 1473–1485.

Quaia, C., Lefevre, P. and Optican, L.M. (1999) Model of the control of saccades by superior colliculus and cerebellum. *J. Neurophysiol.*, 82: 999–1018.

Robinson, D.A. (1975) Oculomotor control signals. In: G. Lennerstrand and P. Bach-y-Rita (Eds.), *Basic Mechanisms of Ocular Motility and Their Clinical Implications*. Pergamon Press, Oxford, pp. 337–374.

Robinson, D.L. and McClurkin, J.W. (1989) The visual superior colliculus and pulvinar. In: R.H. Wurtz and M.E. Goldberg (Eds.), *The Neurobiology of Saccadic Eye Movements*. Elsevier, Amsterdam, pp. 337–360.

Schall, J.D. (1997) Visuomotor areas of the frontal lobe. In: K.S. Rockland (Ed.), *Cerebral Cortex*. Plenum Press, New York, pp. 527–638.

Schall, J.D. and Thompson, K.G. (1999) Neural selection and control of visually guided eye movements. *Annu. Rev. Neurosci.*, 22: 241–259.

Scudder, C.A. (1988) A new local feedback model of the saccadic burst generator. *J. Neurophysiol.*, 59: 1455–1475.

Scudder, C.A., Kaneko, C.R.S. and Fuchs, A.F. (2002) The brainstem burst generator for saccadic eye movements. *Exp. Brain Res.*, 142: 439–462.

Stampe, D.M. and Reingold, E.M. (2002) Influence of stimulus characteristics on the latency of saccadic inhibition. In: J. Hyönä, D.P. Munoz, W. Heide and R. Radach (Eds.), *The Brain's Eye: Neurobiological and Clinical Aspects of Oculomotor Research*. Progress in Brain Research, Vol. 140, Elsevier, Amsterdam, pp. 73–87.

Stein, B.E. and Meredith, M.A. (1993) *The merging of the senses*. MIT, Cambridge, MA.

Tinsley, C.J. and Everling, S. (2002) Contribution of the primate prefrontal cortex to the gap effect. In: J. Hyönä, D.P. Munoz, W. Heide and R. Radach (Eds.), *The Brain's Eye: Neurobiological and Clinical Aspects of Oculomotor Research*. Progress in Brain Research, Vol. 140, Elsevier, Amsterdam, pp. 61–72.

Van Essen, D.C., Newsome, W.T. and Maunsell, J.H. (1984) The visual field representation in striate cortex of the macaque monkey: asymmetries, anisotropies, and individual variability. *Vision Res.*, 24(5): 429–448.

Wurtz, R.H. and Goldberg, M.E. (Eds.) (1989) *The Neurobiology of Saccadic Eye Movements*. Elsevier, Amsterdam.

Zambarbieri, D. (2002) The latency of saccades toward auditory targets in humans. In: J. Hyönä, D.P. Munoz, W. Heide and R. Radach (Eds.), *The Brain's Eye: Neurobiological and Clinical Aspects of Oculomotor Research*. Progress in Brain Research, Vol. 140, Elsevier, Amsterdam, pp. 51–59.

SECTION II

Change blindness and transsaccadic integration

Section Editor: J. Hyönä

CHAPTER 7

Converging evidence for the detection of change without awareness

Ian M. Thornton [1,*] and Diego Fernandez-Duque [2]

[1] Max Planck Institute for Biological Cybernetics, Spemannstrasse 38, 72076 Tübingen, Germany
[2] Cognitive Neurology Unit, A421, Sunnybrook and Women's College Health Science Centre, University of Toronto, Toronto, ON M4N 3M5, Canada

Abstract: In this chapter, we explore the possibility that changes can be registered by the visual system and can influence behavior even in the absence of conscious awareness. We begin by describing the basic phenomenon of *change blindness*, introduce a framework for discussing some of the key issues relating to change detection as a whole, and then examine the main lines of evidence that point to the existence of *implicit change detection*.

Change detection

Change detection has very quickly become one of the most powerful and flexible experimental tools available to the vision researcher. While the long-term significance of this paradigm will almost certainly rest with the emphasis it places on the temporal aspects of vision — change is, after all, something that has to take place over time — its immediate appeal and success lies mainly with the striking phenomenology associated with one specific task, the flicker paradigm (Rensink et al., 1997).

In the flicker paradigm, which is illustrated in Fig. 1, two views of a complex scene are separated by a blank masking field and are alternated in the sequence: scene 1, blank, scene 2, blank, scene 1, blank, scene 2, and so on. The two scenes are identical, except for the presence of one changing item or scene location. Once the changing item has been detected it is clearly visible and often appears very 'obvious'. What is so compelling about this phenomenon is the extreme difficulty most observers usually have in locating the change, often taking many seconds of intense search, and sometimes failing to locate the change at all! (Rensink et al., 1997; Simons and Levin, 1997; Rensink, 2002a).

A crucial factor in making the change hard to detect appears to be the masking field. In addition to the blank field described above, other types of distracting events can be used, including blinks (e.g., O'Regan et al., 2000), saccades (e.g., Bridgeman et al., 1975; Grimes, 1996), movie cuts (Levin and Simons, 1997) and multiple small masking elements called 'mud splashes' (O'Regan et al., 1999). Subsequent work has also shown that the detection of change can also be difficult during virtual reality simulations (e.g., Wallis and Bülthoff, 2000), dynamic animation sequences (e.g., Scholl and Pylyshyn, 1999), side-by-side comparisons of images (the old 'spot the difference' game, Shore and Klein, 2000) and even real-world, face to face, interactions (Simons and Levin, 1998).

---

* Correspondence to: I.M. Thornton, Max Planck Institute for Biological Cybernetics, Spemannstrasse 38, 72076 Tübingen, Germany.
E-mail: ian.thornton@tuebingen.mpg.de

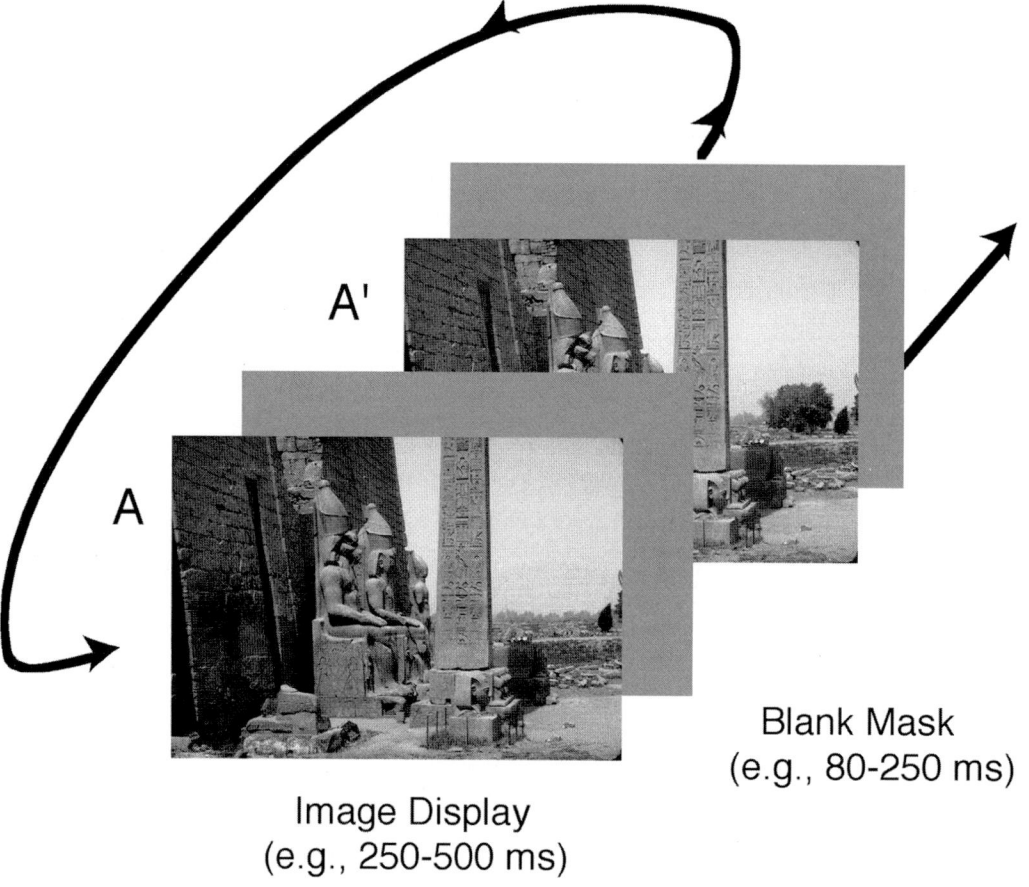

Fig. 1. An example of a flicker paradigm display (Rensink et al., 1997). Two views of a complex scene (A and A′) are separated by a blank masking field and are alternated in the sequence scene 1, mask, scene 2, mask, scene 1, mask, scene 2, and so on. These two scenes differ from one another only with respect to a single changing item or scene location. In this example, taken from the Cambridge Basic Research database, a large tree suddenly appears on the right of the screen in the second image.

Change blindness

In all of the above studies, the observer is asked to report the occurrence of a change. *Change blindness*, then, is operationally defined as a failure to become *explicitly aware* that a change is or was taking place. The main theme of this chapter is that such explicit reports of awareness underestimate the true impact of change. For now, however, we can ask 'why might an observer fail to report a change?'

Fig. 2 provides the framework within which we will explore this question, and other issues relating to change detection, during the current chapter. In later sections we provide a more detailed discussion, but here we note a few keys points:

- the separation of the visual registration of change, from the behavioral consequences of change;
- the creation of parallel attentional and non-attentional processing streams;
- the suggestion that awareness is only one of many behavioral consequences that might follow the registration of change.

A clear assumption in Fig. 2 is that both implicit and explicit detection of change are logically possible via either processing stream. As discussed in more detail below, this reflects a belief that spatiotemporally coherent representations — prerequisites for any form of change detection — can be constructed and maintained both with and without the involvement of attention during the registration

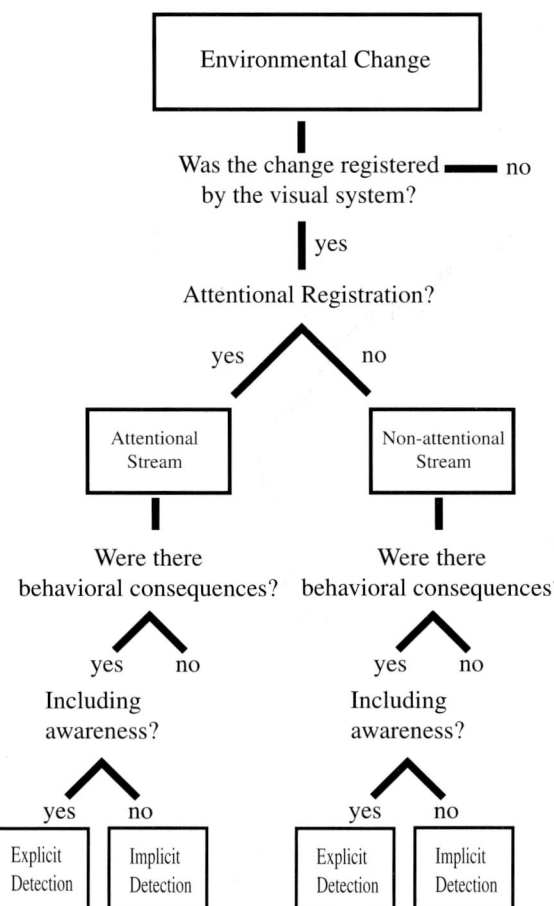

Fig. 2. A framework for exploring change detection. This simplified view of the stages involved in the explicit and implicit detection of change reflects the organization of the sections in the current chapter. Key points include: the separation of the visual registration of change, from the behavioral consequences of change; the creation of parallel attentional and non-attentional processing streams; the separation of the role attention may play in the formation of spatiotemporally coherent representations from its role in the modulation of awareness; the suggestion that awareness is only one of many behavioral consequences that might follow the registration of change. See text for more details.

of change. Furthermore, awareness is not seen as an unavoidable consequence of this registration process in either stream. That is, in the current framework, awareness is assumed to be an attribute which can be 'set' for any representation independent of the method of registration.

Note, that we are not suggesting that the probability of explicit or implicit detection would be equal across these two streams. For example, explicit detection may be much more likely for changes registered in the attentional stream because attention also plays an important part in modulating access to awareness. However, one of the main motivations for proposing this framework is the belief that these two processes — the *formation* of spatiotemporally coherent representations (i.e., registration) and the *modulation* of awareness — may in some sense be separable. We return to this issue later in the chapter.

In any event, the crucial qualitative difference between representations in this framework concerns their manner of registration — with or without attention — not the presence or absence of awareness.

Registration of a change

For an observer to be able to respond to a change in the environment, the visual system must register that change in some way. That is, the visual system must undergo an internal transformation reflecting the change in the environment. The result of such a transformational process is usually conceptualized as some form of *spatiotemporally coherent* mental representation. This concept captures the notion that the individual features or dimensions of a display must be bound together spatially, but also, for the registration of change, they must be connected or linked across time.

The visual system may fail to register a change for a number of reasons. The most obvious one would be a lack of encoding of the pre-change scene. This includes the trivial case in which sensory receptors are not available (e.g., closed eyes, adapted or fatigued receptors, etc.), to theoretically more interesting cases in which failure to encode the pre-change scene may stem from a lack of foveation or attention (e.g., Hollingworth and Henderson, 2002). Even if the pre-change scene is encoded, registration could fail if the blank mask or the changed image were to simply substitute the original image, erasing it from a visual buffer, with no links being maintained across time. These are cases in which the change leaves no trace in the nervous system, so that the observer is truly blind to the change.

Of more interest in the current context are those changes that are registered by the visual system. As can be seen in Fig. 2, we draw an early and important distinction between those changes that may be registered via attentional mechanisms and those registered via non-attentional mechanisms. This distinction reflects a general belief that vision involves multiple processing systems that work together to support our successful interactions with the world. While it seems likely that many forms of processing occur without the direct involvement of attention, there is less agreement as to whether spatiotemporally coherent representations, needed for the registration of change, can exist in the absence of attention.

The dichotomy proposed here is clearly not intended to capture the full complexity of visual processing and visual attention. For example, within the attentional stream we have not distinguished between processing that might involve focused attention from that which involves distributed attention. Likewise, in the non-attentional stream, many candidate systems — each with their own specific form of representation — might operate in parallel, processing aspects of the scene such as its layout, its gist, or the actions it affords.

Attention

Focused attention is considered a key mechanism in establishing representations that are coherent across both space and time (Kahneman et al., 1992; Enns and Di Lollo, 1997; Rensink, 2000a, 2002a). Attention not only binds the individual features of objects or scenes together, but also ensures that identity is maintained across time. Indeed, it has been argued that without attention coherent representations cannot exist. That is, a number of researchers have suggested a general lack of object structure in the absence of attention (e.g., Treisman and Gelade, 1980). Furthermore, because of this, it has been suggested that our subjective impression of a detailed, stable representation of the physical world is little more than a 'Grand Illusion' (O'Regan, 1992). According to this view, we fail to notice that most of our visual world lacks detail and coherence because as soon as we 'look' at a new region of space, we bring that region into the focus of attention (Rensink, 2000b). Studies of change blindness have provided support for such claims (see Noë et al., 2000 for a further discussion).

There is little doubt that attention is crucially involved in the explicit detection of change and theories of change blindness have relied heavily upon it. For example, the 'coherence theory' proposed by Rensink (2000a, 2002a) gives a central role to attention in its account of many empirical observations from the visual search and change blindness literature. The central role of attention in the explicit detection of change is also supported by a wealth of empirical evidence. For example, detection is greatly enhanced when attention is directed to the location of change, either by motion transients, object saliency (Rensink et al., 1997; Shore and Klein, 2000), semantic cues (Rensink et al., 1997), or exogenous cues (Scholl, 2000).

However, one concern with using the above findings to draw general conclusions about the nature of change registration stems from their almost complete reliance on explicit reports of awareness. Such a reliance is problematic for at least two reasons. (1) Awareness — or more precisely explicit report based on awareness — is only one of a whole range of behavioral consequences that could be used to measure the existence and impact of spatiotemporally coherent representations. As we will discuss below, there is increasing reason to believe that at least some of these alternative measures are more sensitive and/or more reliable indicators of change registration than subjective reports. (2) Drawing conclusions about the nature of representations based solely on subjective reports assumes a one-to-one relation between awareness and attention. In the next section, we suggest that this might not be the case.

Awareness

Given the central role that attention occupies in current theories of change blindness, it is important to highlight two possible contributions of attention to change detection. First, as we just noted, attention can be important in establishing and sustaining the representation of change. Second, attention can influence the conscious detection of change (i.e., help the represented change reach visual awareness). Attention almost certainly plays a major role in determining the contents of conscious awareness. Indeed, attention and awareness are so closely linked that they are sometimes used interchangeably. They are not, however, synonymous. Attention has a functional role, modulating information processing. Awareness is perhaps best thought of as an attribute of the represented stimulus (Fernandez-Duque and Johnson, 1999). Attention may help to set this attribute — and indeed attention may prove to be a necessary ingredient — but other factors may also play a role.

These two roles of attention — establishing representations and modulating awareness — frequently coincide. For this reason, they are often confounded. But does one necessarily entail the other? It remains a possibility that representations built or 'bound' by attention will fail to become consciously detected. Similarly, a representation of change may be constructed without attention, only to be affected by attention at a later time.

Recent studies suggest some support for these ideas, as changes to attended objects are sometimes missed. For example, the majority of observers fail to notice when the only actor in a short movie clip is replaced during a camera cut (Levin and Simons, 1997) or when the only partner in a conversation is replaced during a brief interruption (Simons and Levin, 1998; Levin et al., 2002). Similarly, changes made to items that are being monitored in an attentive tracking task (Pylyshyn and Storm, 1988) often go completely unnoticed (Scholl and Pylyshyn, 1999), as do changes to items that are being directly fixated (O'Regan et al., 2000).

These examples lend credibility to the claim that attending to an object, and binding its features across time into a coherent representation, do not always lead to the conscious detection of change. An additional comparison may be needed for the change to reach awareness (e.g., Scott-Brown et al., 2000; Simons, 2000; Hollingworth, 2002). Alternatively, attention may be a graded phenomenon, with awareness of change and representation of change having different thresholds. Another possibility is that attending to an object does not automatically give rise to coherent representations of *all* feature dimensions. Rather, the allocation of attention — and the resulting coherent representations — may be restricted to those feature dimensions that are engaged by the current task or observer strategy. Thus, changes may fail to be consciously detected unless attention has been allocated to the particular dimension or feature that is being updated.

Empirical evidence has also been gathered which relates to the second claim, that changes initially registered without attention can subsequently be affected when attention is allocated to them. If the attentional modulation of awareness is in any way independent from the attentional registration of change, it may be possible to become aware of an unattended change by attending to it *after* it has occurred. To explore this possibility studies have used a cue to direct attention to the location of change after the change has been completed. This post-cueing method suggests that some changes can be reported when a representation of the change — or possibly of the pre-change target — are retrieved from memory by the subsequent allocation of attention (Hollingworth, 2002, but see Becker et al., 2000).

Behavioral consequences

The behavioral consequence that has typically been explored in studies of change detection is the *explicit* report of a change that has reached awareness. In the remainder of this chapter, we explore the possibility that other behavioral consequences can also provide useful markers of change. When these additional consequences occur in the absence of awareness, then *implicit* detection of change has occurred.

Considering awareness as simply one possible behavioral consequence, rather than as the *only* indicator of spatiotemporally coherent representations, is important for several reasons. First, it motivates the search for additional ways to measure the impact of change. For example, various other aspects of behavior might be affected by a registered change, such as the speed and accuracy of direct responses (e.g., the speed with which the presence/absence judgements are made), the speed and accuracy of indirect responses (how the presence of a change might influence performance on a secondary task), or the patterns of eye and hand movements. Second, weakening the theoretical link between awareness and the representation of change allows for the possibility that such implicit effects arise either with or without the involvement of attention during the registration of change (see Fig. 2).

However, it also becomes clear that additional, independent methods for establishing the involvement of attention during change registration become necessary. That is, if we reject the notion that spatiotemporally coherence per se is a hallmark of attention, and we advocate a weakening of the attention–awareness link, then how can we establish when attention is involved in representing change? Clearly, when exploring the role of attention in this context, additional indirect measures, such as behavioral signatures (e.g., spatial cueing effects), neural markers, and/or visuo-motor patterns (e.g., saccade targeting) should also be taken into account.

Implicit processing

The notion that changes may be detected without the involvement of conscious awareness receives credibility from similar findings in other domains. There is a rich literature showing that information can be represented in the brain and have an impact on behavior, without such processing leading to awareness. Classic studies of amnesic patients (Milner et al., 1968) first raised the possibility that memory representations could affect performance in the absence of explicit recall or recognition of stored information (see also, Jacoby et al., 1993; Schacter, 1995 for studies with normal observers). The sequence learning literature (see Clegg et al., 1998, for a review) also demonstrated that complex patterns of behavior could be adopted without explicit awareness (Curran and Keele, 1995; Destrebecqz and Cleeremans, 2001). Similar claims have come from studies of perception/action dissociations (Goodale, 1996).

There is also a growing body of work demonstrating that perceptual processing can often proceed outside of awareness (e.g., Marcel, 1983; Graves and Jones, 1992; Kolb and Braun, 1995; Luck et al., 1996; McCormick, 1997; Moore and Egeth, 1997; Bar and Biederman, 1998; Chen, 1998; Mack and Rock, 1998). In a classic study by Marcel (1983), two probes were presented following a masked word. Observers reported whether or not a word preceded the mask (detection task), which probe most closely resembled the masked word (graphic task), and which probe was semantically closest to the word (semantic task). Even when observers could not consciously detect the presence of the word, they could 'guess' at better than chance levels in the graphic and semantic tasks. These findings indicate that form and meaning can be processed without awareness. Furthermore, the presence of an unaware prime congruent with a target can facilitate responses during lexical decision (Marcel, 1983) and naming tasks (Carr et al., 1982), and these effects are sometimes as large as when subjects are fully aware of the prime (Fowler et al., 1981; Carr et al., 1982).

More recently, Dehaene et al. (2001) have used ERP and fMRI techniques to examine the neural processing that accompanies such implicit effects. They found that masked stimuli engaged a fairly high-level processing stream, including extrastriate cortex, left fusiform gyrus and the precentral sulcus, suggesting fairly sophisticated implicit processing. In a second experiment a repetition priming paradigm was used to show that these identified regions could be selectively adapted, indicating that the meaning of the word had been extracted without awareness.

Implicit perception is not restricted to word processing. Similar findings have also be reported with number processing (Dehaene et al., 1998) and object recognition. For instance, Bar and Biederman (1998) used a backwards masking procedure to present pictures of objects outside of observers' explicit awareness. Lack of awareness was established using an objective criterion of chance performance in a four-alternative forced-choice (4AFC) recognition task. In the test phase, 15 minutes later, priming was found when the exact same objects were presented (identity prime) and this effect was even larger when the objects were presented at the same location (location prime). Objects with the same name but different shape were not primed. This absence of implicit semantic priming in the presence of implicit identity priming may hint at differences in the type of content that can be implicitly represented. Alternatively, the absence of semantic priming in this study may be due to the fact that the semantic effects of unaware primes are usually short lived (Greenwald et al., 1996).

Finally, Chun and Nakayama (2000) have suggested that successful visual interactions with the world could not proceed unless implicit visual memory mechanisms were helping us to select and retain information across space and time. They discuss two such mechanisms, *priming of pop-out* (Maljkovic and Nakayama, 1994, 1996), and *contextual cueing* (Chun and Jiang, 1998). Priming of pop-out is thought to be a transient mechanism that uses implicit traces of previously attended features or locations to help guide attention and eye movements.

Contextual cueing refers to the fact that previously viewed distractor layouts can speed later target responses when the distractor arrays are repeated. This is true as long as the distractor layouts contain invariant configurations that are predictive of target location. Importantly, for both priming of pop-out and contextual cueing, control experiments have demonstrated that observers have no explicit access to the perceptual information that is guiding their behavior.

Behavioral evidence for implicit detection of change

In line with general claims for implicit perceptual effects, several recent studies have begun to examine whether *change* could also be registered in the absence of awareness. Recently, we have used simplified change blindness displays, such as those shown in Fig. 3, to explore both the implicit localization and identification of change (Fernandez-Duque and Thornton, 2000; Thornton and Fernandez-Duque, 2000).

Observers were shown arrays containing 8, 12, or 16 rectangles (half horizontal, half vertical). An array was displayed for 250 ms, after which the screen went blank for 250 ms, then the array reappeared with one of the items in a new orientation, having rotated about its center by 90°.

In one series of studies (Fernandez-Duque and Thornton, 2000), the second display of the array was followed (after a 250 ms delay) by a two-alternative forced-choice (2AFC) task in which two items were highlighted, the item that changed and a diametrically opposite distractor item. Observers were required to indicate which of the two items they thought had changed. If they were aware of the change, this would be an easy decision. If they had no awareness, they were instructed to guess. Following the localization response, observers indicated whether they had seen the item change. The interesting finding was that even in the absence of awareness, observers consistently performed above chance in this 2AFC localization task.

Interestingly, in control experiments we attempted to ascertain the contribution of attention to this implicit localization effect by pairing the same simplified flicker display to various forms of cueing paradigm. Instead of attempting to localize the change, observers simply responded to a target item which was placed either at the location of change or at the location of the diametrically opposite item. While standard cueing effects were found for changes that were explicitly detected, we found no evidence of attentional costs or benefits when observers were unaware of the change, leading us to conclude that a reorienting of the attentional focus was not involved in this form of implicit change detection.

In another series of studies (Thornton and Fernandez-Duque, 2000), we paired rectangle change displays with a speeded orientation discrimination task. The idea here was to explore congruency effects between the changed item and the subsequent probe item, as a function of awareness. Observers were presented with a ring of eight rectangles that appeared briefly, was replaced by a blank screen, and then reappeared. On change trials (66%), one of the items changed orientation between the first and second presentations, say from horizontal to vertical. This change constituted the 'prime phase' for the congruency task, where the salience of the final orientation, vertical, would be raised.

Following the change sequence one of the rectangles in the ring was highlighted and observers were instructed to make a speeded response based on this 'probe' item's orientation. We found that for trials in which observers were aware of the change, probes with an orientation incongruent to the changed item were reported more slowly and less accurately than congruent probes. When observers were unaware of the change, their speed of response was identical to the catch trials, suggesting that the change had not been registered. However, a robust congruency effect was still present in the error rates, suggesting that undetected change had primed the appropriate orientation and that this priming then influenced the response to subsequent probes.

Smilek et al. (2000) used a different approach to explore the impact of implicitly detected changes. They combined the flicker paradigm with a standard visual search task (see also Rensink, 2000b). Observers were asked to search through displays of digits to detect the one item that was changing identity across the blank interval. Individual digits were created by turning the elements of an 8-segment array on and off. Large and small changes were cre-

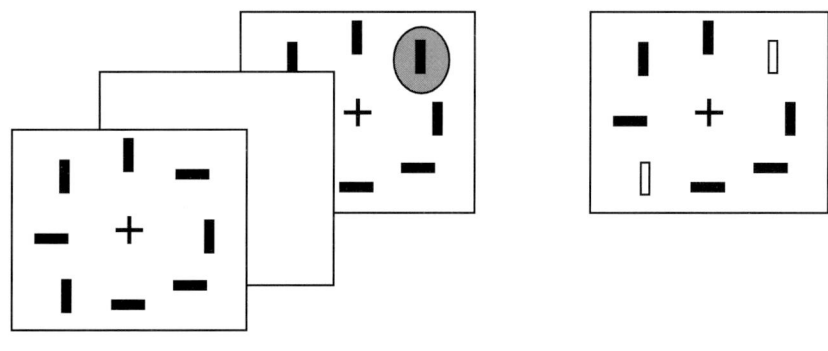

a) Implicit Localization Task

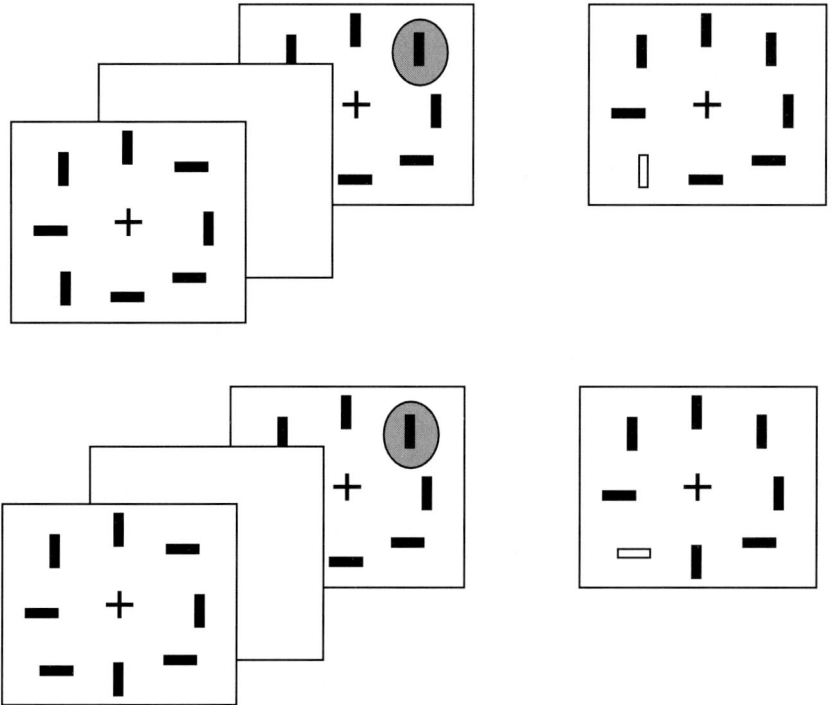

b) Implicit Identification Task

Fig. 3. The studies of the implicit localization and identification of change reported by Fernandez-Duque and Thornton (2000) and Thornton and Fernandez-Duque (2000) used simplified change detection paradigms coupled with a secondary task. In the initial portion of each trial, shown on the left, the two rectangle frames were identical except for a single object which changed orientation during the blank interstimulus interval (ISI). Change was equiprobable at any location and here involves the rectangle located between 12 and 3 o'clock. The gray oval is added here for illustrative purposes and was not present during experiments. (a) In localization studies, this initial portion of the trial was followed by a probe display in which two items, the changed rectangle and its diametrically opposite partner, were highlighted. Observers were asked to click on the item they thought had changed. (b) In identification studies, the change display was followed by the highlighting of a single probe item to which observers made a speeded orientation response. The critical trials, shown here, were when the probe item was opposite the change location and its orientation was either congruent with (top) or incongruent with (bottom) the final orientation of the changed item.

ated by varying the number of elements that were switched on or off during the blank. For example, a large change could be a 2 alternating with a 4 (a change involving 5 elements) and a small change could be a 2 alternating with an 8 (2 elements).

Smilek et al. (2000) measured the efficiency with which large and small changes were found by examining the target present search slopes. They found that the slopes for larger changes were consistently shallower. As the observers' expectations and the nature of the distractors were identical across both types of trial, they concluded that the as-yet-undetected changes were able to guide focal attention to their location. Thus, some form of non-attentional registration of change may have been guiding attention. The suggestion that attention can be implicitly guided to the location of the change contrasts with the results of Fernandez-Duque and Thornton (2000) in which evidence was found for implicit localization of change, but these effects did not appear to be mediated by a covert orienting toward the undetected change. One factor that may account for these different results is the duration of the mask, which was considerably longer in Fernandez-Duque and Thornton (2000) than in the studies by Smilek et al. (2000). In line with this suggestion, Smilek et al. (2002) replicated and extended their original findings, but also revealed that the effect was critically dependent on the duration of the blank. Specifically, when the duration of the blank period was increased from 80 ms to 300 ms, the effect disappeared.

Driver et al. (2001) report two studies from their group which also seem to provide evidence for the implicit processing of change. In one study (Turatto, Russell and Driver, unpubl. data) observers were presented with a simplified flicker display and were asked to report changes in luminance which could occur either within a set of target dots or within a set of background stripes. In some conditions, the well known simultaneous contrast illusion (see Palmer, 1999) was used to create a situation in which a large physical change to the background luminance — alternate stripes changed from light gray to dark gray or vice versa — caused a small illusory change in the luminance of one of the target dots. Observers consistently failed to report the large background change but did sometimes report the illusory change to the target dot. As the illusory dot change completely depended on the background change, this suggests that the unreported modulation of the background stripes was being processed at some level in the visual system.

In another study (Driver, Russell and Howlett, unpubl. data), observers were asked to judge whether two sequentially presented random square patterns were the same or different. In addition to the target patterns, each display also contained a background pattern of dots, which could be organized into regular columns/rows or could have a random organization. The crucial manipulation was that on some trials the organization of the background dots remained constant across the two presentations of the target pattern and on some trials it changed. While a surprise retrospective question, as used in studies of inattentional blindness (Mack et al., 1992; see below), indicated that observers could not explicitly report changes to the organization of the background, both the speed and accuracy of the central task were affected by that organization. Specifically, target-different responses were faster and more accurate when the background also changed and target-same responses were faster and more accurate when the background did not change.

Williams and Simons (2000) used response time measures to identify another example of implicit detection. On each trial of their study, observers were asked to detect feature changes to one of a family of novel complex objects called Fribbles (Williams, 1997). On each trial a single object was briefly shown, occluded and then redisplayed with 0, 1, 2, or 3 of its features modified. Even though only a single object was present on each trial, observers were generally quite poor at reporting changes, with performance generally increasing as a function of the number of changed features. Williams and Simons (2000) also noted, however, that the speed with which observers responded 'same' (i.e., that no change had occurred) varied depending on whether a physical change had taken place. That is, even when observers did not explicitly notice the change, it appeared to implicitly affect another aspect of their behavior, speed of response. Williams and Simons (2000) suggested that such implicit effects might arise simply because explicit reports are a less sensitive measure of change registration than other behavioral consequences.

Two other phenomena closely related to change blindness are worthy of mention in this section, as both have provided evidence for implicit effects involving a spatiotemporal component. In studies of inattentional blindness (Mack et al., 1992; Rock et al., 1992; Mack and Rock, 1998) observers are asked to perform an attentionally demanding primary task — for example, judging the length of two similar line segments — for an extended period of time. On a critical trial, a suprathreshold change is made to the background of the display. For example, random dot patterns may become grouped in some way (Mack et al., 1992), or completely new items, such as dot patterns (Moore and Egeth, 1997) or connecting contours (Chen, 1998) may be added. Even though the unexpected event completely changes the overall display, observers are very often unaware of it and appear to have no explicit access to the nature of the change.

Nevertheless, several studies have now shown that these undetected changes are registered by the visual system and can affect subsequent behavior. For example, Moore and Egeth (1997) introduced flanking patterns to the background of their displays which evoked either the Ponzo illusion or the Müller–Lyer illusion. Both of the these manipulations affected behavior on the primary task, line length judgement, even though the changes were rarely explicitly reported. Similarly, Chen (1998) had observers make size discrimination judgements and then introduced additional features on a critical trial. Very few observers were able to explicitly report the change to the display; however, response times on the primary task were significantly slower when the change was present.

The unexpected events introduced in these studies undoubtedly produce a transient change to the nature of an ongoing display, and thus the failure to report such events is a form of change blindness. As the traditional interpretation of inattentional blindness assumes that such failures arise due to a lack of attention, the implicit effects described by Moore and Egeth (1997) and Chen (1998) are perhaps best attributed to the non-attentional stream shown in Fig. 2. However, as also shown in Fig. 2, and as noted above, a lack of awareness may not always equal a lack of attention during the registration of a change. Further studies will be needed to more clearly determine the origin of these effects.

Another paradigm to show behavioral consequences of change other than explicit *visual* awareness is what Rensink (2002b) has termed 'mindsight'. This involves a standard flicker paradigm and two explicit responses. In addition to indicating when a change has been 'seen', observers were also asked to indicate when they can first 'sense' the presence of a change. Patterns of reaction times indicated that a subset of observers could reliably sense the presence of a change — where sensing can be thought of as conscious, non-visual awareness — several seconds before they were visually aware of the change. Rensink (2002b) suggests that sensing and seeing are qualitatively distinct processes, with only the latter relying directly on focused attention.

The need for converging evidence

As the previous section demonstrates, there are now several lines of independent behavioral evidence to support the notion that change can be represented outside of awareness. However, some studies have failed to show implicit representation of change. Those findings are important in the current context because they help define the necessary conditions for implicit representation of change.

For example, unpublished studies from our lab found no evidence of implicit localization when attention was focused away from the changing array on a demanding secondary task. Similarly, when observers have the opportunity to actively search, using their eyes to scan through a complex display with multiple flickers, no implicit localization effects were found (Mitroff and Simons, 2002). These findings could be reconciled under a proposal that some level of *distributed attention* is needed for implicit localization of change. This proposal makes the prediction that implicit localization of change should be evident when attention is distributed over the whole display but not when attention is being focused *away* from the change onto other display details. One way to explore this prediction, and more generally to resolve conflicting behavioral findings, would be to seek converging evidence from other methodologies (e.g., eye movement studies or neuroimaging).

Another motivation for moving beyond strictly behavioral paradigms relates to the generally agreed importance (and difficulty) of ruling out the contribution of explicit processes when making claims about potential implicit effects (Reingold and Merikle, 1990). Such concerns have given rise to a lively debate about the existence of implicit representation of change.

For example, in the study by Smilek et al. (2000) which was described in the previous section, large changes lead to shallower search slopes than smaller changes. This finding was originally interpreted as suggesting that attention was guided to the location of large changes more effectively than to the location of the small changes. More recently, this interpretation has been challenged on the grounds that slope differences may stem from increased difficulty in detecting small changes (Mitroff et al., 2002). According to this alternative interpretation, the size of change is not a factor in guiding attention. Instead, attention is allocated to every item with equal probability, but attended items with a small change are more likely to be missed than attended items with a large change. Such misses lead to disproportionately slow search times, and in this way disproportionately increase the duration of search for small changes.

This alternative proposal is compelling in that it explains the original findings by Smilek et al. (2000). However, it is challenged by follow-up studies showing that the advantage for large changes depends on the duration of the global mask (Smilek et al., 2002). More specifically, when the duration of the mask is increased from 80 ms to 300 ms, the bias toward large changes disappears. An account based on small changes being missed more often than large changes would need to pose different target detection mechanisms for short and long intervals. Indeed, some researchers have adopted this approach, arguing that longer durations favor object-based processing while short durations favor feature-based processing (Richards et al., 2001).

The findings of Smilek et al. (2000) also depend on spatial proximity. When the displays are presented side-by-side, increasing the spatial disparity, large changes do not benefit relative to small changes (Smilek et al., 2002). This finding again poses a challenge to interpretations based on the small changes being missed more often than large changes as it is not clear why such mechanisms would apply only to the flicker paradigm, and not to the side-by-side paradigm.

Mitroff et al. (2002) also raised concerns about the interpretation of the reaction time data of Williams and Simons (2000). Here 'same' responses on undetected change trials had been slower than 'same' responses on catch trials when no physical change had occurred. Rather than reflecting an independent implicit effect, Mitroff et al. suggest that slower response times could be an indication of lower confidence, which in turn reflects explicit detection. In line with this suggestion, in a control experiment which replicated the main finding of Williams and Simons (2000), a weak positive correlation ($r = 0.282$) was found between speed of response and confidence. Nevertheless, an explanation of speed differences based on reduced confidence in explicit reports rests on the further assumption that implicit detection of change has no influence on subjects' level of confidence. The resolution of this issue would require a clearer understanding of the relationship between awareness and confidence in the context of change.

Claims for the implicit localization (Fernandez-Duque and Thornton, 2000) and identification (Thornton and Fernandez-Duque, 2000) of change have also been questioned. Mitroff et al. (2002) have suggested that these reports of implicit processing can be explained by explicit mechanisms. Elsewhere, we discuss in detail why these specific criticisms do not appear to be justified (Fernandez-Duque and Thornton, 2002). However, such criticisms highlight the difficulty in providing irrefutable behavioral evidence for implicit processing of change. That is, although it is possible to define criteria for establishing indisputable implicit measures (e.g., Holender, 1986; Reingold and Merikle, 1990), and some researchers have adopted them in the context of change detection (Mitroff et al., 2002; Simons and Silverman, 2002), such criteria are often so strict that they place an undue burden of proof on the researcher given the realistic constraints of most experimental scenarios.

A more productive approach involves the realization that any single methodology is unlikely to provide irrefutable evidence. Instead, we should seek converging evidence from multiple methodologies, accepting that each individual approach has its strengths and weaknesses. In this way we may be able to develop criteria that are still conservative enough to minimize false discoveries while at the same time ensuring that genuinely new phenomena are not impossible to establish. In the remainder of this chapter, we review several existing lines of evidence that, when combined with behavioral findings, may provide us with useful, practical tools for exploring the implicit detection of change.

Evidence from eye movement studies

The use of eye movement patterns to study aspects of changing displays considerably pre-dates the current interest in change detection and change blindness (e.g., Bridgeman et al., 1975; McConkie and Zola, 1979). In particular, the question of information processing before, during and after saccadic eye movements has generated a great deal of research (see Verfaillie and De Graef, 2001 for an overview). It has been well-established that while the eye is making its frequent (e.g., 3–4 per second) short (e.g., 40 ms), rapid (up to 1000°/s) saccadic movements during natural viewing, no information uptake is possible (e.g., Matin, 1974). We thus acquire visual information about the world during pre- and post-saccadic fixations. What has been less clear is the extent to which information from pre- and post-saccadic information can be integrated. To help answer this question researchers began to study saccade-contingent changes.

Saccade-contingent changes are display alterations that are triggered by the detection of high-velocity eye movements. Much of the earlier work on saccade-contingent changes involved alterations to written texts during reading (e.g., McConkie and Zola, 1979; Pollatsek and Rayner, 1992), displacement detection in simple displays (e.g., Bridgeman et al., 1975; Li and Matin, 1990) or the integration of information in random visual patterns (e.g., Irwin et al., 1983). The general finding from this early work was that saccade-contingent changes were rarely noticed and thus it was concluded that little or no integration had taken place.

More recent investigations of transsaccadic object and scene memory have favored the use of natural scenes. These studies also find that transsaccadic changes are sometimes very hard to detect (e.g., Grimes, 1996; McConkie and Currie, 1996; Hollingworth and Henderson, 2002). However, there is less agreement on whether this necessarily implies a general lack of integration. Some researchers have claimed complete integration of pre- and post-saccadic views (e.g., McConkie and Rayner, 1976; Feldman, 1985) while others have argued for the complete absence of such transsaccadic integration (e.g., O'Regan, 1992). Most likely, the truth lies somewhere in between, with some information being maintained across views, but only if it is 'selected and coded' in some way (Verfaillie and De Graef, 2001). Selection appears to depend on a number of factors including the particular demands of the task (Ballard et al., 1998; Hayhoe et al., 1998; Land et al., 1999) and the nature of the stimulus (Pollatsek and Rayner, 2001; Gysen et al., 2002). Coding appears to involve some form of consolidation from sensory representations into more stable short-term (e.g., Irwin and Andrews, 1996) or long-term memory representations (e.g., Hollingworth and Henderson, 2002).

The techniques developed for studying transsaccadic changes are very useful in the context of implicit change detection as they provide a useful alternative to simply asking observers what they saw. More specifically, examination of fixation frequency, duration and overall patterning can be used to infer whether unreported changes nevertheless had some impact on the visual system.

Hollingworth et al. (2001a,b), for example, asked observers to examine line drawings of complex, naturalistic scenes for a later memory test. Observers were also told that changes might be introduced to the scenes as they were scanning them and that they should immediately report any detected changes by pressing a key. On critical trials, objects were replaced as the eyes moved away from them. When the eyes returned to a changed object after several seconds, fixation durations were consistently longer (749 ms) than when no change was made to the object (499 ms), even in the absence of explicit detection.

Similar implicit effects on fixation duration have been found in other studies (e.g., Hayhoe et al., 1998; Henderson and Hollingworth, 2002; Hollingworth and Henderson, 2002). The study of Hayhoe et al., is particularly interesting for at least two reasons. First, not only the fixation duration, but the frequency of saccades was affected by the undetected changes. Second, changes only occurred on a small number of trials (10%) and observers were engaged in a demanding primary task (block copying), factors that minimize the use of explicit strategies.

While the previous two studies reveal implicit processing of change within a short time interval, other eye movement studies have shown that changes can be implicitly detected even when an interval of several minutes is presented between the pre- and post-change scene (Ryan et al., 2000). In this experiment, subjects saw a series of complex scenes twice. When presented for the second time, each scene could be either an exact repetition or a modified version of the original scene. Normal subjects revealed increased viewing of the changed region, even when unaware of the change, a finding that provides convergent support for implicit representation of change, in this case over a longer period of time.

The studies reviewed in this section demonstrate that eye movement patterns can provide a more sensitive measure of change registration than verbal reports. Future studies will have to address whether these implicit effects originate in separate, non-attentional mechanisms, or depend on below-threshold attentional registration (see Fig. 2).

Evidence from motor control

There has been considerable debate in the literature as to whether perception and action share common representational mechanisms. Some researchers have proposed a clear separation of processing (e.g., Goodale, 1993; Milner and Goodale, 1995), while others have suggested that they share a 'common code' (e.g., Hommel et al., 2001). Of interest here, are claims that perception and action might sometimes be differentially affected by visual illusions and display manipulations. For example, Aglioti et al. (1995) and Brenner and Smeets (1996) suggested that grasping movements might be immune, respectively, to the Ebbinghaus (or Tichener) illusion and the Ponzo illusion, both of which lead to large perceptual distortions (but see Franz et al., 2000, 2001 for conflicting evidence). Abrams and Landgraf (1990) showed how distance estimates (thought to involve perceptual/cognitive planning) could be affected by an induced motion illusion while location estimates (more related to action) were not.

While the proposed dissociation between perception and action representations remains controversial, it may still prove useful to explore within the context of change detection. This is particularly true in the light of patient work suggesting accurate behavioral responses in the absence of conscious awareness, either to the presence of an object (e.g., blindsight, Weiskrantz, 1986; Cowey and Stoerig, 1991) or to the action typically associated with an object (e.g., some forms of agnosia, Goodale and Milner, 1992).

Of course, the eye movement studies reviewed above clearly relate to motor control. More directly, a number of researchers have suggested at least a temporal dissociation between manual responses to a change and conscious awareness of the change. For instance, when the size or location of a rod is changed as an observer attempts to grasp it, manual adjustments occur several hundred milliseconds before observers can indicate awareness of the change with a verbal report (Castiello et al., 1991; Castiello and Jeannerod, 1991). Importantly, control experiments showed that these effects did not arise due to inherent differences in speed between the two methods of responding (Castiello et al., 1991).

More directly, several studies have demonstrated motor sensitivity to change in the complete absence of explicit report. For example, Bridgeman et al. (1979) and Goodale et al. (1986) both showed that pointing movements towards a target were often corrected when the position of an object was changed during a saccade, even though observers were unaware of the change. More recently, Repp (2000) has used perceptual–motor synchronization tasks to demonstrate implicit detection of change. In these tasks observers were required to press a key in response to a sequence of auditory tones. Repp found that subliminal changes to the timing of the tone sequence, that is, variations "that were well below the explicit detection threshold", nevertheless "led to effective adjustments in the timing of the motor response" (Repp, 2000; see also Thaut et al., 1998; Koch, 1999; Repp, 2001).

Cognitive neuroscience

Since the 1980s there has been a steady increase in the number of brain imaging techniques that have become available for helping to explore the nature of mental processes. The field of Cognitive

Neuroscience (see Gazzaniga et al., 1998 for an introduction), evolved largely in response to these innovations and aims to bring together various disciplines, including neurology, psychology, physiology and imaging.

While there has been a great surge in the number of behavioral studies relating to change blindness over the last 5 years, there are still relatively few that have taken a cognitive neuroscience approach. In this section, we review those imaging studies and also discuss what might be learned from examining relevant patient populations. Imaging, in particular, has the potential to reveal measures of implicit change and to track the formation of 'registered' changes, even if they lack measurable behavioral consequences (see Fig. 2).

Functional magnetic resonance imaging (fMRI)

Functional magnetic resonance imaging (fMRI) is a technique that relies on monitoring patterns of blood flow associated with neural activity. As the magnetic properties of blood changes as a function of oxygenation levels, it is possible to distinguish areas which are receiving fresh, oxygenated blood, — due to metabolic activity in response to some 'functional' stimuli — from those whose activity level is stable. As changes in blood flow occur over the course of seconds, rather than milliseconds, fMRI is a good technique for establishing the locus of neural mechanisms but less useful for establishing the time course of such activity.

Huettel et al. (2001) provide an initial picture of the various processes associated with change detection using a flicker paradigm very similar to that originally employed by Rensink et al. (1997). Post-hoc event-related analysis was used to divide patterns of activation into three task-related categories: transient responses to the flickering stimuli, sustained activation related to the visual search for change, and transient responses due to target detection.

Stimulus-dependent transient responses to flicker onset/offset were found mainly in primary visual areas. Sustained activations were found in areas known to participate in visual search and spatial orienting, including intraparietal sulcus, and frontal and supplementary eye fields. This type of responses declined following target detection. As observers were free to move their eyes during this task, such patterns of activation could have been driven due to the attentional demands of the task or, more directly, by the overt eye movements known to be closely associated with them (e.g., Andersen et al., 1992; Corbetta, 1998). Finally, the transient activation associated with the identification of the change involved several areas known to be associated with target detection (e.g., anterior cingulate) and response execution (e.g., basal ganglia and cerebellum).

Huettel et al.'s study demonstrates how an ongoing search process, such as those required in the flicker paradigm, can be decomposed into components previously identified in short-duration visual attention tasks. However, their study was not designed to probe differences between change detection and change blindness.

Beck et al. (2001) used fMRI to directly examine such differences. They combined a simplified flicker paradigm with an attentionally demanding baseline letter detection task. The change detection task involved reporting a change in two peripherally presented images of either faces or houses, which were flickered for only two cycles. The difficulty of the letter detection task was adapted for each observer to ensure that a roughly equal number of changes were missed as were detected.

As the main goal of Beck et al.'s study was to explore the brain regions that might differentiate change detection from change blindness, their main comparison was between trials in which a change was detected and trials in which the change was missed. Conscious detection of change led to activation of separate category-specific ventral regions (Kanwisher et al., 1997; Epstein and Kanwisher, 1998), as well as a common network of dorsal frontoparietal areas.

More importantly, for some subjects, the pattern of activation for undetected changes was different from the pattern of activation in trials with no change. This result suggests that unreported changes were processed by the visual system. Furthermore, the loci of activation for these unreported changes did not overlap with the areas active during conscious change detection, consistent with the hypothesis of separate mechanisms for implicit and explicit detection of change. However, a more definitive answer must await further research, as in this study activations by implicit changes were only present in a subset of subjects (6 out of 10) for one type of stimulus (faces).

Event-related potentials (ERPs)

Neural activity in large populations of cells gives rise to electrical potentials that can be detected by electrodes placed on the surface of the scalp. Event-related potentials (ERPs) are waveforms associated with a particular task that can be extracted from the overall pattern of neural activity by averaging across multiple trials. The main strength of ERPs is their excellent temporal resolution, which allows them to distinguish two events occurring 4 ms apart. This temporal resolution allows scientists to inquire about the stage of information processing at which attentional effects first occur and offers the possibility of determining when (i.e., how long after the stimulus onset) implicit and explicit processes first diverge.

Niedeggen et al. (2001) used ERPs to explore the detection of a single changing item (position change or identity change) in arrays of alphanumeric characters which were flickered for up to five cycles. The main finding of this study was that target detection was accompanied by a large positive deflection in the 200–800 ms range which was most pronounced over central and parietal sites. This waveform, known as the P3, is a well established finding in the ERP literature (for a review, see Donchin and Coles, 1988). It typically accompanies the conscious detection of low-probability targets (Johnson, 1986) and is thought to reflect a range of cognitive processes, including the updating of working memory, the making of binary decision, as well as various forms of recognition and identification judgements (Donchin and Coles, 1988).

A more interesting finding comes from the trials preceding the detection of the change. In these trials, there was an effect of similar distribution but smaller magnitude than the target detection effect. It is possible that this effect stems from some implicit detection of change, which precedes the explicit detection. Indeed, this effect might help to interpret a finding by Mitroff and Simons (2002) that when implicit localization responses are required on each successive image in a flicker paradigm, performance only improves in the image immediately preceding detection. However, other interpretations need to be ruled out first. It is possible that detected changes sometimes go unreported because the subject waits until the next cycle for confirmation. Similarly, the effects may reflect a lack of confidence on the detection, a possibility that receives support from studies showing that magnitude of the P3 component increases with increased confidence (Hillyard et al., 1971).

Niedeggen et al. (2001) also looked directly for indications of implicit change detection by comparing waveforms from trials in which a change was present but was not reported to those in which a change was absent, the catch trials. They were unable to establish any difference between these two types of trial, suggesting that implicit mechanisms were not operating. However, it is unclear whether such a design has enough power to detect possible implicit effects, given that there were only about 15% of trials with undetected change. Furthermore, subjects in this task were allowed to move their eyes freely. This, combined with the quite long stimulus displays (1500 ms) may have masked implicit effects as ERPs are exquisitely sensitive to eye movements, and in the presence of eye movements, other signals are often hard to detect.

Markers for implicit representation of change were found in a second ERP study that used a flicker paradigm with complex scenes and required subjects to keep their eyes fixated at the center of the screen (Fernandez-Duque et al., 2002). In this task, a within-trial design was used in which a change appeared and disappeared during different phases of each trial, and observers performed several tasks designed to control the distribution of attention. The design ensured that each trial contained periods in which the observer was unaware of change and then later became aware of the change, consciously attending to the change for several seconds after detection. Additionally, task demands ensured that attention was sometimes focused at the change location and sometimes distributed across the whole display.

The analysis proceeded in the following manner. First, markers associated with focusing attention in the absence of a change were identified. Relative to active search, focusing attention in the absence of a change enhanced an ERP-negative component over frontal sites around 100–300 ms after stimulus onset, and in posterior sites at the 150–300 ms window. These effects were then compared to markers elicited by an explicit awareness of change. Being aware of a change replicated the attentional effects in frontal and posterior sites. This is to be expected, as awareness of change depends on focusing attention at the location of change. More importantly, being aware of a change also produced a unique positive deflection in the 350–600 ms window, broadly distributed with its epicenter in medio-central areas. The unique topography and time course of this latter modulation, together with its dependence on the aware perception of change, distinguishes this 'awareness of change' electrophysiological response from the electrophysiological effects of focused attention.

Of more interest to the current topic, was a comparison between phases in which a change was present and the subject was unaware, relative to the stage in which a subject was looking for an absent change. This comparison revealed that undetected changes were accompanied by a bilateral positive deflection in anterior sites which reached significance at 240 ms and remained significant until 300 ms. Interestingly, both the time course and the topography of this deflection were different from those associated with focused attention or awareness. If this deflection proves to be an 'implicit marker' of change — as opposed to a reflection of incidental explicit or strategic processing — then these differences in time course and topography suggest that implicitly detected changes may be registered by different neural systems than those responsible for explicitly detected changes.

Change blindness in special populations

Recently, researchers have started to use change blindness paradigms to explore attention and memory processes in special populations.

In one study, Harp and Rensink (1999) compared the ability of older and younger adults to perform visual search for change (Rensink, 2000b). They found that while older adults were able to filter out irrelevant stimuli just as effectively as younger adults, there was a general slow down in the speed of attention with increasing age. Consistent with this finding, Pringle et al. (2001) found that older adults took longer to detect changes than young subjects. They suggest that this reduced ability to detect changes may be attributable in part to a narrowing of attentional breadth. As both of these studies only probed explicit detection, it may be informative to examine whether aging is also accompanied by a similar decline in the implicit detection of change.

Neglect patients, who have severe problems in spatial attention, may be another special population particularly suited for exploring implicit and explicit representation of change. It has been well established that neglect patients process physical, semantic, and emotional information of objects presented to their neglected field, for which they lack subjective awareness. It is not known whether information about changes would also be encoded without awareness in the neglect field. Clearly, studies of this kind may reveal much about the role of spatial attention in the representation of change.

Studies with special populations could be informative not only about the role of attention in the representation of change, but also about the role of memory in holding those representations. For example, one recent study has used eye movement methodology to explore implicit and explicit detection of change in amnesic patients (Ryan et al., 2000). Both amnesic patients and normal adults saw a series of complex scenes twice. When presented for the second time, each scene could be either an exact repetition or a modified version of the original scene. Normal subjects revealed increased viewing of the changed region, even when unaware of the change, a finding that provides convergent support for implicit representation of change. Interestingly, amnesic patients did not show such an effect, providing evidence of their failure in relational memory.

Conclusions

In this chapter we have explored the notion of *implicit change detection*. We suggest that when an observer fails to explicitly report a change, such events may still sometimes be registered by the visual system and, furthermore, influence subsequent behavior. Two key theoretical issues relating to this possibility concern the role of attention in creating spatiotemporally coherent representations and the relationship between attention and awareness. In the framework described in Fig. 2, we raised the theoretical possibility that change may be represented both with and without the aid of attention, and that the role of attention in modulating awareness is at least partially independent from questions of representation. Several empirical studies have provided evidence that behavioral consequences other than aware detection can accompany the presence of a change. While such behavioral studies are a useful starting point, we argue that it is only by seeking converging evidence from a range of other methodologies, such as eye movements, neuroimaging, and patient populations, that a clear picture will emerge. Here, we have reviewed the current state of the art in this ongoing, interdisciplinary research effort, and have outlined some possible new directions.

Acknowledgements

The authors would like to thank Andrew Hollingworth, Jukka Hyönä and two anonymous reviewers for useful comments and suggestions on earlier drafts of this chapter. During the preparation of this work Diego Fernandez-Duque was supported by a postdoctoral fellowship from the Rotman Research Institute, a fellowship from the Heart and Stroke Foundation of Ontario, and a grant from the Center for Consciousness Studies of the University of Arizona.

References

Abrams, R.A. and Landgraf, J.Z. (1990) Differential use of distance and location information for spatial localization. *Percept. Psychophys.*, 47(4): 349–359.

Aglioti, S., DeSouza, J.F.X. and Goodale, M.A. (1995) Size–contrast illusions deceive the eye but not the hand. *Curr. Biol.*, 5: 679–685.

Andersen, R.A., Brotchie, P.R. and Mazzoni, P. (1992) Evidence for the lateral intraparietal area as the parietal eye field. *Curr. Opin. Neurobiol.*, 2: 840–846.

Ballard, D., Hayhoe, M., Pook, P. and Rao, R. (1998) Deictic codes for the embodiment of cognition. *Behav. Brain Sci.*, 20: 723–767.

Bar, M. and Biederman, I. (1998) Subliminal visual priming. *Psychol. Sci.*, 9(6): 464–469.

Beck, D.M., Rees, G., Frith, C.D. and Lavie, N. (2001) Neural correlates of change detection and change blindness. *Nat. Neurosci.*, 4(6): 645–650.

Becker, M.W., Pashler, H. and Anstis, S.M. (2000) The role of iconic memory in change detection tasks. *Perception*, 29: 273–286.

Brenner, E. and Smeets, J.B.J. (1996) Size illusion influences how we lift but not how we grasp an object. *Exp. Brain Res.*, 111: 473–476.

Bridgeman, B., Hendry, D. and Stark, L. (1975) Failure to detect displacements of the visual world during saccadic eye movements. *Vision Res.*, 15: 719–722.

Bridgeman, B., Lewis, S., Heit, G. and Nagle, M. (1979) Relation between cognitive and motor-oriented systems of visual position perception. *J. Exp. Psychol. Hum. Percept. Perform.*, 5: 692–700.

Carr, T.H., McCauley, C., Sperber, R.D. and Parmelee, C.M. (1982) Words, pictures, and priming: on semantic activation, conscious identification, and the automaticity of information processing. *J. Exp. Psychol. Hum. Percept. Perform.*, 8(6): 757–776.

Castiello, U. and Jeannerod, M. (1991) Measuring time to awareness. *Neuroreport*, 2: 797–800.

Castiello, U., Paulignan, Y. and Jeannerod, M. (1991) Temporal dissociation of motor responses and subjective awareness. *Brain*, 114: 2639–2655.

Chen, Z. (1998) Inattentional amnesia: evidence of perception without awareness. *Invest. Ophthalmol. Vis. Sci.*, 39(4): S629.

Chun, M.M. and Jiang, H. (1998) Contextual cueing: implicit learning and memory of visual context guides spatial attention. *Cognit. Psychol.*, 36: 28–71.

Chun, M.M. and Nakayama, K. (2000) On the functional role of implicit visual memory for the adaptive deployment of attention across scenes. *Vis. Cognit.*, 7: 65–81.

Clegg, B.A., DiGirolamo, G.J. and Keele, S.W. (1998) Sequence learning. *Trends Cogn. Sci.*, 2: 275–281.

Corbetta, M. (1998) Frontoparietal cortical networks for directing attention and the eye to visual locations: identical, independent, or overlapping neural systems? *Proc. Natl. Acad. Sci. USA*, 95: 831–838.

Cowey, A. and Stoerig, P. (1991) Reflections on blindsight. In: A.D. Milner and M.D. Rugg (Eds.), *The Neuropsychology of Consciousness*. Academic Press, London, pp. 11–39.

Curran, T. and Keele, S.W. (1995) Attentional and nonattentional forms of sequence learning. *J. Exp. Psychol. Learn. Mem. Cogn.*, 19: 189–202.

Dehaene, S., Naccache, L., Le Clec'H, G., Koechlin, E., Mueller, M., Dehaene-Lambertz, G., van de Moortele, P.F. and Le Bihan, D. (1998) Imaging unconscious semantic priming. *Nature*, 395: 597–600.

Dehaene, S., Naccache, L., Cohen, L., Le Bihan, D., Mangin, J.F., Poline, J.B. and Riviére, D. (2001) Cerebral mechanisms of word masking and unconscious priming. *Nat. Neurosci.*, 4(7): 752–758.

Destrebecqz, A. and Cleeremans, A. (2001) Can sequence learning be implicit? New evidence with the processes dissociation paradigm. *Psychon. Bull. Rev.*, 8(2): 343–350.

Donchin, E. and Coles, M.G.H. (1988) Is the P300 component a manifestation of context updating? *Behav. Brain Sci.*, 11: 357–374.

Driver, J., Davis, G., Russell, C., Turratto, M. and Freeman, E. (2001) Segmentation, attention and phenomenal visual objects. *Cognition*, 80: 61–95.

Enns, J.T. and Di Lollo, V. (1997) Object substitution: a new form of masking in unattended visual locations. *Psychol. Sci.*, 8: 135–139.

Epstein, R. and Kanwisher, N. (1998) A cortical representation of the local visual environment. *Nature*, 392: 598–601.

Feldman, F.A. (1985) Four frames suffice: a provisional model of vision and space. *Behav. Brain Sci.*, 8: 265–289.

Fernandez-Duque, D. and Johnson, M.L. (1999) Attention metaphors: how metaphors guide the cognitive psychology of attention. *Cognit. Sci.*, 23(1): 83–116.

Fernandez-Duque, D. and Thornton, I.M. (2000) Change detection without awareness: do explicit reports underestimate the representation of change in the visual system? *Vis. Cognit.*, 7: 324–344.

Fernandez-Duque, D. and Thornton, I.M. (2002) Explicit mechanisms do not account for implicit localization and identification of change: a reply to Mitroff et al. (2002). *J. Exp. Psychol.*, under revision.

Fernandez-Duque, D., Grossi, G., Thornton, I.M. and Neville, H.J. (2002). Representing change with and without awareness: an event-related brain potentials study. *J. Cogn. Neurosci.*, in press.

Fowler, C.A., Wolford, G., Slade, R. and Tassinary, L. (1981) Lexical access with and without awareness. *J. Exp. Psychol. Gen.*, 110: 341–362.

Franz, V.H., Gegenfurtner, K.R., Bülthoff, H.H. and Fahle, M. (2000) Grasping visual illusions: no evidence for a dissociation between perception and action. *Psychol. Sci.*, 11: 20–25.

Franz, V.H., Fahle, M., Bülthoff, H.H. and Gegenfurtner, K.R. (2001) Effects of visual illusions on grasping. *J. Exp. Psychol. Hum. Percept. Perform.*, 27: 1124–1144.

Gazzaniga, M.S., Ivry, R.B. and Mangun, G.R. (1998) *Cognitive Neuroscience. The biology of the mind (2nd Edition)*. W.W. Norton & Co., New York, NY.

Goodale, M.A. (1993) Visual routes to knowledge and action. *Biomed. Res.*, 14: 113–123.

Goodale, M.A. (1996) One visual experience, many visual systems. In: T. Inui and J.L. McClelland (Eds.), *Attention and Performance XVI: Information Integration in Perception and Communication*. MIT Press, Cambridge, MA, pp. 369–393.

Goodale, M.A. and Milner, A.D. (1992). Separate visual pathways for perception and action. *Trends Neurosci.*, 15(1): 20–25.

Goodale, M.A., Pelisson, D. and Prablanc, C. (1986) Large adjustments in visually guided reaching do not depend on vision of the hand or perception of target displacement. *Nature*, 320: 748–750.

Graves, R.E. and Jones, B.S. (1992) Conscious visual perceptual awareness vs. non-conscious visual spatial localisation examined with normal subjects using possible analogues of blindsight and neglect. *Cogn. Neuropsychol.*, 9(6): 487–508.

Greenwald, A.G., Draine, S.C. and Abrams, R.L. (1996) Three cognitive markers of unconscious semantic activation. *Science*, 273: 1699–1702.

Grimes, J. (1996) On the failure to detect changes in scenes across saccades. In: K. Akins (Ed.), *Perception, Vancouver Studies in Cognitive Science*. Vol. 5, Oxford University Press, New York, pp. 89–109.

Gysen, V., De Graef, P. and Verfaillie, K. (2002) Detection of intrasaccadic displacements and depth rotations of moving objects. *Vision Res.*, 42: 379–391.

Harp, C.J. and Rensink, R.A. (1999) A comparison of attentional processing in younger and older observers. *Invest. Ophthalmol. Vis. Sci.*, 40(4): S270.

Hayhoe, M., Bensinger, D. and Ballard, D.H. (1998) Task constraints in visual working memory. *Vision Res.*, 38: 125–137.

Henderson, J.M. and Hollingworth, A. (2002) Eye movements and visual memory: detecting changes to saccade targets in scenes. *Percept. Psychophys.*, in press.

Hillyard, S.A., Squires, K.C., Bauer, J.W. and Lindsay, P.H. (1971) Evoked potential correlates of auditory signal detection. *Science*, 172: 1357–1360.

Holender, D. (1986) Semantic activation without conscious identification in dichotic listening, parafoveal vision, and visual masking: a survey and appraisal. *Behav. Brain Sci.*, 9: 1–23.

Hollingworth, A. (2002). Failures of retrieval and comparison constrain change detection in natural scenes. *J. Exp. Psychol. Hum. Percept. Perform.*, in press.

Hollingworth, A. and Henderson, J.M. (2002) Accurate visual memory for previously attended objects in natural scenes. *J. Exp. Psychol. Hum. Percept. Perform.*, 28: 113–136.

Hollingworth, A., Schrock, G. and Henderson, J.M. (2001a) Change detection in the flicker paradigm: the role of fixation position within the scene. *Mem. Cognit.*, 29: 296–304.

Hollingworth, A., Williams, C.C. and Henderson, J.M. (2001b) To see and remember: visually specific information is retained in memory from previously attended objects in natural scenes. *Psychon. Bull. Rev.*, 8: 761–768.

Hommel, B., Müsseler, J., Aschersleben, G. and Prinz, W. (2001) The theory of event coding (TEC): a framework for perception and action planning. *Behav. Brain Sci.*, 24: 849–937.

Irwin, D.E. and Andrews, R. (1996) Integration and accumulation of information across saccadic eye movements. In: T. Inui and J.L. McClelland (Eds.), *Attention and Performance XVI: information Integration in Perception and Communication*. MIT Press, Cambridge, MA, pp. 125–155.

Irwin, D.E., Yantis, S. and Jonides, J. (1983) Evidence against visual integration across saccadic eye movements. *Percept. Psychophys.*, 34: 35–46.

Jacoby, L.L., Toth, J.P. and Yonelinas, A.P. (1993) Separating conscious and unconscious nfluences of memory: Measuring recollection. *J. Exp. Psychol. General*, 122: 139–154.

Johnson, R.J. (1986) A triarchic model of P300 amplitude. *Psychophysiology*, 23: 367–384.

Kahneman, D., Treisman, A.M. and Gibbs, B. (1992) The reviewing of object files: object-specific integration of information. *Cognit. Psychol.*, 24: 175–219.

Kanwisher, N., McDermott, J. and Chun, M.M. (1997) The fusiform face area: a module in human extrastriate cortex specialized for face perception. *J. Neurosci.*, 17: 4302–4311.

Koch, R. (1999) Detection of asynchrony between click and tap. *Paper 1/1999*, Max Planck Institute for Psychological Research, Munich.

Kolb, F.C. and Braun, J. (1995) Blindsight in normal observers. *Nature*, 377: 336–338.

Land, M., Mennie, N. and Rusted, J. (1999) Eye movements and the role of vision in activities of daily living: making a cup of tea. *Perception*, 28: 1311–1328.

Levin, D.T. and Simons, D.J. (1997) Failure to detect changes to attended objects in motion pictures. *Psychon. Bull. Rev.*, 4(4): 501–506.

Levin, D.T., Simons, D.J., Angelone, B.L. and Chabris, C.F. (2002) Memory for centrally attended changing objects in an incidental real-world change detection paradigm. *Br. J. Psychol.*, in press.

Li, W. and Matin, L. (1990) The influence of saccade length on the saccadic suppression of displacement detection. *Percept. Psychophys.*, 48(5): 453–458.

Luck, S.J., Vogel, E.K. and Shapiro, K.L. (1996) Word meanings can be accessed but not reported during the attentional blink. *Nature*, 382: 616–618.

Mack, A. and Rock, I. (1998) *Inattentional Blindness*. MIT Press, Cambridge, MA.

Mack, A., Tang, B., Tuma, R., Kahn, S. and Rock, I. (1992) Perceptual organization and attention. *Cognit. Psychol.*, 24: 475–501.

Maljkovic, V. and Nakayama, K. (1994) Priming of pop-out I. Role of features. *Mem. Cognit.*, 22: 657–672.

Maljkovic, V. and Nakayama, K. (1996) Priming of pop-out II. Role of position. *Percept. Psychophys.*, 58: 977–991.

Marcel, A.J. (1983) Conscious and unconscious perception: experiments on visual masking and word recognition. *Cognit. Psychol.*, 15: 197–237.

Matin, E. (1974) Saccadic suppression: a review and analysis. *Psychol. Bull.*, 81: 899–917.

McConkie, G.W. and Currie, C.B. (1996) Visual stability across saccades while viewing complex pictures. *J. Exp. Psychol. Hum. Percept. Perform.*, 22: 563–581.

McConkie, G.W. and Rayner, K. (1976) Identifying the span of the effective stimulus in reading: literature review and theories of reading. In: H. Singer and R.B. Ruddell (Eds.), *Theoretical Models and Processes in Reading*. International Reading Institute, Newark, DE, pp. 137–162.

McConkie, G.W. and Zola, D. (1979) Is visual information integrated across successive fixations in reading? *Percept. Psychophys.*, 25: 221–224.

McCormick, P.A. (1997) Orienting attention without awareness. *J. Exp. Psychol. Hum. Percept. Perform.*, 23(1): 168–180.

Milner, A.D. and Goodale, M.A. (1995) *The Visual Brain in Action*. Oxford University Press, Oxford.

Milner, B., Corkin, S. and Teuber, H. (1968) Further analysis of the hippocampal amnesic syndrome: 14 year follow-up study of H.M.. *Neuropsychologia*, 6: 215–234.

Mitroff, S.R. and Simons, D.J. (2002) Changes are not localized before they are explicitly detected. *Vis. Cognit.*, in press.

Mitroff, S.R., Simons, D.J. and Franconieri, S.L. (2002) The siren song of implicit change detection. *J. Exp. Psychol. Hum. Percept. Perform.*, 28(4): 798–815.

Moore, C.M. and Egeth, H. (1997) Perception without attention: evidence of grouping under conditions of inattention. *J. Exp. Psychol. Hum. Percept. Perform.*, 23(2): 339–352.

Niedeggen, M., Wichmann, P. and Stoerig, P. (2001) Change blindness and time to consciousness. *Eur. J. Neurosci.*, 14(10): 1719–1726.

Noë, A., Pessoa, L. and Thompson, E. (2000) Beyond the Grand Illusion: what change blindness really teaches us about vision. *Vis. Cognit.*, 7: 93–106.

O'Regan, J.K. (1992) Solving the 'real' mysteries of visual perception: the world as an outside memory. *Can. J. Psychol.*, 46(3): 461–488.

O'Regan, J.K., Rensink, R.A. and Clark, J.J. (1999) 'Mudsplashes' causes blindness to large scene changes. *Nature*, 398(6722): 34.

O'Regan, J.K., Deubel, H., Clark, J.J. and Rensink, R.A. (2000) Picture changes during blinks: looking without seeing and seeing without looking. *Vis. Cognit.*, 7: 191–212.

Palmer, S.E. (1999) *Vision Science: photons to Phenomenology*. MIT Press, Cambridge, MA.

Pollatsek, A. and Rayner, K. (1992) What is integrated across fixations? In: K. Rayner (Ed.), *Eye Movements and Visual Cognition: Scene Perception and Reading*. Springer, New York, pp. 166–191.

Pollatsek, A. and Rayner, K. (2001) The information that is coded across fixations may be different for static and moving objects. *Psychol. Belg.*, 41: 75–87.

Pringle, H.L., Irwin, D.E., Kramer, A.F. and Atchley, P. (2001) The role of attentional breadth in perceptual change detection. *Psychon. Bull. Rev.*, 8: 89–95.

Pylyshyn, Z.W. and Storm, R.W. (1988) Tracking multiple independent targets: evidence for a parallel tracking mechanism. *Spat. Vis.*, 3: 179–197.

Reingold, E.M. and Merikle, P.M. (1990) On the interrelatedness of theory and measurement on the study of unconscious processes. *Mind Lang.*, 5: 9–28.

Rensink, R.A. (2000a) The dynamic representation of scenes. *Vis. Cognit.*, 7: 17–42.

Rensink, R.A. (2000b) Visual search for change: A probe into the nature of attentional processing. *Vis. Cognit.*, 7: 345–376.

Rensink, R.A. (2002a) Change detection. *Annu. Rev. Psychol.*, 53: 245–277.

Rensink, R.A. (2002b) Visual sensing without seeing. *Psychol. Sci.*, manuscript under review.

Rensink, R.A., O'Regan, K. and Clark, J.J. (1997) To see or not to see: the need for attention to perceive changes in scenes. *Psychol. Sci.*, 8: 368–373.

Repp, B.H. (2000) Compensation for subliminal timing perturbations in perceptual–motor synchronization. *Psychol. Res.*, 63: 106–128.

Repp, B.H. (2001) Phase correction, phase resetting and phase shifts after subliminal timing perturbations in sensorimotor synchronization. *J. Exp. Psychol. Hum. Percept. Perform.*, 27: 600–621.

Richards, E., Jolicoeur, P., Stolz, J.A. and Vogel-Sprott, M. (2001) The transition from feature-based to object-based processing. Poster presented at the 42nd Annual Meeting of the Psychonomic Society, Orlando, FL.

Rock, I., Linnet, C.M., Grant, P. and Mack, A. (1992) Perception without attention: results of a new method. *Cognit. Psychol.*, 24: 502–534.

Ryan, J.D., Althoff, R.R., Whitlow, S. and Cohen, N.J. (2000) Amnesia is a deficit in relational memory. *Psychol. Sci.*, 11(6): 454–461.

Schacter, D.L. (1995) Implicit memory: a new frontier for cognitive neuroscience. In: M.S. Gazzaniga (Ed.), *The Cognitive Neurosciences*. MIT Press, Cambridge, MA, pp. 815–824.

Scholl, B.J. (2000) Attenuated change blindness for exogenously attended items in a flicker paradigm. *Vis. Cognit.*, 7: 377–396.

Scholl, B.J. and Pylyshyn, Z.W. (1999) Tracking multiple items through occlusion: Clues to visual objecthood. *Cognit. Psychol.*, 38(2): 259–290.

Scott-Brown, K.C., Baker, M.R. and Orbach, H.S. (2000) Comparison blindness. *Vis. Cognit.*, 7: 253–267.

Shore, D.I. and Klein, R.M. (2000) The effects of scene inversion on change blindness. *J. Gen. Psychol.*, 127(1): 27–43.

Simons, D.J. (2000) Current approaches to change blindness. *Vis. Cognit.*, 7: 1–16.

Simons, D.J. and Levin, D.T. (1997) Change blindness. *Trends Cognit. Sci.*, 1: 261–267.

Simons, D.J. and Levin, D.T. (1998) Failure to detect changes to people during a real-world interaction. *Psychon. Bull. Rev.*, 5(4): 644–649.

Simons, D.J. and Silverman, M. (2002) Neural and behavioral measures of change detection. In: L.M. Chalupa and J.S. Werner (Eds.), *The Visual Neurosciences*. MIT Press, Cambridge, MA, submitted.

Smilek, D., Eastwood, J.D. and Merikle, P.M. (2000) Does unattended information facilitate change detection? *J. Exp. Psychol. Hum. Percept. Perform.*, 26(2): 480–487.

Smilek, D., Eastwood, J.D. and Merikle, P.M. (2002) The role of unattended information in change detection: A reply to Mitroff, Simons and Franconeri (in press). *J. Exp. Psychol. Hum. Percept. Perform.*, Manuscript submitted for publication.

Thaut, M.H., Tian, B. and Azimi-Sadjadi, M.R. (1998) Rhythmic finger tapping to cosine–wave modulated metronome sequences: evidence of subliminal entrainment. *Hum. Mov. Sci.*, 17: 839–863.

Thornton, I.M. and Fernandez-Duque, D. (2000) An implicit measure of undetected change. *Spat. Vis.*, 14(1): 21–44.

Treisman, A.M. and Gelade, G. (1980) A feature-integration theory of attention. *Cognit. Psychol.*, 12: 97–136.

Verfaillie, K. and De Graef, P. (2001) Keeping a transsaccadic record of objects: Introduction to a special issue on object perception across saccadic eye movements. *Psychol. Belg.*, 41: 1–8.

Wallis, G. and Bülthoff, H.H. (2000) What's scene and not seen: influences of movement and task upon what we see. *Vis. Cognit.*, 7: 175–190.

Weiskrantz, L. (1986) *Blindsight: A Case Study and Implications*. Oxford University Press, Oxford.

Williams, P. (1997) *Prototypes, Exemplars, and Object Recognition*. Unpublished PhD thesis, Yale University.

Williams, P. and Simons, D.J. (2000) Detecting changes in novel, complex three-dimensional objects. *Vis. Cognit.*, 7: 297–322.

CHAPTER 8

Blinks, blanks and saccades: how blind we really are for relevant visual events

Sascha M. Dornhoefer [1,*], Pieter J.A. Unema [2] and Boris M. Velichkovsky [1]

[1] *Department of Psychology III, Dresden University of Technology, Mommsenstrasse 13, 01062 Dresden, Germany*
[2] *Department of Experimental Psychology, Maastricht University, P.O. Box 616, 6200 MD Maastricht, The Netherlands*

Abstract: We report on a study in which subjects viewed color video stills of natural traffic situations while eye movements were recorded. A display change could occur randomly during three different occlusion modes — blinks, blanks and saccades — or during a fixation. These changes could be either relevant or irrelevant with respect to the traffic safety situation. Furthermore we contrasted insertions and deletions. All occlusion modes appeared equivalent concerning detection rate and detection time, and only differed from the fixation condition. The results also show that the detection of relevant changes was more likely and faster than that of irrelevant ones. However, even relevant insertions, which were almost always detected, were around 180 ms longer to report when they occurred during an occlusion. Furthermore, the detection of relevant changes was fairly stable across a wide range of the visual field, whereas irrelevant changes were less well detected, the further away from the fovea they occurred. We close with an outlook on a follow-up study where only relevant insertions and the blank occlusion were used in a driving simulator environment. Surprisingly, we found an advantage in change detection rate and time with blanks compared to the control condition. Change detection was also good during blinks, but not in saccades.

Introduction and overview

The variety of functional blindness phenomena

When viewing a scene we actually see far less than we think (e.g. Dennett, 1991; Wolfe, 1999a). Although this fact can be demonstrated with any crowded picture, it is particularly pronounced if there are some changes in either observed or in background events. The first demonstration of functional change blindness goes back to the 19th century (Baxt, 1871). For decades, it was studied in the context of *masking effects*: a target that is clearly visible when briefly presented alone can be rendered invisible by the subsequent presentation of a non-target object in the nearby spatial location (see Enns and Di Lollo, 2000).

Ulric Neisser (1979) contributed to a better ecological validity of the experiments by proposing the 'selective looking' paradigm, an analogue to the 'dichotic listening' from investigations of selective attention. He presented a video with superimposed films of two different teams playing basketball. When monitoring only passes of one team and ignoring passes made by the other team, observers often failed to perceive a continuous irrelevant event — a woman with an umbrella walking across the scene (see also Simons and Chabris, 1999). In another famous study, professional pilots were instructed to land an aircraft in a flight simulator under conditions of poor visibility using a head-up display (Haines, 1991). Two of ten tested pilots were not aware of a

* Correspondence to: S.M. Dornhoefer, Department of Psychology III, Dresden University of Technology, Mommsenstrasse 13, 01062 Dresden, Germany. Tel.: +49-351-4633-3990; Fax: +49-351-4633-7741; E-mail: dornhoefer@applied-cognition.org

large airplane on the runway although it was clearly visible and located directly ahead of them. Being functionally blind to the unexpected obstacle, they simply landed their aircrafts 'through' it.

This inability to perceive unexpected events has been labeled *'inattentional blindness'* (Mack and Rock, 1998). Wolfe (1999b) however argues that these phenomena are rather evidence of *'inattentional amnesia'*, because the changes might have been perceived, but not remembered (in the direct, explicit sense of the word). These change detection failures have recently been investigated in studies focusing primarily on a phenomenon known as *'change blindness'*, which we discuss and investigate in this chapter. There are a few other variants of the change blindness phenomenon worth mentioning, though we will not specifically address them: they include the *'attentional blink'* (Shapiro et al., 1997), *'repetition blindness'* (Kanwisher, 1987) and *'comparison blindness'* (Scott-Brown et al., 2000).

A review of the current explanations (Simons, 2000) demonstrates that the field is in need of more systematic experimental studies before a theoretical synthesis can be provided. Noticing a changing object may be an automatic achievement with respect to detection and localization, but it assumes focused attention and effortful encoding of features if identification is demanded (Velichkovsky, 1982; Rensink et al., 1997). A lack or a re-direction of attention therefore often causes failure to perceive changes to scenes.

How to produce change blindness

Change blindness typically occurs when a global disruption of the retinal image, such as *saccades* (due to saccadic suppression) or *eyeblinks*, obscure the local transient caused by a change. Grimes (1996), for example, demonstrated that people often do not detect large changes to scenes occurring during saccades. In his experiments, observers studied everyday scenes presented on a computer monitor for a later recognition. While they freely explored the scenes, some details were changed in a gaze-contingent manner (e.g. two people exchanging heads or a prominent building in a skyline becoming 25% larger). A considerable number of changes (67%), that could cover one fourth of the picture, sometimes in the center of visual field, were missed. The same changes were easily detected when they occurred during a fixation. These striking results are consistent with earlier studies on the failure to integrate information across saccades (e.g. Irwin et al., 1983; Rayner and Pollatsek, 1983). O'Regan et al. (2000) obtained similar effects when they changed aspects in everyday visual scenes every time an eye blink occurred.

Change blindness is not specifically related to saccades or blinks, however: it can also occur during an artificial global occlusion, such as a *blank screen*, where the disruption of the retinal image by an eye movement is simulated by a brief *blank screen* that is inserted between the original and the modified picture — using either a 'one-shot' (Pashler, 1988; Blackmore et al., 1995; Simons, 1996) or a 'flicker' paradigm (Rensink et al., 1997). In one-shot tasks, the original and the modified picture are each presented for one view before the observers have to guess whether a change has occurred. In the flicker paradigm (it has a less natural character and may interfere with different aspects of perceptual processing, e.g. Macknik et al., 1991), the original picture A alternates with the modified picture A′, each time separated by a brief blank field. A random order of presentation is often used to create temporal uncertainty about the change.

Other global disruptions that have been used in investigations of change blindness are *picture shifts* (Blackmore et al., 1995), *film cuts* in motion pictures (Levin and Simons, 1997) or *physical occluders* in real world situations (Simons and Levin, 1998). Furthermore, change blindness can also occur when the change takes place in full view, namely if a multitude of distracting local transients (often called *'mudsplashes'*) are presented parallel to that produced by the change (O'Regan et al., 1996; Enns and Di Lollo, 2000), or when *gradual changes* occur slow enough not to give rise to the activation of the visual transient channels (Simons et al., 2000).

Factors affecting change blindness

Various factors have been found to modulate change detection. In particular, recent studies have shown that the *relevance* of a change plays an important role in the detection probability. According to Rensink et al. (1997) and O'Regan et al. (1999), changes to objects of central interest (as determined in independent ratings) are detected more readily than changes to objects of marginal interest. Even when eccentricity relative to the eye position is controlled, an advantage in detectability for objects of central interest remains (O'Regan et al., 2000). In a driving simulator study, however, Shinoda et al. (2001) found that task variables interfere with relevance and can modulate detection probability: the highly traffic-relevant replacement of a No-Parking sign by a Stop sign during a blank screen was rarely detected if subjects were asked to follow a lead car and keep a constant distance.

In their elaboration of the classical Neisser experiments, Simons and Chabris (1999) showed that unexpected changes are more likely to be detected the higher the *similarity* between the currently attended and the unexpected events is. In an attempt to replicate these results, Most et al. (2001) demonstrated that the change detection has to be attributed not as much to similarity with attended events, but rather to dissimilarity with the unattended, to-be-ignored stimuli. According to data from the investigations of picture memory, schema-inconsistent changes are more likely to be detected than schema-consistent ones, albeit only in recognition, not in recall tasks (Friedman, 1979; Henderson, 1992).

Focused *attention* may be the single most important factor in change blindness studies. Newby and Rock (1998) found that detection is the better the closer an unexpected stimulus is to the center of attention — not necessarily to the center of fixation. The position that attention mediates change detection is further supported by the findings that verbal (e.g. Rensink et al., 1997) or spatial (Enns and Di Lollo, 2000) cueing improves detection rate. Considering the support for the notion of attention as a necessary condition for change detection, it seems reasonable to assume that, in fact, relevant objects simply are more likely to attract attention than irrelevant ones. This would be in line with Henderson and Hollingworth (1999), who found that fixating an object immediately before or after a change correlates with detection rate. Nevertheless, several recent studies provide evidence that change detection can take place *without awareness* (Hayhoe et al., 1998; Fernandez-Duque and Thornton, 2000; Smilek et al., 2000; Henderson and Hollingworth, 2002), causing Rensink (2000) to point towards the hypothesis, that "conscious visual experience of change is mediated by focused attention, whereas unconscious perception of change is not".

Change detection is further a function of *knowledge* and *expertise* of observers. Archambault et al. (1999) report that the *level of categorization* at which an object has been learned (general vs. specific) interacts with change detection. In an expert–novice comparison of change detection in football images, Werner and Thies (2000) showed that domain-specific expertise attenuates change blindness. Reingold et al. (2001) found experts' advantages in detection of changes to meaningful chess configurations and proved the long-lasting hypothesis that experts work with larger cognitive templates. These findings are consistent with studies showing that the visual scanning strategies evolve with expertise (in the case of road traffic see, e.g., Mourant and Rockwell, 1972; Crundall and Underwood, 1998): experts search a larger visual area more efficiently and with fewer eye movements than novices.

As still another group of factors, the spatial–temporal variables of presentation have to be mentioned. According to Henderson and Hollingworth (1999), change detection decreases with the *foveal distance* from the location of change. They assume that there is a significant role for fixation position in the maintenance of information processing across discrete views of a scene, and that allocation of attention cannot be the sole determinant of detection performance. O'Regan et al. (2000) showed that beyond 2° of visual angle, detection rate remains fairly stable up to at least 8°, with a slight advantage for changes of central interest. With respect to time, the longer an occlusion lasts, the worse subjects perform at change detection: Rensink et al. (2000) report that performance deteriorated as blank durations increased from 40 ms to 320 ms. Phillips and Singer (1974) found a non-monotonous influence of the interstimulus interval (ISI): with a zero-length ISI, changes were detected easily, growing increasingly difficult as the ISI approached 80 ms, beyond which detection became stable up to ISI of over 300 ms (see also Enns and Di Lollo, 2000). Rensink et al. (2000) examined whether extended viewing time of the initial image improves change detection. They provided an uninterrupted preview of the original image of 8 s before starting an AAA'A'-flicker sequence (with following image durations of 240 ms each). Observers were asked to remember as much of the image as possible. A comparison with a study using the same flicker sequence without an additional preview (Rensink et al., 1997) revealed no effect of previewing time. Rensink et al. (2000) therefore conclude that change blindness is not caused by an insufficient time to construct a coherent representation.

Finally, the *type of change* seems to play a role. According to Simons (1996), the appearance of an object in a previously empty array is more likely to be detected than the replacement of one object by another. Phillips and Singer (1974) as well as Stelmach et al. (1984) also found that adding an item to the visual array was more likely to be detected than deleting one. Henderson and Hollingworth (1999) found better detection rates for deletions compared to rotations. In the study, a 90° rotation was detected only 10% of the time, when neither the prenor the post-saccadic fixation landed on the change location, while deletions were detected in the same conditions 40% of the time. In Grimes' experiment (1996), changes to object properties (color, rotations) were detected more easily than layout and semantic category changes.

An experiment on variation of relevance and type of occlusion

In the light of the discussed data, which demonstrate an abundance of situations and factors inducing change blindness (saccades, blinks, blanks, mudsplashes, gradual changes), the question arises how serious these effects are in everyday life. Let us consider the mere number of blinks and saccades made during the day: someone who makes an average of 12–15 blinks per minute (Barbato et al., 2000) lasting 150 ms on average while making an average of 4 saccades per second with an average duration of 35 ms, experiences a global occlusion 17–18% of the time. Thus, although it has well been established that blanks, blinks and saccades are effective in eliciting change blindness, a direct comparison is necessary to determine whether the respective influences are comparable. Considering this, we were interested to find out to what extent the types of occlusion occurring in everyday life may contribute to the failure of detecting relevant and irrelevant changes in realistic traffic scenes.

Method

Stimuli and design

The experiment involved 60 digitized color stills taken from a video containing a variety of real traffic scenes recorded from the vantage point of the driver through the windshield of a car. The stills were digitized to 800×600 pixel bitmaps with a color resolution of 24 bits per pixel. To each of the images, four different manipulations could occur, resulting in a set of 240 trials.

A complete-within-subjects design was used to study the effects of occlusion type and relevance on detection probability and detection latency. Stimuli were presented in random order in three sets of 100 trials, each containing an equal number of trials of each condition. The changes could be executed during either of four conditions: a screen blanking, which lasted 112 ms, an eye blink, a saccade or a fixation (as non-occlusion condition). Subjects were asked to respond by pressing a button as soon as they noticed a change. In contrast to the endogenous occlusions (blinks and saccades) external blanks may serve as a cue. Therefore, in order to avoid guessing, 60 blank screen catch trials were added to the 240 trials, i.e. no changes were made. Presentation of the 300 trials occurred in any of four predetermined quasi-random orders. A trial started with a blank screen for 1500 ms. The unchanged image was shown for 4000, 4500, 5000, 5500 or 6000 ms before a change was initiated. In the blank condition, this meant that the image was changed at the end of the above-mentioned period. In the blink, saccade, and fixation conditions, the image was changed immediately upon next occurrence of the event. When a blink trial was up and no blink occurred during the following 6 s, the trial was aborted and discarded from further analysis. The trial ended when the button was pressed or when it was not pressed within 5 s following the change. Reaction times were measured from the moment of de-occlusion. Thus, in the blank- and the fixation-condition, reaction time was measured from the moment of image change, in the saccade condition reaction times were measured from the start of the next fixation, and in the blink-condition reaction times were measured either from the moment the blink was over (when the blink occurred during a fixation) or from the start of the next fixation in case the blink occurred during a saccade.

We contrasted two classes of change (Fig. 1). *Driving-relevant* changes were such changes that the driver of a vehicle in that situation would have to take action in order to avoid a dangerous or potentially dangerous situation. These changes included objects (e.g. pedestrians, vehicles or bicycles) that appeared or disappeared in front of the driver or changes within such objects — e.g. the (dis)appearance of braking lights. *Driving-irrelevant* changes could be any other kind of change — e.g. the (dis)appearance of a tree or a house's window. Five independent judges determined whether a change should be rated as driving-relevant or driving-irrelevant. Overall inter-rater agreement was better than 95%. Furthermore two kinds of changes, namely insertions and deletions were contrasted. Size, distance (with respect to the focus of extension) and color contrast of the changes were counterbalanced across all changes.

Subjects

Twenty-four subjects, 13 female and 11 male aged 20 to 30 years (mean = 23.25, SD = 2.64), volunteered for the study. All subjects were students of psychology at Dresden University of Technology and

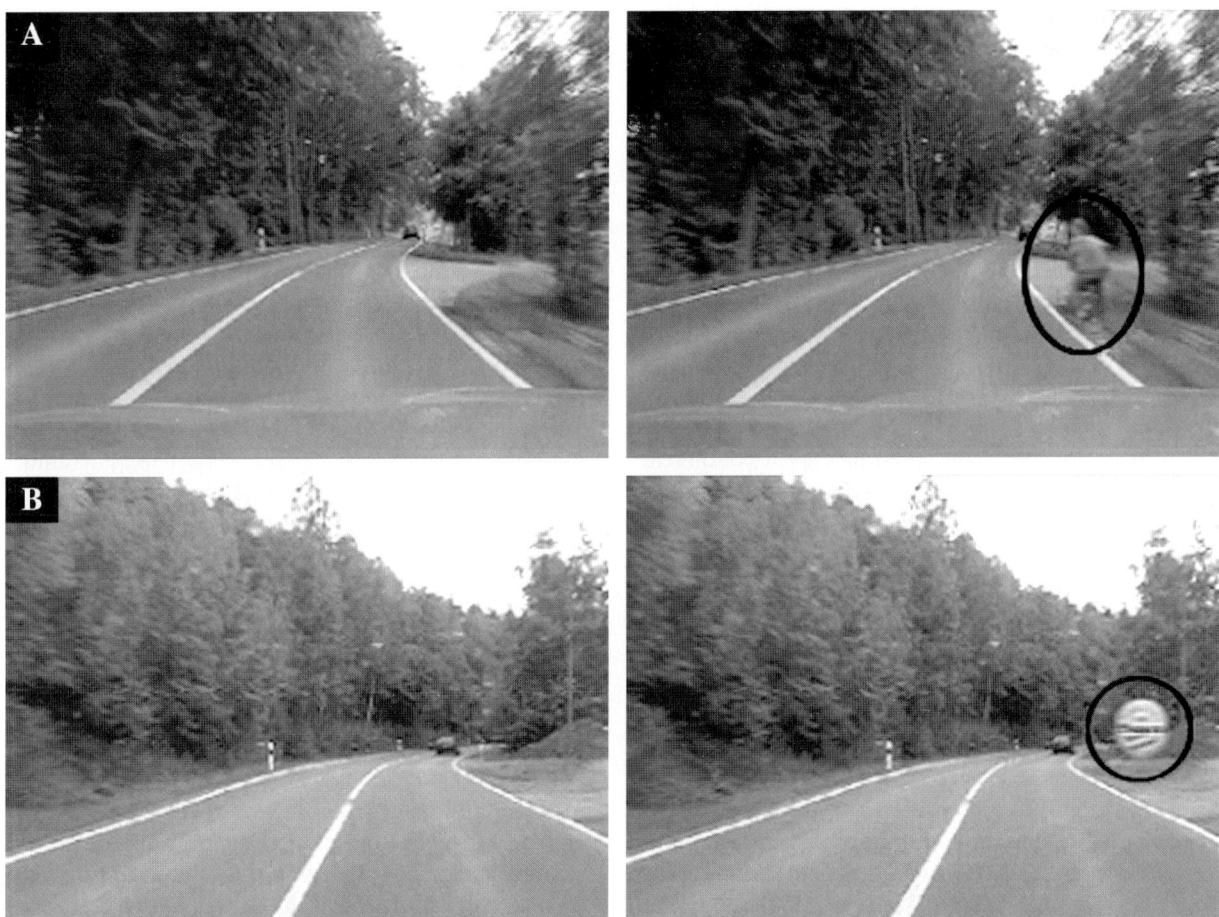

Fig. 1. Sample image-pairs used in the experiment. (A) Relevant change: a bicyclist appears on the right side. (B) Irrelevant change: an advertisement object appears on the right side.

reported normal or corrected to normal vision. None of the subjects had participated in a change blindness study before. Furthermore all subjects were holders of a driving license.

Procedure

Subjects were seated in front of a 17" ViewSonic color monitor running at a vertical refresh rate of 100 Hz. Viewing distance was approximately 60 cm from the screen surface, resulting in a viewing angle of ~30° horizontally and 20° vertically. Subjects were instructed to watch the scenes while trying to imagine being the driver of a car approaching the scene and to press the left mouse-button as soon as they noticed a change. They were also asked not to be bothered by a blank screen that could sometimes appear. Before the eye tracking equipment was fitted to the subjects, a series of 20 test trials was presented to familiarize them with the procedure. After fitting and calibration of the eye tracker, subjects proceeded with the experiment. An automatic drift correction was performed every 5th trial, a recalibration took place every 30th trial. Subjects had a 5-min break after 100 and 200 trials. All participants saw the trials in one of four random orders of presentation. The whole experiment lasted approximately 75 min, including preparation and two 5-min breaks.

Apparatus

In order to perform eye-movement-contingent changes to the scenes, the SR-Research Eyelink™ I eyetracker was used. The system uses a headband holding a camera to compensate for head movements and one camera for each eye. Eye movements were recorded monocularly using the dominant eye, with an accuracy of less than 1°, sampled at 250 Hz. The eye tracking PC was interfaced by means of an Ethernet connection to a stimulus-presenting Pentium PC, which received the eye position data with an approximate delay of 8 ms. Eye movements larger than 0.3° per sample were considered to be saccades and detected by an online algorithm using four samples, resulting in a total delay of 24 ms. Fixations were identified as the absence of a saccade, unless missing pupil data indicated a blink — both, fixations and blinks, were also detected within 24 ms.

To avoid flicker, changes of the scenes were always performed during the vertical retrace and synchronized to the next vertical refresh (100 Hz), resulting in a potential further delay of 0 to 10 ms — thus an eye contingent display change was executed within 24 to 34 ms. The avoidance of flicker was considered to be more important than minimizing the delay, while choosing a relatively high cutoff criterion for minimal saccadic velocity to ensure that changes could be performed before a saccade was terminated. All stimulus data (scene, change location, change type, occlusion type and size) as well as all subject responses were sent time-stamped to the eyelink system in order to enable a retrospective in-depth analysis.

Results

Data analysis

All received data were inspected offline to decide whether they were recorded correctly or should be discarded. Trials were discarded when at the time of image change the eliciting event (saccade, fixation, blink) was over or when (e.g. due to noise) the detection algorithm had proven incorrect with respect to the event. In particular when a blink was used as the intended occlusion and the maximal wait time of 6 s was exceeded, the trial was discarded in order to avoid systematic differences in exposure time. Five subjects with less than ten observations in any of six cells (occlusion types by relevance) were excluded from further analysis, resulting in a final data set of 19 subjects with a total of 4461 valid trials. Guessing did not to play a significant role in the blank condition: the average false alarm rate in the 'no change' condition was 5.3%, the highest individual rate among all subjects was 8.3%. The blink rate over all subjects was 14 per minute on average with an average duration of 140 ms. Saccades were made four times per second on average with an average duration of 43 ms. Two $3 \times 2 \times 2$ (occlusion × relevance × change-type) repeated measures anova's were performed to test significances of the experimental factors on detection rate and detection time, respectively. Fixation was used as a control condition. Since the occurrence of saccades, blinks and fixations cannot be exactly predicted, exposure times

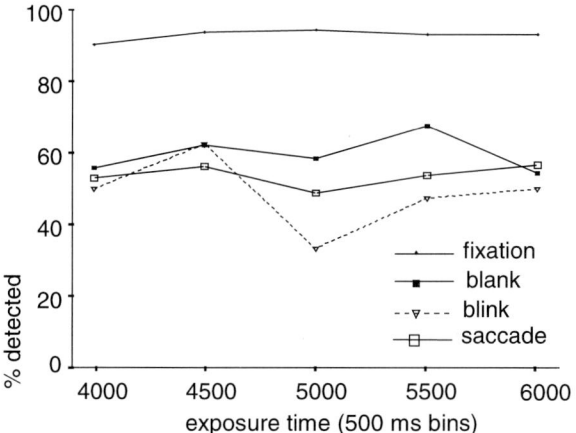

Fig. 2. Detection rate as a function of exposure time.

were not exactly matched. In order to test whether the analyses were possibly biased due to differences in exposure time, detection rate was plotted against exposure times in 500 ms bins per occlusion condition (Fig. 2).

Exposure time was measured as the time elapsed between first appearance of the original image and the initiation of the occlusion. As the figure shows, there is no systematic increase in detection rate as a function of exposure time. Analysis of variance using five bins of exposure time (4000 to 6000 ms) showed no effect of exposure time ($F = 1.076$, df $= 4$, $p = 0.369$) nor any interaction with occlusion mode ($F = 0.609$, df $= 8$, $p = 0.771$).

Occlusion type

The probabilities of detecting changes as a function of the type of occlusion are shown in Fig. 3A. Repeated measurement analysis of variance over the three occlusions showed no effect of occlusion on the detection probability ($F_{2,18} = 1.371$, $p = 0.257$). Pair-wise comparison using Bonferroni adjustment for multiple comparisons showed that the occlusion conditions only differed significantly from the (fixation) control condition (for all comparisons, $p < 0.001$).

Average reaction times were calculated from those trials in which a change was detected. Reaction times were measured as the interval between de-occlusion of the change and the button press. Fig. 3B shows the mean reaction times for each occlusion type and the control condition. The analysis of variance showed no effect of occlusion type ($F_{2,18} = 3.997$, $p = 0.116$). Pair-wise comparison showed that the differences between the occluded conditions and the fixation condition are highly significant (for all comparisons, $p < 0.001$), whereas none of the other comparisons yields significant differences.

Relevance

The probabilities of detecting relevant and irrelevant changes are shown in Fig. 4A for each occlusion condition, bar colors indicating the two levels of relevance. Relevance of change proves to have a large and significant ($F_{1,18} = 133.81$, $p < 0.001$)

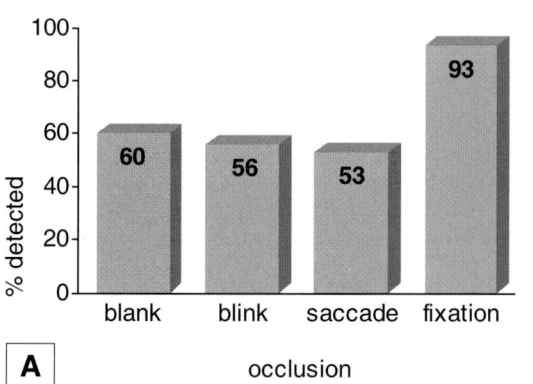
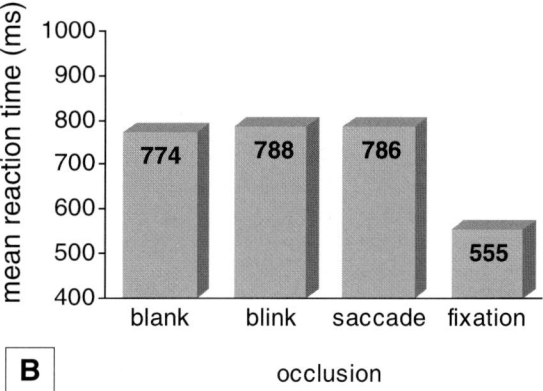

Fig. 3. (A) Mean percent detected by types of occlusion over all subjects and all images. (B) Mean reaction time by types of occlusion over all subjects and all images.

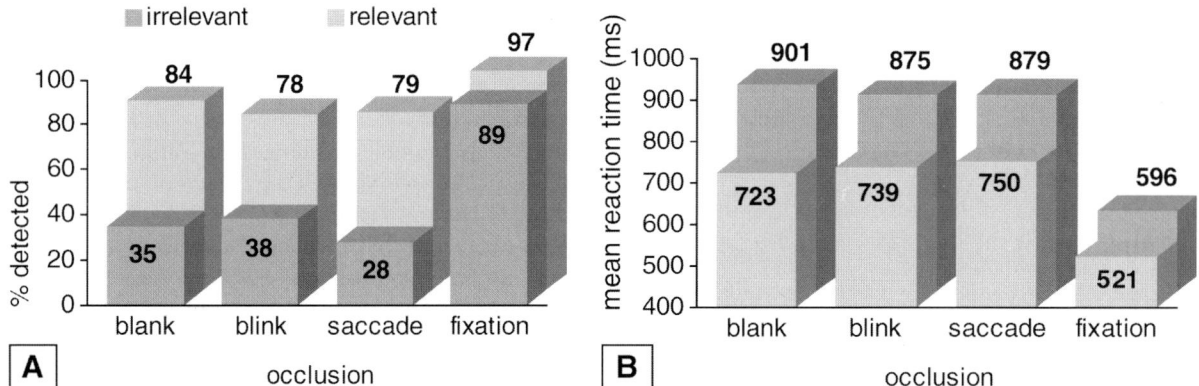

Fig. 4. (A) Mean percent detected by types of occlusion and relevance over all subjects and all images. (B) Reaction time by types of occlusion and relevance over all subjects and all images.

effect on detection rate in the expected direction. No further interactions were found.

Fig. 4B shows the estimated means of reaction times for each occlusion type, bar colors indicating the two levels of relevance. Analysis of variance showed a significant effect of relevance ($F_{1,18} = 24.22$, $p = 0.008$) on reaction time, but no further interactions.

Foveal distance

As visual acuity drops with increasing distance from the fovea, it seems reasonable to try to account for the decay of performance by a lack of visual resolution in the periphery. The distance from the fovea to the center of the change location was calculated at the moment of de-occlusion. In all cases, the average eye position during the fixation was taken as the point of reference. Fig. 5 shows the detection rate as a function of foveal distance and occlusion type, for relevant and irrelevant changes. Since the distance to change parameter was determined post hoc, the number of observations per distance category was not equal for all subjects, so a statistical analysis would contain the hazard of capitalizing on chance. There are, however, a number of stable tendencies in the data that we want to discuss.

In the first place, as can be seen in Fig. 5A, relevant

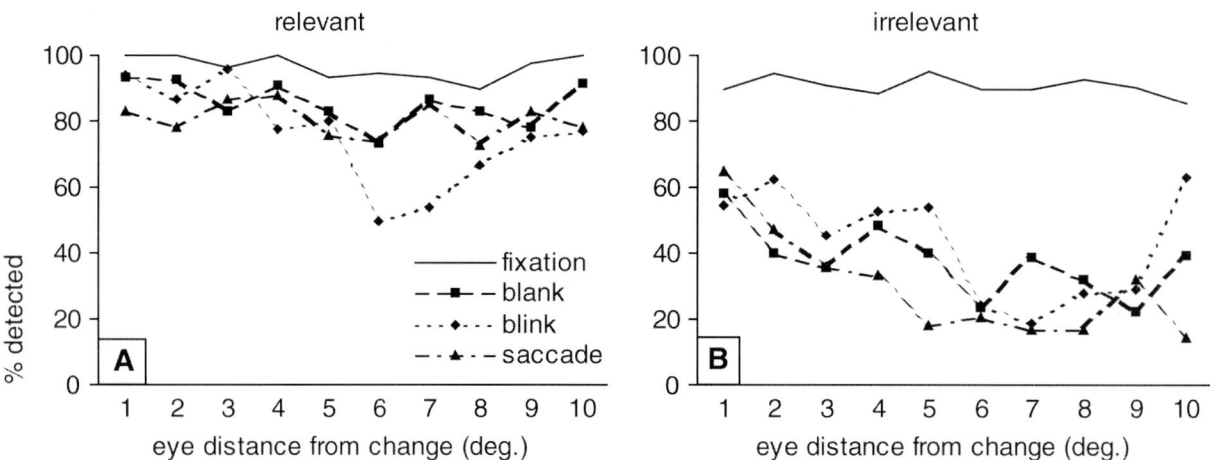

Fig. 5. Mean percent detected as a function of foveal distance and occlusion type over all subjects and all images: (A) relevant changes; (B) irrelevant changes.

changes (both occluded and unoccluded) are detected largely independent from the distance of the change location to the fovea over a range of 0 to 10°. In the case of irrelevant changes (Fig. 5B), detection rate is equally unaffected by change distance from the fovea if the change occurs during a fixation. However, if the change happens during a blink, blank or a saccade, it seems to be of advantage when the change occurs in the (para)foveal area.

Type of change

In line with several previous reports (e.g. Stelmach et al., 1984) we found that occluded insertions were detected significantly more often ($F_{1,18} = 633.22$, $p < 0.001$) and faster ($F_{1,18} = 12.94$, $p = 0.001$) than deletions (see also Velichkovsky et al., 2002). In particular we were interested to see if such differences would apply only to changes within the foveal range, or rather over the whole retinal array.

Fig. 6 clearly shows that insertions are detected considerably more often than deletions in our study. Moreover, the data also demonstrate that insertions are detected almost equally well over a large range of distances from the fovea, whereas detecting deletions gets worse as the distance between the fovea and the locus of a changing event increases.

General discussion and outlook

Blinks, blanks or saccades: it doesn't really matter

In the present study, we tested whether change blindness occurs equally often in three different situations containing a global temporary occlusion during which a change takes place. Our results show that all occlusion types have an essentially equal effect on change detection, also with respect to their interaction with other independent and dependent variables. This conclusion has an important implication for our understanding of change-blindness phenomena.

As a matter of fact, blanks, blinks and saccades represent different degrees of the subject's endogenous control over the global disruptions of visual stimulation. Recently, Shore and Klein (2000) compared a change detection study using the simultaneous inspection paradigm (a pair of photographic images presented next to each other) with a flicker study. Both paradigms showed an advantage for detection of central interest changes when the images were presented upright. When the images were inverted the advantage disappeared in the simultaneous condition — in the flicker condition, the center-of-interest effect remained intact. This difference, however, may be related to the highly specific conditions

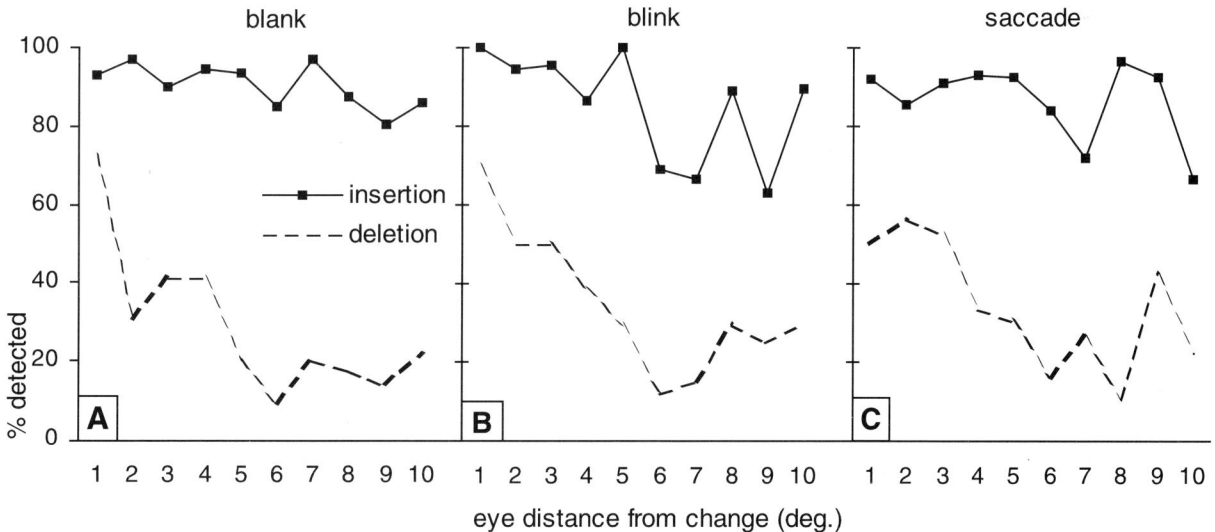

Fig. 6. Mean percent detected as a function of foveal distance and change type over all subjects and all images: (A) blank condition; (B) blink condition; (C) saccade condition.

of the flicker paradigm. We will discuss similarly deviating results obtained in dynamic presentation conditions at the end of the chapter. As Rensink (2002) points out, it is also of importance to distinguish between change and difference: a change refers to a transformation or modification of a single structure over time, whereas a difference refers to a lack of similarity in the properties of two structures. Thus detecting a difference in the simultaneous inspection study and detecting a change in the flicker study represent two different kinds of activities. In our study a single transition instead of a flicker paradigm was used and there appears to be no significant difference, neither in change detection rate nor in change detection latency, between changes occurring during endogenously induced occlusions and exogenous screen disruptions imposed on the subject. Furthermore, the difference between relevant and irrelevant changes remained the same in all occlusion settings.

Similar to O'Regan et al. (2000), we found that overall occluded changes were detected well when they took place within the foveal range. We furthermore found this to be true for blanks, blinks as well as for saccades. Beyond the foveal range — in all occlusion conditions — there was a decrease in performance for irrelevant changes. Relevant changes were almost equally likely to be detected anywhere in the visual field.

Relevance and type of change: what is left of change blindness?

Our basic motivation in conducting this study was to find out to what degree saccades and blinks may create difficulties in visual processing of naturalistic scenes from traffic situations. Our experimental results show that the occlusion method has no effect on detection rate and reaction time, so that naturally occurring blinks and saccades lead to the same functional blindness effects as laboratory blank displays. Thus, although most of the change-blindness paradigms are irrelevant to everyday life events, it has to be borne in mind that a simple natural event like a blink or a saccade may severely hamper detection of changes to the environment. On first sight, this conclusion seems to be impressive and even frightening with respect to driving, because the overall change detection rate is as low as 55%.

In line with a recent proposal "to cure change blindness" (Henderson and Hollingworth, 2002), we would prefer a more differential analysis here. First of all, the detection of relevant changes is considerably better than that of irrelevant changes, though subjects continue to miss about 20% of the changes and even when the changes are detected, reaction times are still almost 220 ms slower than when the change occurs during a fixation. Due to our traffic-related definition of relevance we want to stress that these differences may not be comparable to those found by Rensink et al. (1997) and others. The next step in the dismantling of change blindness is to consider the detection difference due to the types of change. Insertions are likely to be detected almost always. Obviously, the sudden insertion (not disappearance) of relevant objects is of particular importance in real world situations.

What is left of the change-blindness effects, however, is the exceptionally long reaction time. Despite the nearly perfect detection rate, relevant insertions were reported with a delay of approximately 180 ms in comparison to the fixation condition (Velichkovsky et al., 2002). This delay cannot be dismissed on practical reasons, i.e. with respect to road-traffic safety. Perhaps it is also of theoretical significance as the label 'ceiling effect' says nothing about underlying processing. We suspect that the contrast of a high detection rate and still rather slow motor responses is related to the fact that global disruptions of image can induce rudimentary startle and orienting states with their inhibitory consequences for sensorimotor processes (Schlenoff, 1985; Velichkovsky and Pannasch, 2002). A more endogenous cause for the delay (e.g. in the sense of re-entrant processes in masking and change-blindness phenomena) also seems to be feasible in view of the recent reports that both change blindness and motor inhibition can be produced by purely cognitive factors such as task switching (Pannasch et al., 2001; Enns et al., 2002).

Insertions were detected almost equally well anywhere in the periphery, up to distances of 10° from the fovea. Simons' (1996) proposal, that the difference in detection of insertions and deletions results from adding an object to a 'previously empty array' does not explain this if we take the 'previously empty array' literally, since in the present experiment there were hardly any previously empty arrays —

rather, objects were superimposed on an articulated background. In a more figurative sense, however, a deletion may be considered as the removal of visual information from the environment resulting in the inability to relate any stored knowledge to it, and hence as a physical implementation of inattentional amnesia as implied by Wolfe (1999b): if an object is removed from the physical environment while it is not currently attended, there is no way of retrieving any information about it from visual memory. Contrary, if an object is inserted that has neither been encoded nor discarded, then it is likely that the insertion advantage lies in its novelty, rather than in memory for features of the superimposed region. We are inclined to consider the data on insertions in the framework of current studies of expertise (in particular, Reingold et al., 2001) rather than as a manifestation of low-level ambient vision (Trevarthen, 1968) because the detection performance strongly interacts with semantic relevance of the changes across the visual field.

Change detection in dynamically changing displays

Due to the fact that we worked with static scenes the ecological validity of our results remains somewhat unclear. To provide further evidence about the extent of change blindness in road traffic, we conducted a follow-up driving simulator study (Velichkovsky et al., 2002). This time we used only traffic-relevant inserted changes that occurred during blanks or fixations. As in the present experiment, a one-shot detection paradigm was used. Against our expectations, we found systematic differences between occlusion modes. If considered in terms of a speed-accuracy trade-off, the results can be summarized by the following conclusion: as the modes of occlusion, blinks and blanks are related to the best performance in change detection, saccades to the worst, the detection in the control fixation condition is lying somewhere in-between.

What is the reason for this astonishing reversal of 'change blindness'? One could suppose that in the dynamic setting blanks serve as a cue telling the subject if not *where* then at least *when* to search for change. There is compelling evidence against such explanation, however. Firstly, false alarm rate was extremely low in blanks. Secondly and more important, the cuing hypothesis cannot explain a perfect change detection with blinks. We prefer another approach by stressing one similarity of otherwise so different blanks and blinks in one parameter: the duration of occlusion. This parameter also differentiates blinks and blanks as a whole from saccades. With their duration of about 40 ms, saccadic occlusions lead to a relatively low rate of change detection as well as slow reaction times. The question is then, what may happen on the continuum of occlusion durations from 40 to 150 ms that interact with dynamics of the situation and overturn the 'change blindness' effect? A preliminary answer can be found in research on visual motion and causality perception (Michotte, 1946/1963) that demonstrates that occlusions of about 100 ms and more disrupt the perceptual continuity of visual events, transforming them to a short static snapshot. In a static environment, global occlusions obscure the local transient caused by a change and thereby prevent attention from being attracted to it. A dynamic situation is changing constantly. In contrast to static scenes, the multitude of distracting transients (in motion fields but perhaps also in the flicker condition) makes it likely that attention is equally driven to all potential regions of change. Hence, any interruption that is sufficiently long can counteract the attentional load imposed by the flow of moving gradients and contours and thus enables subjects to see that a change has taken place (see also Kourtzi and Nakayama, 2002).

Further empirical studies on change detection errors in the real world (Levin and Simons, 1997), simulated environments (Wallis and Bülthoff, 2000; Shinoda et al., 2001) and motion pictures (Simons and Levin, 1998) can surely provide a better understanding of change blindness in dynamically changing displays. Current studies on change blindness in dynamic settings, however, differ largely with respect to their methods (e.g. Saiki, 2002, this volume). Although the nature of the effects discovered in our experiments clearly needs further investigation, we meanwhile recommend great caution in extrapolating results from static 'change blindness' studies to dynamic situations.

Acknowledgements

Major part of the work described in this chapter was supported by research grants of the BMW-AG, Munich. We would like to thank Alexandra Rothert and Jens Helmert for their help in conducting the experiment. We also thank one anonymous reviewer, Jun Saiki and Eyal Reingold for helpful comments on an earlier draft.

References

Archambault, A., O'Donnell, C. and Schyns, P.G. (1999) Blind to object changes: when learning the same object at different levels of categorization modifies its perception. *Psychol. Sci.*, 10(3): 249–255.

Barbato, G., Ficca, G., Muscettola, G., Fichele, M., Beatrice, M. and Rinaldi, F. (2000) Diurnal variation in spontaneous eye-blink rate. *Psychiatry Res.*, 93(2): 145–151.

Baxt, N. (1871) Ueber die Zeit, welche noethig ist, damit ein Gesichtseindruck zum Bewusstsein kommt und ueber die Groesse (Extension) der bewussten Wahrnehmung bei einem Gesichtseindrucke von gegebener Dauer [On the time that a visual impression needs to come to consciousness and on the extension of the conscious perception for a visual impression of a given duration]. *Pfluegers Arch. Gesamte Physiol.*, 4: 274–311.

Blackmore, S.J., Brelstaff, G., Nelson, K. and Troscianko, T. (1995) Is the richness of our visual world an illusion? Transsaccadic memory for complex scenes. *Perception*, 24: 1075–1081.

Crundall, D.E. and Underwood, G. (1998) Effects of experience and processing demands on visual information acquisition in drivers. *Ergonomics*, 41: 448–458.

Dennett, D.C. (1991) *Consciousness Explained*. Little, Brown and Company, Boston, MA.

Enns, J.T. and Di Lollo, V. (2000) What's new in visual masking? *Trends Cogn. Sci.*, 4(9): 345–352.

Enns, J.T., Visser, T.A.W., Kawahara, J. and Di Lollo, V. (2002) Visual masking and task switching in the attentional blink. In: K. Shapiro (Ed.), *The Limits of Attention: Temporal Constraints on Human Information Processing*. Oxford University Press, New York, NY, pp. 65–81.

Fernandez-Duque, D. and Thornton, I.M. (2000) Change detection without awareness: do explicit reports underestimate the representation of change in the visual system? *Vis. Cognit.*, 7(1–3): 324–344.

Friedman, A. (1979) Framing pictures: the role of knowledge in automatized encoding and memory for gist. *J. Exp. Psychol. Gen.*, 108: 316–355.

Grimes, J. (1996) On the failure to detect changes in scenes across saccades. In: K. Akins (Ed.), *Perception (Vancouver Studies in Cognitive Sciences)*. Vol. 2, Oxford University Press, New York, NY, pp. 89–110.

Haines, R.F. (1991) A breakdown in simultaneous information processing. In: G. Obrecht and L. Stark (Eds.), *Presbyopia Research*. Plenum, New York, NY, pp. 171–175.

Hayhoe, M.M., Bensinger, D.G. and Ballard, D.H. (1998) Task constraints in visual working memory. *Vision Res.*, 38: 125–137.

Henderson, J.M. (1992) Object identification in context: the visual processing of natural scenes. *Can. J. Psychol.*, 46: 319–341.

Henderson, J.M. and Hollingworth, A. (1999) The role of fixation position in detecting changes across saccades. *Psychol. Sci.*, 10(5): 438–443.

Henderson, J.M. and Hollingworth, A. (2002) A cure for change blindness. *Behav. Brain Sci.*, 24(5): in press.

Irwin, D.E., Yantis, S. and Jonides, J. (1983) Evidence against visual integration across saccadic eye movements. *Percept. Psychophys.*, 34(1): 49–57.

Kanwisher, N.G. (1987) Repetition blindness: type recognition without token individuation. *Cognition*, 27: 117–143.

Kourtzi, Z. and Nakayama, K. (2002) Distinct mechanisms for the representation of moving and static objects. *Vis. Cognit.*, 9: 248–264.

Levin, D.T. and Simons, D.J. (1997) Failure to detect changes to attended objects in motion pictures. *Psychon. Bull. Rev.*, 4(4): 501–506.

Mack, A. and Rock, I. (1998) *Inattentional Blindness*. MIT Press, Cambridge, MA.

Macknik, S., Fisher, B. and Bridgeman, B. (1991) Flicker distorts visual space constancy. *Vision Res.*, 31: 2057–2064.

Michotte, A. (1946/1963) *The Perception of Causality* (T.R. Miles and E. Miles, Transl.), Methuen, London.

Most, S.B., Simons, D.J., Scholl, B.J., Jimenez, R., Clifford, E. and Chabris, C.F. (2001) How not to be seen: the contribution of similarity and selective ignoring to sustained inattentional blindness. *Psychol. Sci.*, 12(1): 9–17.

Mourant, R.R. and Rockwell, T.H. (1972) Strategies of visual search by novice and experienced drivers. *Hum. Factors*, 14: 325–335.

Neisser, U. (1979) The control of information pickup in selective looking. In: A.D. Pick (Ed.), *Perception and its Development: A Tribute to Eleanor J. Gibson*. Lawrence Erlbaum, Hillsdale, NJ, pp. 201–219.

Newby, E.A. and Rock, I. (1998) Inattentional blindness as a function of proximity to the focus of attention. *Perception*, 27: 1025–1040.

O'Regan, J.K., Rensink, R.A. and Clark, J.J. (1996) Mudsplashes render picture changes invisible. *Invest. Ophthalmol. Vis. Sci.*, 37: 213.

O'Regan, J.K., Rensink, R.A. and Clark, J.J. (1999) Change-blindness as a result of 'mudsplashes'. *Nature*, 398(6722): 34.

O'Regan, J.K., Deubel, H., Clark, J.J. and Rensink, R.A. (2000) Picture changes during blinks: looking without seeing and seeing without looking. *Vis. Cognit.*, 7(1–3): 191–211.

Pannasch, S., Dornhoefer, S.M., Unema, P.J.A. and Velichkovsky, B.M. (2001) The omnipresent prolongation of visual fixations: saccades are inhibited by changes in situation or subject's activity. *Vision Res.*, 41(25–26): 3345–3351.

Pashler, H. (1988) Familiarity and visual change detection. *Percept. Psychophys.*, 44(4): 369–378.

Phillips, W.A. and Singer, W. (1974) Function and interaction of on and off transients in vision, I. Psychophysics. *Exp. Brain Res.*, 19: 493–506.

Rayner, K. and Pollatsek, A. (1983) Is visual information integrated across saccades? *Percept. Psychophys.*, 34(1): 39–48.

Reingold, E.M., Charness, N., Pomplun, M. and Stampe, D.M. (2001) Visual span in expert chess players: evidence from eye movements. *Psychol. Sci.*, 12(1): 48–55.

Rensink, R.A. (2000) When good observers go bad: change blindness, inattentional blindness, and visual experience. *Psyche*, 6(9).

Rensink, R.A. (2002) Change detection. *Annu. Rev. Psychol.*, 53: 245–277.

Rensink, R.A., O'Regan, J.K. and Clark, J.J. (1997) To see or not to see: the need for attention to perceive changes in scenes. *Psychol. Sci.*, 8: 368–373.

Rensink, R.A., O'Regan, J.K. and Clark, J.J. (2000) On the failure to detect changes in scenes across brief interruptions. *Vis. Cognit.*, 7(1–3): 127–145.

Saiki, J. (2002) Multiple-object permanence tracking: limitation in maintenance and transformation of perceptual objects. In: J. Hyönä, D. Munoz, W. Heide and R. Radach (Eds.), *The Brain's Eye: Neurobiological and Clinical Aspects of Oculomotor Research*. Progress in Brain Research, Vol. 140, Elsevier, Amsterdam, pp. 133–148.

Schlenoff, D.H. (1985) The startle responses of blue jays to Catocala (Lepidoptera: Noctuidae) prey models. *Anim. Behav.*, 33: 1057–1067.

Scott-Brown, K.C., Baker, M.R. and Orbach, H.S. (2000) Comparison blindness. *Vis. Cognit.*, 7(1–3): 254–267.

Shapiro, K.L., Arnell, K.M. and Raymond, J.E. (1997) The attentional blink. *Trends Cogn. Sci.*, 1(8): 291–296.

Shore, D.I. and Klein, R.M. (2000) The effects of scene inversion on change blindness. *J. Gen. Psychol.*, 127(1): 27–43.

Shinoda, H., Hayhoe, M.M. and Shrivastava, A. (2001) What controls attention in natural environments? *Vision Res.*, 41(25-26): 3535–3545.

Simons, D.J. (1996) In sight, out of mind: when object representations fail. *Psychol. Sci.*, 7(5): 301–305.

Simons, D.J. (2000) Current approaches to change blindness. *Vis. Cognit.*, 7(1-3): 1–16.

Simons, D.J. and Chabris, C.F. (1999) Gorillas in our midst: sustained inattentional blindness for dynamic events. *Perception*, 28: 1059–1074.

Simons, D.J. and Levin, D.T. (1998) Failure to detect changes to people in a real-world interaction. *Psychon. Bull. Rev.*, 5(4): 644–649.

Simons, D.J., Franconeri, S.L. and Reimer, R.L. (2000) Change blindness in the absence of visual disruption. *Perception*, 29: 1143–1154.

Smilek, D., Eastwood, J.D. and Merikle, P.M. (2000) Does unattended information facilitate change detection? *J. Exp. Psychol. Hum. Percept. Perform.*, 26(2): 480–487.

Stelmach, L.B., Bourassa, C.M. and Di Lollo, V. (1984) Detection of stimulus change: the hypothetical roles of visual transient responses. *Percept. Psychophys.*, 35(3): 245–255.

Trevarthen, C. (1968) Two visual systems in primates. *Psych. Fo.*, 31: 321–337.

Velichkovsky, B.M. (1982) Visual cognition and its spatial–temporal context. In: F. Klix, J. Hoffmann and E. van der Meer (Eds.), *Cognitive Research in Psychology*. North-Holland, Amsterdam, pp. 112–134.

Velichkovsky, B.M. and Pannasch, S. (2002) In search of the ultimate evidence: the fastest visual reaction adapts to environment, not retinal locations. *Behav. Brain Sci.*, in press.

Velichkovsky, B.M., Dornhoefer, S.M., Kopf, M., Helmert, J. and Joos, M. (2002) Change detection and occlusion modes in road-traffic scenarios. *Transport Res. F*, 5(2): 99–109.

Wallis, G. and Bülthoff, H.H. (2000) What's in scene and not seen. *Vis. Cognit.*, 7(1-3): 175–190.

Werner, S. and Thies, B. (2000) Is 'change blindness' attenuated by domain-specific expertise? An expert–novices comparison of change detection in football images. *Vis. Cognit.*, 7(1-3): 163–173.

Wolfe, J.M. (1999a) Visual experience: less than you think, more than you know. In: C. Taddei-Ferretti and C. Musio (Eds.), *Neuronal Basis and Psychological Aspects of Consciousness*. Vol. 8, World Scientific, Singapore, pp. 165–185.

Wolfe, J.M. (1999b) Inattentional amnesia. In: V. Coltheart (Ed.), *Fleeting Memories*. MIT Press, Cambridge, MA, pp. 71–94.

CHAPTER 9

Multiple-object permanence tracking: limitation in maintenance and transformation of perceptual objects

Jun Saiki *

Graduate School of Informatics, Kyoto University, Yoshida-Honmachi, Sakyo-ku, Kyoto, 606-8501 Japan

Abstract: Research on change blindness and transsaccadic memory revealed that a limited amount of information is retained across visual disruptions in visual working memory. It has been proposed that visual working memory can hold four to five coherent object representations. To investigate their maintenance and transformation in dynamic situations, I devised an experimental paradigm called multiple-object permanence tracking (MOPT) that measures memory for multiple feature–location bindings in dynamic situations. Observers were asked to detect any color switch in the middle of a regular rotation of a pattern with multiple colored disks behind an occluder. The color-switch detection performance dramatically declined as the pattern rotation velocity increased, and this effect of object motion was independent of the number of targets. The MOPT task with various shapes and colors showed that color–shape conjunctions are not available in the MOPT task. These results suggest that even completely predictable motion severely reduces our capacity of object representations, from four to only one or two.

Introduction

Our visual world is dynamic, multidimensional, and contains multiple objects. Objects have various perceptual features such as color, texture, shape, and size; and they are moving and changing their perceptual properties across time. Therefore, to perceive and understand visual scenes and events, we need to make correspondences of feature values to multiple objects, and to keep track of them as they move.

Recently, some researchers suggest that our perception of stable and coherent scenes may be an illusion, and that our internal representation of visual objects and scenes is much less than we think (O'Regan, 1992; Ballard et al., 1997; Horowitz and Wolfe, 1998). One of the most striking demonstrations is 'change blindness' (Levin and Simons, 1997; Rensink et al., 1997; Simons and Levin, 1998; and many others), which has a close relation to the literature of transsaccadic memory (Irwin et al., 1983; Irwin, 1991, 1992; Deubel et al., 1996; McConkie and Currie, 1996; and many others). Although change blindness and transsaccadic memory research revealed that our visual cognition might be functioning with rather schematic representations of the environment, we still do not know what they are and how they are formed and maintained. This chapter first reviews the change blindness research and its implications, then focuses on the issue of maintenance and transformation of episodic representation of multiple objects, and introduces some experimental work with multiple-object permanence tracking (MOPT) paradigm. The study with the MOPT paradigm revealed that the capacity of visual working memory strongly depends on spatiotemporal characteristics of objects.

---

* Correspondence to: J. Saiki, Graduate School of Informatics, Kyoto University, Yoshida-Honmachi, Sakyo-ku, Kyoto, 606-8501 Japan. Tel.: +81-75-753-3147; Fax: +81-75-753-3147; E-mail: saiki@i.kyoto-u.ac.jp

Change blindness and its implications

The important question shared by both change blindness and transsaccadic memory literature is the visual stability problem: how does the visual world appear stable despite the discontinuities caused by saccades and other visual disruptions? Eye movement research has revealed that the visual system is not superposing pre- and post-saccadic images (Irwin et al., 1983), but retaining a limited amount of abstract visual information (Irwin, 1992). Based on these findings, saccade target theory has been proposed as a theory of visual stability (Deubel et al., 1996; McConkie and Currie, 1996). The saccade target theory assumes that critical features of the saccade target are used to maintain transsaccadic stability.

Change blindness is considered as an extension of the transsaccadic stability problem to more general visual cognition. A number of studies show that even without saccade-contingent changes, people are often blind to changes across discontinuities in scenes, motion pictures, and social interactions (Levin and Simons, 1997; Rensink et al., 1997; Simons and Levin, 1998). In the context of change blindness, the saccade target objects appear to correspond to attended objects (Rensink et al., 1997), though there are some data suggesting that attention is not sufficient to detect changes (Levin and Simons, 1997).

What is common to the change blindness and transsaccadic memory literature is that despite our subjective stability of visual cognition, only a limited amount of information is retained across visual disruptions. Visual attention in a broader sense (including eye fixation) appears to be an important determinant of information to be retained. As for the amount of retained information, visual short-term memory (VSTM) or visual working memory (VWM) appears to be an underlying mechanism, because VSTM or VWM is postulated as storing a limited amount (sometimes claimed to be four objects) of abstract visual information. Indeed, Irwin (1991) suggested that transsaccadic memory is equivalent to VSTM. Thus, in order to understand how the visual system solves the visual stability problem in general, we should investigate visual attention and visual working memory.

To establish the visual stability, some kind of representation of the external scene should be formed, where visual attention and working memory appear to be playing key roles. Since scene representation needs to bind object features to space and time, such representation is often called episodic representation. In the following section, I will discuss the episodic representation in visual cognition.

Episodic representation in visual cognition

Episodic representation can be defined as mental representation whose featural information is bound to its spatiotemporal properties. This feature–location binding is important in visual cognition. If you are to reach some object among many distractors, you need to know the target location in addition to the target identity. In the dynamic world with multiple objects, formation of episodic representation is an indispensable ability for successful interaction with the external world.

For episodic representation to be adaptive, there seem to be two important properties: retention and transformation. Because input to our visual system is quite often disrupted by internal (such as blink, and saccade) and external (such as occlusion) causes, we need to keep information about the environment at least for a short period. At the same time, because objects in the environment are moving around and changing, we need to keep the object information by transforming internal representations.

Retention and transformation of episodic representation have been studied with these two paradigms: change detection paradigm and multiple-object tracking (MOT), respectively. The change detection paradigm is originally used to investigate visual short-term memory (Phillips, 1974; Pashler, 1988), and recently used for the evaluation of visual working memory (Luck and Vogel, 1997). Typically, a display with multiple items is briefly presented followed by a retention interval. After the interval, a second display that may contain some change from the first display, and observers' task is to judge whether the two displays are the same or different. Using the change detection paradigm, Luck and Vogel (1997) investigated the functional unit and the capacity of visual working memory. They used multiple objects defined by multiple dimensions such as color, orientation, and size. Participants' change detection performance was determined by the number of objects, not by the number of visual features, and the change detection performance was quite accurate up to four objects. Luck and Vogel interpreted this finding as showing that a functional unit of visual working memory is the representation of perceptual objects where multidimensional information is integrated, and its capacity is about four. The change detection task is suitable for investigating the retention of visual information.

In contrast, the MOT paradigm focuses on the transformation of episodic representations. The MOT was devised by Pylyshyn and Storm (1988), and studies using the MOT showed that people are able to mentally track four to five moving objects concurrently. Participants were presented a set of 10–12 items (crosses or dots) randomly placed on the display, and asked to track some of them. Then, the dots slowly moved in random directions for several seconds, followed by a test to discriminate whether a probed dot is the one they were tracking or not. Participants' performance was quite accurate as long as the number of dots to be tracked is below four or five, suggesting that the visual system can transform spatiotemporal information of four to five objects concurrently.

These two lines of research show an interesting coincidence: for both retention and transformation, the capacity limit happens to be about four. However, to make any firm conclusions from these findings, we need to investigate the relation between retention and transformation in visual working memory. There are few studies in such a direction (e.g., Scholl and Pylyshyn, 1998), and they are still not so systematic. This study is one of the first attempts to systematically investigate the relation between retention and transformation of episodic representations. Before reporting the experiments, I first discuss the implications of these experiments for the major theoretical frameworks of episodic representation.

Theories of episodic representation

There are some theoretical proposals on episodic representation, which can be classified into two broad types: object files and visual indexes. Kahneman and Treisman (1984) proposed the notion of object files. Object files are temporary episodic representations of real world objects, which are separate from the representations stored in a long-term recognition network (Kahneman et al., 1992). Each object file contains information about a particular object in a scene, and is addressed by its location at a particular time (hereafter I call this spatiotemporal location), not by any feature or identifying label. An object file collects sensory information, updates it as the sensory situation changes, and may be discarded when the object disappears from the view. Kahneman et al. assume that there is some limit to the number of object files to be stored concurrently, and some limit in the spatial/temporal gap that can be bridged. The second type is visual indexes (Pylyshyn, 1989, 1994; Ballard et al., 1997). Pylyshyn's (1989) FINST theory is an example. Pylyshyn (1989) proposed capacity-limited preattentive visual indexes called FINST (Finger of INSTantiation). FINST is a reference to a particular feature or feature cluster, and keeps pointing the same feature cluster as the cluster moves (Pylyshyn, 1989). One important property of FINST is that it does not encode any properties of the feature in question, but that it merely makes it possible to locate the feature in order to examine it further if needed. Thus, FINST can be considered as a spatiotemporal index of feature clusters, which can be constructed preattentively, but there is a capacity limit to the number of FINSTs to be activated concurrently. Pylyshyn and Storm (1988) suggested that the capacity limit is four to five by multielement tracking paradigm.

Although the object files and visual indexes share properties as episodic representation of the visual world, they have an important difference. Object file theory assumes that multiple representations of integrated features can be formed, whereas the visual index theory assumes the formation of multiple indexes, not integrated representation. This difference leads to different interpretations of the current data suggesting the capacity limit of four objects in both retention and transformation. A natural interpretation by object file theory is that we can form four object files concurrently, and they can be retained and transformed when necessary. By contrast, visual index theory interprets the finding from the MOT paradigm as concurrent maintenance of four visual indexes, but the finding from the change detection paradigm (Luck and Vogel, 1997) as successful reference of feature information via indexes. The dynamic maintenance of multiple indexes, and feature reference via indexes are separate processes, and do not necessarily have the same capacity limit.

To evaluate the plausibility of the accounts by object file theory and visual index theory, the investigation of the relation between retention and transformation of episodic representations is necessary. To this end, I devised an experimental paradigm called multiple-object permanence tracking (MOPT), where feature–location binding needs to be retained over the occlusion duration while actively transforming the binding. According to the object file theory, the observer should show the same capacity limit of about four objects, because feature–location binding itself is the functional unit. According to the visual index theory, on the other hand, it is quite likely that the capacity limit of visual working memory will be substantially reduced when retention and transformation are both necessary. This is because transformation of indexes and feature extraction via indexes are separate processes.

General method: multiple-object permanence tracking

The idea behind the multiple-object permanence tracking (MOPT) paradigm is the mixture of multiple-object tracking and change detection tasks, especially the object-permanence test used in the infant development literature (Leslie et al., 1998). In the MOT paradigm, observers do not need to maintain the binding of features (e.g., colors) and its spatiotemporal location, because the features of objects are irrelevant (usually homogeneous). On the other hand, the typical change detection task does not require tracking of objects. By combining these two paradigms, the MOPT task can investigate the maintenance and transformation of feature–location binding (see Fig. 1). Observers were shown a pattern of four colored disks and an occluder on top. By smooth rotation of the pattern and the occluder with constant angular velocities, the pattern appeared and disappeared alternately. The sequence was either regular clockwise or counterclockwise rotation throughout, containing one visible period in which the locations of two colors were switched (color switch). Observers were required to judge whether a sequence contains a color switch. Notice that detection of a color switch needs memory for conjunction of each circle's color and spatiotemporal location. Thus the performance for the color-switch condition is the critical measure of memory for the color–location binding in this paradigm. Note that as shown in Fig. 1, when a change occurs, the post-change frames go back to normal. This is because the single frame irregularity eliminates participants' strategy to memorize the color order (most likely verbally) for first some frames and to compare it with the later frames.

Procedure

At the beginning of the experiment, participants were given the instruction with the diagram similar to Fig. 1. The differences between the two sequence types and response mappings were fully explained using the diagram. Then, participants had a block of six to eight practice trials to familiarize with the procedure. Experimental trials were made up of blocks of 24 to 30 trials, and participants could take a rest between blocks. Throughout this study, the experimental conditions were mixed randomly from trial to trial. In the main experiments, the instruction allowed participants to move their eyes to achieve their best performance. Their eye movements were not monitored.

Part I: spatiotemporal characteristics of multiple-object permanence tracking

Experiment 1: effect of angular velocity

Method

All stimuli were four colored circles with 1.2° in visual angle in diameter configured as a square. Each circle was placed at 3.6° in visual angle from the center of the occluder. Four equiluminant colors (red, green, blue, and yellow) were used, and the combinations of displayed colors were counterbalanced across trials. The occluder has four openings of 25°, through which the colored pattern was seen. The color-switch event occurred between the 4th and 7th occluded periods. The time and location of color switch were unpredictable to the observers. Observers judged whether a sequence contained any irregularity without correct feedback. The main in-

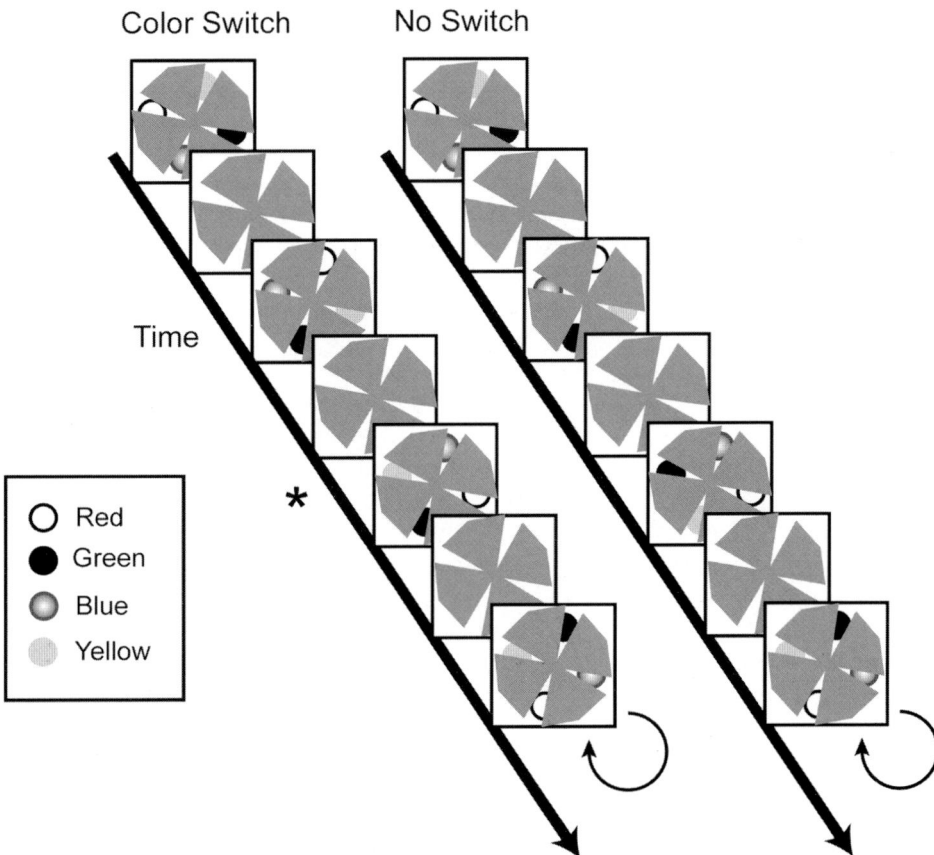

Fig. 1. Schematic illustration of the multiple-object permanence tracking task. In this example, rotation direction is clockwise, and irregularity occurs in the second frame. For the visibility the background was white but for real stimuli, background was always black. Colors were denoted by different shadings in figures in this chapter, but real stimulti were colored.

dependent variable was the angular velocity of the pattern. In order to keep the exposure duration of the pattern equivalent, the angular velocity was manipulated by the relative motion of the pattern and the occluder (Fig. 2). In the condition of 126°/s, only the pattern smoothly moved, thus the angular velocity was 126°/s. By contrast, in the condition of 0°/s, the pattern was stationary, and the occluder rotated in the opposite direction with the angular velocity of 126°/s. In the conditions of 42 and 84°/s, the pattern and the occluder rotated in the opposite directions with the velocity ratio of 1 : 2 and 2 : 1, respectively. Note that all conditions had exactly the same durations of visible period (360 ms) and occluded period (360 ms). Each condition had 24 regular trials, and 48 irregular trials, thus there were 288 experimental trials. Experimental programs were written in MATLAB, using Psychophysics Toolbox extensions (Brainard, 1997; Pelli, 1997). There were seven observers including the author, and all had normal color vision.

Results and discussion

Fig. 3 shows corrected hit rates as a function of angular velocity. Corrected hit rate was obtained by $1 - (1 - \text{hit})/(1 - \text{FA})$, following Pelli (1985). As shown in Fig. 3, mean hit rate declined monotonically as the angular velocity increased, $F(3, 18) = 20.53$, $p < 0.001$. In the 0°/s condition, the hit rate was above 0.9, which is consistent with the findings of Luck and Vogel (1997). In the other conditions, the accuracy was analogous to Saiki (1999) using flicker displays. The impairment in these conditions was

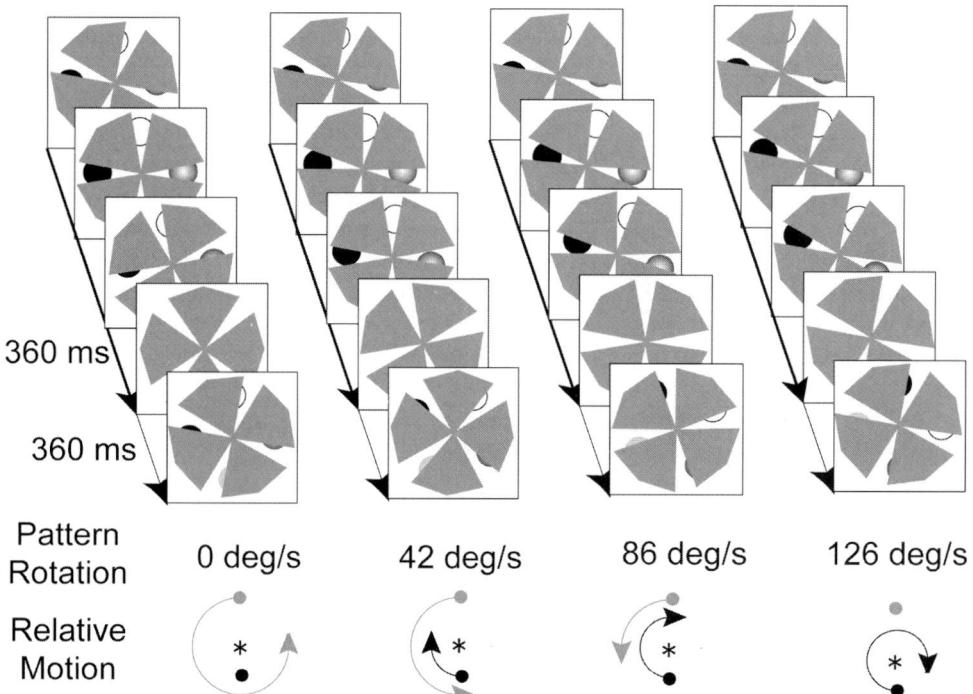

Fig. 2. Schematic illustration of the manipulation of angular velocity in Experiment 1.

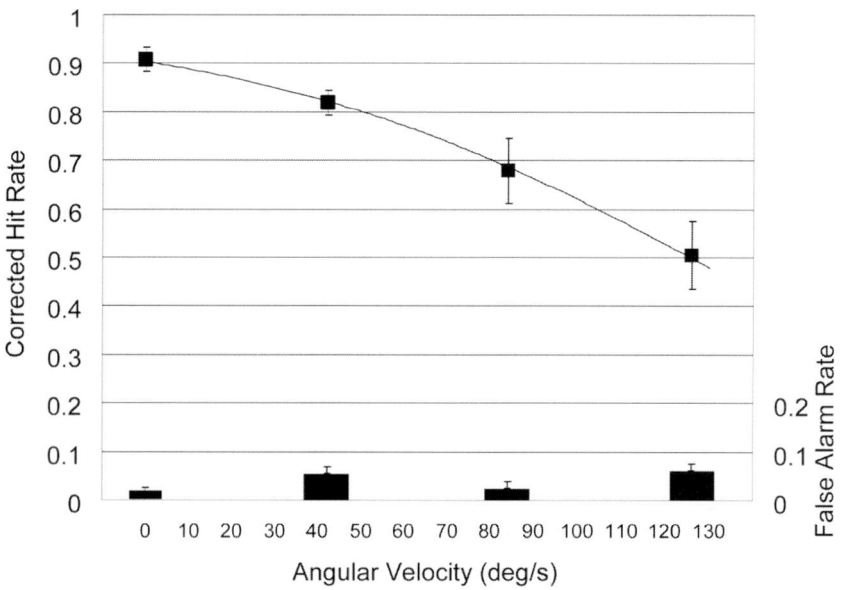

Fig. 3. Mean corrected hit rates in Experiment 1. Error bars denote the standard errors. Bars are false alarm rates. A fitting curve was obtained from the uncertainty model.

not due to tracking failure, because pattern motion was three to four times slower than the known speed limit of attentive tracking of visible patterns (about 360° rotation per second, see Verstraten et al., 2000). Furthermore, the impairment was not due to the failure in perceiving colors in motion displays, because previous experiments showed that observers had no difficulty in detecting the replacement of one color with a new one (Saiki, 1999). False alarm rates are denoted by bars in Fig. 3; they were low in all angular velocity conditions.

Experiment 2: effect of occlusion duration

Experiment 1 showed that our performance of color-switch detection impaired as the angular velocity of the pattern increased. Because of the constant occlusion duration, it is unclear whether the determinant of color-switch detection is the amount of angular displacement during the occluded period (spatial displacement), or the angular velocity (spatiotemporal displacement). To address this issue, Experiment 2 manipulated the duration of occlusion in addition to the angular velocity.

Method

The materials were the same as those in Experiment 1, except for the following changes. There were two independent variables, angular velocity and occlusion duration. Angular velocity conditions were 0, 63 and 126°/s. In the condition of 63°, the pattern and occluder rotated with a velocity ratio of 1:1. Occlusion duration conditions were 520 ms, 360 ms, 200 ms and 40 ms. Duration of one cycle (visible and occlusion period) was fixed to 720 ms. Occlusion duration was manipulated by the opening of the occluder (Fig. 4). There were 576 experimental trials. There were six observers including the author, and all had normal color vision.

Results and discussion

Fig. 5 shows the mean corrected hit rates as a function of occlusion duration for each angular velocity condition. The hit rate declined as a function of occlusion duration in all three angular velocity conditions, $F(3, 15) = 49.55$, $p < 0.0001$, and again the angular velocity had significant effects on detection performance, $F(2, 10) = 25.81$, $p < 0.0005$.

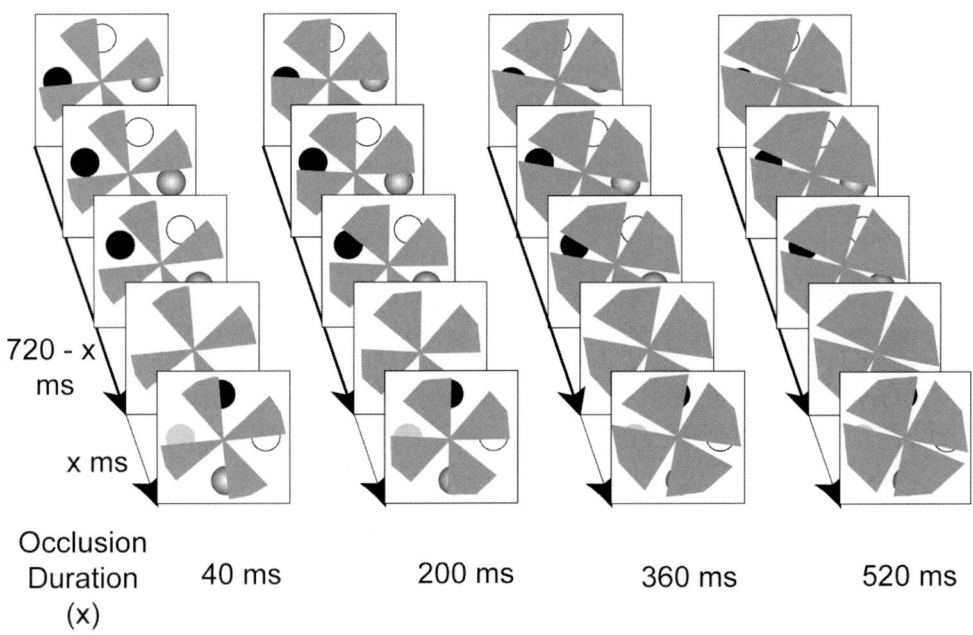

Fig. 4. Schematic illustration of the manipulation of the occlusion duration in Experiment 2.

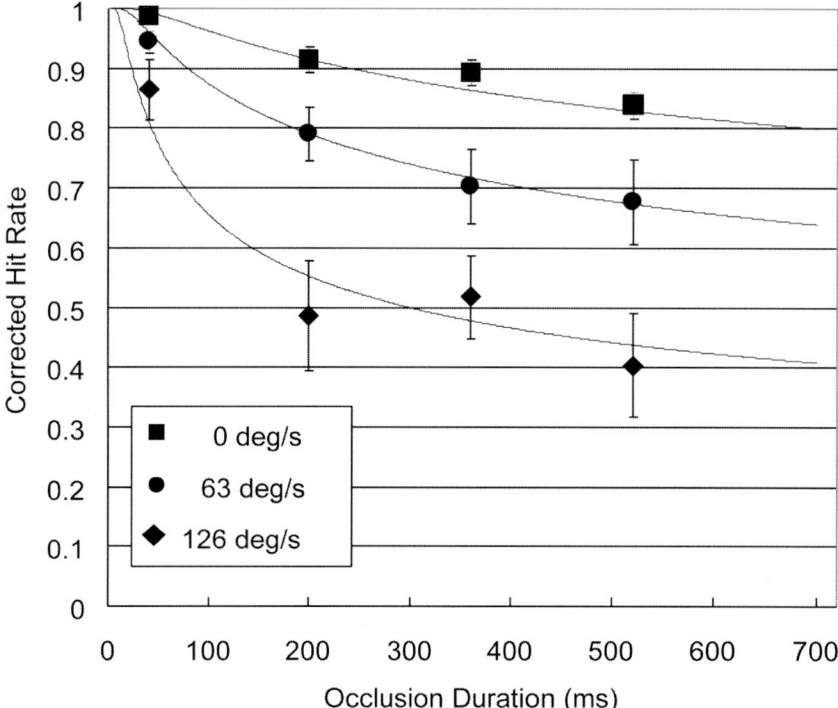

Fig. 5. Mean corrected hit rates in Experiment 2. Fitting curves were obtained from the uncertainty model.

An ANOVA revealed the significant interaction of angular velocity and occlusion duration as well, $F(6, 30) = 4.99$, $p < 0.005$. As detailed below, however, the model-based analysis revealed that the interaction could be accounted for by the modulation of the threshold of the forgetting curves by the angular velocity.

Experiment 3: capacity in terms of the number of targets

Experiments 1 and 2 showed that our performance of color-switch detection impaired as a function of angular velocity and occlusion duration. In the framework of the working memory literature, the effect of angular velocity can be considered as the processing cost. According to the influential view of resource sharing, cognitive processing and retention systems share a limited resource, implying the trade-off between retention and processing (Daneman and Carpenter, 1980; Just and Carpenter, 1992). If there is a trade-off between processing and retention, the processing cost should be substantially reduced as the retention cost decreases. Experiment 3 addressed this issue by examining the interaction between the processing and retention costs manipulated by the angular velocity and the number of targets, respectively.

Method

The material was the same as in Experiment 1, except for the following changes. There were two independent variables, angular velocity and the number of targets. Angular velocity conditions were 0 and 126°/s. The number of targets was manipulated by precuing flash as in the MOT task. This experiment used six disks with different equiluminant colors, and at the beginning of each trial, target objects to be tracked were cued by flashing (Fig. 6). Observers were asked to detect color switch between cued targets, and ignore any switches between distractors. Color switch between a target and a distractor never occurred. The intrusion errors (respond to the color switch between distractors) were used as the indicator of accuracy in location tracking. The number

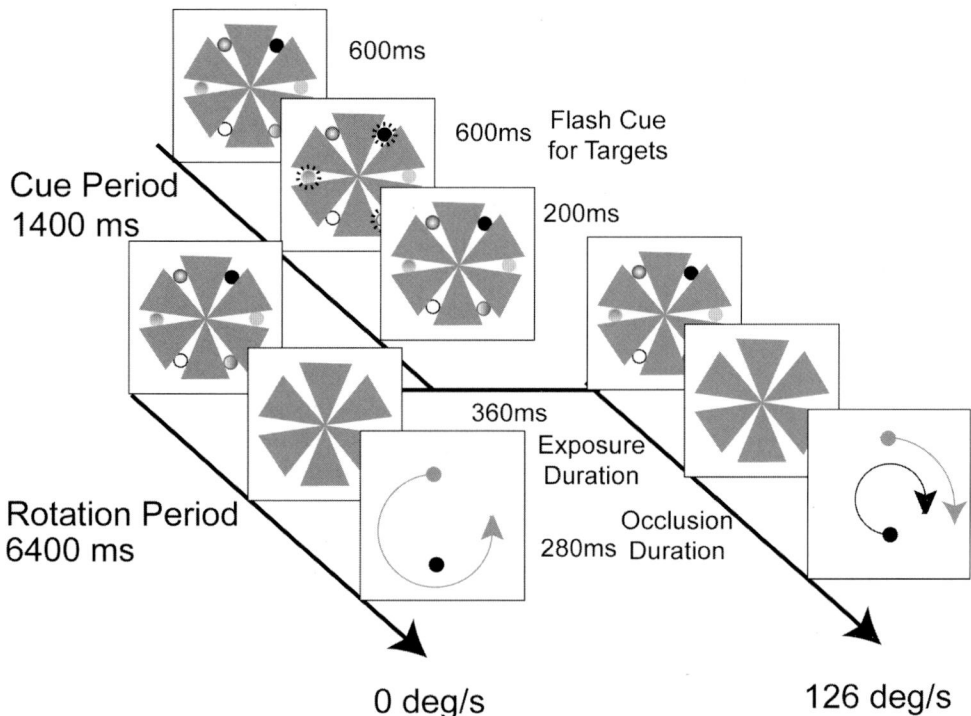

Fig. 6. Schematic illustration of the procedure in Experiment 3.

of targets was 2, 3, 4, or 6. There were 576 experimental trials. There were six observers including the author, and all had normal color vision.

Results and discussion

Fig. 7 shows the mean corrected hit rates as a function of the number of targets for each angular velocity condition, and the rates of intrusion errors and false alarms. The frequency of intrusion errors was not significantly different from false alarms (Fig. 7) ($F(1,5) = 5.67$, $p > 0.05$), confirming that the performance of MOPT tasks mainly reflects memory for color–location binding, not location memory per se. The hit rates (Fig. 7) showed significant main effects of the number of targets, $F(3,15) = 31.66$, $p < 0.0001$, and of the angular velocity ($F(1,5) = 53.07$, $p < 0.001$), but the lack of the significant interaction ($F(3,15) = 2.84$, $p > 0.05$) suggests the independent influence of the number of objects, and their angular velocity, to color-switch detection. The model assuming the independent effects of angular velocity and the number of targets also confirms the independence of retention cost and transformation cost.

Model-based analysis of the spatiotemporal characteristics of color–location binding

To understand the spatiotemporal characteristics of dynamic color–location binding, the corrected hit rates for the three experiments were fitted by an uncertainty model in the form of a Weibull function (Pelli, 1985). The model had the following form:

$$P_c^*(t) = 1 - \exp\left[-\left(\frac{\alpha N^{1/\beta}\exp(-\gamma^\omega/\beta)}{\log(t)}\right)^\beta\right] \quad (1)$$

where t is the occlusion duration, N is the number of targets, and ω is the angular velocity. α, β, γ are the parameters of the model. P_c^* is the hit rate corrected for guessing.

Simply put, the model operates with a number of independent task-relevant detectors by taking the maximum of their output. The proposed model assumes that (1) the effective number of detectors is a decreasing function of the number of targets, (2) it

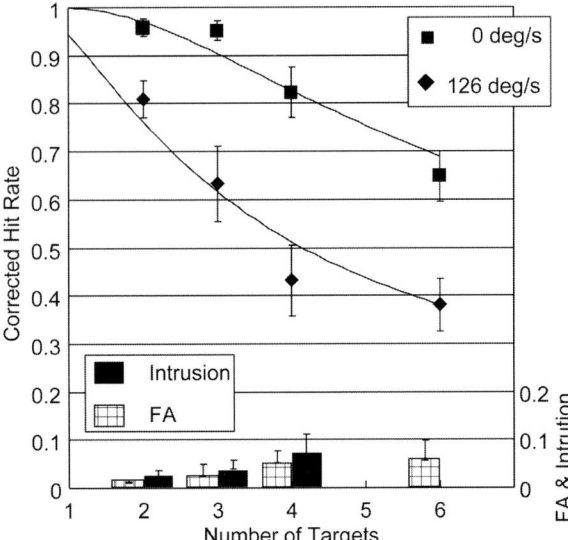

Fig. 7. Mean corrected hit rates in Experiment 3. Filled and striped bars were mean proportion of intrusion errors and false alarms, respectively. Fitting curves were obtained from the uncertainty model.

decays exponentially with the angular velocity, and (3) performance of each detector is a Weibull function of the occlusion duration with the fixed slope parameter. Overall, the model could account for the data of all experiments quite well (R^2: 0.999, 0.972 and 0.961 for Experiments 1, 2 and 3, respectively) with similar parameter values (ranges: α 19.31–19.33; β 1.83–2.14; γ 1.34–1.44). The curves in Figs. 3, 5 and 7 are those fitted by the models for the data of Experiments 1, 2, 3, respectively. For comparison with other work, the conventional 75% threshold level showed that the angular velocity threshold was 66°/s (Experiment 1), life-span of object working memory in the conditions of 0°/s, 63°/s and 126°/s was 1159 ms, 276 ms and 56 ms, respectively (Experiment 2), and the capacity in terms of the number of targets for the 0°/s and 126°/s were 5.1 and 2.1 targets, respectively (Experiment 3). Note that the stationary conditions (0°/s) had threshold values consistent with the previous work. The model's assumption of the independent influences of the number of objects and their spatiotemporal properties (angular velocity) on the threshold thus suggests that these factors affect dynamic feature binding independently.

Part II: feature interactions in MOPT

Part I investigated the maintenance and transformation of color–location binding. The results showed that color–location binding is vulnerable to the objects' movements. Since the color was the only distinguishing feature of objects in Part I, it is unclear whether the impairment observed in Part I reflects the binding of location with a single feature, or the binding of location with higher-level object representation. Kanwisher (1987, 1991) proposed a type/token representational system, where type is representation of an object not bound to space and time, presumably located in long-term memory (LTM). Henderson (1994) proposed a similar dual-route model of transsaccadic object perception. According to these accounts, a relatively abstract representation of objects is available to the visual system, and if so, in the context of the MOPT task, there are some cases where feature switch can be detected without binding features to their locations. Part II addressed this issue by investigating the feature-switch detection with multiple-feature objects. Objects in Experiments 4 and 5 were defined by color and shape, and color and color, respectively. In the case of color–shape conjunction stimuli, there were four possible events: object switch, color switch, shape switch, and no switch. Observers were asked to identify the event occurring in the sequence.

There were two signatures of memory for location-independent feature conjunctions: first, color switch and shape switch are easer to detect than object switch, and second, error analysis should reveal that there are more confusions between color switch and shape switch, than other combinations. This is because color switch and shape switch contain new shape–color combinations in switch periods, whereas object switch does not. Analogous to the easy detection of color replacement (Saiki, 1999), if color–shape conjunction functions as a higher-level feature, color-switch and shape-switch detection is simply a feature detection without binding the feature to the location. At the same time, because the detection of a new color–shape combination itself cannot distinguish color switch and shape switch, there should be more confusion errors between them.

Experiment 4: MOPT with color–shape defined objects

Method

The method was identical to that of Experiment 1, except for the following changes. There were four shapes (circle, square, pentagon, and triangle) as shown in Fig. 8a. Combinations of displayed colors and shapes were counterbalanced across trials. Each object was placed at 3.2° in visual angle from the center of the occluder. There were four possible events: object switch, color switch, shape switch, and no switch. Observers were asked to identify the type of event. Each angular velocity condition had 192 trials, 48 trials for each event type, thus there were 768 experimental trials. There were five observers including the author, and all had normal color vision.

Results and discussion

Fig. 9a shows accuracy as a function of angular velocity for each event type. In general, as in Part I, there was a strong effect of angular velocity ($F(3,12) = 21.57$, $p < 0.0001$). However, the feature conjunction hypothesis was not supported. First, there was no significant advantage of color switch and shape switch over object switch. In fact, the accuracy of the object-switch condition was significantly higher than that of the shape switch ($F(1,4) = 11.33$, $p < 0.05$) and showed a marginal tendency to be higher than that of the color switch ($F(1,4) = 5.36$, $p < 0.1$). Second, the error analysis (Fig. 9b) showed that there were few confusion errors between color switch and shape switch. As shown in Fig. 9b, the mean rate of confusion errors was not significantly different from the mean false alarm rate ($F(1,4) = 2.36$). Most errors were misses.

Experiment 5: MOPT with color–color defined objects

Method

The method was identical to that of Experiment 4, except for the following changes. Instead of colored shapes, this experiment used squares with two different colors, their combinations being randomly assigned. Objects were made up of two concentric squares with different sizes, 1.4° and 0.8° of each side (Fig. 8b). Therefore, the four event types were object switch, outer switch, inner switch, and no switch. The outer and inner colors were always different. There were five observers including the author, and all had normal color vision. All observers

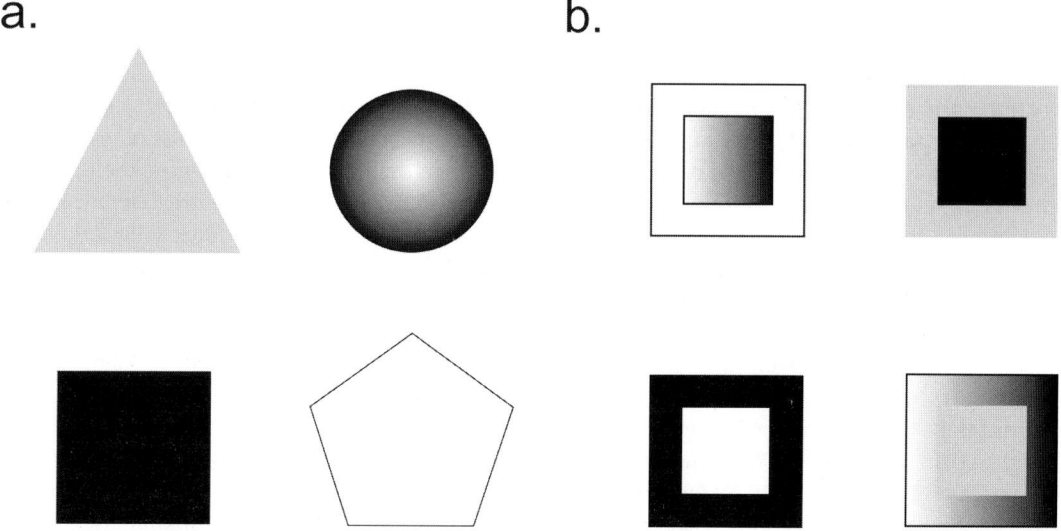

Fig. 8. Examples of objects used in Experiments 4 and 5. (a) Objects in Experiment 4. (b) Objects in Experiment 5.

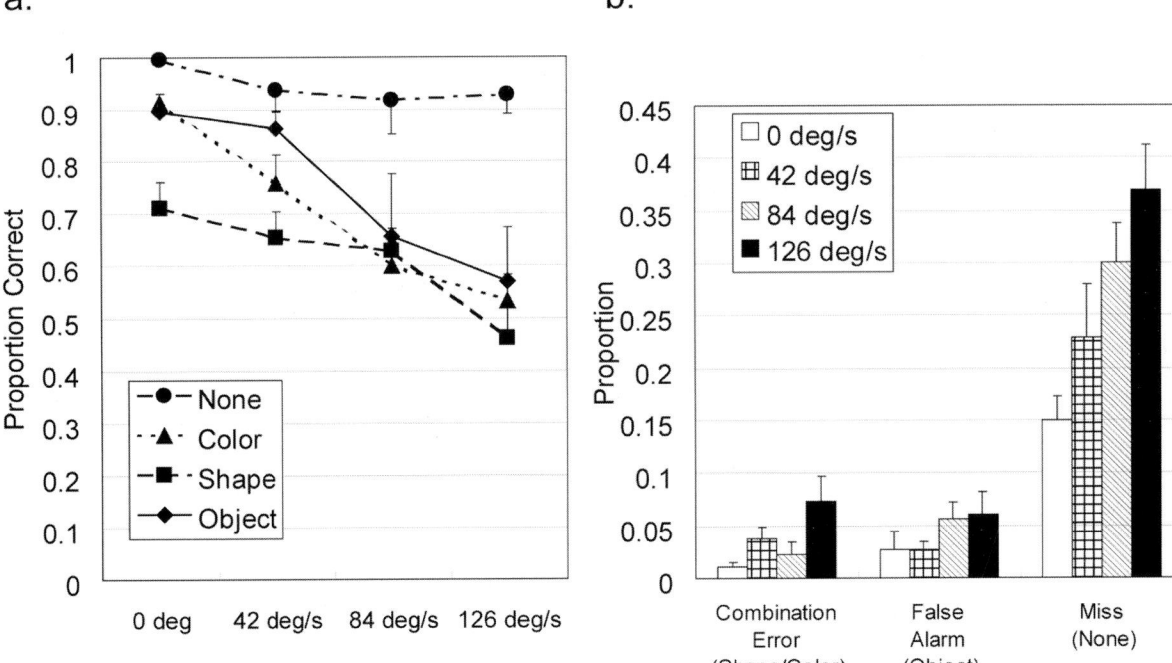

Fig. 9. (a) Mean accuracy as a function of the angular velocity for each event type in Experiment 4. (b) Distribution of errors for color- and shape-switch trials.

participated in Experiment 4, and the order of the two experiments was counterbalanced.

Results and discussion

Fig. 10a shows mean accuracy as a function of angular velocity for each event type. As in Experiment 4, the effect of angular velocity was significant ($F(3,12) = 11.24$, $p < 0.001$). Again, there was no evidence for the feature conjunction hypothesis: the object-switch condition showed higher accuracy than the inner-switch condition ($F(1,4) = 8.56$, $p < 0.05$), and no significant difference from the outer-switch condition ($F(1,4) = 2.01$, $p > 0.1$). Error analysis (Fig. 10b) again showed that confusion errors between inner and outer switch was not significantly different from the false alarm rate ($F(1,4) = 4.26$, $p > 0.05$). Compared with Experiment 4, one notable difference is that even the stationary condition showed many errors, which is inconsistent with the findings of Luck and Vogel (1997). Accuracy in the 0°/s condition was significantly higher in Experiment 4 than in Experiment 5 ($F(1,4) = 73.89$, $p < 0.001$).

General discussion

It has been widely believed that the capacity of the visual working memory is about four objects, based on the change-detection task measuring the retention, and on the multiple-object-tracking task measuring the transformation. If these findings reflect the characteristics of the coherent representation of objects such as object files, we should expect that the same capacity estimate will be obtained in the situation where objects information should be retained and transformed simultaneously. The MOPT task was created to answer this question, and the results cast doubt on the plausibility of the object file account. Our ability of retaining feature–location binding is greatly impaired as the cost of spatial transformation increases, even when the transformation cost is

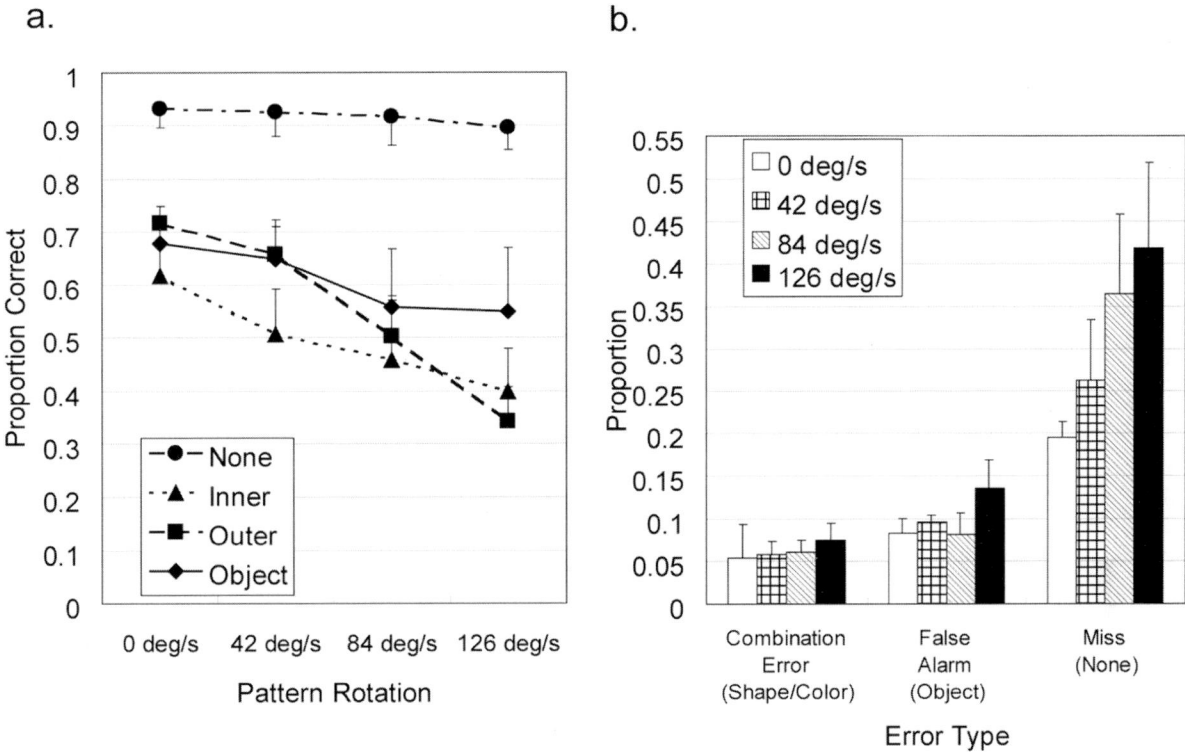

Fig. 10. (a) Mean accuracy as a function of the angular velocity for each event type in Experiment 5. (b) Distribution of errors for inner- and outer-switch trials.

well within the range of successful tracking in the attentive tracking paradigm (Verstraten et al., 2000). Thus, it is unlikely that a set of coherent representations, where feature and spatiotemporal information is tightly bound, is maintained and transformed in a dynamic situation.

Spatiotemporal characteristics of episodic representation

The results of Part I revealed that the observers' performance in the MOPT task could be accounted for by a modified uncertainty model where the number of objects and angular velocity independently affect the accuracy. The estimated life-span of object representation over occlusion was only 56 ms when the angular velocity of the pattern was 126°/s. From Experiment 3, the estimated capacity (number of targets) was only 2.1 objects. The processing cost manipulated by the spatial transformation has such profound effects on the retention of episodic representation that object files, if any, cannot survive even a small spatiotemporal discontinuity. They can function as memory only when there is no spatial transformation, which is inconsistent with the widely assumed function of the visual working memory.

This study revealed that feature–location binding of multiple objects becomes quickly unavailable in dynamic situations. From the object file account, it can be explained that multiple-object files constructed during the visible period are destroyed quickly. By contrast, the visual index account can explain the result by separate mechanisms of tracking and feature extraction. Even during the visible period, the number of objects whose features are bound to the index depends on the processing cost. In other words, the object file account postulates the common capacity limit of object files during the visible period (presumably four), whereas the visual index account assumes that the number of object files depends on the transformation cost, even if they are visible. This study cannot provide the answer to this problem, and further study of estimating the number of object files during dynamic visible scenes is necessary.

Feature interactions in episodic representation

In Part II, I investigated the possible functional roles of feature conjunctions in the MOPT task. If the shape–color conjunction or color–color conjunction is retained in visual working memory, then switch of a single feature can be detected without binding features to spatiotemporal locations. Two signatures of such conjunction coding, viz. higher accuracy in the feature-switch conditions and more confusion errors between two feature-switch conditions, were not observed in Experiments 4 and 5, suggesting that such location-independent feature conjunctions are not available in the MOPT task. There are some possible reasons for this result. First of all, color–shape and color–color conjunctions used in this study were not represented in LTM, because they are arbitrary combinations of feature values. Second, the effects of type representation or object detectors are not sensitive to the explicit detection tasks such as the MOPT. Indeed, these effects are usually obtained by implicit tasks such as preview benefit and priming. In any case, in the explicit detection and identification where episodic representation plays a key role, location information appears to play a critical role in the formation of feature conjunctions. This is consistent with some theoretical proposals of the special role of location information (Treisman, 1988; Tsal and Lavie, 1993). For example, Treisman's Feature Integration Theory assumes that feature bindings are mediated by spatial locations, and Tsal and Lavie (1993) provided some evidence that attending to object features such as color and shape entails attention directed to their location.

Relation to transsaccadic memory research

The results of this study showed the importance of spatiotemporal location information in forming feature–location binding. An important issue for further study is what coordinate systems the visual working memory uses. A preliminary study conducted in our lab suggests that the accurate memory for the multiple feature–location binding in the stationary condition is mediated by retinotopic coordinates. Observers either fixated to a stationary point or pursued a rotating point while running the MOPT task with 0°/s and 126°/s conditions. Pilot data showed that in the 0°/s condition, the performance in the fixation and pursuit conditions were markedly different. The color-switch detection in the pursuit condition was extremely difficult, even though the pattern was stationary in the environment-centered coordinates. This impairment does not seem to be merely the cost of pursuit eye movement, because in the 126°/s condition, the pursuit condition showed better color-switch detection than the fixation condition. However, it is possible that fast saccade and slow pursuit may play different roles in multiple-object permanence, thus it is premature to conclude the retinotopic coordinates based on the comparison between fixation and pursuit conditions. Further systematic investigation is necessary to resolve this issue.

Finally, the severe cost of object motion in the maintenance of feature–location binding appears to be contradictory to some findings of transsaccadic memory showing that motion information is in fact better maintained (Verfaillie and De Graef, 2000). Verfaillie and De Graef (2000) showed that, using a point-light walker stimulus, observers are sensitive to transsaccadic changes related to the in-depth rotation of the figure, but not sensitive to the changes in its image-plane location. The apparent discrepancy does not reflect the role of motion information per se, but the role of motion in extracting some abstract visual information. In the case of point-light walker display, motion is necessary to recover the 3-D structure of human body that is maintained across saccade. By contrast, the moving pattern in the MOPT task does not provide any abstract structure. Furthermore, in the MOPT task, spatial configuration of component objects is irrelevant to the feature–location binding, thus the motion only imposes the transformation costs on the maintenance of binding. Therefore, this study and Verfaillie and De Graef (2000) investigate different aspects of roles of motion in visual cognition.

Relation to real life situations

In real life settings, many objects are moving independent of the viewer. Thus, when many objects are moving and one needs to monitor their identity and locations (e.g., air traffic control), a situation similar to the multiple-object permanence tracking occurs. Of course, in the physical world, a change of object identity during the short visual disruption is extremely rare, but such unusual and experimental settings allowed us to reveal the severe limitation of our ability to hold the identity of multiple objects. The findings from the MOPT paradigm have important implications for the monitoring of a complex visual scene such as air traffic control. It is quite dangerous for one officer to monitor four aircrafts simultaneously, because it imposes a high cognitive load that may lead to fatal error.

Another issue on the relation to the real life setting is the specificity of rotation in the findings of the present work. We may be particularly vulnerable to the rotation in the MOPT setting. Further investigation is necessary to understand the type of motion with which the visual system has difficulty in dealing in the MOPT situation. More systematic studies with careful control and monitoring of eye movements and with various types of visual motion should reveal the basic operation of the visual system in the dynamic world.

Conclusion

As a general answer to the visual stability problem, attentional construction of episodic representation of multiple objects in visual working memory has been postulated. Contrary to the assumption of stability and coherence of episodic representation, this study revealed that it is extremely vulnerable to transformation costs, and that the feature binding becomes quickly unavailable. When objects are moving, integrated representation of only one or two objects can be maintained. To achieve the visual stability with such limited internal representation, the visual system appears to utilize the visual indexing mechanism (Pylyshyn, 1989, 1994; Ballard et al., 1997), and the efficient feature extraction mechanism with attention. Probably, for most cases with visual disruption, this small system is just enough to achieve visual stability, except for some physically unrealistic situations created by visual cognition researchers for the change blindness and transsaccadic memory experiments.

Acknowledgements

I thank Toshio Inui, Masayoshi Nagai, Ben Tatler, Jukka Hyönä, and an anonymous reviewer for helpful comments for the earlier drafts and technical assistance. This work was supported by Grants-in-Aid for Scientific Research for the Japanese Ministry of Education, Science, and Culture (Nos. 11610075, 12551001, 13610084, and 14019053), The Research for the Future Program from the Japan Society for the Promotion of Science (JSPS-RFTF99P01401), and Toyota High-Tech Research Grant Program.

References

Ballard, D.H., Hayhoe, M.M., Pook, P.K. and Rao, R.P.N. (1997) Deictic codes for the embodiment of cognition. *Behav. Brain Sci.*, 20: 723–767.

Brainard, D.H. (1997) The psychophysics toolbox. *Spat. Vis.*, 10: 443–446.

Daneman, M. and Carpenter, P.A. (1980) Individual differences in working memory and reading. *J. Verb. Learn. Verb. Behav.*, 19: 450–466.

Deubel, H., Schneider, W.X. and Bridgeman, B. (1996) Post-saccadic target blanking prevents saccadic suppression of image displacement. *Vision Res.*, 36: 985–996.

Henderson, J.M. (1994) Two representational systems in dynamic visual identification. *J. Exp. Psychol. Gen.*, 123: 410–426.

Horowitz, T.S. and Wolfe, J.M. (1998) Visual search has no memory. *Nature*, 394: 575–577.

Irwin, D.E. (1991) Information integration across saccadic eye movements. *Cognit. Psychol.*, 23: 420–456.

Irwin, D.E. (1992) Perceiving and integrated visual world. In: D.E. Meyer and S. Kornblum (Eds.), *Attention and Performance XIV*. MIT Press, Cambridge, MA, pp. 121–142.

Irwin, D.E., Yantis, S. and Jonides, J. (1983) Evidence against visual integration across saccadic eye movements. *Percept. Psychophys.*, 34: 49–57.

Just, M.A. and Carpenter, P.A. (1992) A capacity theory of comprehension: individual differences in working memory. *Psychol. Rev.*, 99: 122–149.

Kahneman, D. and Treisman, A. (1984) Changing views of attention and automaticity. In: R. Parasuraman and D.A. Davis (Eds.), *Varieties of Attention*. Academic Press, New York, NY.

Kahneman, D., Treisman, A. and Gibbs, B.J. (1992) The reviewing of object files: object specific integration of information. *Cognit. Psychol.*, 24: 175–219.

Kanwisher, N.G. (1987) Repetition blindness: type recognition without token individuation. *Cognition*, 27: 117–143.

Kanwisher, N.G. (1991) Repetition blindness and illusory conjunction: errors in binding visual types with visual tokens. *J. Exp. Psychol. Hum. Percept. Perform.*, 17: 404–421.

Leslie, A.M., Xu, F., Tremoulet, P.D. and Scholl, B.J. (1998) Indexing and the object concept: developing 'what' and 'where' systems. *Trends Cogn. Sci.*, 2: 10–18.

Levin, D.T. and Simons, D.J. (1997) Failure to detect changes to attended objects in motion pictures. *Psychon. Bull. Rev.*, 4: 501–506.

Luck, S.J. and Vogel, E.K. (1997) The capacity of visual working memory for features and conjunctions. *Nature*, 390: 279–281.

McConkie, G.W. and Currie, C.B. (1996) Visual stability across saccades while viewing complex pictures. *J. Exp. Psychol. Hum. Percept. Perform.*, 22: 563–581.

O'Regan, J.K. (1992) Solving the 'real' mysteries of visual perception: the world as an outside memory. *Can. J. Psychol.*, 46: 461–488.

Pashler, H. (1988) Familiarity and visual change detection. *Percept. Psychophys.*, 44: 369–378.

Pelli, D.G. (1985) Uncertainty explains many aspects of visual contrast detection and discrimination. *J. Opt. Soc. Am. A*, 2: 1508–1532.

Pelli, D.G. (1997) The video toolbox software for visual psychophysics: transforming numbers into movies. *Spat. Vis.*, 10: 437–442.

Phillips, W.A. (1974) On the distinction between sensory storage and short-term visual memory. *Percept. Psychophys.*, 16: 283–290.

Pylyshyn, Z.W. (1989) The role of location indexes in spatial perception: a sketch of the FINST spatial-index model. *Cognition*, 32: 65–97.

Pylyshyn, Z.W. (1994) Some primitive mechanisms of spatial attention. *Cognition*, 50: 363–384.

Pylyshyn, Z.W. and Storm, R. (1988) Tracking multiple independent targets: evidence for both serial and parallel stages. *Spat. Vis.*, 3: 179–197.

Rensink, R.A., O'Regan, J.K. and Clark, J.J. (1997) To see or not to see: the need for attention to perceive changes in scenes. *Psychol. Sci.*, 8: 368–373.

Saiki, J. (1999) Relation blindness? Difficulty in detecting violation of spatial relations in regular rotations of a triangular pattern. *Invest. Ophthalmol. Visual Sci.*, 41: Suppl. 796.

Scholl, B.J. and Pylyshyn, Z.W. (1998) Tracking multiple items through occlusion: clues to visual objecthood. *Cognit. Psychol.*, 38: 259–290.

Simons, D.J. and Levin, D.T. (1998) Failure to detect changes to people in a real-world interaction. *Psychon. Bull. Rev.*, 5: 644–649.

Treisman, A. (1988) Features and objects: the fourteenth Bartlett memorial lecture. *Q. J. Exp. Psychol. Hum. Exp. Psychol.*, 40A: 201–237.

Tsal, Y. and Lavie, N. (1993) Location dominance in attending to color and shape. *J. Exp. Psychol. Hum. Percept. Perform.*, 19: 131–139.

Verfaillie, K. and De Graef, P. (2000) Transsaccadic memory for position and orientation of saccade source and target. *J. Exp. Psychol. Hum. Percept. Perform.*, 26: 1243–1259.

Verstraten, F.A.J., Cavanagh, P. and Labianca, A.T. (2000) Limits of attentive tracking reveal temporal properties of attention. *Vision Res.*, 40: 3651–3664.

CHAPTER 10

What information survives saccades in the real world?

Benjamin W. Tatler *

Sussex Centre for Neuroscience, School of Biological Sciences, University of Sussex, Brighton BN1 9QG, UK

Abstract: Recent change detection research demonstrates impressively that we do not retain and fuse the pictorial content of successive fixations. This raises two distinct issues: (1) when and how is point-by-point information lost or replaced? and (2) might more abstract information be extracted and retained from fixations? In this chapter I explore both of these issues. I consider the evidence for a very short-term richly detailed visual representation of the current target of fixation that survives the saccade but is overwritten by the content of each new fixation shortly after it begins. The possibility of abstract representations of the visual surroundings is then discussed. Under conditions of competitive, parallel processing, as are present in real life situations, multiple types of information are extracted and retained from complex natural scenes. Time courses for extraction vary between different types of information. The inclusion of eye movement data reveals a crucial role for fixations in information extraction. The data suggest that information assimilation into the representations tested here is dominated by the fovea and is integrated and accumulated from multiple foveations. From these studies we are able to construct a rudimentary framework, in which representational faithfulness and richness depend upon fixation history of that part of the visual scene, thus producing an efficient and potentially task-specific representation.

The puzzle of visual perception

In the ten years since Grimes famously demonstrated how bad we are at detecting changes to natural images that occur during eye movements (later published as Grimes, 1996), the debate about perceptual stability has been re-ignited and our views of visual perception have had to be radically overhauled.

It has long been a puzzle how the brain constructs the continuous and seemingly completely detailed visual percept. This became particularly enigmatic once we began to understand the nature of eye movements (since Helmholtz, 1867) and the non-uniformity of retinal sampling (Østerberg, 1935). These areas of research showed that the input that the eyes supply to the brain is in the form of a series of relatively static images of the world separated by brief periods of effective blindness. In the second half of the last century formal explanations of perceptual stability across eye movements began to appear in the literature. These ideas built upon the long-running assumption that there must reside in the brain point-by-point pictures of the world that we view (e.g. Berkeley, 1709, 1710, 1713; Hume, 1739, 1748). It was proposed that an 'Integrative Visual Buffer' exists in the visual system in which point-by-point copies of the retinal images from each fixation are retained and fused (McConkie and Rayner, 1976; Rayner, 1978). In this way, over a number of fixations a complete and detailed internal representation of the visual surroundings could be constructed. These ideas remained a popular component of explanations of visual perception, despite some evidence that pictorial details might not be retained (e.g. Bridgeman et al., 1975).

The case for point-by-point representations in the visual system was significantly weakened during the 1980s and early 1990s by the work of researchers including Irwin, Pollatsek and Rayner (e.g. Irwin et al., 1983; Rayner and Pollatsek, 1983; Irwin, 1991, 1993; Pollatsek and Rayner, 1992), who consistently

---

* Correspondence to: B.W. Tatler, Sussex Centre for Neuroscience, School of Biological Sciences, University of Sussex, Brighton BN1 9QG, UK. Tel.: +44-1273-872765; Fax: +44-1273-678535; E-mail: b.w.tatler@sussex.ac.uk

demonstrated lack of transsaccadic integration of information. Grimes' (1996) use of natural images to demonstrate how profoundly unaware observers can be of changes in scenes, provided those changes occur during saccades, ignited widespread interest in the debate and gave rise to the new field of *change blindness* research. The findings of change blindness studies raise two questions about the visual system. Firstly, might it be that the point-by-point pictorial content of each fixation is not retained? Secondly, if this pictorial detail is not retained, what is the nature of the information (if any) that is extracted and retained from fixations? In this chapter I will consider each of these issues in turn. A combination of real world experimentation and viewing of images presented on computer screens has allowed me to test the availability of pictorial information and to assess the extent of information extraction and retention from fixations.

Pictorial content of fixations

In the last ten years, a large number of studies has demonstrated failure of observers to detect changes if those changes are timed to coincide with saccades (McConkie and Currie, 1996), blinks (O'Regan et al., 2000), or brief interruptions to viewing in the form of artificially inserted black screens between presentations of images (Rensink et al., 1995, 1997, 2000). This impressive *change blindness* has been used to suggest that we do not retain the point-by-point pictorial content of fixations, but instead that this detail is lost every time we move our eyes.

One of the compelling aspects of this research has been the emphasis on naturalness in the experimental protocols: many studies have used natural images as the stimuli. In this way it is often hoped that potential pitfalls encountered in the use of artificial stimuli, such as phosphor persistence (e.g. Jonides et al., 1982), will be avoided (for a discussion of these problems see Bridgeman and Mayer, 1983) and that the conclusions drawn from change detection studies will be more closely applicable to the operation of the visual system in real life. While change detection experiments bring the situation closer to real life, viewing images presented on a computer screen may not be equivalent to unconstrained activity in the real world. Simons and colleagues have extended change detection protocols to encompass more realistic situations. The detection of changes during movie sequences observed by participants, is one such extension of change detection protocols (Simons and Levin, 1997; Simons and Chabris, 1999). These studies found impairments in the detection of changes made during editorial cuts to movie sequences, similar to those that had been suggested by change detection studies using static scenes. Simons and Levin also carried out a real world analog of the change detection paradigm, whereby changes occurred to the visual scene during an induced interruption to the participant's viewing (Simons and Levin, 1998). 8 out of 15 participants in this experiment failed to notice that the experimenter, with whom they were engaged in conversation, swapped with another experimenter during an interruption to viewing, so that they were talking to a different person in the latter portion of the conversation. This finding offers real world support for laboratory-based change detection findings.

In a recent study (Tatler, 2001), I attempted to investigate some of the implications of change detection research under real world conditions, without the use of the induced change paradigm. My aim was to assess the availability of information about the precise content of fixations at and before the moment of visual interruption to a natural, everyday task; in this case making a cup of tea. From these data I hoped to investigate the suggestion arising from change detection studies that rich pictorial information is lost each time we move our eyes.

The results of this tea making study showed that participants were able to access richly detailed and accurate information about the content of their fovea for the interrupted fixation, but such detail was unavailable for previous fixations. Such a finding is consistent with the suggestion that veridical visual information from fixations is lost each time we move our eyes. Hence this study offered support for change detection findings, under real world conditions and in the absence of artificially induced change.

The ability to access rich information for the current fixation, but not for prior fixations might suggest that participants are reporting the content of their retinas. However, an interesting finding from this tea making study was the occurrence of two pieces of evidence that suggested that this could not be the case. Firstly, on the occasions in which the visual interruption coincided with a saccade, participants still reported what was at the center of the fixation before the saccade in 55% of trials, despite the fact that the retinal image at the moment of the interruption would no longer have been of this fixation. The second piece of evidence came from consideration of the errors made by participants when they were attempting to report the content of the fixation occurring at the moment of the interruption. In 31% of these incorrect trials (the equal most common type of error) participants mistakenly reported the foveal content of the fixation immediately preceding the interrupted fixation (i.e. the 'penultimate fixation'). This type of error was only possible if participants were reporting the content of a visual store rather than the retina itself. These two pieces of evidence were used to argue that participants were reporting the content of a visual buffer in which richly detailed information about the content of a fixation is retained until it is overwritten soon after the start of each new fixation. Support for the possibility of a store with the properties described has been provided by other recent studies (Deubel et al., 1996, 1998; Becker et al., 2000; De Graef and Verfaillie, 2002, this volume; Deubel et al., 2002, this volume).

Having implicated a visual store in which details of the current fixation are stored briefly, we should now consider the possible nature of the store and the information within. In the published manuscript I suggested that the store must be a low-level visual store in which a veridical copy of the retinal image is held. To claim that the data describe a low-level, pre-categorical store when the experimental measure is explicit and necessarily post-categorical might appear to be an over-interpretation of the data. I will now consider in slightly more detail the rationale for my proposition. The reports given by participants are undoubtedly post-categorical. However, I would argue that they could be drawn from a post-categorical literal translation of the content of a pre-categorical buffer. If there is no selection during translation then the post-categorical memory trace can be used to describe the properties of the pre-categorical, richly detailed store from which they were translated. The rationale for suggesting a literal, non-selective translation of information is based mainly on the richness of detail contained in the reports given by participants. These reports were precise enough to localize a position in space usually defined to within 1° and correctly described the content of the foveal image in 81% of trials. It remains, however, that from the data in the tea making study alone, it is difficult to determine whether the post-categorical memory trace from which the reports are drawn contains a reflection of a pre-categorical store or instead contains a direct reflection of the retinal image (i.e. no intermediary pre-categorical store). In the case of the latter then the temporal properties of the store described in Tatler (2001) would be those of the post-categorical information store, rather than a pre-categorical store from which the post-categorical information is drawn. Further investigation would be necessary to dissect these possibilities. However, while there might be some question as to whether the store characterized is truly pre- or post-categorical in nature, this does not weaken the main arguments and conclusions drawn from the tea making data. Whatever the precise nature of the store, the information contained within is a richly detailed representation of the target of fixation and the data can be used to characterize the timing of information replacement in the store (discussed more fully below).

The suggestion of a richly detailed visual memory store bears similarities to the old ideas of iconic memory (Sperling, 1960; Neisser, 1967) and appears to contradict the many recent studies that have argued against such a store (e.g. Haber, 1983). However, recent studies have implicated similar stores. Findings by Deubel and colleagues (Deubel et al., 1996, 1998, 2002, this volume) implicate transsaccadic retention (but not fusion) of low-level visual information. Becker et al. (2000) suggest transsaccadic persistence of an iconic trace of an individual fixation. De Graef and Verfaillie (2002, this volume) interrogate and characterize a low-level transsaccadic informational persistence in the form of a visual analog rather than icon. While both the visual icon and analog are pre-categorical, richly detailed representations, they are proposed to exist in slightly different forms. One such difference is that the icon is retinotopically organized, whereas the analog is spatiotopically organized. The details of the buffer proposed in Tatler (2001), do not agree entirely with descriptions of either memory store, and indeed may describe a post-categorical representation of the target of fixation. However, they are perhaps most consistent with the idea of the visual icon, because the high precision and accuracy of reporting foveal targets implies retinotopic rather than spatiotopic organization.

Inspection of the durations of interrupted fixations on trials in which the penultimate fixation was mistakenly reported clearly suggested that the overwrite within the proposed buffer could occur at any time within the first 400 ms of each fixation (see fig. 6, Tatler, 2001). 400 ms is a large potential window during which replacement might occur. However, the data show that many of the overwrites occur much earlier in the fixation, with the majority occurring during the first 100 ms and almost all by 250 ms into the fixation. Hence although overwriting in the buffer may occur as late as 400 ms after the end of the saccade, most occur much closer to the initiation of fixation.

Persistence of visual information until after the start of the new fixation is supported by Becker et al.'s recent study (2000). That information is taken up from the new fixation in a window near the start of the fixation (typically within the first 100 ms) is supported by several other studies. Rayner et al. (1981) proposed that in reading information is taken up within the first 50–70 ms of each fixation. De Graef and Verfaillie (2002, this volume) use post-saccadic masking to suggest that overwriting of the content of fixations occurs within the first 50 ms of fixations. Deubel et al. (2002, this volume) find a similar 50 ms period of sensitivity for information uptake at the start of fixations. The suggestion that overwrites may occur as late as 400 ms into the fixation implies a surprisingly large time window, but is supported by the time window of information utilization found by Blanchard et al. (1984) in reading tasks.

While the conclusions of change detection studies are undoubtedly correct in proposing that richly detailed information from fixations is not retained and fused from successive fixations, it is now becoming increasingly clear that to extend this argument to propose that point-by-point information is never internalized (O'Regan and Noë, 2002) is perhaps less sound. Accumulating evidence suggests that within a fixation we are able to access a highly detailed representation of the retinal image that resides in a visual store, the content of which is overwritten each time we re-fixate our surroundings.

Observations of eye movements in real world experiments show that we direct our eyes at what we are manipulating (e.g. Ballard et al., 1992; Land et al., 1999; Hayhoe, 2000; Land and Hayhoe, 2001). These observations are consistent with the framework outlined above, in which point-by-point pictorial information is available within the timescale of a single fixation, but is lost each time we relocate our gaze. They are also consistent with the proposition that the world can itself act as an 'outside memory' (O'Regan and Lévy-Schoen, 1983), negating the necessity to internalize information about the visual world from multiple fixations. Consideration of this issue brings us to the second question raised by change detection studies. Arguments against the existence of a point-by-point pictorial representation built up over multiple fixations are sometimes extended to assume that there is no transsaccadic information retention of any sort (O'Regan and Noë, 2002). However, in the real world we can make single and reasonably accurate gaze shifts of up to 140° (e.g. Grealy et al., 1999; Land et al., 1999). Accurate gaze targeting over these distances cannot be explained easily in terms of peripheral vision and would seem to require the assistance of some internally available information about the surroundings. Similar implications arise from the study of memory-guided saccades (e.g. Karn et al., 1997; Karn and Hayhoe, 2000) whereby accurate eye movements are made when there are no currently available visual cues for targeting. It is to the question of what type of information might survive eye movements that this chapter now turns.

Information extraction from fixations

Many researchers have considered the possibility of the retention of more abstract information about visual stimuli (e.g. Hochberg, 1968; Irwin, 1991, 1993; Pollatsek and Rayner, 1992; Henderson, 1994, 1997). Indeed the possibility of non-pictorial representation has much older roots and can be seen in the proposition of Hobbes (1651, 1656) that mental representations might take the form of language-like symbols. In the light of recent change detection studies it seems that we must consider in more detail the possibility of abstract transsaccadic representation since point-by-point visual information is lost over the course of multiple fixations.

An abstract representation might take the form of any type of information about the world that is not point-by-point pictorial information. Several candidates for the type of information that might be retained and used to construct a non-pictorial representation have been considered over the years. Particular attention in the literature has been paid to two: gist and spatial layout. Gist refers to the overall meaning or nature of a scene or image (e.g. whether a scene is of a kitchen or an office) and is independent of explicit knowledge of the scene's content, layout or other detail. This type of information can be extracted very rapidly from scenes (e.g. Intraub, 1980, 1981) even for presentation times as brief as 120 ms (Biederman, 1981). Spatial layout refers to the overall arrangement and positioning of items and features within a scene. Layout information can be independent of semantics and properties of objects (e.g. Hochberg, 1968). Gibson (1979) proposed that spatial layout information is internally represented as a matter of course by the visual system and does not rely on effortful extraction. Similar suggestions of the existence of abstract spatial representations that survive multiple eye movements can be found frequently in the literature (e.g. Simons, 1996; Rensink, 2000).

Spatial layout and gist need not be the only types of information extracted. Object properties, such as color and shape, offer potential candidates for representation. Note that object shape is not the same as object identity: while identity information might specify that the object is a kettle, there are many possible forms that the kettle may take. Retention of abstracted object properties has been proposed on several occasions in the scene perception literature (e.g. Henderson, 1994; Henderson and Siefert, 1999; Hollingworth and Henderson, 2002). Aginsky and Tarr (2000) found enhanced performance for detecting surface properties in change detection experiments when relevantly cued, suggesting the possibility that representation of color might be built up during the pre-cue period and used in the subsequent detection task.

Knowledge of the content of a scene in terms of a catalogue of objects and features present offers another prospective form of extracted information. Henderson and Hollingworth (1999) concluded that there is strong evidence for encoding object presence or object identity information over multiple fixations when participants view naturalistic scenes. Recently, Melcher (2001) found that the number of objects recalled improved steadily as presentation times were increased from one to four seconds, for computer-generated complex scenes. This result was used to propose a medium-term visual memory for scene content, persisting for a period between several seconds and several minutes. The very existence of an extensive body of literature on object recognition suggests that information about presence and identity is extracted from scenes. The form of retained information about objects that is used in their identification is a matter of some debate. However, while reports of viewpoint-dependent object recognition might suggest image-like object representation (e.g. Bulthoff and Edelman, 1992; Humphrey and Khan, 1992; Tarr, 1995), others find viewpoint-independence in object identification studies and use this to propose a more abstract form of object representation (Biederman, 1987; Biederman and Gerhardstein, 1993, 1995). Thus there is evidence for the possibility that object identity (and hence a catalogue of scene contents) might be implicated in abstract representation of the visual surroundings.

While there have been numerous studies of the types of information that might be extracted from visual stimuli, most have investigated only one of the possible candidates in isolation (except, for instance, Aginsky and Tarr, 2000). Such an approach might weaken the conclusions drawn by removing another aspect of naturalness from the experimental protocol. In the real world it is likely that we extract multiple types of information in parallel and so a thorough description of information extraction should account for this possibility. By isolating a single type of information, the potential arises for the observer to allocate unnaturally high attentional resources to the extraction of that type of information, thus misrepresenting the extent to which that type of information is normally retained by the visual system.

The second set of experiments that I will discuss attempts to address some of these issues in the study of visual representations. Several candidates for the type of information that might be extracted and retained from scenes were tested. These candidates were: *gist*, *scene content* (the objects or features present in the scene), *absolute spatial layout* (where items are located in the scene), *relative spatial layout* (spatial relations between items in the scene), object *shape* (the specific form of an item) and object *color*. The extraction of the different types of information is tested under conditions of competitive, parallel processing, as are present in real life situations.

Based on previous studies, we can make a number of predictions about what we might expect to find in these experiments. Gist information is likely to be encoded rapidly and effectively (e.g. Biederman, 1981). Information about the presence (or absence) of objects within a scene might be expected to be achieved rapidly and to be assimilated to a relatively high extent. This is because object identification can be achieved within very brief presentation times even for complex natural scenes (Delorme et al., 2000). Previous studies of transsaccadic memory suggest relatively poor encoding of absolute position information (Pollatsek et al., 1990; Deubel et al., 1996; Verfaillie and De Graef, 2000). Aginsky and Tarr (2000) suggest that object presence and positional information have higher priorities in representations than object color information. From these studies we might expect to see highest performance for gist questions with increasingly poor performances for presence information, position information and finally color.

The data presented and discussed below are excerpts from two forthcoming studies of abstract visual representation (Tatler et al., 2002a,b). Since these manuscripts are presently unpublished, I will describe relevant methodology and present key results below, upon which the subsequent discussion is based.

Methods

Participants

14 participants took part in the experiment. All had normal or corrected-to-normal vision and had not previously taken part in eye movement studies.

Procedure

Each participant viewed 48 photographic images of everyday, familiar, real world scenes. Images were displayed on a 17″ color monitor, positioned at a viewing distance of 60 cm. Consequently, visual stimuli subtended 30° by 22° of each participant's visual field. Image presentation time varied randomly between 1 and 10 s, during which time participants were free to view the scene as they wished. Following each image presentation two questions were asked, each requiring a four-alternative forced-choice response. These questions were drawn from questions covering the six types of information tested: gist, content, absolute layout, relative layout, object shape and object color. Questions were counterbalanced between participants. The response options for absolute position and shape questions were pictorial, for the other questions the options were written words. Gist questions did not relate to specific items or features in the scenes, but the other five question types did. Items tested varied in size from 0.04 to 32% of the total screen area. The position of the item tested was also varied between questions and scenes, although more of the tested items occurred centrally in the images than at the margins. By testing a wide range of aspects of the scene regarding a wide variety of object and feature sizes and positions, it was hoped that viewing strategies by the participants would be kept as general as possible and that the inspection period would be analogous to the initial survey upon entering a new scene or visual environment.

There are some limitations to the protocol used here to assess the content and nature of representations. Primarily, the use of explicit questioning might limit our ability to probe any implicit form of represented information. While I acknowledge this limitation, I would point out that this might not be too much of a problem, because questions were asked in the form of a four-alternative forced choice. The use of forced-choice questioning allows for the possibility that responses may reflect implicitly encoded information. Unfortunately, the extent to which responses were drawn from implicit knowledge cannot be assessed here, but could have been estimated if participants had been asked to give a confidence rating after each response.

Results and discussion

Responses of all participants to each question type suggest that performance was above chance for all types of information tested (Fig. 1). One sample *t*-tests confirm above-chance performance in each question (gist: $t_{13} = 15.22$, $p < 0.05$; presence: $t_{13} = 7.75$, $p < 0.05$; shape: $t_{13} = 5.75$, $p < 0.05$; color: $t_{13} = 9.25$, $p < 0.05$; absolute position: $t_{13} = 5.79$, $p < 0.05$; relative position: $t_{13} = 3.94$, $p < 0.05$). Hence when participants view the natural scenes, they are extracting information about the overall gist of the scene, the items and features contained in it, their absolute and relative positions and details about the shape and color of items. The retention of multiple types of information about scenes is consistent with suggestions in various studies (De Graef, 1992; Henderson, 1992; Rayner and Pollatsek, 1992; Aginsky and Tarr, 2000; Rensink, 2000; Hollingworth and Henderson, 2002). However, while these researchers propose representation of more than one type of information, each only goes as far as adding one or two extra types of information. Rensink (2000) proposed a representation comprising gist, layout and long-term scene schema (an amalgamation of long-term memories of similar scenes and expectations based on previous experience). Aginsky and Tarr (2000) proposed that representations include scene layout and object surface properties. Hollingworth and Henderson (2002) suggested that representations contain local object details indexed to scene layout. De Graef (1992) and Rayner and Pollatsek (1992) described representations comprising primarily object identity and layout information. Based on the data presented in this chapter, the above ideas can be extended and integrated by proposing an abstract representation in which all of these types of information are included.

Participants do not perform equally on the six different types of questions tested (Fig. 1). This observation implies that within the time scale of one to ten seconds of viewing images, not all types of information are given equal priority. Participants perform highly in questions about the nature of the scenes, suggesting that gist information is extracted effectively within the 10-s viewing time. Participants perform at much lower levels in the other five questions implying that these types of information are not extracted or retained as precisely or extensively as gist information during the time scale of viewing. The different relative extents of extraction might imply different degrees of prominence in the representa-

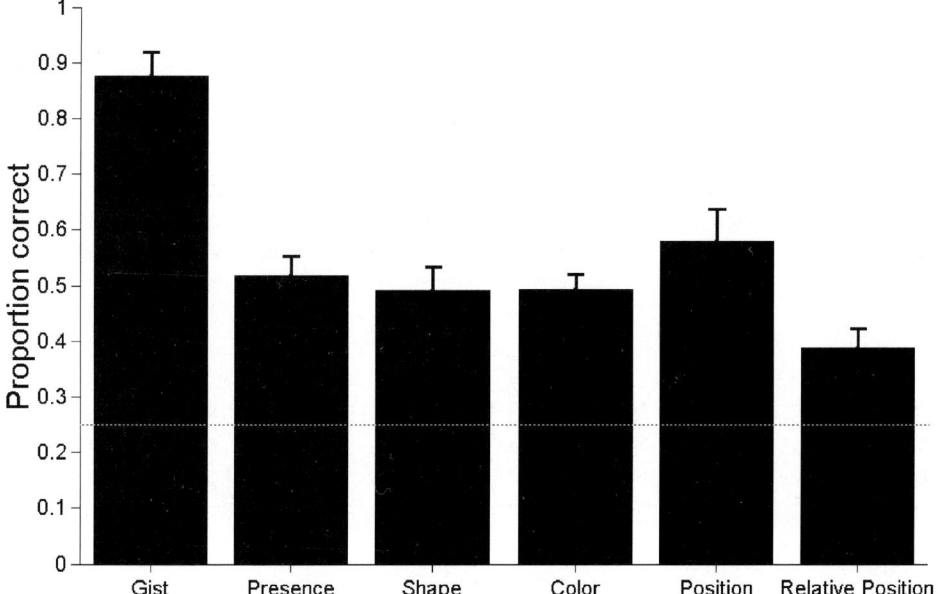

Fig. 1. Performance by all participants in answering questions covering the six categories of information tested in this experiment ($N = 1306$ responses). Responses were in the form of a four-alternative forced choice, thus chance performance would be 25% in this experiment. Responses were above chance in all questions, with highest performance in response to gist questions and poorest performance in response to questions testing the relative positions of items in the images. The dotted line shows chance (25%). Error bars indicate standard error between participants.

tions constructed. The suggestion that different types of information have differing prominences in the representation is consistent with conclusions drawn by Aginsky and Tarr (2000). They suggested that color information is not as important in representations as item presence or position. The observed data do not appear to fit the predictions detailed earlier, based upon previous studies of transsaccadic memory. However, before considering this point further, it is important to consider the data more carefully.

As stated earlier, presentation times for images were varied between trials. Consequently, we were able to monitor the effect of viewing time upon the extraction of each of the types of questions asked. Fig. 2 depicts performance in response to questions as a function of inspection time for scenes. Linear regression showed that performance in response to gist questions did not vary with viewing time (slope $(\beta) = -8.3 \times 10^{-4}$, intercept $(\alpha) = 0.87$, $t_{114} = 0.09$, $p(\beta = 0) > 0.05$). Performance increased significantly with presentation time for presence ($\beta = 4.5 \times 10^{-2}$, $\alpha = 0.29$, $t_{111} = 3.36$, $p(\beta = 0) < 0.05$) and shape ($\beta = 4.3 \times 10^{-2}$, $\alpha = 0.29$, $t_{105} = 3.26$, $p(\beta = 0) < 0.05$) questions. While overall the trend in color performance was insignificant ($\beta = 2.1 \times 10^{-2}$, $\alpha = 0.37$, $t_{108} = 1.41$, $p(\beta = 0) > 0.05$), if only the first 6 s of viewing are considered, there appears to be a trend of increasing performance with viewing time. Trends in performance for absolute position ($\beta = 2.0 \times 10^{-2}$, $\alpha = 0.47$, $t_{114} = 1.40$, $p(\beta = 0) > 0.05$) and relative position ($\beta = 2.1 \times 10^{-2}$, $\alpha = 0.28$, $t_{104} = 1.56$, $p(\beta = 0) > 0.05$) were both non-significant. From these data we can suggest details of the time course of abstract representation.

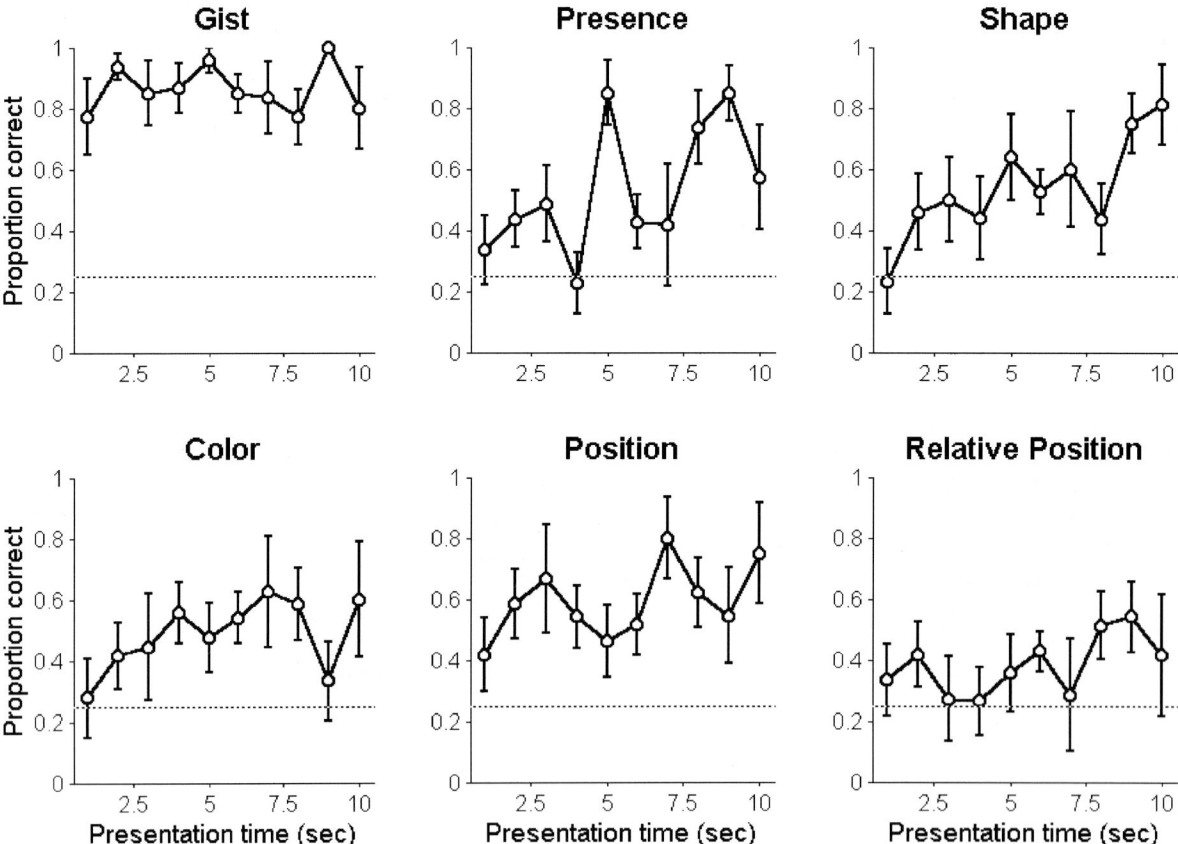

Fig. 2. The effect of presentation time upon the proportion of questions answered correctly by participants for each of the six types of question. Performances in response to different types of information were affected by presentation time in different ways. Dotted lines indicate chance. Error bars indicate standard error between participants.

After one second, performance for gist questions is above chance ($t_{10} = 4.22$, $p < 0.05$), is near maximal and does not change significantly with prolonged exposure, suggesting that assimilation of gist information into representations is accomplished within this short time scale. This time course is consistent with previous studies of the extraction of gist information from scenes, which have suggested that gist can be extracted fully within hundreds of milliseconds (e.g. Biederman, 1981). In contrast, performance for all other questions is at chance after one second, requiring prolonged exposure to accumulate (presence: $t_{13} = 0.73$, $p > 0.05$; shape: $t_{12} = 0.18$, $p > 0.05$; color: $t_{11} = 0.22$, $p > 0.05$; position: $t_{11} = 1.38$, $p > 0.05$; relative position: $t_{10} = 0.71$, $p > 0.05$).

After two seconds, performance in response to questions testing absolute position — but not for presence ($t_{12} = 1.99$, $p > 0.05$), shape ($t_{10} = 1.66$, $p > 0.05$), color ($t_{12} = 1.55$, $p > 0.05$) or relative position ($t_{12} = 1.56$, $p > 0.05$) — is significantly above chance ($t_{12} = 2.94$, $p < 0.05$). Consequently, we might propose early construction of a sketch of gist and rudimentary spatial layout upon exposure to a new visual scene. Prominence of gist and layout information in representations is consistent with the suggestion by Rensink (2000) and with conclusions drawn by Aginsky and Tarr (2000) who suggest that position and presence are more 'salient' in the representational system than surface properties such as color.

Prolonged exposure to scenes results in the assimilation of additional information to the representation, in the form of encoding details of object presence, shape, color and relative position as well as increasing the faithfulness of overall spatial information. Continued assimilation of information over the course of several seconds is consistent with a recent report by Melcher (2001). Melcher found that for viewing complex computer-generated scenes, as viewing time was increased from 1 to 2 and then 4 s, the number of items recalled by participants increased.

The overall performances in each question type shown in Fig. 1 are an under-estimation of the potential extent of extraction of each of the categories of information. After ten seconds, presence, shape and absolute position information have all reached performance levels of around 70–80% correct, whereas performance in color questions is 60% and relative position questions are only answered correctly in 45% of cases. At this point we can return to the predictions for these experiments outlined earlier. The data confirm highest priority for gist information and its rapid extraction. Similarly, presence and absolute position appear to be represented more faithfully than color. However, the data do not support the predicted rapid assimilation of object presence information, based upon rapid object identification in previous studies. This may be due to the added complexity of the scenes used in the present experiments compared with some of the object identification studies. Similarly, observers may have different priorities (due to different experimental requirements) and this might account for the extended time course of presence information extraction reported here.

So far in our discussion of the possibility of abstract representation of visual stimuli, we have neglected the role of the eye in the extraction process. If we consider retinal non-homogeneity of sampling it seems reasonable to suggest that efficacy of information extraction might vary with eccentricity in the retinal image. Furthermore, the fovea is not directed equally to every position on the visual stimulus either for viewing complex images (e.g. Buswell, 1935; Yarbus, 1967) or in the real world (Ballard et al., 1992; Land et al., 1999). Given these constraints, it seems logical and indeed necessary to consider the role of eye movements in any studies of information extraction. In a classic review of perception and the approaches to its study, Bevan (1958) made a similar observation. He argued that the faithfulness with which a percept matches the environment must depend critically upon the mechanism employed to scan and encode the input. Indeed, during free viewing it has been found that details of scenes are preferentially encoded if they lie near to the fovea during fixation compared to more peripheral targets (Parker, 1978; Nelson and Loftus, 1980; Henderson and Hollingworth, 1999). Perhaps, then, it is surprising that many studies of information extraction from visual scenes do not take into account the movements of the eyes.

The role of fixation position in information extraction

When participants viewed the 48 natural images in the experiments described earlier, eye movements were recorded throughout viewing. A SensoMotoric Instruments (SMI) EyeLink eye tracker was used to collect eye position data at a sampling rate of 250 Hz to an average spatial accuracy of ±0.40° in all trials of this experiment. From these records, the positions of foveations on the images were extracted and related to the positions of the items tested in the questions that followed each image presentation.

The first and most obvious measure of the role of the eye in information extraction is to compare performance in response to questions regarding items that had been foveated during viewing, to items that had not been foveated (Fig. 3). This approach cannot be employed for gist questions, because there was no target object. However, this analysis is applicable to the remaining five (item-specific) question types. For the purposes of this study, items were deemed to have been fixated if the center of gaze, specified by the SMI eye tracker data, fell within 1.5° of the item tested. The 1.5° cut-off is based on estimates of effective fovea size in naturalistic tasks (Johansson et al., 2001). There is a large increase in performance for items that had been fixated during viewing, over items that were not fixated for all five item-specific question types except relative position (Fig. 3), showing that there is an advantage to information extraction if the item was

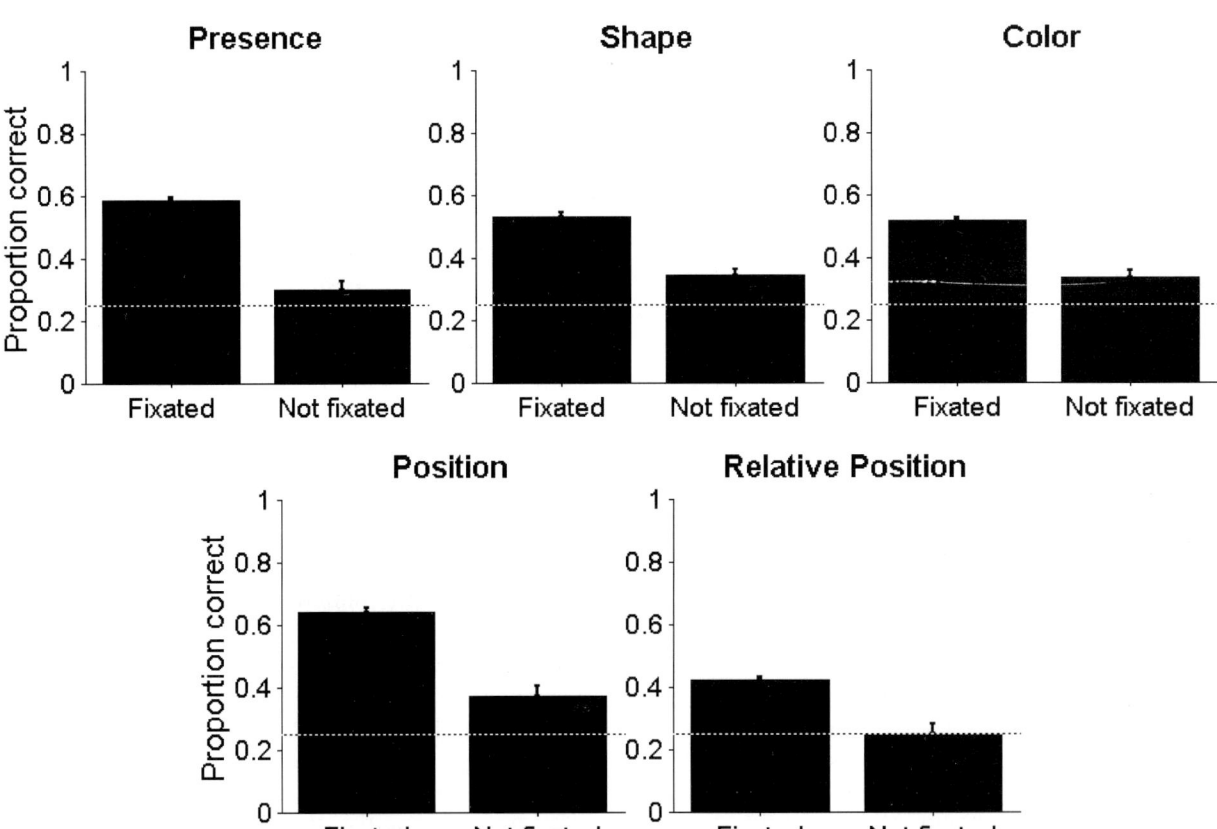

Fig. 3. Responses of all participants for all item-specific question categories according to whether or not the item tested was fixated during viewing. An item was deemed to have been fixated if the center of gaze indicated by the SMI eye tracker record was brought within 1.5° of any part of the item at any point during viewing. Performance was much enhanced when items had been fixated. If items were not fixated during viewing performance was near chance. The dotted line shows chance (25%). Error bars indicate between-participant standard errors.

foveated at any time during viewing (presence: $t_{23} = 2.67$, $p < 0.05$; shape: $t_{23} = 2.35$, $p < 0.05$; color: $t_{23} = 2.30$, $p < 0.05$; absolute position: $t_{22} = 2.50$, $p < 0.05$; relative position: $t_{22} = 1.69$, $p > 0.05$). This simple finding immediately demonstrates that it is essential to consider eye movements in the study of information extraction. Foveation of an item enhances performance to such an extent that to neglect consideration of where the fovea is directed during information extraction is to overlook a key aspect of the extraction process itself. Hollingworth and Henderson (2002) have reported a similar effect of fixation position for a change detection paradigm, showing that detection rates increased dramatically if changes were made to an item after it had been fixated compared to changes made to items that had not yet been fixated. Performance in response to questions testing items that had not been fixated during the experiments that I present here are near chance (presence: $t_{11} = 0.12$, $p > 0.05$; shape: $t_{11} = 0.41$, $p > 0.05$; color: $t_{11} = 0.30$, $p > 0.05$; absolute position: $t_{10} = 0.34$, $p > 0.05$; relative position: $t_{10} = 7.7 \times 10^{-17}$, $p > 0.05$). This result suggests that the accurate extraction of information for integration into the form of representation of the viewed scene tested in this experiment is largely confined to the fovea. The data show that directing the center of gaze to within 1.5° of an item greatly enhances the effective extraction of useful information from items in the scene. Loftus et al. (1983) have provided support for localized information extraction around the center of fixation during viewing visual scenes. Similarly, Henderson (1992) proposed a model of scene perception based upon localized processing, whereby information extraction is spatially limited to the locus of attention.

Fixating an item has a clear effect on performance, but the above measure is too crude for a full consideration of the role of fixation in information extraction. An obvious extension is to consider the role of re-fixation. By comparing the number of times an item was fixated to subsequent performance in the questions, it is clear that there is an advantage of re-fixation (Fig. 4). Linear regression of performance levels across all question types shows a significant increase with increasing number of foveations of the relevant item ($\beta = 6.9 \times 10^{-2}$, $\alpha = 0.36$, $t_{63} = 4.89$, $p(\beta = 0) < 0.05$). This result is important because it clearly demonstrates that information from multiple fixations is retained and combined cumulatively. Here we see at once a compelling argument for the supposition that some forms of abstract information are extracted and retained by the visual system and that representations are constructed via the accumulation of information over multiple fixations. These on-item fixations may be separated by multiple intervening fixations. Hence any or all fixations on any positions in the image potentially involve the simultaneous extraction of multiple types of information from that location. Support for the accumulation of information about an object over successive, separated fixations can be found in a recent change detection study (Hollingworth and Henderson, 2002).

While viewing complex images of natural scenes participants are able to extract multiple types of information in parallel. The processes of information extraction are determined crucially by the locations to which the fovea is directed within the image during the course of viewing. Multiple visits to an item by the fovea allow information to be accumulated about the object, increasing the faithfulness of the representation of that item. Bevan's (1958) argument that explanations of perception must encompass the scanning and encoding processes undoubtedly applies to the investigation of visual representation.

General discussion

From the data discussed in this chapter we are able to construct a rudimentary working hypothesis about the processes of information extraction from each fixation as we view natural scenes, and its integration into visual representations. With each new fixation as the eyes are moved around the visual surroundings, a richly detailed pictorial representation of the retinal image is routinely established in a visual store. Concurrently, information is being extracted and retained from the retinal image (or perhaps the visual store). This information extraction is largely localized to the fovea. When the eyes are subsequently moved to a new position in the scene (typically after about 1/3 of a second), a new richly detailed representation overwrites the content of the visual buffer and abstract information about the content of this new position begins to be extracted.

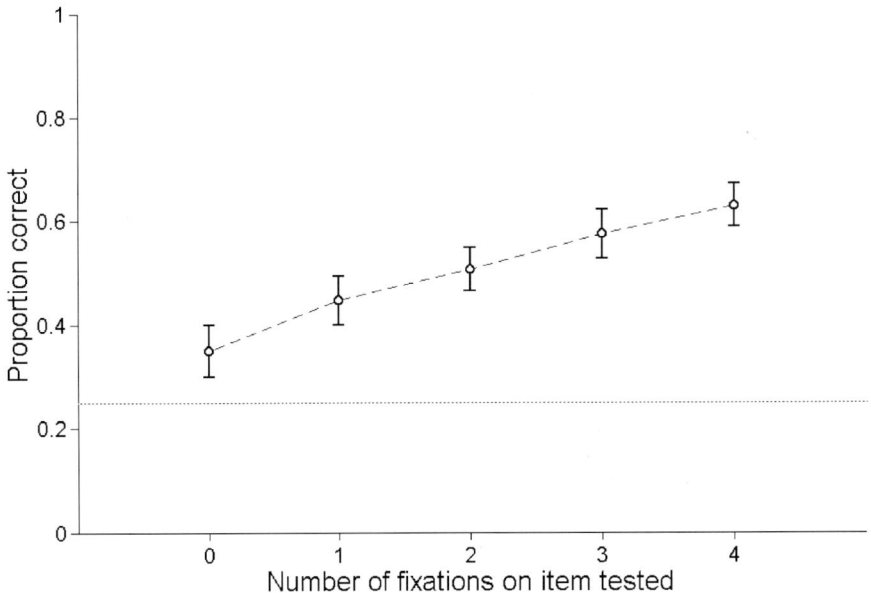

Fig. 4. The effect of the number of times an item was fixated during viewing upon performance in response to questions about that item. There was a clear and steady increase in performance with increasing number of fixations on the item tested. Data for items fixated more than four times during viewing are excluded due to small numbers of trials. The dotted line shows chance (25%). Error bars indicate between-participant standard errors.

Consideration of the role of eye movements in the construction of representations shows that each fixation serves to add localized detail to the overall representation of the scene, adding information primarily from the foveal image. Hence global representations of scenes are built up locally and the richness of different portions of the representation will vary according to the fixation history of the corresponding location in the visual scene. Participants do not direct their eyes to all parts of a natural scene, and there are large variations in fixation densities on different regions of scenes. The implication therefore is that an abstract representation of the current visual surroundings will vary greatly in richness over its extent. There will be regions that were not fixated and hence little or no local detail will be represented. Conversely some regions will be fixated a number of times and so the representation of these locations will be richly detailed.

Local variability in representational faithfulness increases efficiency, by having little or no detail in the representation of areas that are rarely foveated. Conversely, areas of 'interest' in the scene (Buswell, 1935) are represented richly. Consequently, the processes of information extraction for retention by the visual system work to effectively weight the resultant representation according to how the eyes are directed around the scene. In real life tasks, it is clear that in general the eye is directed to areas according to the requirements of the current task, with a general strategy of looking at what you are doing (Ballard et al., 1992; Land et al., 1999). Hence such a fixation-weighted representational system will produce a representation with rich detail of the areas and items used in a task, while avoiding the inefficiency of encoding less relevant regions of the visual environment.

The ideas presented in this chapter describe the beginnings of a framework for representation in the visual system and highlight the need for further exploration of the issues raised from these data collected under viewing conditions that were designed to be close to natural. Ten years on from the inception of change detection research, we are still some way from understanding visual representation and perception. While there remain many unanswered questions, we are perhaps beginning to understand more about what we need to be asking and how to approach our questioning.

Acknowledgements

I thank Michael Land and Jenny Rusted for their comments on the manuscript and Iain Gilchrist for the use of his SMI eye tracker for collection of the behavioral data. I also thank Peter De Graef and an unnamed reviewer for their helpful and constructive comments on an earlier version of this chapter.

References

Aginsky, V. and Tarr, M.J. (2000) How are different properties of a scene encoded in visual memory? *Vis. Cognit.*, 7: 147–162.

Ballard, D.H., Hayhoe, M.M., Li, F., Whitehead, S.D., Frisby, J.P., Taylor, J.G. and Fisher, R.B. (1992) Hand–eye coordination during sequential tasks. *Philos. Trans. R. Soc. Lond. B Biol. Sci.*, 337: 331–339.

Becker, M.W., Pashler, H. and Anstis, S.M. (2000) The role of iconic memory in change-detection tasks. *Perception*, 29: 273–286.

Berkeley, G. (1709) An essay towards a new theory of vision. Re-published in: A.D. Lindsay (Ed.), *A New Theory of Vision and Other Writings*. Dent, London (1910).

Berkeley, G. (1710) A Treatise Concerning the Principles of Human Knowledge. Re-published in: K.P. Winkler (Ed.), *A Treatise Concerning the Principles of Human Knowledge*. Hackett Publishing Co., Indianapolis (1982).

Berkeley, G. (1713) Three Dialogues between Hylas and Philonous, in Opposition to Sceptics and Atheists. Re-published in: A.D. Lindsay (Ed.), *A New Theory of Vision and Other Writings*. Dent, London (1910).

Bevan, W. (1958) Perception: evolution of a concept. *Psychol. Rev.*, 65: 34–55.

Biederman, I. (1981) On the semantics of a glance at a scene. In: M. Kubovy and J.R. Pomerantz (Eds.), *Perceptual Organization*. Lawrence Erlbaum Associates, Hillsdale, NJ, pp. 213–253.

Biederman, I. (1987) Recognition-by-components — a theory of human image understanding. *Psychol. Rev.*, 94: 115–147.

Biederman, I. and Gerhardstein, P.C. (1993) Recognizing depth-rotated objects — evidence and conditions for 3-dimensional viewpoint invariance. *J. Exp. Psychol. Hum. Percept. Perform.*, 19: 1162–1182.

Biederman, I. and Gerhardstein, P.C. (1995) Viewpoint-dependent mechanisms in visual object recognition — Reply to Tarr and Bulthoff (1995). *J. Exp. Psychol. Hum. Percept. Perform.*, 21: 1506–1514.

Blanchard, H.E., McConkie, G.W., Zola, D. and Wolverton, G.S. (1984) Time course of visual information utilization during fixations in reading. *J. Exp. Psychol. Hum. Percept. Perform.*, 10: 75–89.

Bridgeman, B. and Mayer, M. (1983) Failure to integrate visual information from successive fixations. *Bull. Psychon. Soc.*, 21: 285–286.

Bridgeman, B., Hendry, D. and Stark, L. (1975) Failure to detect displacement of the visual world during saccadic eye movements. *Vision Res.*, 15: 719–722.

Bulthoff, H.H. and Edelman, S. (1992) Psychophysical support for a 2-dimensional view interpolation theory of object recognition. *Proc. Natl. Acad. Sci. USA*, 89: 60–64.

Buswell, G.T. (1935) *How People Look at Pictures: A Study of the Psychology of Perception in Art*. University of Chicago Press, Chicago.

De Graef, P. (1992) Scene-context effects and models of real-world perception. In: K. Rayner (Ed.), *Eye Movements and Visual Cognition: Scene Perception and Reading*. Springer, New York, pp. 243–259.

De Graef, P. and Verfaillie, K. (2002) Transsaccadic memory for visual object detail. In: J. Hyönä, D.P. Munoz, W. Heide and R. Radach (Eds.), *The Brain's Eye: Neurobiological and Clinical Aspects of Oculomotor Research*. Progress in Brain Research, Vol. 140, Elsevier, Amsterdam, pp. 181–196.

Delorme, A., Richard, G. and Fabre-Thorpe, M. (2000) Ultra-rapid categorisation of natural scenes does not rely on colour cues: a study in monkeys and humans. *Vision Res.*, 40: 2187–2200.

Deubel, H., Schneider, W.X. and Bridgeman, B. (1996) Postsaccadic target blanking prevents saccadic suppression of image displacement. *Vision Res.*, 36: 985–996.

Deubel, H., Bridgeman, B. and Schneider, W.X. (1998) Immediate post-saccadic information mediates space constancy. *Vision Res.*, 38: 3147–3159.

Deubel, H., Schneider, W.X. and Bridgeman, B. (2002) Transsaccadic memory of position and form. In: J. Hyönä, D.P. Munoz, W. Heide and R. Radach (Eds.), *The Brain's Eye: Neurobiological and Clinical Aspects of Oculomotor Research*. Progress in Brain Research, Vol. 140, Elsevier, Amsterdam, pp. 165–180.

Gibson, J.J. (1979) *The Ecological Approach to Visual Perception*. Houghton Mifflin, Boston, MA.

Grealy, M.A., Craig, C.M. and Lee, D.N. (1999) Evidence for on-line visual guidance during saccadic gaze shifts. *Proc. R. Soc. Lond. B Biol. Sci.*, 266: 1799–1804.

Grimes, J. (1996) On the failure to detect changes in scenes across saccades. In: K. Atkins (Ed.), *Perception: Vancouver Studies in Cognitive Science*. Vol 2, Oxford University Press, New York, pp. 89–110.

Haber, R.N. (1983) The impending demise of the icon — a critique of the concept of iconic storage in visual information-processing. *Behav. Brain Sci.*, 6: 1–11.

Hayhoe, M.M. (2000) Vision using routines: a functional account of vision. *Vis. Cognit.*, 7: 43–64.

Helmholtz, H.v. (1867) *Handbuch der Physiologischen Optik*. 1st Voss, Hamburg.

Henderson, J.M. (1992) Object identification in context — the visual processing of natural scenes. *Can. J. Psychol.*, 46: 319–341.

Henderson, J.M. (1994) Two representational systems in dynamic visual identification. *J. Exp. Psychol. Gen.*, 123: 410–426.

Henderson, J.M. (1997) Transsaccadic memory and integration during real-world object perception. *Psychol. Sci.*, 8: 51–55.

Henderson, J.M. and Hollingworth, A. (1999) The role of fixation position in detecting scene changes across saccades. *Psychol. Sci.*, 10: 438–443.

Henderson, J.M. and Siefert, A.B.C. (1999) The influence of enantiomorphic transformation on transsaccadic object integration. *J. Exp. Psychol. Hum. Percept. Perform.*, 25: 243–255.

Hobbes, T. (1651) Elements of Philosophy. Re-published in: W. Molesworth (Ed.), *The English works of Thomas Hobbes of Malmesbury*. John Bohn, London (1839–45).

Hobbes, T. (1656) Leviathan. Re-published in: W. Molesworth (Ed.), *The English works of Thomas Hobbes of Malmesbury*. John Bohn, London (1839–45).

Hochberg, J. (1968) In the mind's eye. In: R.N. Haber (Ed.), *Contemporary Theory and Research in Visual Perception*. Holt, New York, pp. 309–331.

Hollingworth, A. and Henderson, J.M. (2002) Accurate visual memory for previously attended objects in natural scenes. *J. Exp. Psychol. Hum. Percept. Perform.*, 28: 113–136.

Hume, D. (1739) A treatise of human nature. Re-published in: L.A. Selby-Bigge and P.H. Nidditch (Eds.), *Hume's Treatise*. 2nd ed., Clarendon Press, Oxford (1978).

Hume, D. (1748) An Enquiry Concerning Human Understanding. Re-published in: A.G.N. Flew (Ed.), *An Enquiry Concerning Human Understanding*. Open Court, La Salle (1988).

Humphrey, G.K. and Khan, S.C. (1992) Recognizing novel views of 3-dimensional objects. *Can. J. Psychol.*, 46: 170–190.

Intraub, H. (1980) Presentation rate and the representation of briefly glimpsed pictures in memory. *J. Exp. Psychol. Hum. Learn. Mem.*, 6: 1–12.

Intraub, H. (1981) Rapid conceptual identification of sequentially presented pictures. *J. Exp. Psychol. Hum. Percept. Perform.*, 7: 604–610.

Irwin, D.E. (1991) Information integration across saccadic eye-movements. *Cognit. Psychol.*, 23: 420–456.

Irwin, D.E. (1993) Perceiving an integrated visual world. In: D.E. Meyer and S. Kornblum (Eds.), *Attention and Performance XIV: Synergies in Experimental Psychology, Artificial Intelligence and Cognitive Neuroscience*. MIT Press, Cambridge, MA, pp. 121–142.

Irwin, D.E., Yantis, S. and Jonides, J. (1983) Evidence against visual integration across saccadic eye-movements. *Percept. Psychophys.*, 34: 49–57.

Johansson, R.S., Westling, G.R., Backstrom, A. and Flanagan, J.R. (2001) Eye–hand coordination in object manipulation. *J. Neurosci.*, 21: 6917–6932.

Jonides, J., Irwin, D.E. and Yantis, S. (1982) Integrating visual information from successive fixations. *Science*, 215: 192–194.

Karn, K.S. and Hayhoe, M.M. (2000) Memory representations guide targeting eye movements in a natural task. *Vis. Cognit.*, 7: 673–703.

Karn, K.S., Moller, P. and Hayhoe, M.M. (1997) Reference frames in saccadic targeting. *Exp. Brain Res.*, 115: 267–282.

Land, M.F. and Hayhoe, M.M. (2001) In what ways do eye movements contribute to everyday activities? *Vision Res.*, 41: 3559–3565.

Land, M.F., Mennie, N. and Rusted, J. (1999) The roles of vision and eye movements in the control of activities of daily living. *Perception*, 28: 1311–1328.

Loftus, G.R., Nelson, W.W. and Kallman, H.J. (1983) Differential acquisition rates for different types of information from pictures. *Q. J. Exp. Psychol. A Hum. Exp. Psychol.*, 35: 187–198.

McConkie, G.W. and Currie, C.B. (1996) Visual stability across saccades while viewing complex pictures. *J. Exp. Psychol. Hum. Percept. Perform.*, 22: 563–581.

McConkie, G.W. and Rayner, K. (1976) Identifying the span of the effective stimulus in reading: literature review and theories of reading. In: H. Singer and R.B. Buddell (Eds.), *Theoretical Models and Processes of Reading*. International Reading Association, Newark, NJ, pp. 137–162.

Melcher, D. (2001) Persistence of visual memory for scenes — a medium-term memory may help us to keep track of objects during visual tasks. *Nature*, 412: 401–401.

Neisser, U. (1967) *Cognitive Psychology*. Appleton Century Crofts, New York.

Nelson, W.W. and Loftus, G.R. (1980) The functional visual field during picture viewing. *J. Exp. Psychol. Hum. Learn. Mem.*, 6: 391–399.

O'Regan, J.K. and Lévy-Schoen, A. (1983) Integrating visual information from successive fixations — does trans-saccadic fusion exist. *Vision Res.*, 23: 765–768.

O'Regan, J.K. and Noë, A. (2002) A sensorimotor account of vision and visual consciousness. *Behav. Brain Sci.*, 24, in press.

O'Regan, J.K., Deubel, H., Clark, J.J. and Rensink, R.A. (2000) Picture changes during blinks: looking without seeing and seeing without looking. *Vis. Cognit.*, 7: 191–211.

Østerberg, G. (1935) Topography of the layer of rods and cones in the human retina. *Acta Ophthalmol., Suppl.*, 6: 1–103.

Parker, R.E. (1978) Picture processing during recognition. *J. Exp. Psychol. Hum. Percept. Perform.*, 4: 284–293.

Pollatsek, A. and Rayner, K. (1992) What is integrated across fixations? In: K. Rayner (Ed.), *Eye Movements and Visual Cognition: Scene Perception and Reading*. Springer, New York, pp. 166–191.

Pollatsek, A., Rayner, K. and Henderson, J.M. (1990) Role of spatial location in integration of pictorial information across saccades. *J. Exp. Psychol. Hum. Percept. Perform.*, 16: 199–210.

Rayner, K. (1978) Foveal and parafoveal cues in reading. In: J. Requin (Ed.), *Attention and Performance*. Vol 7, Lawrence Erlbaum Associates, Hillsdale, NJ, pp. 149–162.

Rayner, K. and Pollatsek, A. (1983) Is visual information integrated across saccades. *Percept. Psychophys.*, 34: 39–48.

Rayner, K. and Pollatsek, A. (1992) Eye-movements and scene perception. *Can. J. Psychol.*, 46: 342–376.

Rayner, K., Inhoff, A.W., Morrison, R.E., Slowiaczek, M.L. and Bertera, J.H. (1981) Masking of foveal and parafoveal vision during eye fixations in reading. *J. Exp. Psychol. Hum. Percept. Perform.*, 7: 167–179.

Rensink, R.A. (2000) The dynamic representation of scenes. *Vis. Cognit.*, 7: 17–42.

Rensink, R.A., O'Regan, J.K. and Clark, J.J. (1995) Image

flicker is as good as saccades in making large scene changes invisible. *Perception*, 24: 26–27.

Rensink, R.A., O'Regan, J.K. and Clark, J.J. (1997) To see or not to see: the need for attention to perceive changes in scenes. *Psychol. Sci.*, 8: 368–373.

Rensink, R.A., O'Regan, J.K. and Clark, J.J. (2000) On the failure to detect changes in scenes across brief interruptions. *Vis. Cognit.*, 7: 127–145.

Simons, D.J. (1996) In sight, out of mind: when object representations fail. *Psychol. Sci.*, 7: 301–305.

Simons, D.J. and Chabris, C.F. (1999) Gorillas in our midst: sustained inattentional blindness for dynamic events. *Perception*, 28: 1059–1074.

Simons, D.J. and Levin, D.T. (1997) Change blindness. *Trends Cogn. Sci.*, 1: 261–267.

Simons, D.J. and Levin, D.T. (1998) Failure to detect changes to people during a real-world interaction. *Psychon. Bull. Rev.*, 5: 644–649.

Sperling, G. (1960) The information available in brief visual presentations. *Psychol. Monogr.*, 74: 1–29.

Tarr, M.J. (1995) Rotating objects to recognize them — a case-study on the role of viewpoint dependency in the recognition of 3-dimensional objects. *Psychon. Bull. Rev.*, 2: 55–82.

Tatler, B.W. (2001) Characterising the visual buffer: real-world evidence for overwriting early in each fixation. *Perception*, 30: 993–1006.

Tatler, B.W., Gilchrist, I.D. and Rusted, J. (2002a) The time course of abstract visual representation. In prep.

Tatler, B.W., Gilchrist, I.D. and Land, M.F. (2002b) The role of fixation in abstract representation of visual scenes. In prep.

Verfaillie, K. and De Graef, P. (2000) Transsaccadic memory for position and orientation of saccade source and target. *J. Exp. Psychol. Hum. Percept. Perform.*, 26: 1243–1259.

Yarbus, A.L. (1967) *Eye Movements and Vision*. Plenum Press, New York.

CHAPTER 11

Transsaccadic memory of position and form

Heiner Deubel [1,*], Werner X. Schneider [1] and Bruce Bridgeman [2]

[1] *Department of Psychology, Ludwig-Maximilians-Universität, Leopoldstrasse 13, 80802 Munich, Germany*
[2] *Department of Psychology, University of California, Social Sciences 2, Santa Cruz, CA 95064, USA*

Abstract: Why and how people perceive the visual world as continuous and stable, despite the gross changes of its retinal projection that occur with each saccade, is one of the classic problems in perception. In the present paper, we argue that an important factor of visual stability and transsaccadic perception is formed by the reafferent visual information, i.e., the visual display that is present when the eyes land. After a review of some of the relevant theoretical, behavioural and physiological research on space constancy, saccadic suppression and transsaccadic memory, three experiments are presented. In a first experiment, we study the effect of an extended horizontal bar covering the target area for a short period after the saccade on saccadic suppression of image displacement. The results show that the bar acts just like a temporary blanking of the saccade target, leading to a strong reduction of saccadic suppression. In the second experiment, we show that any object that is present immediately after the saccade can establish a spatial reference, even if it is dissimilar to the saccade target. In a third experiment we study, with a similar approach, the effect of blanking and postsaccadic information on transsaccadic integration of form information. The data demonstrate that a localized postsaccadic object tends to replace the content of transsaccadic memory.

Theoretical background

Introduction

Visual information exists all around us, but physiological constraints prevent us from seeing it all at once. When the eye fixates an area, high resolution is limited to a narrow region around the central fovea. Therefore, saccades are required that bring different regions of the world into view. However, such eye movements induce several problems that the perceptual system must solve. A first problem is that, because of the high eye velocity during a saccade, the visual input is reduced or eliminated during the time of a saccade. Nevertheless, we do

---

* Correspondence to: H. Deubel, Department of Psychology, Ludwig-Maximilians-Universität, Leopoldstrasse 13, 80802 Munich, Germany. Tel.: +49-89-2180-5282; Fax: +49-89-2180-5211; E-mail: deubel@psy.uni-muenchen.de

not perceive repetitive 'wipe-outs' of the visual information. Second, the images of the objects in the world drastically change their retinal positions during each saccade. Nevertheless, we do not remain disoriented with each saccade. Space constancy is normally perfect, the world does not appear to jump in the slightest when the eye moves. By contrast, a comparable retinal image motion, produced externally by having the observer tap on his eyeball, produces an alarming percept of instability.

Why and how people perceive the visual world as continuous and stable, despite the gross changes of its retinal projection that occur with each saccade, is certainly one of the classic problems in perception. In the present paper, we want to argue that an important factor of visual stability and transsaccadic perception is formed by the reafferent visual information, i.e., the visual display that is present when the eyes land. But before we present our own data, we will review some of the relevant theoretical, behavioural and physiological research on space constancy, saccadic suppression and transsaccadic memory.

Space constancy and the role of efference copies during saccadic eye movements

One of the first accounts of the problem of space constancy was provided by Helmholtz (see Helmholtz, 1963). He assumed that retinal image motion due to eye or body movements is sensed, but not perceived. Constancy of visual direction is maintained by combining the image motion and the "effort of will involved in trying to alter the effort of will". Closely related, more modern attempts to account for space constancy were mainly cancellation theories, in which the sensory effects of an eye movement are compensated by a simultaneous, equal and opposite extraretinal signal about the position of the eyes in the orbit (Sperry, 1950; von Holst and Mittelstaedt, 1954). The retinal and extraretinal signals cancel each other somewhere in the brain, resulting in a space-constant representation of visual space. In these theories an oculomotor efference copy, proprioception, or some combination of both subtracts from the disturbing effects of a displaced retinal image following a saccade.

Cancellation theories cannot support space constancy unaided, however, because the extraretinal signals are not exact copies of the actual eye movement. First, their gain (ratio of extraretinal signal to actual eye movement) is usually less than one (Grüsser et al., 1987), so they are too small to afford complete compensation. Also dynamically, extraretinal signals of eye position are far from perfect. Direction constancy for flashed stimuli in darkness is grossly disturbed in the vicinity of the saccade. Leonard Matin and colleagues (e.g., Matin, 1972) and Bischof and Kramer (1968) were among the first to study errors in the localization of flashed objects around the time of saccadic eye movements. These and a large number of subsequent studies (e.g., Honda, 1989; Schlag and Schlag-Rey, 1995) analyzed the perception of short localized flashes before, during or after a saccade. The general finding was that these stimuli are systematically mislocalized. Mislocalization starts about 100 ms before the eyes begin to move, where flashes have a tendency to be seen as displaced in the direction of the saccade. Perceived displacement reaches a maximum around the time of the onset of the saccadic movement. These perceptual displacements are presumably a reflection of the mechanisms that compensate for the actual shift in retinal position brought about by the movement of the eye.

In a more detailed account of saccadic mislocalization, recent research has demonstrated that the mislocalization of flashes before and during saccades is not spatially homogeneous. Ross et al. (1997) showed that targets are not simply perceived as displaced in the direction of the saccade. Rather, objects that are closer than the saccade target are perceived as being displaced into the direction of the saccade, and those that are further away than the target are perceived as closer. In other words, targets flashed before and during saccades tend to converge towards the saccade target which results in an apparent 'compression' of the visual world around the saccade target. This compression can even be perceived for natural images presented shortly during the saccade (Ross et al., 1997). Lappe et al. (2000) recently studied saccade-induced mislocalization under various conditions. Interestingly, they found that compression of visual space only occurs when visual references were available after the saccade. Other studies have shown that visual references also modify the gain of the pre-saccadic mislocalization (Honda, 1999).

Thus it seems that extraretinal information about eye position is notoriously imprecise, statically and dynamically. However, even a small error of the extraretinal signal should result in a disturbance of constancy. One compelling solution to this problem is that the visual system has the built-in assumption that the world as a whole does not change during an eye movement. A mechanism that becomes important here is saccadic suppression; indeed, it has been suggested that saccadic suppression 'bridges the errors' that remain due to the imperfect cancellation mechanism (Bridgeman et al., 1994). Therefore, let us next look at saccadic suppression.

Saccadic suppression

Saccadic suppression is a reduction of the visual sensitivity to events occurring before, during, and immediately after saccadic eye movements. Two separate types of saccadic suppression should be distinguished. First, there are many studies on the visual sensitivity to short flashes presented around the time of the saccade (for a review, see, e.g., Matin, 1974). Typically, these studies have reported a moderate threshold elevation (two to threefold) for detecting spots of light flashed briefly during saccades. Other researchers used gratings that were briefly presented during saccades. Their results demonstrate that saccadic suppression is strongest for the low spatial frequencies (below 1 cycle per degree), while higher spatial frequencies remain largely unaffected (Wolf et al., 1978, 1980; Burr et al., 1994). This selectivity of suppression to the magnocellular pathway strongly suggests that this type of suppression is specific to motion signals (see, e.g., Ross et al., 2001).

The second type of saccadic suppression, more relevant in the context discussed here, concerns the detection of image displacement that occurs during saccadic eye movements. During fixation, the sensitive motion detectors of the visual system allow to perfectly perceive even very small displacements of visual objects. Due to the high retinal velocity during a saccade, however, these signals are basically 'wiped-out' with each eye movement. This leads to a strong reduction in sensitivity (by three to four log units) for detecting displacements during saccades (Bridgeman et al., 1975). Magnocellular pathways are also implicated in saccadic suppression of displacement (Bridgeman and Macknik, 1995).

The threshold increase for image jumps during saccades is much larger than the threshold increase for other changes such as brightness increments. In the context of recent work, saccadic suppression of image displacement can be interpreted as a special case of 'change blindness' (Rensink et al., 1997; Rensink, 2002, this volume), the inability of human subjects to identify changes that take place in a visual scene from one fixation to the next, or even within a single fixation if a blank interval prevents direct motion perception.

Without the direct evidence for a target jump from motion detectors, detection of intrasaccadic image displacement requires the comparison of pre- and postsaccadic target locations. Saccadic suppression of image displacement therefore seems to imply either that the required precise comparison is normally not performed, or that transsaccadic memory about the location of objects is not available to the visual system, or is very poor. Indeed, Bridgeman et al. (1994) in their theoretical account of visual stability assumed that there is no need for transsaccadic memory of object positions, rather, the spatial positions are calculated anew after each saccade. This raises the question of the nature of transsaccadic memory, and of what and how much information is contained in this store.

Transsaccadic memory

At the core of most accounts of visual stability is the assumption that some information is stored from one fixation to the next. In its extreme version, this assumption would suggest that presaccadic and postsaccadic information are integrated into a very detailed, high-capacity spatial buffer that combines information from one fixation to the next. Such a mechanism of spatiotopic superposition has indeed been proposed by several authors (e.g., McConkie and Rayner, 1976; Wolf et al., 1980; Jonides et al., 1982; Breitmeyer, 1984). However, despite the intuitive appeal of this hypothesis, ample empirical evidence has demonstrated that it is probably wrong. Several investigators have found that subjects are unable to fuse pre- and postsaccadic patterns in successive fixations to obtain an integrated composite pattern (e.g., Irwin, 1983; O'Regan and Levy-Schoen, 1983; Rayner and Pollatsek, 1983; for a comprehensive overview see also Irwin, 1993a). Moreover, it has been shown that changing the visual characteristics of words and pictures, such as object size or letter case, has no disruptive effect on word or picture naming (e.g., McConkie and Zola, 1979; Rayner et al., 1980). More importantly, it has also no consequences on eye movements in reading. McConkie and Zola (1979) have used cAsE AlTeRnAtIoNs from one fixation to another and found that readers did not notice these changes, and that they did not affect eye movements.

But if the successive 'snapshots' of the world are not fused into a transsaccadic buffer, how can the visual system then produce a stable and continuous representation of a scene? The current assumption is that transsaccadic memory exists but is less image-like in form, containing instead more abstract representations of the information present in each fixation. Rayner et al. (1980) found that a word presented in one fixation speeded the naming of the word in the next fixation, irrespective of an intrasaccadic change of the letter case. Pollatsek et al. (1984) demonstrated that visual and conceptual similarity facilitated the identification of objects across saccades, regardless of changes in object size. So, it seems that abstract visual features and identity codes are combined across fixations. More recent work has also emphasized that while memory for absolute spatial positions across saccades is poor, relational information is well retained from one fixation to the next (e.g., Carlson-Radvansky, 1999; Verfaillie and De Graef, 2000).

In addition to the question of the level of the transsaccadic representations, another important aspect concerns the amount of information that is stored across the saccade. Irwin, 1992 (see also below) found that subjects could remember between three and four letters across an eye movement. Memory capacity for visual elements was estimated to be between three and six elements (Irwin, 1993b).

In summary, there is now agreement that information integration across saccades is carried out at an abstract level. Transsaccadic memory seems to be an undetailed, limited-capacity memory. It is relatively long-lasting (more than several seconds, Irwin, 1991) and is not strictly tied to spatial position. When transsaccadic memory capacity is measured in number of items, it is estimated that three to six memory items survive the saccade. In all these properties transsaccadic memory is similar to, if not identical with, visual short-term memory (Irwin, 1991). For recent and comprehensive overviews of further various aspects of transsaccadic memory see, e.g., Rayner (1998) and De Graef and Verfaillie (2001, 2002, this volume).

Is there a special role for the saccade target?

A number of theories have emphasized a special role of the processing of the saccade target for perceptual stability and transsaccadic memory. Deubel et al. (1984) were probably the first to propose that a transsaccadic memory representation of the saccade target may serve to relocate visual objects across saccades. In more recent work, we (Deubel and Schneider, 1994; Deubel et al., 1996, 1998) developed a 'reference object theory' that assumes that pre- and postsaccadic visual 'snapshots' are linked by means of the saccade target which is assumed by the visual system as being stable. In a very similar theoretical approach, the 'saccade target theory' (McConkie and Currie, 1996; Currie et al., 2000) also assigns a privileged status to the object that constitutes the target for the saccade. Both theories assume that with each new fixation the visual system runs through a sequence of processing steps which starts with the selection of one object as the target for the next saccade. Particular features about the saccade target are selected and stored in a transsaccadic memory to facilitate the re-identification of the target at the start of the next fixation. Then the saccade is executed that brings the target object into central vision. After the eye has landed, the visual system searches for the critical target features within a limited region around the landing site. If the target object is found, the relationship between its retinal location and its mental representation is compared in order to coordinate these two types of information. If the postsaccadic target localization fails (e.g., because the intrasaccadic target shift was too large), however, the assumption of visual stability is abandoned. As a consequence, a target displacement is perceived.

There is some empirical evidence that supports the assumption of a preferential transsaccadic processing of the saccade target. In a study by Irwin (1992) subjects were presented an array of letters while they fixated a central fixation point; the onset of a peripheral stimulus indicated the saccade target. The letters disappeared with the saccade, following the eye movement, the subjects were required to report one of the letters in a partial report paradigm. Irwin found that subjects could remember only 3–4 letters, and that report of the letters near the saccade target was much more accurate than of the other letters in the array. This suggests that information near the saccade target is more likely to be encoded in transsaccadic memory than information from more distant locations. McConkie and Currie (1996) used full-colour pictures of natural scenes which changed during the saccade. In their Experiment 2, the scene expanded or contracted during the eye movement. McConkie and Currie found that the detectability of these image changes was a direct function of the displacement size at the location where the eyes landed, confirming the importance of the local region around the saccade target. Finally, Currie et al. (2000), also using full-colour pictures of natural scenes, studied the detectability of intrasaccadic displacements of objects in the display. They found that displacements of the saccade target object were much easier to detect than displacements of the background (with the saccade target object remaining stationary).

A strong version of the 'saccade target theory' would predict that only information about the saccade target would be stored across the saccade, while intrasaccadic changes of other objects would remain imperceptible. There is clear empirical evidence against this conjecture, however. So, Deubel et al. (1998) presented a simple configuration of a saccade target and a nearby distractor, one of both objects was displaced by a small amount during the saccade. The data revealed no systematic preference for the displacement of the saccade target to be detected. Verfaillie and De Graef (2000) made subjects saccade from one biological motion walker at the fixation position to another in the visual periphery. During the saccade, either the walker at the launch site or the walker which was the saccade target changed in depth orientation or in location. The results show that change detection for the walker at the saccade target was not more accurate than for the walker at the presaccadic fixation.

An important factor to consider in this context is visual attention. A number of investigators have shown that attention movements obligatorily precede saccadic eye movements, leading to a selective improvement of the detection and identification of items presented at the saccade target location, and to a deterioration of performance at other stimulus locations (e.g., Hoffman and Subramaniam, 1995; Kowler et al., 1995; Deubel and Schneider, 1996). This is so even if subjects are instructed to attend to a location other than the saccade target. Irwin and Gordon (1998) manipulated attention in a transsaccadic letter recognition task. Subjects were encouraged to attend to one region in a display while they moved their eyes either to the region they were attending or to another region. The results show that accuracy was high at positions that subjects were asked to attend to, but it was about equally high for positions close to the saccade target, even if the subjects were asked to attend elsewhere. So, the effect of making a saccade to a location produced as much benefit as biasing the subject to attend to a location. Irwin and Gordon (1998) also found, as did Irwin (1992), that subjects were able to remember about four items of the letter display, supporting the argument that the capacity of transsaccadic memory is approximately four objects.

The findings that attention precedes eye movements and that transsaccadic memory capacity is about four items combined may solve the seeming contradictions in the research described above. It has been frequently suggested that the encoding of a visual stimulus in working memory requires selective attention (e.g., Schneider, 1999). In scenes consisting of only two objects like in the experiments of Deubel et al. (1996) and Verfaillie and De Graef (2000) it is likely that both objects are attended before the saccade, so both stimuli are encoded with sufficient accuracy in transsaccadic memory. The more complex stimuli of Irwin (1992), McConkie and Currie (1996) and Currie et al. (2000), however, exceed the capacity of the visual memory; hence only a selected subset of the stimuli, preferentially around the saccade target area, will be still in memory for further processing after the saccade.

The role of reafferent information: the blanking effect

The previous paragraphs discussed the question of what is contained in transsaccadic memory, and why it is encoded. However, an important, but often neglected aspect of memory performance arises only at the moment when memory is probed, which is here when the saccade lands. Then, a comparison has to take place of the contents of transsaccadic memory and the actual reafferent visual information. The question arises how this comparison works and to what extent the stored information content may be affected, and possibly, overwritten, by the new retinal information.

We here propose that the effect of the postsaccadic information on the contents of transsaccadic memory is indeed an important factor for both transsaccadic memory and perceived visual stability. Evidence for our conjecture comes from our experiments on saccadic suppression of image displacement with simple targets (Deubel and Schneider, 1994; Deubel et al., 1996). In these experiments, we demonstrated that saccadic suppression largely disappears with a stunningly simple manipulation, namely by blanking the target with saccade onset and restoring it only 50–300 ms after the eyes stop at the end of a saccade; we called this effect the 'blanking effect'. The blanking effect occurs even for targets in darkness, meaning that displacement detection under this condition relies on extraretinal signals rather than on retinal information from the structured environment. It has been argued that saccadic suppression of image displacement implies that transsaccadic information about spatial positions is poor. However, the considerable accuracy with which subjects can judge transsaccadic displacements in the 'blanking' condition clearly requires both the maintenance of high-quality information about presaccadic target position across the saccade, and a precise extraretinal signal! Thus, it follows from our findings that precise information about the presaccadic target position and a precise extraretinal signal are indeed available for stimulus localizations after the saccade, but they ordinarily are not used in perception. We have suggested that this is because the visual system assumes, as a null-hypothesis, the stability of any object that is continuously available both before and after the saccade. Only a very large discrepancy between eye movement magnitude and image position is able to break this assumption. This assumption is also broken, however, when the presaccadic object is not present immediately after the saccade. Only under this condition are precise transsaccadic information and extraretinal signals used to achieve displacement detection. Because of its strong effect in unveiling information available transsaccadically, target blanking presents a tool for studying visual stability and the nature of spatial information transferred across the saccade.

While the absence of a postsaccadic target eliminates saccadic suppression, its presence largely determines whether other stimuli in the field are seen as stable. We demonstrated this in the experiments with two stimuli (a target and a distractor) already described above (Deubel et al., 1998). One of the manipulations in these experiments included a postsaccadic blanking of one of the stimuli, while the other stimulus was displaced during the saccade. Even when the postsaccadic blank was very short (e.g., 50 ms), the blanked object was invariably perceived as moving across the saccade, while the moved (but continuously present) object was perceived as stable. The fact that this striking illusion even occurred for object displacements of up to half of the size of the saccade illustrates that under this condition perceptual stability is determined not by extraretinal signals but by the object that is found when the eyes land.

This research showed that an object is perceived as stable if it is visible at the end of the eye movement. If the target is blanked even for only 50 ms after the saccade, the visual system fails to find it and the assumption of target stability is broken. In natural visual environments, the stabilization system works well because objects almost never disappear across saccades. However, objects of fixation frequently become obscured briefly by other objects, such as blowing leaves or snow. If the period of occlusion is brief, the object is still perceived, but it is perceived to be behind the occluding object. The effect has been called amodal completion by Michotte (1963), who has described many of its properties. Amodal completion is so effective that we are normally unaware that an object of attention has been briefly obscured. The question arises whether the space constancy system can also tolerate such temporary absence of a saccade target. In other words, is amodal completion as effective as the continuous presence of the target for maintaining constancy? For this purpose, in Experiment 1 the target region is covered, for 250 ms after a saccade, with a bar that provides no information about target location. If the space constancy system is capable of amodal completion, as in perception of occluded objects, this bar should have no effect on the perceived continuity of target location, and detection of an intrasaccadic displacement should be poor. If space constancy requires actual physical presence of the target, however, detection of the displacement should be good, just as with the blanking effect when the target is extinguished and later reappears. In Experiment 2 we provide a pattern during the blanking interval that has no configurational similarity or spatial overlap with the saccade target, but specifies the potential location of the target. The experiment investigates whether any object that is present immediately after the saccade can establish a spatial reference, even if it is dissimilar to the saccade target. Experiment 3 studies, with a similar approach, the effect of blanking and postsaccadic information on transsaccadic integration of form information.

Experiments

Experiment 1: occluding the stimulus

Methods

Seven paid subjects participated in this experiment. They were naïve with respect to the object of the study, but were experienced with the equipment from other eye-movement-related tasks, and had normal visual acuity. Each subject performed at least three separate sessions in each paradigm. For each experiment, the results shown are based on 100–200 trials per condition from each subject. Stimuli were presented on a 21″ video monitor at a frame rate of 100 Hz. Screen background luminance was 2.2 cd/m^2; the luminance of the saccade target and of other stimuli was 25 cd/m^2. The subjects viewed the screen binocularly from a distance of 80 cm. Head movements were restricted by a bite board and a forehead rest. Eye movements were measured with an SRI Generation 5.5 Purkinje-image eyetracker (Crane and Steele, 1985) and sampled at a rate of 500 Hz. Further details of computer control, calibration and triggering are given in Deubel et al. (1996).

The visual target consisted of a small white cross subtending a visual angle of 0.2°. The subject's task was to maintain fixation on the target, and to track it with a saccade if it jumped across the visual field. At the start of each trial the target jumped left or right 6° or 8° to elicit a saccade. The two amplitudes and directions were randomized and equally probable to minimize anticipation and adaptation effects. Saccades beginning earlier than 140 ms or later than 400 ms after the target step were discarded. The computer triggered a second displacement when it detected the saccade elicited by the first target step (see Fig. 1A). The size of the second target displacement was 0.6°, and it was elicited either into the same or into the opposite direction of the first step. At the end of each trial, in a two-alternative forced-choice procedure, the subject's task was to report the direction of the second target shift with respect to the direction of the primary saccade ('forward' vs. 'backward').

The different sequences of stimulus presentations of this experiment are sketched in Fig. 1A. Four different experimental conditions were included. In a first control condition, the target was displaced during the primary saccade, but no blanking occurred ('No blank' condition). In a second condition, the primary saccade triggered a blanking of the target which lasted 250 ms ('blank' condition); then the displaced target reappeared. A blanking time of 250 ms was found to fully elicit the blanking effect in a previous study (Deubel et al., 1996). In the third condition, a horizontal bar, 28° long, extending across the entire width of the screen, appeared during the 250 ms period ('Occluding bar' condition). While the target was not present, from the detection of the saccade until 250 ms thereafter, the bar was displayed at the horizontal level of the target, covering both the previous target position and the various possible post-blanking target positions. Finally, in an additional control condition ('Masking bars' condition), two bars identical to the occluding bar were presented above and below the target region. Like the single long bar, they provided no information about the eventual (horizontal) position of the target, but this configuration did not cover the position of the target. Here the target was not occluded behind another object but clearly had disappeared during the blanking interval. The bars were each 28° long and 0.56° high. They were displayed only during the 250 ms blank period.

Results

Fig. 1B gives the discrimination performance in the four experimental conditions as percent correct; chance level is 50%. First, the data replicate the blanking effect described in our previous work: while the discrimination of intrasaccadic displacements is close to chance level for the non-blanked condition in which the target is continuously present, performance is dramatically enhanced by the introduction of the 250 ms blanking period, reaching about 92% correct. This means that subjects can correctly report the target displacements when the target is absent for a short period immediately after the saccade. Second, the data show that detectability of a target jump is also improved considerably (with respect to the 'No blank' condition) when the target's possible

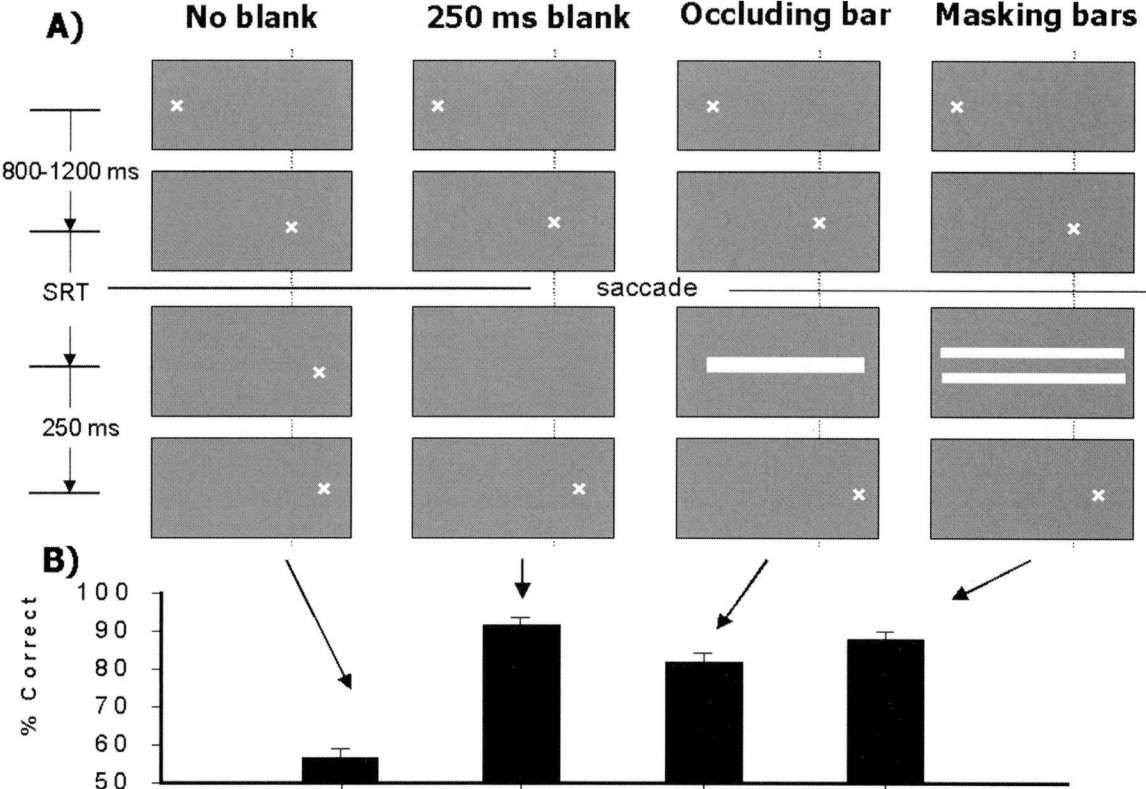

Fig. 1. (A) Experimental conditions in Experiment 1. The open rectangles show the appearance of the screen in successive time intervals. The small 'x' represents the saccade target. SRT = saccadic reaction time. First column from left: 'no blank' control condition. Second column: condition with 250 ms postsaccadic target blanking. Third column: stimulus sequence with a long bar covering the target area during the blanking interval. Rightmost column: comparison condition with two bars that do not obscure the location of the saccade target. (B) The data show percent correct displacement discrimination with no blank, a 250 ms blanking, with a long occluding bar present throughout the 250 ms blank, and with two long bars present throughout the blank interval. Error bars indicate between-subject standard errors.

post-blanking positions are occluded by the long bar. In this case performance is intermediate between the blanking and the non-blanking detectabilities. The target displacement detectability with the occluding bar is significantly better than in the no-blank condition ($t(6) = 4.99$; $p < 0.01$), but also significantly worse than detectability in the 250 ms blank condition ($t(6) = 4.1$; $p < 0.01$). Finally, detectability of the target displacements in the two-bar condition, where the target disappears during the blanking interval, is only about 4% worse than detectability with the blanked target but no other stimuli in the field. This difference is not significant ($p > 0.05$). The results show that, in order to induce the 'blanking' effect, the screen has not necessarily to be blank.

Rather, the critical feature of the blanking effect seems to be the temporary absence of the (localized) target. But is it critical that the postsaccadic object is identical to the presaccadic target?

Experiment 2: target substitution

Experiment 1 studied the possible effect of amodal completion on space constancy and the blanking effect. In this experiment, the postsaccadic occluder (the bar) was neither localized in the horizontal dimension nor did target and occluder share featural properties. In Experiment 2 we examined the effect of presenting a well-localized spatial pattern, visually very dissimilar to the target, during the blanking interval. If the postsaccadic object must be geometrically similar to the original target in order to be accepted as a spatial reference, the visual system should simply ignore the stimulus. However, if the space constancy system accepts a highly dissimilar alternative pattern as a 'place holder' for the reference object, the location of this pattern should strongly affect displacement perception of the target.

Methods

Six naïve subjects participated in this experiment. Again, four different conditions were included in the experiment. Typical sequences of stimulus presentations are given in Fig. 2A. As in the previous experiment, there was a 'No blank' and a '250 ms blank' condition, without presentation of any other stimuli (Fig. 2A, first and second columns), In the critical conditions, additional stimuli were presented. Note that concerning the target, the stimuli were identical to the '250 ms blank' condition. During the blanking interval a pattern appeared consisting of two rectangles, 0.4° wide × 0.56° high. They were 0.94° apart, positioned vertically above and below the eventual position of the post-blanking target. Thus the two rectangles replaced the original target for 250 ms postsaccadically. The rectangles did not overlap the target spatially, but their horizontal position was well-defined. At the same time, the empty region in the centre of the substituted stimulus clearly revealed that the original saccade target had disappeared, and there were no common elements between the original target and the substituted target. Concerning the location of the substitute target, two

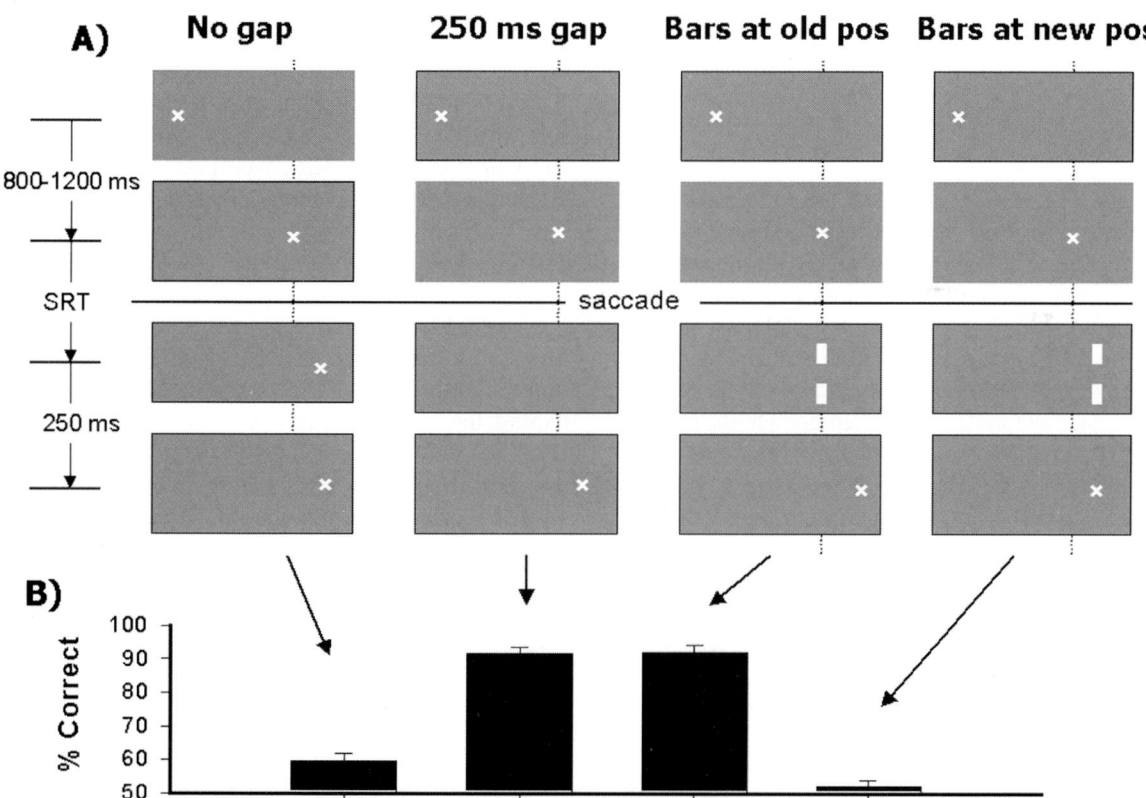

Fig. 2. (A) Stimulus conditions in Experiment 2. Display format as in Fig. 1. The two leftmost columns again represent the 'no blank' and the '250 ms blank' control conditions. In the third condition, two short rectangles appear for 250 ms at the horizontal (presaccadic) location of the blanked target. In the fourth condition, the bars are presented at the new (displaced) position of the blanked target. (B) Discrimination performance in control conditions and with presentation of a pattern of two short rectangles at the old and at the new target position during the blanking interval.

different conditions were applied. In a first condition, the rectangles appeared at the location of the old (presaccadic) target (Fig. 2A, third column). In a second condition, the rectangles appeared at the location where the displaced target would appear after the blanking period (Fig. 2A, rightmost column).

If the absence of visual information about target position alone is sufficient to yield the detectability of target displacement, discrimination performance should be independent of the rectangle pattern presentation, and should be as good as in the blanking condition. If the rectangle pattern present immediately after the saccade is accepted as a spatial reference, however, the perception of target displacement should be determined by the pattern location in a well-predictable way: in the condition where the pattern appears at the old target position, displacement detection for the saccade target should be perfect. When the pattern appears at the new target position, however, no displacement should be perceived because the short rectangles specify the future position of the target as the new spatial reference.

Results

Discrimination performance in this experiment is presented in Fig. 2B. While performance is at chance for the 'No blank' control condition, displacement detection is close to perfect for the '250 ms blank' condition, reproducing the blanking effect. The more interesting cases however are the situations in which the additional rectangles are presented. These stimuli are irrelevant for the subject's task, and the sequence of presentation of the target is identical to the 'blank' condition. Nevertheless, the location of the rectangle pattern now determined whether the subject perceived stability or displacement of the target. When the pattern of rectangles appeared at the presaccadic target location, discrimination of the target jumps was perfect, whereas discrimination with the pattern appearing at the new, displaced target location was similar to the non-blanking condition. Thus, in the latter case, the pattern did not enable the subjects to do any better than they had done in the no-blanking condition; they behaved as though the target had always been present. Thus, the results demonstrate that any localized object found at saccade end is taken as a spatial reference, even if obviously different from the target.

Experiment 3: perception of transsaccadic form changes

The two previous experiments demonstrated (1) that the absence of a target immediately after the saccade improves displacement detection and (2) that the postsaccadic presence of any localized stimulus, even if clearly not identical to the target, affects the localization of the target across the saccade. Experiment 3 investigates whether similar manipulations lead to similar effects if the detection of form changes rather than location is probed. With this experiment we intended to investigate, first, whether a temporal blanking of the stimulus immediately after the saccade also subserves the perception of transsaccadic changes of form, second, whether an occluding bar also acts like a blanking, and third, whether an irrelevant stimulus (a mask) present for a short period of time after saccade end leads to a deterioration of performance. The stimuli we used consisted of a rectangular, checkerboard-like array of small bright squares. We call these stimuli 'Phillips-patterns', since Phillips (1974) and Phillips and Christie (1977) introduced patterns of this kind for the study of visual short-term memory.

Methods

Four naïve subjects participated in the experiment. The four different sequences of stimulus presentations are depicted in Fig. 3A. The subject initially fixated the fixation cross. After a random delay, a 'Phillips-pattern' appeared, 6 or 8°, to the left or to the right of fixation. This pattern was composed of an array of dark and bright small rectangles, each 0.27° wide. As to the complexity of the pattern, two different levels of difficulty were used. In the 'Easy' condition the pattern was 4 squares high and 4 squares wide. In the 'Difficult' condition, the pattern was 4 squares high and 5 squares wide (see Fig. 3A). The subject was instructed to saccade to the appearing pattern. Triggered by the onset of the saccade, in all four conditions a bright horizontal bar covering the width of the display appeared for 10 ms (1 frame). This bar served to wipe-out all remains of phosphor persistence.

Again four different stimulus conditions were used. In the first (non-blanked) condition, the bar

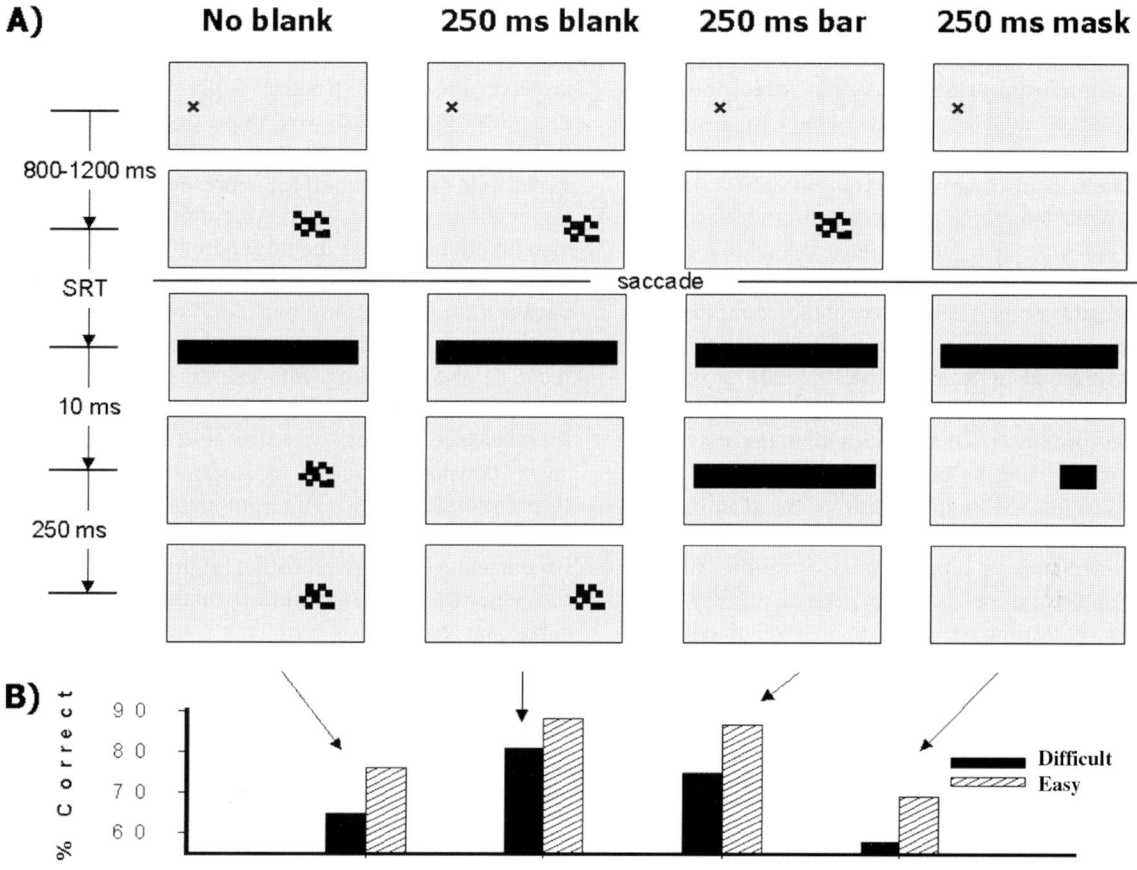

Fig. 3. (A) Stimulus conditions in Experiment 3. Display format as in Fig. 1. Here, subjects are asked to indicate, in a 2AFC task, whether the upper or the lower half of the postsaccadic pattern was different from the presaccadic target pattern. (B) Percent correct discrimination for the four experimental conditions. Both levels of difficulty are presented separately ('Easy': light bars; 'Difficult': dark bars).

was replaced, still during the saccade, by a slightly changed version of the presaccadic pattern. In this postsaccadic pattern, one of the squares constituting the pattern had changed location. This change occurred, in 50% of the trials, in the upper half of the pattern, in the other 50% of the trials, in the lower half of the pattern. The subject had to indicate, in a 2AFC task, whether the change had occurred in the upper or the lower part of the pattern. The second 'blanked' condition was similar to the first except that a blank period of 250 ms was introduced, starting during the saccade. In the third condition, a long horizontal bright bar was presented for 250 ms that completely covered the stimulus area ('bar' condition). Only then did the changed pattern appear. Finally, in the forth condition ('mask' condition), the presaccadic pattern was replaced, for 250 ms, by a homogeneous, bright rectangle covering the same area as the presaccadic target pattern, before the changed pattern appeared.

Results

Fig. 3B depicts the percentages of correct discrimination for the four different conditions, plotted separately for the 'Easy' (light bars) and the 'Difficult' (dark bars) conditions. As a general data pattern the results show, not surprisingly, that the 'Easy' conditions lead to a better performance than the 'Difficult' conditions ($F(1,4) = 108.6$; $p < 0.001$). More interestingly, however, the different experimental conditions also lead to significantly different performance

($F(3,12) = 14.3$; $p < 0.001$). We tested this by post-hoc pairwise comparisons (Bonferroni correction). As a first interesting result, the data reveal that the introduction of a 250 ms blank leads to a significant improvement of performance with respect to the no-blank control condition ($p = 0.029$). As for displacement detection, perception of transsaccadic changes is improved substantially by taking away target information at the end of the saccade, i.e., by a postsaccadic blank. The 250 ms 'bar' condition is not different from the 'blank' condition. Even if the target is replaced by a high-contrast (non-localized) bar, this is very helpful for transsaccadic discrimination performance. This implies that the essential aspect for the blanking effect is the absence of a localized stimulus. Most interesting is the result from the 'mask' case. Here, the visual system finds, when the saccade lands, a homogeneous stimulus of the same size as the presaccadic pattern. Under this condition, performance drops to a level that is as low as, if not worse than, the 'no-blank' condition (comparisons with the 'blank' and the 'bar' conditions yield highly significant differences, $p < 0.001$). This suggests that the postsaccadic mask replaces the memory representation of the presaccadic stimulus, but only if the postsaccadic stimulus is a localized, object-like pattern.

General discussion

Postsaccadic visual information affects the use of transsaccadic memory

This study represents a continuation of our previous work on the blanking effect. The central result of our previous investigations was that when a saccade target is blanked even for a short interval during and after a saccade, its transsaccadic displacement becomes much more visible than when the target is continuously present (Deubel et al., 1996). A second important finding was that the object that is found by the visual system immediately after the saccade is normally perceived as stable, and it is taken as a spatial reference for judging whether other (blanked) objects had moved (Deubel et al., 1998).

The main objective of Experiment 1 was to investigate whether the postsaccadic presentation of a non-localized stimulus occluding the target area can produce an enhancement of displacement detection. The data of Fig. 1 confirm that when the saccade target is absent for a short temporal interval after the primary saccade, even small displacements that go otherwise undetected become obvious to the observer. This blanking effect is present when only the target disappears for a few hundred ms, but it can also be elicited when the target area is covered by an occluding stimulus. The difference in performance between the 'Occluding bar' condition and the '250 ms blank' condition means that the beneficial effects of the blanking interval are not completely transferred when the target is occluded, as though the occluded 'target' was still able to influence the space constancy system to suspend the search for the reference object. Thus amodal presence of the target, even in the absence of any information about its current position, is sufficient to elicit some of the benefit to space constancy that normally occurs across saccades.

The results of the second experiment help to clarify one of our previous results (Deubel et al., 1998). In that paper, we found that the reference object need not be the saccade target, but could be another nearby pattern under some conditions. We presented two geometrically dissimilar targets, one the saccade goal and the other a distractor. If they were displaced relative to one another during a saccade, and one object had a blank, the visual system nearly always accepted the continuously present object as the reference object and perceived it to have remained at the same spatial position during the saccade. This was true whether the new reference object had originally been defined as the saccade goal or the distractor. Whether that object had actually been displaced during the saccade was irrelevant to this assigning of stability, and whether the newly accepted stable reference object was geometrically similar to the original saccade goal was also irrelevant. In our Experiment 2 we now asked for the effect of substituting the target, for a short interval after the saccade, with an otherwise irrelevant, but well localized pattern. It turned out that the continuous availability of information about object position in this condition determined whether the target was seen as stable or as jumping, even though the bar pattern was very different from the target. This finding is consistent with the assumption that the location of the short rectangles, present when the eyes land after the primary saccade, are taken by the visual system as the position of the (presaccadic) target. Obviously, the system detecting target position after the end of a saccade is not particularly selective about the geometric characteristics of the target. Visual form-related features of the reference object are unimportant in searching for the postsaccadic pattern, as long as the location is specified. As long as something appears in about the right place at the right time, according to our hypothesis the space constancy algorithm is satisfied that the reference object has been found, and no further computations are performed; the intrasaccadic displacement of the pattern goes unnoticed.

We conclude from this combination of results that the location of the target forms a major image feature used by the visual system in order to establish space constancy. If one of two objects is blanked, as was the case in our earlier experiments, then only the other object is available to become the reference object. Since the system is not selective about visual features, this distractor becomes the reference object by default, provided the location of the distractor is sufficiently close to the saccade goal object. By the time the blanked target reappears, the system is already committed to the other object as the reference object. The blanked target is then seen as displaced because its position is judged relative to the reference object, whose position is assumed to be stable.

Taken together, the present findings, as well as our previous results with the blanking effect (Deubel et al., 1996, 1998), support the idea that the visual system normally assumes that objects have not been displaced during saccadic eye movements, unless it is overwhelmed with contrary evidence, hence the high threshold for detecting simple image displacements during saccades. The present data can be interpreted in terms of the theories of visual stability described previously. The blanking effect demonstrates the importance of the stimuli that are present immediately after a saccade. According to our theoretical interpretation, the visual system searches for the presaccadic object of attention within a spatiotemporal 'constancy window', comparing the stored features with the new image around the saccade goal immediately after a saccade (Deubel et al., 1984; Irwin et al., 1994). If this target is found within a certain spatial and temporal window, the visual system assumes it to have remained stable during the saccade, and the target becomes a 'reference object' to determine the positions of other objects and textures (Deubel et al., 1996; McConkie and Currie, 1996). According to this theory, then, extraretinal signals are not used for transsaccadic integration under normal circumstances, because the reference object usually is found. The constancy mechanism concentrates on the region near the saccade target, with only secondary influence from other locations. Only changes in the saccade goal and possibly a few other attended objects are transferred accurately across saccades (Irwin et al., 1994). In other words, the structure of the postsaccadic visual scene plays a key role in the process of re-establishing visual direction following a saccade.

If the target is not found (as with target blanking), the assumption of stationarity is broken. Both extraretinal signals, such as efference copy and proprioception, and retinal signals from the visual context are used to compute the new target location. Only in this case does the system use information about sensory conditions before the saccade, ultimately leading to the detection of transsaccadic object displacements. This presaccadic information is stored across the saccade, but normally, when an object is present at the moment the primary saccade lands, it is discarded as soon as the reference object is found.

The tendency to discard, or substitute, the presaccadic information with the postsaccadic visual reafference is also obvious in the results from our Experiment 3 where we studied the effect of postsaccadic information on transsaccadic detection of form changes. Amazingly, the visual systems seems to obey very similar rules in this task, as it does for the task of displacement detection. First, our data demonstrate that postsaccadic blanking, as well as the presentation of a non-localized bar covering the target area leads to a strong improvement of transsaccadic perception of form change. This implies that more (form) information is contained in transsaccadic memory than normal (non-blank) tasks would suggest. Second, the condition with the postsaccadic mask shows that stimuli found after the saccade tend to replace the memory information, making the perception of transsaccadic changes very difficult. However, this effect requires that the postsaccadic stimulus is an object-like, localized item.

The present experiments also provide some characterization of the timing of the transsaccadic integration process. The results suggest that the presence or absence of an object at the moment when the eye lands is an essential determining factor for that object to become a spatial reference. This implies that the reference object need not be the saccade target: another nearby object can take that role, if the saccade target is blanked in a critical postsaccadic period so that it is unavailable for establishing a new calibration. This demonstrates that temporal continuity of an object is more important even than selection as a saccade target in establishing a reference object.

Our results necessitate some modification of the reference object theory that we described earlier (Deubel et al., 1996; McConkie and Currie, 1996). The visual system need not be committed to a single identified reference object before the saccade begins, for a task-irrelevant non-target object can become the reference object, and the system does not know in advance which object will be appropriate as the reference object. Whether an object is defined as target or distractor before the saccade seems to play little role in the postsaccadic determination of the reference object. Nevertheless, there is some independent evidence that the saccade goal target may be more important than other objects for postsaccadic visual calibration. Bischof and Kramer (1968), for instance, found perceived locations to be corrected more quickly near the saccadic goal than at other retinal positions. In a saccadic suppression experiment in which either the saccade target or another visual object such as the previous fixation target moved during the saccade, Heywood and Churcher (1981) showed that subjects often misattribute an intrasaccadic displacement of the saccade goal to a displacement of the other object, tending to preserve space constancy preferentially for the saccade goal. Finally, an important role of the saccade target is suggested by Ross et al. (1997), demonstrating that stimuli flashed shortly before a saccade are mislocalized such that they are perceived closer to the saccade target. Whether this 'spatial attraction' by the saccade target is related to the effect of our 'reference object' mechanism that tries to anchor presaccadically attended objects on the target found after the saccade must be clarified by further research (Lappe et al., 2000).

Possible physiological mechanisms of visual stability across saccadic eye movements

The mechanisms proposed above are based on the assumption that presaccadic information is remapped over the saccade in order to interact with the postsaccadic visual reafference. Neurons in lateral intraparietal cortex (LIP) described by Duhamel et al. (1992) may be performing some of the computations required by our theory. Receptive fields in this area shift to compensate for a saccade about 80 ms before the start of the movement. Thus the LIP seems to store presaccadic, visual information across the saccades and possesses quantitative spatial information about the saccade. The receptive fields are large, however, and would not be able to hold details of the features of a reference objects. Similar properties have been reported from neurons in the superior colliculus (Walker et al., 1995).

Further evidence for transsaccadic storage of saccade target features come from a recent study by Moore et al. (1998). They studied the visual selectivity of saccade-related responses of area V4 neurons in monkeys making delayed eye movements to receptive field stimuli of varying orientation. The neurons exhibit a selective presaccadic enhancement, quite separate from the response to the stimulus onset. The presaccadic enhancement appears to provide a strengthening of a decaying featural representation immediately before an eye movement is directed to visual targets. The authors suggest that this reactivation provides a mechanism by which a clear perception of the saccade goal can be maintained during the execution of the saccade, possibly for the purpose of establishing perceptual continuity across eye movements.

Acknowledgements

This study was supported by the Deutsche Forschungsgemeinschaft (SFB 462).

References

Bischof, N. and Kramer, E. (1968) Untersuchungen und Überlegungen zur Richtungswahrnehmung bei willkürlichen sakkadischen Augenbewegungen. *Psychol. Forsch.*, 32: 185–218.

Breitmeyer, B.G. (1984) *Visual Masking: An Interactive Approach.* Oxford University Press, New York, NY.

Bridgeman, B. and Macknik, S.L. (1995) Saccadic suppression relies on luminance information. *Psychol. Res.*, 58: 163–168.

Bridgeman, B., Hendry, D. and Stark, L. (1975) Failure to detect displacement of the visual world during saccadic eye movements. *Vision Res.*, 15: 719–722.

Bridgeman, B., van der Heijden, A.H.C. and Velichkovsky, B.M. (1994) A theory of visual stability across saccadic eye movements. *Behav. Brain Sci.*, 17: 247–292.

Burr, D.C., Morrone, M.C. and Ross, J. (1994) Selective suppression of the magnocellular visual pathway during saccadic eye movements. *Nature*, 371: 511–513.

Carlson-Radvansky, L.A. (1999) Memory for relational information across saccadic eye movements. *Percept. Psychophys.*, 61: 919–934.

Crane, H.D. and Steele, C.M. (1985) Generation V dual-Purkinje-image eye-tracker. *Appl. Opt.*, 24: 527–537.

Currie, C.B., McConkie, G.W., Carlson-Radvansky, L.A. and Irwin, D.E. (2000) The role of the saccade target object in the perception of a visually stable world. *Percept. Psychophys.*, 62: 673–683.

De Graef, P. and Verfaillie, K. (2001) Special issue: transsaccadic object perception. *Psychol. Belg.*, 41: 1–114.

De Graef, P. and Verfaillie, K. (2002) Transsaccadic memory for visual object detail. In: J. Hyönä, D.P. Munoz, W. Heide and R. Radach (Eds.), *The Brain's Eye: Neurobiological and Clinical Aspects of Oculomotor Research*. Progress in Brain Research, Vol. 140, Elsevier, Amsterdam, pp. 181–196.

Deubel, H. and Schneider, W.X. (1994) Can man bridge a gap? *Behav. Brain Sci.*, 17: 259–260.

Deubel, H. and Schneider, W.X. (1996) Saccade target selection and object recognition: Evidence for a common attentional mechanism. *Vision Res.*, 36: 1827–1837.

Deubel, H., Wolf, W. and Hauske, G. (1984) The evaluation of the oculomotor error signal. In: A.G. Gale and F. Johnson (Eds.), *Theoretical and Applied Aspects of Eye Movement Research*. Elsevier–North-Holland, Amsterdam, pp. 55–62.

Deubel, H., Schneider, W.X. and Bridgeman, B. (1996) Postsaccadic target blanking prevents saccadic suppression of image displacement. *Vision Res.*, 36: 985–996.

Deubel, H., Bridgeman, B. and Schneider, W.X. (1998) Immediate post-saccadic information mediates space constancy. *Vision Res.*, 38: 3147–3159.

Duhamel, J.R., Colby, C. and Goldberg, M. (1992) The updating of the representation of visual space in parietal cortex by intended eye movements. *Science*, 225: 90–92.

Grüsser, O.-J., Krizic, A. and Weiss, L.-R. (1987) Afterimage movement during saccades in the dark. *Vision Res.*, 27: 215–226.

Helmholtz, H.v. (1963) *Handbuch der Physiologischen Optik (1866)*. Dover.

Heywood, S. and Churcher, J. (1981) Direction-specific and position-specific effects upon detection of displacements during saccadic eye movements. *Vision Res.*, 21: 255–261.

Hoffman, J.E. and Subramaniam, B. (1995) The role of visual attention in saccadic eye movements. *Percept. Psychophys.*, 57: 787–795.

Honda, H. (1989) Perceptual localization of visual-stimuli flashed during saccades. *Percept. Psychophys.*, 45: 162–174.

Honda, H. (1999) Modification of saccade-contingent visual mislocalization by the presence of a visual frame of reference. *Vision Res.*, 39: 51–57.

Irwin, D.E. (1983) Evidence against visual integration across saccadic eye movements. *Percept. Psychophys.*, 34: 49–57.

Irwin, D.E. (1991) Information integration across saccadic eye movements. *Cognit. Psychol.*, 23: 420–456.

Irwin, D.E. (1992) Memory for position and identity across eye movements. *J. Exp. Psychol. Learn. Mem. Cogn.*, 18: 307–317.

Irwin, D.E. (1993a) Perceiving an integrated visual world. In: D.E. Meyer and S. Kornblum (Eds.), *Attention and Performance XIV: Synergies in Experimental Psychology*. MIT Press, Cambridge, MA, pp. 121–142.

Irwin, D.E. (1993b) Memory for spatial position across saccadic eye movements. In: G. d'Ydewalle and J. van Rensbergen (Eds.), *Perception and Cognition: Advances in Eye Movement Research*. North Holland, Amsterdam, pp. 323–332.

Irwin, D.E. and Gordon, R.D. (1998) Eye movements, attention and trans-saccadic memory. *Vis. Cognit.*, 5: 127–155.

Irwin, D.E., McConkie, G.W., Carlson-Radvansky, L.A. and Currie, C. (1994) A localist evaluation solution for visual stability across saccades. *Behav. Brain Sci.*, 17: 265–266.

Jonides, J., Irwin, D.E. and Yantis, S. (1982) Integrating visual information from successive fixations. *Science*, 215: 192–194.

Kowler, E., Anderson, E., Dosher, B. and Blaser, E. (1995) The role of attention in the programming of saccades. *Vision Res.*, 35: 1897–1916.

Lappe, M., Awater, H. and Krekelberg, B. (2000) Postsaccadic visual references generate presaccadic compression of space. *Nature*, 403: 892–895.

Matin, L. (1972) Eye movements and perceived visual direction. In: D. Jameson and L. Hurvitch (Eds.), *Handbook of Sensory Physiology 7*. Springer, Berlin, pp. 331–380.

Matin, E. (1974) Saccadic suppression: A review and an analysis. *Psychol. Bull.*, 81: 899–917.

McConkie, G.W. and Currie, C.B. (1996) Visual-stability across saccades while viewing complex pictures. *J. Exp. Psychol. Hum. Percept. Perform.*, 22: 563–581.

McConkie, G.W. and Rayner, K. (1976) Identifying the span of the effective stimulus in reading: literature review and theories of reading. In: H. Singer and R. Ruddell (Eds.), *Theoretical Models and Processes of Reading*. International Reading Institute, Newark, DE, 2nd ed., pp. 137–162.

McConkie, G.W. and Zola, D. (1979) Is visual information integrated across successive fixations in reading? *Percept. Psychophys.*, 25: 221–224.

Michotte, A. (1963) *The Perception of Causality*. (T.R. Miles and C. Miles, Transl.) Methuen, London.

Moore, T., Tolias, A.S. and Schiller, P.H. (1998) Visual representations during saccadic eye movements. *Proc. Natl. Acad. Sci. USA*, 95: 8981–8984.

O'Regan, J.K. and Levy-Schoen, A. (1983) Integrating visual information from successive fixations: does trans-saccadic fusion exist? *Vision Res.*, 23: 765–768.

Phillips, W.A. (1974) On the distinction between sensory storage and short-term visual memory. *Percept. Psychophys.*, 16: 283–290.

Phillips, W.A. and Christie, D. (1977) Interference with visualization. *Q. J. Exp. Psychol.*, 29: 637–650.

Pollatsek, A., Rayner, K. and Collins, W.E. (1984) Integrating pictorial information across eye movements. *J. Exp. Psychol. Gen.*, 113: 426–442.

Rayner, K. (1998) Eye movements in reading and information processing — 20 years of research. *Psychol. Bull.*, 124: 372–422.

Rayner, K. and Pollatsek, A. (1983) Is visual information integrated across saccades? *Percept. Psychophys.*, 34: 39–48.

Rayner, K., McConkie, G.W. and Zola, D. (1980) Integrating information across eye movements. *Cognit. Psychol.*, 12: 206–226.

Rensink, R.A. (2002) Commentary: Changes. In: J. Hyönä, D.P. Munoz, W. Heide and R. Radach (Eds.), *The Brain's Eye: Neurobiological and Clinical Aspects of Oculomotor Research*. Progress in Brain Research, Vol. 140, Elsevier, Amsterdam, pp. 197–207.

Rensink, R.A., O'Regan, J.K. and Clark, J.J. (1997) To see or not to see: the need for attention to perceive changes in scenes. *Psychol. Sci.*, 8: 368–373.

Ross, J., Morrone, M.C. and Burr, D.C. (1997) Compression of visual space before saccades. *Nature*, 386: 598–601.

Ross, J., Morrone, M.C., Goldberg, M.E. and Burr, D.C. (2001) Changes in visual perception at the time of saccades. *Trends Neurosci.*, 24: 113–121.

Schlag, J. and Schlag-Rey, M. (1995) Illusory localization of stimuli flashed in the dark before saccades. *Vision Res.*, 35: 2347–2357.

Schneider, W.X. (1999) Visual–spatial working memory, attention and scene representation: a neuro-cognitive theory. *Psychol. Res.*, 62: 220–236.

Sperry, R.W. (1950) Neural basis of the spontaneous optokinetic response produced by visual inversion. *J. Comp. Physiol. Psychol.*, 43: 482–489.

Verfaillie, K. and De Graef, P. (2000) Transsaccadic memory for position and orientation of saccade source and target. *J. Exp. Psychol. Hum. Percept. Perform.*, 26: 1243–1259.

Von Holst, E. and Mittelstaedt, H. (1954) Das Reafferenzprinzip. *Naturwissenschaften*, 37: 464–476.

Walker, M.F., Fitzgibbon, E.J. and Goldberg, M.E. (1995) Neurons in the monkey superior colliculus predict the visual result of impending saccadic eye-movements. *J. Neurophysiol.*, 73: 1988–2003.

Wolf, W., Hauske, G. and Lupp, U. (1978) How presaccadic gratings modify postsaccadic modulation transfer function. *Vision Res.*, 18: 1173–1179.

Wolf, W., Hauske, G. and Lupp, U. (1980) Interaction of pre- and postsaccadic patterns having the same coordinates is space. *Vision Res.*, 20: 117–124.

CHAPTER 12

Transsaccadic memory for visual object detail

Peter De Graef* and Karl Verfaillie

Laboratory of Experimental Psychology, Department of Psychology, University of Leuven, B-3000 Leuven, Belgium

Abstract: When we move our eyes around in real-world scenes, we typically have several peripheral previews of an object before we direct our eyes straight at the object. Numerous studies on transsaccadic memory have investigated whether there is any evidence for the integration of peripheral object information acquired presaccadically with foveal object information acquired postsaccadically. We review this evidence to illustrate the currently dominant view that transsaccadic object memory is sparse and contains little visual object detail. However, based on some recent studies of the role of postsaccadic stimulus blanking in transsaccadic change detection, we hypothesize that transsaccadic object memory involves the automatic emergence of a *visual analog*: a high-capacity, non-selective, internal representation of visual object detail. This hypothesis is tested by examining cued detection of intrasaccadic changes in the in-depth orientation of objects in scenes. The data provide preliminary support for the presence of the visual analog, but also show that its functionality is strictly limited by attentional and temporal constraints on the process of reading out information from the visual analog.

Transsaccadic memory: the great interfixational void

Exploration of an everyday visual scene typically involves an alternation between fixations on objects in the scene and saccades bringing peripherally located objects in foveal vision (De Graef et al., 1990; Henderson and Hollingworth, 1999a). Because visual intake is reduced during saccades (Matin, 1974; Matin, 1986; Ross et al., 2001) and the retinal projection of the outside world changes position with every saccade, the result of this scanning behavior is a temporally and spatially discontinuous train of 'snapshots'. To explain the contrast between this characterization of the proximal stimulus during scene exploration and our phenomenological experience of a stable and continuous visual world, numerous studies have addressed the question of whether, and if so, how information acquired on one fixation is stored across saccades and integrated with information from subsequent fixations (for overviews see Pollatsek et al., 1990; Irwin and Andrews, 1996). In other words, is there such a thing as transsaccadic memory and what are its contents?[1]

While only quite recently some attempts have been made to develop a detailed and testable account of the representations involved in transsaccadic object perception (e.g., Henderson, 1994; Irwin, 1996; Germeys et al., 2002) transsaccadic memory for objects has been studied extensively in the past. Two main strategies have been used. The first has

---

* Correspondence to: Peter De Graef, Laboratory of Experimental Psychology, Department of Psychology, University of Leuven, Tiensestraat 102, B-3000 Leuven, Belgium. Tel.: +32-16-32-59-67; Fax: +32-16-32-60-99; E-mail: peter.degraef@psy.kuleuven.ac.be

---

[1] The focus of this chapter is on transsaccadic memory for objects across a single fixation–saccade–fixation cycle bringing a peripherally located object into foveal vision. It is commonly accepted that over the course of the multiple fixation–saccade–fixation cycles viewers use to explore a scene, an internal, episodic model of the contents and spatial layout of that particular scene is developed (Friedman, 1979; De Graef, 1992; Rayner and Pollatsek, 1992; Chun and Nakayama, 2000; Hollingworth and Henderson, 2002). In contrast, the development of an episodic object representation across a single fixation–saccade cycle is a much-debated topic as will become clear in the remainder of the chapter.

been to investigate to what extent postsaccadic processing of an object on fixation n is modulated by presaccadic processing of that object on fixation $n-1$. In this search for *transsaccadic preview effects*, the relation between pre- and postsaccadic object appearance has been systematically manipulated to identify the object features that are integrated across saccades. Specifically, during the critical saccade the presaccadic image was replaced by the postsaccadic image thus selectively altering or preserving particular features of the presaccadic image. Measures of subsequent ease of identification of the postsaccadic object (e.g., naming latency or gaze durations) were collected to determine whether the (violation of) transsaccadic correspondence between pre- and postsaccadic object images had any effect. The prevailing conclusion from this line of research was that transsaccadic memory does not contain a pixel-by-pixel, visually detailed representation of the presaccadic object: identification of the object is not hindered when it is intrasaccadically displaced or changed in size (Pollatsek et al., 1984, 1990), nor when there is no overlap between the specific object contour segments that are displayed pre- and postsaccadically (Henderson, 1997).

The second approach to study transsaccadic memory for objects has been more direct. Viewers are explicitly asked to compare pre- and postsaccadic images and to determine whether or not a change has occurred intrasaccadically. Because saccadic suppression masks the transient associated with intrasaccadic changes, detection of such a change implies that the changed stimulus aspect was presaccadically coded and stored and then compared with the postsaccadic image. As was the case in the transsaccadic preview studies, the *transsaccadic change detection* paradigm revealed a high tolerance for intrasaccadic changes in a stationary object's position (Deubel et al., 1996; McConkie and Currie, 1996), both in egocentric coordinates (Verfaillie et al., 1994) and in allocentric coordinates (Verfaillie and De Graef, 2000; De Graef et al., 2001). In addition, low detection rates were found for intrasaccadic changes of object orientation (Henderson and Hollingworth, 1999b), or of object size and color (Grimes, 1996) in realistic images of real-world scenes. Again, the conclusion drawn from these studies was that transsaccadic memory for objects is not 'iconic', that is, it cannot be characterized as a visual, truthfully detailed rendition of the presaccadic object.

This conclusion in the domain of transsaccadic object perception is consistent with the results of numerous other studies exploring and disproving the notion that transsaccadic integration of fixation contents is achieved on the basis of a point-by-point spatiotopic fusion of pre- and postsaccadic images (for reviews see Irwin, 1991, 1992a; O'Regan, 1992; Pollatsek and Rayner, 1992; O'Regan and Noë, 2001). Further support for the notion that transsaccadic memory is sparse and only contains a post-categorical, verbal summary abstracted away from visual detail, appears to be provided in the recent explosion of *change blindness* studies (for an overview see Simons, 2000; also see Rensink, 2002). All of these studies purport to demonstrate that viewers are blind to change in their visual environment as long as the local transient associated with the change is somehow masked. Such masking can be achieved by simultaneously introducing attention capturing local transients (O'Regan et al., 1999) or a global transient such as a grey-out of the image (Rensink et al., 1997), a blink (O'Regan et al., 2000), or saccade (Henderson and Hollingworth, 1999b). Wolfe et al. (2000) correctly point out that this phenomenon should not be termed *change blindness* because it does not illustrate that viewers are blind to change but rather are amnesic with respect to the situation before the change. However, based on their study of postattentive vision (i.e., the perceptual representation of recently attended objects) they do concur with the conclusion that human vision does not involve a cumulative and visually detailed, internal representation of whatever scene is currently being processed in a series of discrete fixations (for an extensive defense of this view, see O'Regan and Noë, 2001). In other words, whenever we move our eyes from one scene location to the next, the details of what we just viewed seem to disappear in the great void between fixations (but see Fernandez-Duque and Thornton, 2000, for a compelling defense of the view that studies requiring explicit change detection say little about the sparsity or richness of implicit representations).

Transsaccadic object perception: bridging the (not so empty) void

While one would be hard pressed to find modern-day advocates of the idea that pre- and postsaccadic object views are spatiotopically integrated in a pixel-by-pixel fashion, there are numerous recent studies on transsaccadic object perception which indicate that some visual object properties are in fact coded presaccadically and stored across saccades.

In a series of transsaccadic change detection studies, Verfaillie and colleagues (Verfaillie et al., 1994; Verfaillie, 1997; Verfaillie and De Graef, 2000) repeatedly demonstrated that the in-depth orientation in which an object is viewed presaccadically is integrated across saccades. Henderson and Siefert (1999, 2001) found transsaccadic preview benefits when the presaccadic left–right orientation of an object was preserved across a saccade. Carlson-Radvansky and Irwin (1995) and Carlson-Radvansky (1999) documented the transsaccadic maintenance of a structural description of an object, representing not the object's point-by-point details (i.e., the specific line segments making up a pattern) but rather its constituent parts (i.e., organized, connected clusters of line segments) and the relations between them. Earlier, the transsaccadic preservation of visual features such as global object shape had already been noted by Pollatsek et al. (1984). Specifically, they observed transsaccadic preview benefits in identifying an object that had been preceded by another, visually similar object previewed at the same location (e.g., a carrot preceding a baseball bat). That the object description carried across the saccade is indeed visual in nature and not a verbal description of the visual properties of the presaccadic image, can be concluded from Irwin's (1991, 1992) demonstrations that meaningless random-dot patterns can be stored transsaccadically and that letters can be spatiotopically pattern-masked if the postsaccadic mask is presented soon enough after the saccade. Specifically, in one set of studies (Irwin, 1991), viewers were able to make same–different judgments about random-dot patterns when the first pattern was presented as a peripheral saccade target and the second pattern appeared postsaccadically at the location that was now foveated. In a second series of experiments, Irwin (1992b) had viewers make a saccade in an array of letters, removed the array intrasaccadically and presented a small mask indicating which letter had to be reported. If the mask was presented 40 ms after the saccade, it decreased performance for the letter that had presaccadically appeared at the cued location, showing spatiotopic masking of the transsaccadic representation of the array.

Having established the presence of a visual object representation in the transsaccadic void, the question arises as to why we do not routinely access it when faced with the task of detecting stimulus changes during a saccade or other transient-masking discontinuities of the visual stimulus. We will first discuss two possible answers to this question: (1) transsaccadic object representations are selectively limited to information that helps object identification, and (2) transsaccadic object representations are rich and non-selective, but are carried by a volatile medium that quickly loses all information that is not selectively attended. Following our discussion of these two alternatives we will present new data collected to test the latter hypothesis.

First, transsaccadic object perception in scenes can be regarded as a basic, functional routine that has evolved in our everyday visuo-motor interaction with the world (Hayhoe, 2000; Verfaillie et al., 2001). The purpose of this routine is to take advantage of the fact that generally we are allowed more than one fixation on a given scene. For the objects in that scene this provides us with the opportunity to integrate object information sampled from a sequence of initially peripheral and ultimately foveal glimpses. Thus, foveal object identification can be jumpstarted by preliminary peripheral processing. In other words, while a single fixation may in principle be sufficient to identify an object, the preferred modus operandi is to increase speed and reliability of object identification by transsaccadic integration of foveal and extrafoveal evidence from multiple fixations.

Under the assumption that the default purpose of transsaccadic object perception is to expedite object identification, we hypothesize that only object properties that are relevant for object identification, will be entered into transsaccadic memory. This would explain why object orientation, part-structure, and global shape, were found to be an integral part of transsaccadic object memory (see above), while poor transsaccadic memory was observed for object position (e.g., Bridgeman et al., 1975; Li and Matin, 1990; Verfaillie et al., 1994; De Graef et al., 2001), object size (Pollatsek et al., 1984), or specific object contour segments (Henderson, 1997). [2]

A second explanation of the sparse nature of transsaccadic object memory does not invoke the notion of purposeful, presaccadic buffering of object-diagnostic information. Instead, it assumes that during every fixation the visual system automatically takes a high-capacity, non-selective snapshot of the scene (Becker et al., 2000; Rensink et al., 2000; Tatler, 2001, 2002, this volume). However, as soon as the fixation ends the snapshot starts decaying. Moreover, it is highly susceptible to masking by the new snapshot coming in during the next fixation. Only when information in the snapshot is selectively attended can it be insulated from the detrimental effects of decay and masking. Hence, the sparsity of transsaccadic object memory is not due to a functional presaccadic selection of object-diagnostic properties, but to the impossibility of simultaneously attending to every aspect of the richly detailed internal scene representation that is in principle available after every fixation.

Note that this account is quite similar to the model of informational persistence proposed by Irwin and Yeomans (1986). According to this model, the visual display not only gives rise to an iconic, sensory trace that is time-locked to stimulus onset, but also to a *visual analog*, a maskable internal representation of the form and location of items in the display, which decays within 150–300 ms after stimulus offset. Only selective attention to specific information in the analog can insulate that information against decay and masking by transferring it to a more durable store such as visual short-term memory (Di Lollo and Dixon, 1988; Gegenfurtner and Sperling, 1993). Irwin and Yeomans (1986) viewed transfer from this visual analog as a parallel mechanism for stimulus processing. Specifically, in addition to the direct translation from volatile iconic traces into nonvisual identity codes fit for storage in short-term memory, the visual analog provides an intermediate and more durable level of stimulus representation from which detailed visual and spatial information can be translated into nonvisual identity codes and abstract spatial coordinates.

Is transsaccadic object memory based on a visual analog?

The notion of a highly volatile, detailed and non-selective representation derived anew from every single fixation on a visual scene has received considerable support in the change blindness literature. In particular the role of selective attention as an insulator for elements in the intrafixational icon has been emphasized in order to explain why certain elements of a visual stimulus are much less susceptible to change blindness than others. Specifically, changes that occur near to the (intended) point of fixation (and the associated attentional focus) are more readily noticed (Henderson and Hollingworth, 1999b; Hollingworth et al., 2001); changes in scene elements that received high a priori interest ratings are noticed faster than changes in low interest elements (Rensink et al., 1997); changes are less noticeable when they occur in scene elements from which attention has been diverted by instructions (Simons and Chabris, 1999) or attention-capturing stimulus manipulations (O'Regan et al., 1999).

The hypothesized interaction between an intrafixational analog and selective attention in change blindness demonstrations, was tested by Becker et al. (2000) in a combination of the flicker paradigm (Rensink et al., 1997) and partial-report procedures (Sperling, 1960). Viewers were presented with an alternating sequence of two circular arrays of items (letter, symbols or colored disks). The two arrays were separated by a variable-duration blank interval and viewers had to determine whether the array had changed across the blank. On some proportion of the trials, the blank interval between the two arrays contained a position cue. This cue indicated the specific

---

[2] Note that the presumed restriction of transsaccadic object memory to object-diagnostic information does not preclude that in specific task settings additional object properties that are usually not instrumental to object identification, can be carried across the saccade. For instance, when color needs to be transsaccadically coded in order to discriminate between objects, color may be represented as an integral part of transsaccadic object memory (Irwin and Andrews, 1996; Carlson et al., 2001). Similarly, when capturing object position is essential for an adequate sensorimotor interaction with the object (e.g., when the object is moving) position will be transsaccadically coded (Pollatsek and Rayner, 2001; Gysen et al., 2002).

item in the array about which subjects had to decide whether it had changed across the blank. Timing of the cue onset relative to the offset of the first array and the onset of the second array was manipulated. Two findings were of interest to the present discussion. First, the study replicated the standard observation from the change blindness studies: when a blank interval between the two arrays masked the local transient accompanying the change, change detection dropped dramatically. Secondly, however, when the blank interval contained a cue marking the location of the item change, change detection improved reliably when the cue was presented sufficiently quickly after offset of the first array and long enough before onset of the second array. Becker et al. (2000) concluded from this that presentation of the first array gave rise to a quickly decaying and maskable representation. By guiding attention to a particular item in that representation before spontaneous decay had gone too far and before masking by the second array could take place, the item was transferred to visual short-term memory and could be successfully compared with the corresponding item in the second array.

The results of Becker et al.'s (2000) change blindness study are quite similar to data obtained with the transsaccadic blanking paradigm (Deubel et al., 1996, 1998, 2002, this volume). In this paradigm, subjects are asked to saccade to a designated target object, and during the saccade the target is blanked for variable durations up to 270 ms, but always extending beyond the end of the saccade. In other words, as the eye lands, the intended saccade target is not there and only reappears later during the fixation. The main result from these studies is that intrasaccadic target displacements that are not detectable under normal conditions, suddenly become quite detectable when a blank is introduced. This result could be interpreted as showing that the blanking manipulation postponed the normal masking of the presaccadic visual analog by the postsaccadic image. Because we can safely assume that selective attention preceded the saccade to the target (Schneider, 1995, 1999), the target was insulated from iconic decay and could be successfully compared with the post-blanking stimulus.

The similarity between Becker et al.'s (2000) partial-report data obtained with the flicker paradigm and the transsaccadic blanking studies by Deubel and colleagues raises the question whether poor change detection and limited transsaccadic object memory can be regarded as caused by the same underlying mechanism: selective transfer of the attended aspects of a non-selective, volatile, visual analog to more durable storage in visual short-term memory or activated entries in long-term memory. The experiment reported below was designed to address that question.

Cued detection of intrasaccadic changes in object orientation

To test whether a visual analog derived from a given scene fixation plays any role in the integration of object features across the subsequent saccade, we had viewers saccade to a designated object in a realistic line drawing of a scene. During the saccade, the display was changed to a blank field containing a location cue that either marked the saccade target or another object that had been present in the scene. The blank + cue display remained on the screen for the first 50, 100, or 250 ms of the postsaccadic fixation. Subsequently, it was replaced by the presaccadic scene in which the object at the cued location had changed its in-depth orientation. In a two-alternative, forced-choice task, subjects were asked to determine whether the cued object had turned to the left or to the right. Performance in this blank + cue condition was compared to a cue-only condition in which the postsaccadic scene already appeared during the saccade (i.e., was not blanked for part of the postsaccadic fixation) and contained a cue marking the changed object.

Our decision to study intrasaccadic orientation changes was inspired by the apparent discrepancy between transsaccadic coding of object orientation in scenes versus in isolation: while the orientation of peripherally presented, isolated objects is stored across saccades (Verfaillie and De Graef, 2000; Henderson and Siefert, 2001), detection of intrasaccadic orientation changes of a saccade target object in a full scene is poor (Henderson and Hollingworth, 1999b). This discrepancy could be taken to show that there are qualitative differences between (transsaccadic) object identification in realistic scenes and (transsaccadic) object identification in vitro. Alternatively, the discrepancy may originate from the fact that isolated objects provide a much better quality peripheral preview, allowing the presaccadic computation of a viewpoint-dependent structural object description, which can then be compared to the object's postsaccadic appearance. For objects in scenes, preview quality is much lower due to lateral masking by other objects and background and the presaccadic object view is masked by the postsaccadic view before it can be processed to the level of a viewpoint-dependent representation. If the latter suggestion holds, then the presence of an unmasked visual analog may provide a sufficient extension of the presaccadic view to achieve a representation of presaccadic object orientation and to detect changes in the postsaccadic object orientation. Hence, we would predict performance in our task to be low in the absence of blanking and to increase when a blank is inserted at the onset of the postsaccadic fixation.

The presence of a visual analog in transsaccadic object perception also predicts that performance should increase with the duration of the blank because longer blanks extend the availability of the visual analog for attentive processing of the cued object. However, previous measurements of the decay function in the visual analog all agree that this internal scene representation decays within 150–300 ms from stimulus offset (Irwin and Yeomans, 1986; Di Lollo and Dixon, 1988; Loftus et al., 1992). Thus, adding an average saccade duration of 50 ms to the blanking intervals which were timed from the end of the critical saccade, availability of the visual analog should be good throughout the 50 and 100 ms blanking intervals but should start decreasing during the 250 ms blank. As a result, performance should improve up to blanking intervals of 100 ms but may then start decreasing because of decay in the analog.

Because non-selectivity is an essential characteristic of the visual analog, we finally hypothesized that it should carry information about the in-depth orientation of every object in the scene. Thus, postponing postsaccadic masking and precueing the location of the changed object should increase performance for both targets and bystanders relative to the cue-only condition in which the changed scene masked the visual analog from the onset of the postsaccadic fixation. However, because the saccade target was at the center of attention just after the saccade, its chances of surviving analog decay and subsequent masking by the postsaccadic scene should initially be better than those of the bystander. Thus, there should be a saccade target superiority which is most pronounced at the shorter blanking intervals: as the postsaccadic masking is delayed by longer blanking intervals and the subjects get time to shift their attention to the cued location of the bystander in the visual analog, its presaccadic orientation should become more accessible for comparison with its postsaccadic orientation and performance for the bystander should approach that for the target. Taking into account the decay function for the visual analog we would expect target and bystander performance curves to approach each other as blanking durations go up to 100 ms and to start separating again at longer intervals: bystander performance should be more susceptible to decay of the visual analog because the attention shift to the bystander location inevitably will occur later than that to the target.

Method

Subjects

Eight subjects from the University of Leuven subject pool took part in the experiment. All had normal or corrected-to-normal vision and were paid 7.5 EUR for their participation.

Stimuli

All stimuli were black-on-grey line drawings of realistic scenes and objects. The scenes measured 16 (width) by 12 (height) degrees of visual angle; average object size was 2.7° by 2.7°. The 16 different scene backgrounds were selected from the sets provided by van Diepen and De Graef (1994) and Hollingworth and Henderson (1998). The objects were selected from a library of line drawings depicting each of 40 objects in 7 different views (Germeys, 2002). For each of the scene backgrounds, two probe objects were chosen which were plausible to appear in that scene and that could be postsaccadically cued to be evaluated for intrasaccadic changes in their in-depth orientation. For each of the 32 probe objects, 3 views were selected: 15°, 45°, and 75° rotations from a frontal view. The 45° view was always the

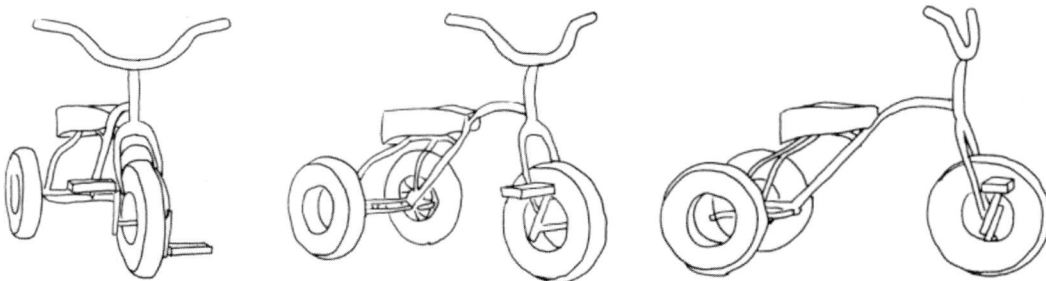

Fig. 1. Example of the three object views used to produce transsaccadic in-depth rotations changes from either a presaccadic 15° view (left), or a presaccadic 75° view (right), to a postsaccadic 45° view (middle).

postsaccadic end orientation of the probe object. Presaccadically, the probe object appeared in either the more frontal 15° or the more sagittal 75° view. As can be seen in Fig. 1, the resulting 30° changes between pre- and postsaccadic views produced quite distinct appearances of the same probe object and can hardly be qualified as too subtle to notice.

For each of the 16 scenes, 2 additional objects were selected to serve as alternate saccade targets in conditions where the intrasaccadically rotated probe object served as a saccade bystander rather than as the saccade target. Probes and alternates were all inserted in the scene (average eccentricity of the probes was 5.1°), with one probe in each hemifield and the corresponding alternate in the opposite hemifield. This is illustrated in Fig. 2 for the probes *baby carriage* and *tricycle* and their alternates *trailer* and *plant*.

Design

The within-subjects factorial combination of 4 blanking durations (0, 50, 100, and 250 ms) and 2 levels of saccadic status for the probe object (target vs. bystander) resulted in 8 conditions. Each of the 32 probe objects was measured once in each condition, producing a total of 256 experimental trials. To avoid any predictable relationship between the direction of the intrasaccadic orientation change of the probe (left turn vs. right turn) and the probe's presaccadic view, postsaccadic view, absolute position on the screen or relative position in the scene, we always used the same 45° postsaccadic view and constructed 4 orientation changes for each probe by factorially combining the presaccadic probe orientation (15° vs. 75°) and the orientation of the whole stimulus (original vs. mirrored). Thus, a 15° to 45° rotation could be a right turn (original stimulus) or a left turn (mirrored stimulus), and 75° to 45° rotation could be a left turn (original stimulus) or a right turn (mirrored stimulus). The 4 types of orientation changes were counterbalanced over probe objects and experimental conditions.

Procedure and apparatus

Upon arrival, subjects were extensively instructed about the phenomenon of blindness to intrasaccadic changes. Through slow-paced demonstration trials, subjects were familiarized with the type of stimuli they would see (i.e., realistic line drawings of oriented objects in scenes) and with the experimental task of having to judge intrasaccadic orientation changes while their eye movements were being measured. Subjects were then seated at 150 cm from a 460 × 300 mm Sony GDM-W900 screen running in non-interlaced NTSC-mode (756 × 486 at 60 Hz). After individual calibration of the eye tracker they received a practice session of 16 trials (2 from each experimental condition). Subsequently, they received all 256 experimental trials in a pseudo-random order, preventing successive presentations of the same probe or scene and ensuring an even distribution of trials from the 8 experimental conditions. The experiment lasted approximately 45–60 min. Subjects were given a rest every 50 trials or whenever they experienced fatigue. No feedback was given until the end of the experiment.

Eye movements were recorded with a Generation 5.5 dual-Purkinje-image eye tracker (Crane and

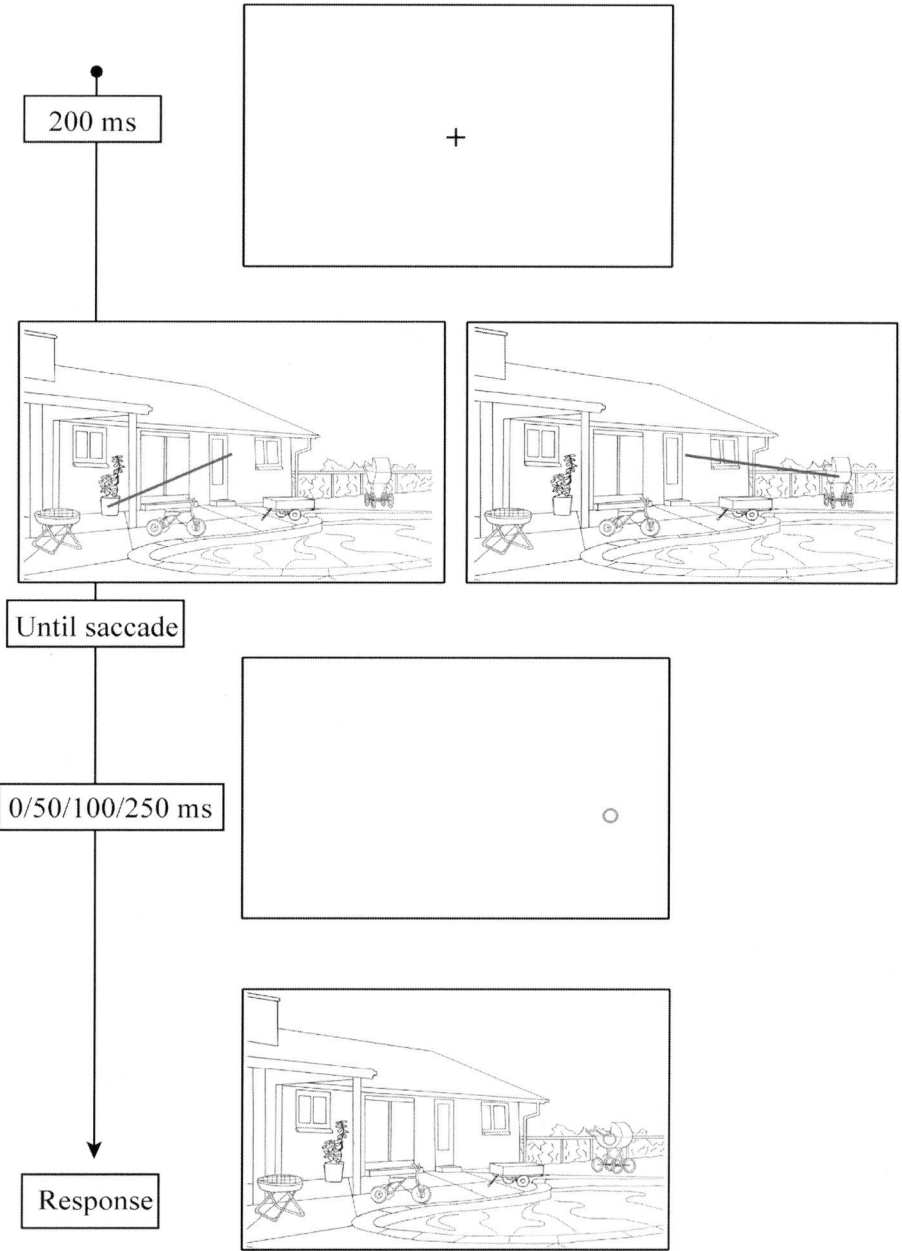

Fig. 2. Illustration of the course of a trial. Following a central fixation (top panel) subjects were presented with a scene in which a red line (here in black) pointed at the intended saccade target. During the ensuing saccade the scene was replaced by a variable-duration blank field containing a red circular cue (here in black), marking the previous location of the saccade target (presaccadic scene on the right) or a saccade bystander (presaccadic scene on the left). After the blank, subjects responded whether the object cued by the circle had turned left or right during the saccade (in this case the baby carriage had turned right).

Steele, 1985). This system has an accuracy of 1 min of arc and a 1000 Hz sampling rate. It was interfaced with a 486 PC, storing every sample of the left eye's position. For each sample, the computer made an on-line decision about the eye state: fixation, saccade, blink, or signal loss. Eye state and position were fed into a second 233 MHz Pentium MMX PC, in control of stimulus presentation (for an extensive description of this dual-PC eye-tracking system see Van Rensbergen and De Troy, 1993; van Diepen, 1998). Intrasaccadic display changes were completed within 21 ms, well inside the average 54 ms saccade duration.

The course of a trial is illustrated in Fig. 2. First, a central fixation cross was presented until the eye tracker detected a steady 200 ms fixation on the fixation cross. At that time a scene appeared containing a red line extending from the central fixation position to the middle of the object that was intended as saccade target. During the saccade, the presaccadic scene was either replaced by a blank field of the same color and luminance as the scene background (50, 100, and 250 ms blank conditions), or it was replaced by the postsaccadic scene (0 ms blank condition). In each of these replacement scenes, a red circle (0.5° in diameter) indicated the location of the probe object about which subjects would have to decide whether it had turned right or left during the saccade. On half of the trials, the cue marked the target of the saccade, on the other half it marked the former location of an object that was present in the opposite hemifield. In the blanking conditions, the onset of the postsaccadic scene containing the rotated probe object was delayed by the designated blanking interval measured from the onset of the postsaccadic fixation on the saccade target. The probe object changed orientation on every trial, subjects simply indicated the direction by pressing a left-hand key for left turns and a right-hand key for right turns. Reaction times were measured from the appearance of the probe object, except in the no-blank condition where the rotated probe appeared intrasaccadically and the reaction time was measured from the onset of the first fixation following this intrasaccadic appearance.

Subjects were allowed a maximum of 400 ms to initiate the designated saccade and a maximum of 3000 ms to respond to the postsaccadic probe. When RTs were too long, or the saccades were too slow or did not end at the intended target object, the trial was interrupted and subjects were cautioned to be faster or more accurate. The interrupted trials were recycled once at the end of the experimental session.

Results

All trials with accurate and timely saccades and responses before the 3000 ms deadline were entered in an analysis of reaction times to eliminate possible outliers. Outliers were defined as responses with RTs below 200 ms or RTs that deviated more than 3 SDs from the mean for that subject in that experimental condition. This procedure resulted in the elimination of 6% of all possible observations, evenly distributed across experimental conditions. The remaining trials were analyzed for response speed and accuracy and for various eye movement parameters.

Reaction times

Correct RTs were entered in a repeated-measures ANOVA with blanking interval (0, 50, 100, 250 ms) and saccadic status (target vs. bystander) as factors. This analysis showed a main effect of saccadic status, $F(1,7) = 113.61$, MSE = 230,840, $p < 0.0001$, with faster RTs for saccade targets (1092 ms) than for saccade bystanders (1404 ms). Neither the effect of blanking nor its interaction with saccadic status approached reliability.

Proportion correct

The blanking × saccadic status repeated-measures ANOVA on the proportion of correct identifications of the direction of intrasaccadic object rotation revealed better performance for the saccade target than for the saccade bystander, $F(1,7) = 12.29$, MSE = 0.017, $p < 0.01$, and an interaction of blanking and saccadic status, $F(3,21) = 4.98$, MSE = 0.003, $p < 0.01$. This interaction is plotted in Fig. 3. Three elements are worth noting.

First, under normal viewing conditions (i.e., in the absence of a postsaccadic blank) viewers cannot do this task: performance did not reliably differ from chance (i.e., 0.50) for either the saccade target, $t(7) = 1.85$, or the saccade bystander, $t(7) = 1.26$.

Second, as soon as a 50 ms postsaccadic blank is introduced, performance for the saccade target increases well above chance level, $t(7) = 5.33$, but fails to increase further as the blanking interval is extended. Performance reaches asymptote with a 50 ms blank and remains completely stable afterwards as

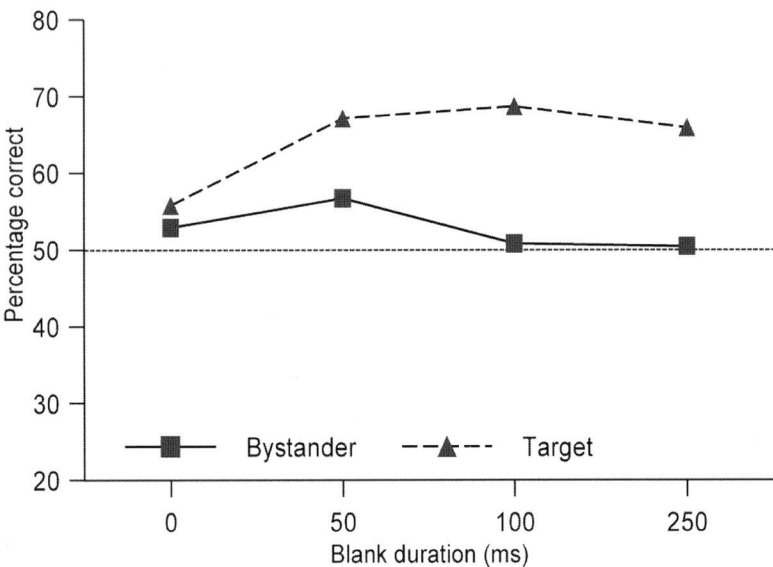

Fig. 3. Proportion correct responses in the rotation discrimination task, as a function of the saccadic status of the rotated object and the duration of the postsaccadic blank. Dotted line indicates chance-level performance.

confirmed by a set of pairwise comparisons between the successive blanking durations for the saccade target condition: only the comparison between 0 ms and 50 ms blanking is reliable, $F(1,7) = 30.62$, MSE $= 0.003$, $p < 0.001$. Comparisons between 50 ms and 100 ms, $F(1,7) < 1$, and between 100 and 250 ms, $F(1,7) = 1.43$, MSE $= 0.004$, $p = 0.27$, reveal no further effects of blanking duration.

Third, performance for the bystander objects is entirely unaffected by the presence of a postsaccadic blank regardless of the duration of the blanking interval. While there appears to be a hint of improvement for the 50 ms blank, performance still does not exceed chance level, $t(7) = 1.77$, nor does it reliably differ from performance in the no-blank condition, $F(1,7) = 1.65$, MSE $= 0.006$, $p = 0.24$. Differences between 50 ms and 100 ms blanking, $F(1,7) = 1.19$, MSE $= 0.023$, $p = 0.31$, and between 100 and 250 ms, $F(1,7) < 1$, also proved to be non-reliable.

Eye movement parameters

To rule out the possibility that differences in response accuracy were incidentally caused by correlated differences in presaccadic processing time, we entered saccade latency (i.e., the time taken to fixate the scene before initiating the critical saccade) in a blanking duration × saccadic status repeated-measures ANOVA. Average saccade latency was 279 ms and none of the effects in this analysis approached reliability (all F values <1.13).

The intended purpose of inserting a blank + cue at the onset of the postsaccadic fixation, is to provide viewers with the opportunity to shift their attention in the visual analog to the representation of the object that was spatially cued. In classic partial-report studies the presence of such shifts is inferred from an increase in performance for objects at the cued location. In the present study, the continuous measurement of eye movements allowed us to look for overt signs of these presumed covert shifts of attention. Specifically, we analyzed postsaccadic target fixation parameters as a function of blanking duration, saccadic status of the probe object, and response accuracy.[3] Not surprisingly, the analysis showed that

---

[3] For each trial, we analyzed the duration of the first fixation on the target, the number of consecutive fixations during the first pass over the target, and the summed duration of first-pass fixations or *gaze*. We only report statistics about the first fixation durations, but the patterns for gaze durations and number of fixations were identical with the exception that these measures also showed an effect of response accuracy with shorter target gazes and fewer target fixations when an orientation change of the target was correctly detected.

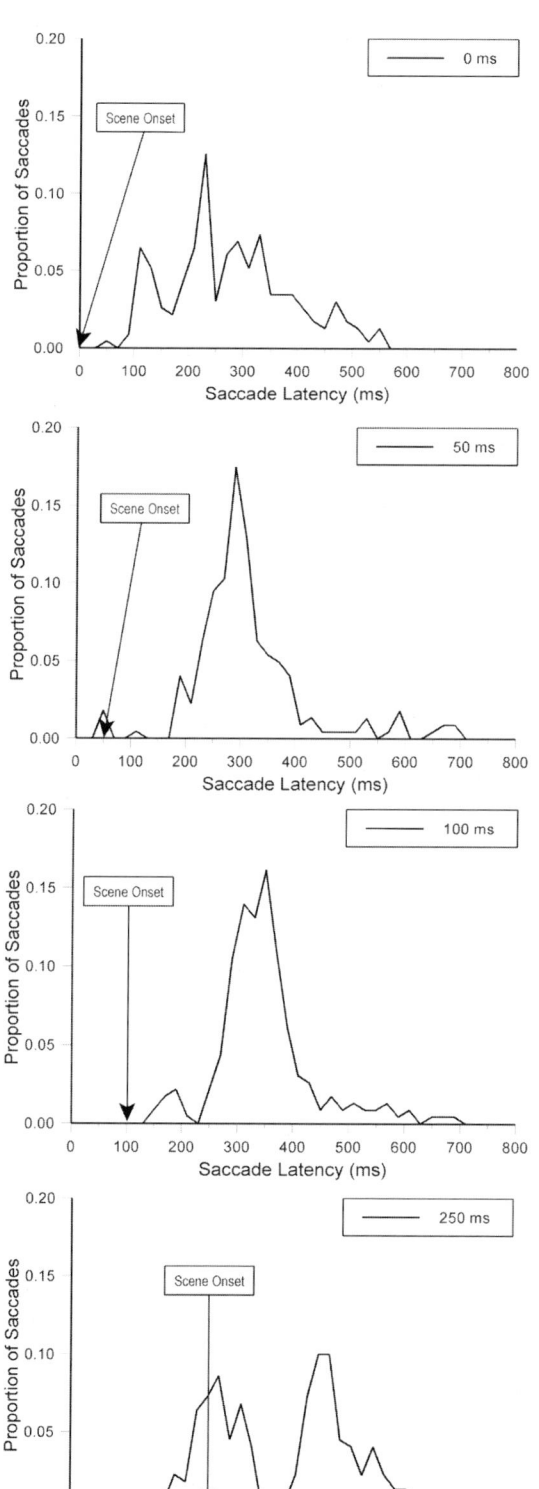

viewers were reliably quicker to move their eyes away from the target when the cue did not appear at the saccade target location but marked the location of a bystander, $F(1,7) = 43.0$, MSE = 296,377, $p < 0.0004$. While this effect suggests responsiveness to the appearance of the cue, a main effect of blanking duration on target fixation times indicates otherwise, $F(1,21) = 9.91$, MSE = 101,198, $p < 0.0003$. Specifically, as blanking duration increased, target fixations became longer, indicating that the saccade away from the target was primarily in response to the appearance of the postsaccadic scene, not the appearance of the postsaccadic cue marking the probe object.

This effect on average target fixation times was confirmed in a more detailed plot of the distribution of saccade latencies away from the target towards the location of the cued bystander object. As can be seen in Fig. 4, the main peak of the distribution shifted in response to an increase of the blanking interval. Thus, saccades were always most frequent at about 230–250 ms after the replacement of the blank by the postsaccadic scene. The latency and time-locked nature of these saccades relative to scene onset, identifies them as voluntary saccades towards the cued probe object in the scene, not towards the cue by itself. Only the distribution for the 250 ms blanking condition shows a first population (peaking at 250 ms after fixation onset) of saccades directed towards the bystander cue in the blank, and a second population (peaking at 450–470 ms after fixation onset) of saccades directed towards the cued bystander in the postsaccadic scene. Of all recorded saccades, this first population is the only overt indication of preceding covert shifts of attention to the cue in the blank and, consequently to the presumed bystander's representation in the visual analog. However, assuming that the delay between attention and gaze shift generally will not be much longer than 100 ms (Henderson, 1992), this implies that attention shifted to the bystander after about 150 ms of blanking at which time the analog might already have decayed

Fig. 4. Distribution of latencies for saccades towards the cue marking the bystander location and away from the target of the critical saccade. Bin size is 20 ms and latencies are measured from the end of the critical saccade.

considerably. Note that our saccade analysis does not exclude the possibility of covert shifts of attention to the bystander during the initial stages of the blank. It is always possible that attention shifted without a subsequent eye movement, although such an uncoupling of attention and gaze is not very likely when the saccade targets are visual onsets (Klein et al., 1992) as is the case in the present study.

Discussion

The obtained results present somewhat of a puzzle. On the one hand, postsaccadic blanking revealed that the information necessary to compute a peripheral object's in-depth orientation in a full scene, is in fact carried across a saccade but is not routinely accessible for explicit comparison with the postsaccadic object orientation. This finding resolves the discrepancy raised by earlier findings of transsaccadic orientation coding for isolated objects (e.g., Verfaillie and De Graef, 2000) that did not generalize to objects in scenes (Henderson and Hollingworth, 1999b). However, we cannot simply conclude from this that the key to detecting transsaccadic changes of object orientation lies in the use of a task that sufficiently strongly demands the use of object orientation. Specifically, if task relevance were the only requirement for observing transsaccadic orientation changes we have to wonder why subjects were at chance in the 0 ms blank condition and suddenly improved when a 50 ms blank was introduced: in both cases the transsaccadic maintenance of the object's orientation was equally crucial to task performance. Hence, the main conclusion to be drawn from these data is that there seems to be a trace of presaccadic visual object detail that survives the saccade, but ordinarily is masked by the object information encoded during the subsequent fixation. Thus, the notion of a visual analog playing a role in transsaccadic object memory appears to be supported.

On the other hand, performance curves for the target and the bystander show little evidence of the properties one would expect such a visual analog to have. First, there was no reliable sign of a decrease in performance as blanking durations extended beyond the point where the visual analog has previously been found to show substantial decay (e.g., Di Lollo and Dixon, 1988). Second, the gain in performance derived from the delay of the postsaccadic scene was all-or-none. It asymptoted with a 50 ms blank and, despite the fact that performance was nowhere near ceiling, it showed no further increase as more time was allowed to selectively attend to the probe object in the unmasked analog. Finally, blanking only affected performance for the saccade target object and had no effect on the detection of orientation changes in the bystander. This runs counter to the idea that the visual analog should be high capacity and nonselective and should contain information about more than one object in the presaccadic scene.

The transsaccadic visual analog revisited

In an attempt to resolve the discrepancy between the apparent presence of a visual analog and the failure to find evidence for that analog's presumed properties, two points require further consideration.

Quickly asymptoting effects of blanking

One way to look at the lack of evolution in target performance after reaching asymptote with a 50 ms blank is to regard it as the net result of two opposing trends that cancel each other out. Specifically, 100 ms after scene offset (i.e., an average saccade duration of 50 ms plus a 50 ms postsaccadic blank) decay of the analog may have set in, driving performance levels down. At the same time, however, the quality of the viewpoint information derived from the target's representation in the visual analog may still be increasing as a result of selective attention, driving performance levels up. To test this hypothesis of two counteracting influences, future research should manipulate the delay between the start of the blank and the onset of the cue marking the location of the probe object. This should reveal whether there is any decay of the target's representation in the analog in the absence of an explicit cue to attend to that representation.

An alternative explanation of the limitation of blanking benefits to a 50 ms blank duration, hinges on the finding that the visual intake of foveal stimulus information appears to be limited to the first 50–75 ms of every new fixation. Using a foveal mask that moved in synchrony with the eyes and appeared at designated delays after the onset of every new fixation, sensitivity to the mask was found to be limited to onset delays up to 50–75 ms, both in reading (Rayner et al., 1981) and in scene exploration (van Diepen et al., 1995). Foveal masks appearing any later during the fixation had no effect on the fluency of the eye movement pattern. Thus, our current failure to find any additional benefit from blanking durations beyond 50 ms may indicate that the visual system treats the visual analog as if it were the visual world itself: foveal information is sampled only during the first 50 ms of a new fixation, regardless of whether the fixated stimulus is internal or external. This estimate of a sensitive period for information sampling at the onset of a new fixations is quite consistent with the Deubel et al. (1996) finding that intrasaccadic object displacement detection is enhanced by postsaccadic blanking for durations up to 100 ms. Because the blank duration in the Deubel et al. studies is measured from its onset during the saccade, actual durations of effective postsaccadic blanks were shorter and are close to our 50–75 ms estimate.

Limitation of blanking effects to saccade targets

Unlike what might be expected from a high-capacity, non-selective, visual analog we found no evidence for the representation in that analog of objects other than the saccade target. Contrary to what Becker et al. (2000) observed in partial-report studies of the internal representation between two alternating images in the flicker paradigm, we found no indications that a spatial cue at the onset of a postsaccadic blank enables selective access to the implicit representation of any object that was present during the previous fixation. Perhaps we should simply conclude from this that there is no stimulus-wide, visual analog carried across a saccade and that this is a fundamental distinction between the *intrafixational* representation which is tapped in the flicker paradigm, and the *interfixational* representation which is tapped in transsaccadic change studies.

Alternatively, one might argue that the failure to find blanking effects for the bystanders does not mean that there is no transsaccadic visual analog but only confirms that the visual system consults it in a manner that is time-locked to the end of the saccade and/or the onset of the fixation. Specifically, only when information in the visual analog can be accessed by attentive processing within 50–75 ms after the end of the saccade, will it be transferred to more durable stores where it can impact subsequent perception or perceptual decisions. Given that our analysis of postsaccadic, overt processing shifts away from the target revealed that the preceding covert attention shifts only occurred after about 150 ms into the postsaccadic fixation, it is clear that in those cases no useful information could be derived from any bystander representations that might have been present in a transsaccadic visual analog. In other words, measuring effects on bystander performance may only serve as a way of testing for the existence of the transsaccadic visual analog if the effects can be measured inside the sensitive period for visual stimulus sampling that is time-locked to the saccade–fixation alternation.

Concluding remarks

The data reported in this chapter bear on the question whether the memory for objects in scenes during a single fixation–saccade–fixation cycle involves the automatic emergence of a high-capacity, non-selective, internal representation of visual object detail. It may seem that this issue has been extensively examined and refuted in earlier work on the integrative visual buffer (e.g., Rayner and Pollatsek, 1983; Irwin, 1991). However, the visual representation we are investigating here is of a different kind: it is not a retinotopic, visible persistence, which is time-locked to presaccadic stimulus onset and somehow needs to be spatially aligned with the postsaccadic image in order to expedite transsaccadic integration of pre- and postsaccadic images (Pollatsek and Rayner, 1992). Rather, it is a spatiotopic, informational persistence, which is time-locked to presaccadic stimulus offset, and which codes visual detail and location of objects in a rapidly decaying and maskable trace (Irwin and Yeomans, 1986; McRae et al., 1987; Di Lollo and Dixon, 1988; Irwin, 1992b).

Based on the present results and very similar data in other transsaccadic blanking studies (Deubel et al., 1996, 1998) we think that it is reasonable to further entertain the hypothesis that transsaccadic object perception involves a visual analog, an informational persistence which is distinct from the limited-capacity and slowly decaying object files in visual short-term memory and activated object representations in long-term memory (Irwin, 1996). However, our results also indicate that access to this visual analog during normal fixation–saccade–fixation sequences is subject to strict temporal limitations: only information that is selectively attended within 50–75 ms after the end of the saccade will be entered into the perceptual equation. This implies that readout from the visual analog will be spatially limited to the region surrounding the target of the saccade, or any other stimulus regions that can be quickly reached by postsaccadic attention. The latter could include stimulus regions for which a presaccadic attentional bias has been installed by way of instructions (Irwin and Gordon, 1998) or stimulus regions that were presaccadically entered into a multi-step saccade program.[4]

One might of course wonder what the functional significance could be of a scene-wide visual analog if only one or two items at most can be transferred from it for further processing. One possibility we speculatively entertain is that the function of the visual analog in transsaccadic perception is to store pre-attentive object files. Germeys et al. (2002) outlined a theory of transsaccadic object identification according to which every fixation produces strictly location-bound representations of peripheral objects that are unattended bystanders to the current saccade target. We think that the purpose of these pre-attentive object files may be to continuously provide the visual system with a spatially distributed set of saccade target choices for the next attention/gaze shift. If the visual analog were to carry these bystander representations, their salience as future saccade targets could ensure the quick attention shifts needed to access their representation in the analog.

Finally, selectivity in reading out from the transsaccadic analog is not only spatial but will also be task-dependent. Much as it is the case for an externally present image, stimulus aspects that are not attended to will not be read out even if attention is spatially allocated to the right location (O'Regan et al., 2000). This implies that the two opposing characterizations of transsaccadic selectivity which we proposed in the abstract of this chapter, may in fact coexist. In other words, transsaccadic object memory is not selective because the visual system presaccadically buffers only functional information, or because it intrasaccadically loses all non-attended visual detail from a decaying analog. Rather it may be selective because it postsaccadically only reads out functional information from the visual analog, to compare and integrate it with the spatially and temporally synchronous information sampled from the external stimulus.

Acknowledgements

This work was supported by Concerted Research Effort Convention GOA 98/01 of the Research Fund K.U. Leuven, the Belgian Programme on Interuniversity Poles of Attraction Contract P4/19, and the Fund for Scientific Research of Flanders. Portions of the data were presented at the 11th European Conference on Eye Movements in Turku, Finland, August, 2001. The authors want to thank Filip Germeys and two anonymous reviewers for their comments on an earlier draft.

References

Becker, M.W., Pashler, H. and Anstis, S.M. (2000) The role of iconic memory in change-detection tasks. *Perception*, 29: 273–286.

Bridgeman, B., Hendry, D. and Stark, L. (1975) Failure to detect displacement of the visual world during saccadic eye movements. *Vision Res.*, 15: 719–722.

Carlson, L.A., Covell, E.R. and Warapius, T. (2001) Transsaccadic coding of multiple objects and features. *Psychol. Belg.*, 41: 9–27.

Carlson-Radvansky, L.A. (1999) Memory for relational information across eye movements. *Percept. Psychophys.*, 61: 919–934.

---

[4] Using a variation of the paradigm introduced in this chapter, we recently presented some new data for conditions where both the bystander and the target were presaccadically cued as potential locations for intrasaccadic orientation changes (De Graef and Verfaillie, 2002). This allowed viewers to set up a rapid two-step saccade program (center-to-target, target-to-bystander). Under these conditions which facilitate quick postsaccadic attention shifts from the target to the bystander, we observed blanking benefits for the bystander. In addition, we found a decay of blanking benefits for the target at blanking durations greater than 50 ms. Both findings support our hypothesis that selective attention governs readout from the analog and that this readout appears to be temporally limited to the initial 50–75 ms of the postsaccadic fixation.

Carlson-Radvansky, L.A. and Irwin, D.E. (1995) Memory for structural information across eye movements. *J. Exp. Psychol. Learn. Mem. Cogn.*, 21: 1441–1458.

Chun, M.M. and Nakayama, K. (2000) On the functional role of implicit visual memory for the adaptive deployment of attention across scenes. *Vis. Cognit.*, 7: 65–81.

Crane, H.D. and Steele, C.M. (1985) Generation-V dual-Purkinje-image eyetracker. *Appl. Opt.*, 24: 527–537.

De Graef, P. (1992) Scene-context effects and models of real-world perception. In: K. Rayner (Ed.), *Eye Movements and Visual Cognition: Scene Perception and Reading*. Springer, New York, pp. 243–259.

De Graef, P. and Verfaillie, K. (2002) *The visual analog in transsaccadic object perception*. Paper presented at the Experimental Psychology Conference, 9–11 April, Leuven.

De Graef, P., Christiaens, D. and d'Ydewalle, G. (1990) Perceptual effects of scene context on object identification. *Psychol. Res.*, 52: 317–329.

De Graef, P., Verfaillie, K. and Lamote, C. (2001) Transsaccadic coding of object position: effects of saccadic status and allocentric reference frame. *Psychol. Belg.*, 41: 29–54.

Deubel, H., Schneider, W.X. and Bridgeman, B. (1996) Postsaccadic target blanking prevents saccadic suppression of image displacement. *Vision Res.*, 36: 985–996.

Deubel, H., Bridgeman, B. and Schneider, W.X. (1998) Immediate post-saccadic information mediates space constancy. *Vision Res.*, 38: 3147–3159.

Deubel, H., Schneider, W.X. and Bridgeman, B. (2002) Transsaccadic memory of position and form. In: J. Hyönä, D.P. Munoz, W. Heide and R. Radach (Eds.), *The Brain's Eye: Neurobiological and Clinical Aspects of Oculomotor Research*. Progress in Brain Research, Vol. 140, Elsevier, Amsterdam, pp. 165–180.

Di Lollo, V. and Dixon, P. (1988) Two forms of persistence in visual information processing. *J. Exp. Psychol. Hum. Percept. Perform.*, 14: 671–681.

Fernandez-Duque, D. and Thornton, I.M. (2000) Change detection without awareness: do explicit reports underestimate the representation of change in the visual system? *Vis. Cognit.*, 7: 323–344.

Friedman, A. (1979) Framing pictures: the role of knowledge in automatized encoding and memory for gist. *J. Exp. Psychol. Gen.*, 108: 316–355.

Gegenfurtner, K.R. and Sperling, G. (1993) Information transfer in iconic memory experiments. *J. Exp. Psychol. Hum. Percept. Perform.*, 19: 845–866.

Germeys, F. (2002) *A new set of 280 black-and-white line drawings of depth-rotated objects* (Psyc. Rep. No. 287). University of Leuven, Laboratory of Experimental Psychology, Leuven.

Germeys, F., De Graef, P. and Verfaillie, K. (2002) Transsaccadic identification of saccade target and flanker objects. *J. Exp. Psychol. Hum. Percept. Perform.*, 28: 868–883.

Grimes, J. (1996) On the failure to detect changes in scenes across saccades. In: K. Akins (Ed.), *Perception*. Vancouver Studies in Cognitive Science, Vol. 5, Oxford University Press, New York, pp. 89–110.

Gysen, V., De Graef, P. and Verfaillie, K. (2002) Detection of intrasaccadic displacements and depth rotations of moving objects. *Vision Res.*, 42: 379–391.

Hayhoe, M.M. (2000) Vision using routines: a functional account of vision. *Vis. Cognit.*, 7: 43–64.

Henderson, J.M. (1992) Visual attention and eye movement control during reading and picture viewing. In: K. Rayner (Ed.), *Eye Movements and Visual Cognition: Scene Perception and Reading*. Springer, New York, pp. 260–283.

Henderson, J.M. (1994) Two representational systems in dynamic visual identification. *J. Exp. Psychol. Gen.*, 123: 410–426.

Henderson, J.M. (1997) Transsaccadic memory and integration during real-world object perception. *Psychol. Sci.*, 8: 51–55.

Henderson, J.M. and Hollingworth, A. (1999a) High-level scene perception. *Annu. Rev. Psychol.*, 50: 243–271.

Henderson, J.M. and Hollingworth, A. (1999b) The role of fixation position in detecting scene changes across saccades. *Psychol. Sci.*, 10: 438–443.

Henderson, J.M. and Siefert, A. (1999) The influence of enantiomorphic transformation on transsaccadic object integration. *J. Exp. Psychol. Hum. Percept. Perform.*, 25: 243–255.

Henderson, J.M. and Siefert, A. (2001). Types and tokens in transsaccadic object identification: effects of spatial position and left–right orientation. *Psychon. Bull. Rev.*, 8: 753–760.

Hollingworth, A. and Henderson, J.M. (1998) Does consistent scene context facilitate object perception? *J. Exp. Psychol. Gen.*, 127: 398–415.

Hollingworth, A. and Henderson, J.M. (2002) Accurate visual memory for previously attended objects in natural scenes. *J. Exp. Psychol. Hum. Percept. Perform.*, 28: 113–136.

Hollingworth, A., Schrock, G. and Henderson, J.M. (2001) Change detection in the flicker paradigm: the role of fixation position within the scene. *Mem. Cognit.*, 29: 296–304.

Irwin, D.E. (1991) Information integration across saccadic eye movements. *Cognit. Psychol.*, 23: 420–456.

Irwin, D.E. (1992a) Memory for position and identity across eye movements. *J. Exp. Psychol. Learn. Mem. Cogn.*, 18: 307–317.

Irwin, D.E. (1992b) Visual memory within and across fixations. In: K. Rayner (Ed.), *Eye Movements and Visual Cognition: Scene Perception and Reading*. Springer, New York, pp. 146–165.

Irwin, D.E. (1996) Integrating information across saccadic eye movements. *Curr. Dir. Psychol. Sci.*, 5: 94–100.

Irwin, D.E. and Andrews, R.V. (1996) Integration and accumulation of information across saccadic eye movements. In: T. Inui and J.L. McClelland (Eds.), *Attention and Performance XVI: Information Integration in Perception and Communication*. Bradford, Cambridge, pp. 125–155.

Irwin, D.E. and Gordon, R.D. (1998) Eye movements, attention, and trans-saccadic memory. *Vis. Cognit.*, 5: 127–155.

Irwin, D.E. and Yeomans, J.M. (1986) Sensory registration and informational persistence. *J. Exp. Psychol. Hum. Percept. Perform.*, 12: 343–360.

Klein, R., Kingstone, A. and Pontefract, A. (1992) Orienting of visual attention. In: K. Rayner (Ed.), *Eye Movements and Visual Cognition: Scene Perception and Reading*. Springer, New York, pp. 46–65.

Li, W. and Matin, L. (1990) The influence of saccade length on the saccadic suppression of displacement detection. *Percept. Psychophys.*, 48: 453–458.

Loftus, G.R., Duncan, J. and Gehrig, P. (1992) On the time course of perceptual information that results from brief visual presentations. *J. Exp. Psychol. Hum. Percept. Perform.*, 18: 530–549.

Matin, E. (1974) Saccadic suppression: a review and analysis. *Psychol. Bull.*, 81: 899–917.

Matin, L. (1986) Visual localization and eye movements. In: K.R. Boff, L. Kaufman and J.P. Thomas (Eds.), *Handbook of Perception and Human Performance*. Vol. 1, Wiley, New York, pp. 20.1–20.45.

McConkie, G.W. and Currie, C.B. (1996) Visual stability across saccades while viewing complex pictures. *J. Exp. Psychol. Hum. Percept. Perform.*, 22: 563–581.

McRae, K., Butler, B.E. and Popiel, S.J. (1987) Spatiotopic and retinotopic components of iconic memory. *Psychol. Res.*, 49: 221–227.

O'Regan, J.K. (1992) Solving the 'real' mysteries of visual perception: the world as an outside memory. *Can. J. Psychol.*, 46: 461–488.

O'Regan, J.K. and Noë, A. (2001) A sensorimotor account of vision and visual consciousness. *Behav. Brain. Sci.*, 24: 939–1031.

O'Regan, J.K., Rensink, R.A. and Clark, J.J. (1999) Change-blindness as a result of 'mudsplashes'. *Nature*, 398: 34.

O'Regan, J.K., Deubel, H., Clark, J.J. and Rensink, R.A. (2000) Picture changes during blinks: looking without seeing and seeing without looking. *Vis. Cognit.*, 7: 191–211.

Pollatsek, A. and Rayner, K. (1992) What is integrated across fixations? In: K. Rayner (Ed.), *Eye Movements and Visual Cognition: Scene Perception and Reading*. Springer, New York, pp. 166–191.

Pollatsek, A. and Rayner, K. (2001) The information that is combined across fixations may be different for static and moving objects. *Psychol. Belg.*, 41: 75–87.

Pollatsek, A., Rayner, K. and Collins, W.E. (1984) Integrating pictorial information across eye movements. *J. Exp. Psychol. Gen.*, 113: 426–442.

Pollatsek, A., Rayner, K. and Henderson, J.M. (1990) Role of spatial location in integration of pictorial information across saccades. *J. Exp. Psychol. Hum. Percept. Perform.*, 16: 199–210.

Rayner, K. and Pollatsek, A. (1983) Is visual information integrated across saccades? *Percept. Psychophys.*, 34: 39–48.

Rayner, K. and Pollatsek, A. (1992) Eye movements and scene perception. *Can. J. Psychol.*, 46: 342–376.

Rayner, K., Inhoff, A.W., Morrison, R.E., Slowiaczek, M.L. and Bertera, J.H. (1981) Masking of foveal and parafoveal vision during eye fixations in reading. *J. Exp. Psychol. Hum. Percept. Perform.*, 7: 167–179.

Rensink, R.A. (2002) Change detection. *Annu. Rev. Psychol.*, 53: 245–277.

Rensink, R.A., O'Regan, J.K. and Clark, J.J. (1997) To see or not to see: the need for attention to perceive changes in scenes. *Psychol. Sci.*, 8: 368–373.

Rensink, R.A., O'Regan, J.K. and Clark, J.J. (2000) On the failure to detect changes in scenes across brief interruptions. *Vis. Cognit.*, 7: 127–145.

Ross, J., Morrone, M.C., Goldberg, M.E. and Burr, D. (2001) Changes in visual perception at the time of saccades. *Trends Neurosci.*, 24: 113–121.

Schneider, W.X. (1995) VAM: a neuro-cognitive model for visual attention, control of segmentation, object recognition, and space-based motor action. *Vis. Cognit.*, 2: 331–375.

Schneider, W.X. (1999) Visual–spatial working memory, attention, and scene representation: A neuro-cognitive theory. *Psychol. Res.*, 62: 220–236.

Simons, D.J. (2000) Current approaches to change blindness. *Vis. Cognit.*, 7: 1–15.

Simons, D.J. and Chabris, C.F. (1999) Gorrilas in our midst: sustained inattentional blindness for dynamic events. *Perception*, 28: 1059–1074.

Sperling, G. (1960) The information available in brief visual presentations. *Psychol. Monogr.*, 74: 1–29.

Tatler, B. (2001) Characterising the visual buffer: real-world evidence for overwriting early in each fixation. *Perception*, 30: 993–1006.

Tatler, B.W. (2002) What information survives saccades in the real world? In: J. Hyönä, D.P. Munoz, W. Heide and R. Radach (Eds.), *The Brain's Eye: Neurobiological and Clinical Aspects of Oculomotor Research*. Progress in Brain Research, Vol. 140, Elsevier, Amsterdam, pp. 149–163.

van Diepen, P.M.J. (1998) New data-acquisition software for the Leuven dual-PC controlled Purkinje eye-tracking system (Psyc. Rep. No. 246). Laboratory of Experimental Psychology, University of Leuven.

Van Diepen, P.M.J. and De Graef, P. (1994) *Line-drawing library and software toolbox* (Psyc. Rep. No. 165). University of Leuven, Laboratory of Experimental Psychology, Leuven.

Van Diepen, P.M.J., De Graef, P. and d'Ydewalle, G. (1995) Chronometry of foveal information extraction during scene perception. In: J.M. Findlay, R. Walker and R.W. Kentridge (Eds.), *Eye Movement Research: Mechanisms, Processes and Applications*. North-Holland, Amsterdam, pp. 349–362.

Van Rensbergen, J. and De Troy, A. (1993) *A reference guide for the Leuven dual-PC controlled Purkinje eyetracking system* (Psyc. Rep. No. 145). University of Leuven, Laboratory of Experimental Psychology, Leuven.

Verfaillie, K. (1997) Transsaccadic memory for the egocentric and allocentric position of a biological-motion walker. *J. Exp. Psychol. Learn. Mem. Cogn.*, 23: 739–760.

Verfaillie, K. and De Graef, P. (2000) Transsaccadic memory for position and orientation of saccade source and target. *J. Exp. Psychol. Hum. Percept. Perform.*, 26: 1243–1259.

Verfaillie, K., De Troy, A. and Van Rensbergen, J. (1994) Transsaccadic integration of biological motion. *J. Exp. Psychol. Learn. Mem. Cogn.*, 17: 649–670.

Verfaillie, K., De Graef, P., Germeys, F., Gysen, V. and Van Eccelpoel, C. (2001) Selective transsaccadic coding of object and event-diagnostic information. *Psychol. Belg.*, 41: 89–114.

Wolfe, J.M., Klempen, N. and Dahlen, K. (2000) Postattentive vision. *J. Exp. Psychol. Hum. Percept. Perform.*, 26: 693–716.

CHAPTER 13

Commentary: Changes

Ronald A. Rensink [*]

Department of Psychology, University of British Columbia, 2136 West Mall, Vancouver, BC V6T 1Z4, Canada

Abstract: It is argued that change perception can provide a powerful way to explore various aspects of vision, such as visual attention and the accumulation of information across saccades. Several studies of change perception are discussed, and their results consolidated with existing knowledge to cast new light on our understanding of the visual system.

"All things change, and nothing stays still. . ."
(Heraclitus, c. 500 BCE)

Introduction

This past decade has seen a great resurgence of interest in the perception of change. Change has, of course, long been recognized as a phenomenon worthy of study, and vision scientists have given their attention to it at various times in the past (for a review, see Rensink, 2002a). But things seem different this time around. This time, there is an emerging belief that instead of being just another visual ability, the perception of change may be something central to our 'visual life', and that the mechanisms that underlie it may provide considerable insight into the operation of much of our visual system.

This development may have been sparked by a number of factors: technology that allowed the easy creation of dynamic displays, a feeling in the air that it was time for something new, or it may have simply been a matter of chance. But once underway, this development was fueled by results, results that included both novel behavioral effects and new theoretical insights. Many of these centered around *change blindness* [1], the failure of observers to see large changes that are made contingent upon some transient event, such as a brief blank, or a saccade (see Rensink, 2000b). Given the strength and robustness of these effects, they provide a powerful way to explore a number of issues, such as the extent to which our behavior is based on nonconscious processing of visual input, the way that attention is (and is not) involved in vision, and the extent to which visual information is accumulated across saccades.

The chapters presented in this section provide excellent illustrations of the success of this approach in providing new insights into the operation of our visual system. In what follows, an attempt will be made to consolidate the results and conclusions obtained by each of these studies with a broader theoretical framework based on earlier work. Such an approach will hopefully show that studies of change

---

[*] Correspondence to: R.A. Rensink, Department of Psychology, University of British Columbia, 2136 West Mall, Vancouver, BC V6T 1Z4, Canada. Tel.: +1-604-822-2579; Fax: +1-604-822-6923;
E-mail: rensink@psych.ubc.ca

[1] It should be emphasized that change blindness is a true *blindness* (failure to see the change), and not an *amnesia* (forgetting a change that was perceived). Although observers may have seen the previous display (and so might be amnesic in regard to its contents), the fact that they are set to report change as soon as it occurs rules out the possibility that they see the change itself and then forget. For a more detailed discussion of this issue, see Rensink (2000a).

perception can help resolve a number of important issues in visual perception, and — even more importantly — raise a number of interesting new questions.

Background

Change blindness

Consider the situation shown in Fig. 1. In this *flicker paradigm*, an original image A alternates with a modified image A′, with brief blank fields between successive images.

Observers have great difficulty noticing most changes under these conditions, even when the changes are large, repeatedly made, and the observer knows they will occur. Such *change blindness* (Rensink et al., 1997) is a very general phenomenon: it can be induced in a variety of ways, such as when changes occur simultaneously with (1) saccades (e.g., Bridgeman et al., 1975); (2) real-world interruptions (Simons and Levin, 1998); (3) brief 'splats' that do not cover the change (Rensink et al., 2000). For a comprehensive review of work on change blindness, see Simons (2000) and Rensink (2000b, 2002a).

The need for attention to perceive change

The generality and robustness of this effect indicates that change blindness involves mechanisms central to our visual experience of the world. In particular, it has been suggested that *focused attention is needed for the conscious perception of change* (Rensink et al., 1997). In this view, attention creates a coherent structure that can support the perception of change. If the transient signal that accompanies the change is swamped via other transients (or is otherwise rendered inoperative), the guidance of attention is lost and change blindness is induced.

Coherence theory

Change blindness can be severe, and remains severe even when observers are given several seconds to try

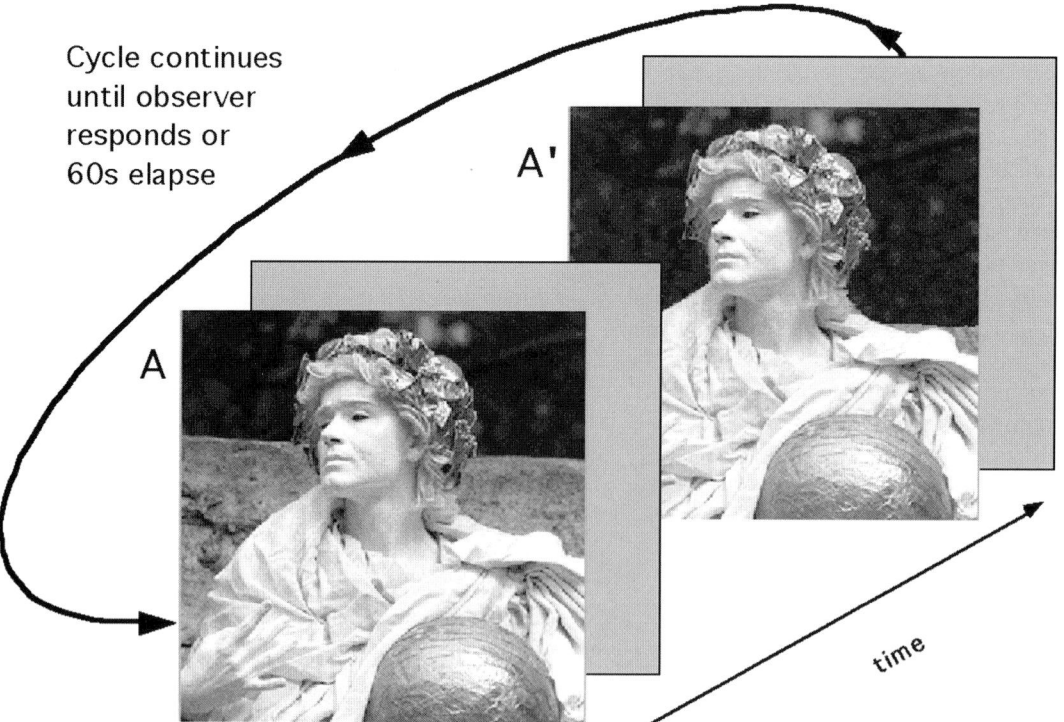

Fig. 1. Flicker paradigm. Original image A (statue with background wall) and modified image A′ (statue with wall lowered) are displayed in the order A, A′, A, A″, ... with gray fields briefly displayed between successive images (Rensink et al., 1997).

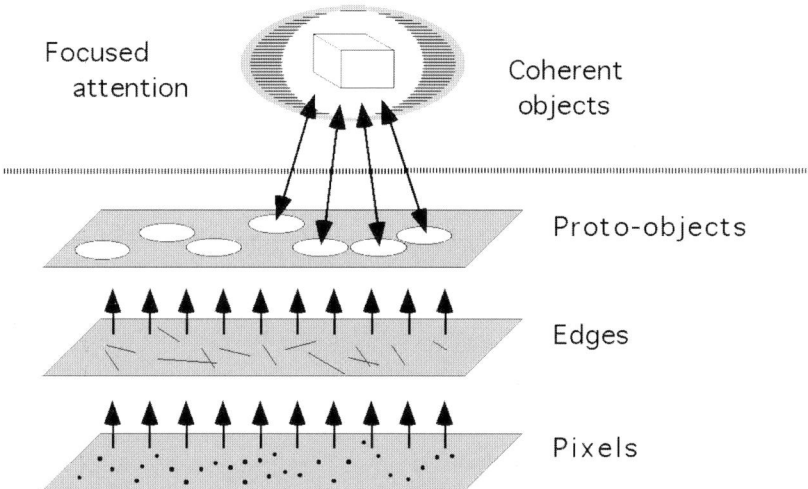

Fig. 2. Coherence theory. Early-level processes create proto-objects rapidly and in parallel across the visual field. Focused attention 'grabs' these volatile proto-objects and stabilizes them. As long as the proto-objects are 'held' in a coherence field, they form an individuated object with both temporal and spatial coherence (Rensink, 2000c).

to memorize the image (Rensink et al., 2000). To account for this, it has been proposed that the coherent structures formed by attention are not long-lasting, but instead exist only as long as attention is directed to them. More precisely, this *coherence theory* of attention (Rensink, 2000c) has three parts (Fig. 2).

(i) Prior to focused attention, low-level *proto-objects* are continually formed rapidly and in parallel across the visual field. These 'preattentive' structures can be quite complex, but are volatile, having no real memory. Thus, they are simply *replaced* when any new stimulus appears at their location.

(ii) Focused attention selects a small number of proto-objects and *stabilizes* them. This is done via links that feed back from a single, higher-level *nexus*; the resultant circuit is referred to as a *coherence field*. This representation has a high degree of coherence over space and time: any new stimulus at that location is treated as the *change* of an existing structure rather than the appearance of a new one.

(iii) After focused attention is released, the object loses its coherence and dissolves back into its constituent proto-objects. There is little or no 'aftereffect' of having been attended.

The limited amount of information that can be attended at any one time explains why observers can fail to detect changes in 'attended' objects (Levin and Simons, 1997). When focused attention is directed to something in the world, it will not generally be possible to represent all of its properties in a coherence field — only a few of its aspects can be represented at any one time. If an aspect being represented is one of the aspects changing in the world, the change will be seen; otherwise, change blindness will again result.

Triadic architecture

Given that attention is limited, it is critical that eye movements and attentional shifts be made to the appropriate object at the appropriate time. One proposal for how this might be carried out is the *triadic architecture* of visual processing (Rensink, 2000c). This is composed with three largely independent systems (Fig. 3):

(i) a high-capacity early-level system that rapidly creates detailed, volatile proto-objects in parallel across the visual field;

(ii) a limited-capacity attentional system that forms these structures into representations of objects with spatiotemporal coherence;

(iii) a limited-capacity nonattentional system that provides a context (or *setting*) to guide attention to the appropriate objects in the scene.

According to this view, a complete representation of the scene is never constructed: only one coherent

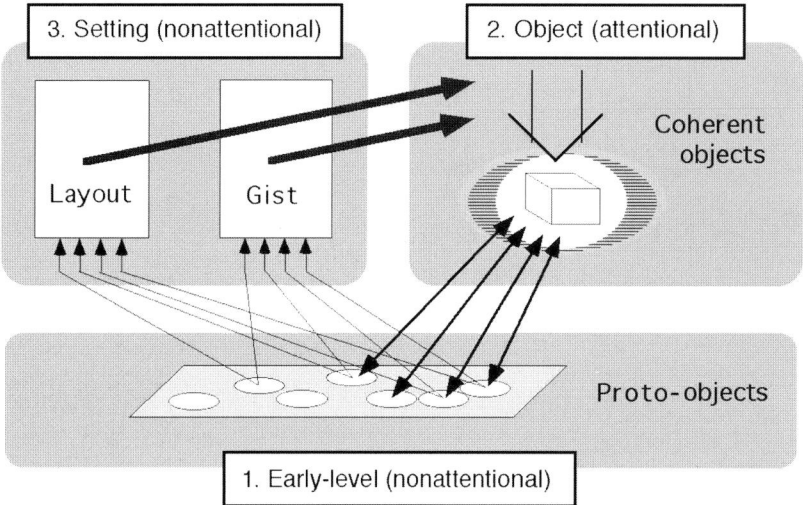

Fig. 3. Triadic architecture. Visual perception may be carried out via the interaction of three systems. (1) Early-level processes create volatile proto-objects. (2) Focused attention acts as a hand to 'grab' these structures and form an object with both temporal and spatial coherence. (3) Setting information — obtained via a nonattentional stream — guides the allocation of focused attention (Rensink, 2000c, 2001).

object is represented at any one time, with the setting providing a context that successfully directs attention so that the right information is made available at the right time. Such an approach uses representations that are stable and representations that contain large amounts of visual detail. But at no point does it use representations that are both stable *and* contain large amounts of detail.

Note that the setting system is subdivided into at least two subsystems, each of which involves a different aspect of scene structure.

(i) The abstract meaning (or *gist*) of a scene, e.g., whether the scene is a harbor, city, or picnic.

(ii) The spatial arrangement (or *layout*) of objects in the scene. Note that although layout information may not be volatile, it is not detailed, with relatively little information stored concerning each item.

However, it is important to mention that nonattentional streams are also possible. The key point in all of this is that the attentional system is only one among many concurrent systems, and that although attention is required for the formation of coherent structure, it is not necessarily a precursor or a partner in the operation of other aspects of visual perception (Rensink, 2000c).

New developments

Implicit perception of change

Given that large changes can take place for extended stretches of time without being (consciously) seen, change blindness can provide a potentially powerful way to investigate whether various aspects of visual processing can occur implicitly, i.e., occur without being accompanied by conscious visual experience. Thornton and Fernandez-Duque (2002, this volume) provide a comprehensive survey of the work that has been done on the implicit detection of change, as well as on related results that support their contention that change can be registered in the absence of visual awareness. Among other things, they make clear the difficulties in establishing the existence of implicit perception. However, they argue that this can be done in a reliable way by looking at consistencies in the patterns of results found via different kinds of tests.

Thornton and Fernandez-Duque make a number of distinctions that are worth keeping in mind, such as those between *visual perception* and *visual registration*, and between *attention* and *awareness*. The first of these is based on the increasing tendency to regard *perception* as being limited to the conscious

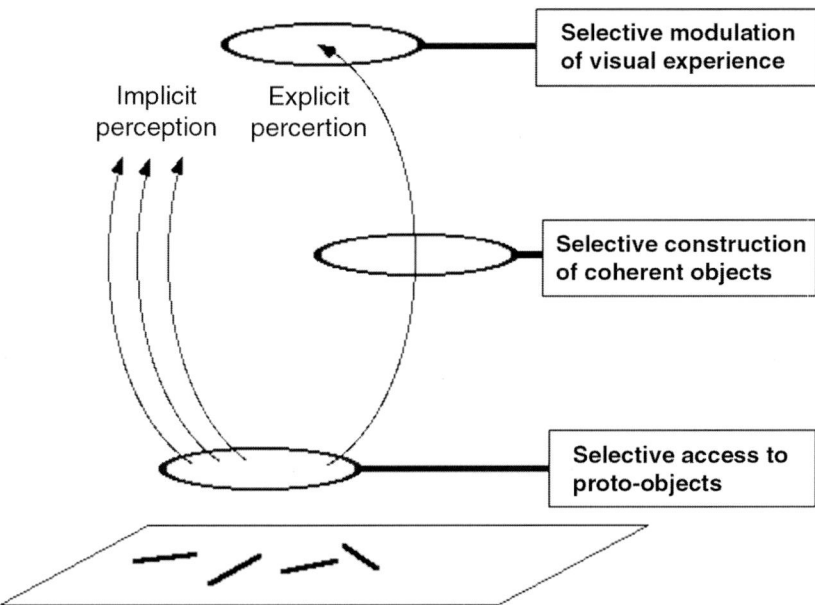

Fig. 4. Possible types of attentional process. Attention (defined as a selective factor that limits processing) can act at least three possible locations. (1) Selective *access* of all processes to the array of early-level proto-objects. (2) Selective *construction* of spatiotemporally coherent representations. (3) Selective *modulation* of conscious awareness. Whether these are aspects of a single process or of different processes remains unknown.

(or at least, non-motoric) aspects of visual processing (cf. Milner and Goodale, 1995; Rensink, 2000c). The term *registration* is therefore a useful way to discuss the visual pickup of information without committing to whether or not the result will be experienced in a conscious way.

It may be important to point out here that even if a change is *registered* (i.e., it has an effect on an organism via visual transmission), this does not imply that it is *represented* as such. For example, an initial view of an object could be placed into long-term memory, and at some time later compared with a new view. From this it might be deduced that a change has occurred. On the other hand, if the new view was simply stored (or combined) with the old, the variability in the resultant representation might weaken the ability of the organism to recognize the object on the next encounter. The change would then be registered, but it would be difficult to say that is represented, at least in any direct way.

Thornton and Fernandez-Duque also make clear the importance of distinguishing between two roles of attention: the *modulation* of awareness (a subjective state) and the *construction* of spatiotemporally coherent representations (Fig. 4). They point out that — conceptually, at least — these are two rather different things. Whether or not they really are correlated is far from certain. One source of confusion is the common belief (mentioned by Thornton and Fernandez-Duque) that if an observer attends to an object, all of its properties would be attended, and thus would be put into coherent form. If this were true, the failure to see changes in attended objects would support the separation of these two aspects. However, as discussed above, this is not the case; a coherence field includes only a selected subset of properties (Rensink, 2000b). Thus, most properties of an attended object would not be in coherent form at any time, and so, would not be seen to change. As such, this leaves unsettled the question of whether modulation and construction are separate processes.

Another distinction worth making in this regard is that between attention as selective *access* and attention as selective *construction* of coherent structure (Rensink, 2002b). Although these two aspects may be part of the same process, it is also possible that they are carried out by separate processes (Fig. 4). If so, this would explain why implicit detection of change would fail when attention is directed elsewhere: although attention-as-construction is not required for implicit perception, visual input still is. Thus, if input to the implicit system is stopped due to a diversion of attention-as-access, it will effectively stop any implicit perception of change (or any other implicit visual process, for that matter), even if no spatiotemporal coherence is involved.

Applicability of change blindness research

Turning now to the more intensively studied explicit detection of change, Dornhöfer et al. (2002, this volume) examine the extent to which change blindness might occur in everyday life, and the extent to which the theoretical conclusions that have been reached would apply to various aspects of vision. Change blindness has already been found to be a surprisingly robust phenomenon (see e.g., Rensink, 2002a): it can, for example, be induced by making changes contingent with brief blank fields (e.g., Rensink et al., 1997), saccades (e.g., Bridgeman et al., 1975), and localized 'splats' that do not cover the item being changed (Rensink et al., 2000). Dornhöfer et al. (2002, this volume) compare the degree of change blindness induced via several different methods (blinks, blanks, and saccades), and find that it does not depend on the particular type of method used, nor on the exposure time of the displays. As such, they provide a useful confirmation of the robustness of change blindness, strengthening the argument that it is not due to some experimental artifact but instead reflects the failure of mechanisms that are important to everyday vision.

Curiously, after confirming that change blindness is an effect that is both strong and robust, Dornhöfer et al. (2002, this volume) argue that we do not need to worry about it much in everyday life, since over 80% of relevant changes were detected. This may not be all that comforting once it is realized that many events (e.g., braking for stopped automobiles ahead) occur many times a day; even one traffic accident a day would be more than most people could endure. More generally, attempting to continually allocate attention to important items is something that is effortful and requires constant vigilance; if anything disturbs this, change blindness could easily result. Indeed, a large number of traffic accidents are caused by drivers engrossed in conversations on their cell phone (e.g., Redelmeier and Tibshirani, 1997), presumably because of attentional diversion.

Following Simons and Levin (1998) and Wallis and Bülthoff (2000), Dornhöfer et al. (2002, this volume) also investigate the nature of change perception on dynamic displays. Interestingly, they find differences in performance on static and dynamic displays. These differences are worth further investigation; not only do they occur in situations similar to activities carried out in everyday life (e.g., automobile driving), but they may also provide new insights into the operation of the change-perception process itself.

The dynamics of change perception

As a step towards understanding the dynamics of the representations involved in change perception, Saiki (2002, this volume) presents several elegant experiments on the perception of changes in controlled dynamic displays. These are based on a new paradigm (multi-object permanence tracking) that combines aspects of the flicker paradigm (Rensink et al., 1997) with the multiple-object tracking task (Pylyshyn and Storm, 1988); viz., detecting changes in a set of tracked items. (See also Scholl and Pylyshyn, 1998.)

Saiki finds that the ability to detect switches in the properties of these items depends strongly on their velocity, and that the cost of tracking a moving item through space can be separated from the cost of binding its properties to their correct locations. Furthermore, he finds that the tracked items contain only individual features, and not their conjunctions, thereby ruling out the model of *object files* proposed by Kahneman et al. (1992), in which features are bound together in local bundles. Instead, he argues, the mechanism involved in attention is much more like the visual indexes proposed by Ballard et al. (1997) or Pylyshyn and Storm (1988).

Saiki makes no mention of coherence fields, but it is worth examining what implications his results have for this model of attention. As mentioned above (or see Rensink, 2001), a *coherence field* is a circuit formed of feedforward and feedback paths that link a set of (attended) *proto-objects* to a higher-level *nexus*. Whereas the upward propagation of information is relatively straightforward, the downward connections can only be established by a correlation

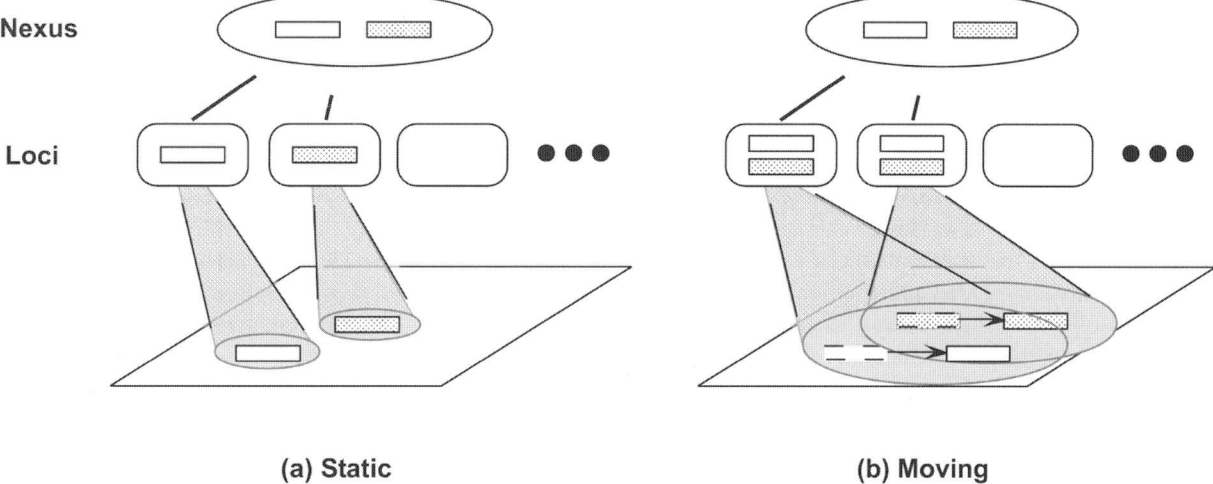

Fig. 5. Dynamics of coherence fields. (a) When proto-objects are static, a feedback circuit (coherence field) is established between a selected proto-object and a locus in the nexus; the contents of these loci are then pooled. (b) When a proto-object is moving, the correlation between the representation at its (actual) position and the representation being sent down the feedback connections deteriorates, since the proto-object is no longer at its expected position. This leads to a delocalization of its spatial linkage, causing the loci to pool properties from several items, and so creating a failure to detect switches among the properties of attended items.

of the nexus signal with that of the proto-object at the target location. (For details on a similar scheme involving a lower-level system of feedforward and feedback connections, see DiLollo et al., 2000.)

Consider now the case where the items are static (Fig. 5a). Since a switch of properties between the attended items can be accurately detected, this supports the idea of *weak aggregation* (Rensink, 2001). Here, the nexus has a separate memory *locus* for each link, with the locus signals then combined into an aggregate description. When the items are static, then, a change or switch in any of their properties could be detected. But if the items are moving, a different situation emerges (Fig. 5b): given that the information traveling along the links is propagated at a finite velocity, a moving proto-object would cause problems with correlations between the expected signal (the signal from the nexus) and the signal at the intended location, and these problems would worsen with increasing velocity. Because of the resultant disturbance, the 'locking on' of the downward path would temporarily fail, along with the spatial link. Until spatial localization could be reasserted, each locus would pool signals from a relatively large area of space, thus impeding the ability to detect switches in properties of the (localized) items that were being tracked.

This account is, of course, rather sketchy, and many more experiments will be needed to supply it with more detail (or cause it to be rejected). The important point here, however, is that the experiments of the kind described by Saiki show how dynamic displays can be used to provide important insights into the nature of the coherent representations underlying the conscious perception of change.

Preservation of nonattended information

Although much of the work on explicit change detection has focused on spatiotemporal continuity, Tatler (2002, this volume) examines the fate of the other systems involved in visual perception, viz., the array of (unattended) volatile proto-objects in early vision, as well as the various kinds of context information. In particular, he examines the extent to which these can be preserved across saccades. Note that in contrast to an exploration of how well observers can perceive dynamic change [2] (which might

---

[2] *Dynamic change* refers to seeing the actual progress of the change itself, and not just seeing that the initial and final states differ. For a more detailed discussion of the various kinds of change that may be distinguished, see Rensink (2002a).

be the hallmark of the spatiotemporal coherence associated with focused attention), the tests used by Tatler involve other aspects of visual perception.

In regard to the elements of early vision, Tatler investigates what can be reported after a saccade is made. His results indicate that the contents of the new fixation overwrite the old, but do not do so immediately. This is consistent with the proposal of Rensink (2000c) that the contents of early vision are volatile, with unattended proto-objects replaced by the proto-objects corresponding to new stimuli appearing at their location. Models of this replacement process based on the phenomenon of common-onset masking (DiLollo et al., 2000) indicate that most of this replacement is achieved by 160 ms, and the remainder by 320 ms. This is reasonably consistent with Tatler's estimate that most of the replacement is achieved by 250 ms, and the remainder by 400 ms.

The conclusions that Tatler draws concerning the nature of this kind of visual memory level are largely consistent with the characteristics of early vision, and is also consistent with the proposal that iconic memory (or *informational persistence*) is just the decaying trace of the proto-object array (Rensink, 2000c). Tatler correctly points out that although there is no need to *maintain* highly detailed information (since the world can be used as an external memory; Stroud, 1955; Dennett, 1991), there is nevertheless a need to *use* (and therefore represent) it. The only real contention here might be his assertion that this level of representation is precategorical, because of the precision involved. However, the formation of proto-objects (either individually or in groups) is highly sensitive to spatial position (Rensink and Enns, 1995), and it may be that the sensitivity to spatial position is simply a consequence of this.

Regarding the kind of information that might be preserved in the setting system, Tatler provides a nice assay of the time course of the development of different possible kinds of information. Results show an early (and almost immediate) development of gist information, followed by a progressive buildup of layout information. This is consistent with the operation of the triadic architecture proposed by Rensink (2000c); indeed, the results argue for layout being constructed by the sequential entry of fixated items into a more durable representation that does not require attention for its maintenance. It is an open issue as to how much information can be accumulated this way. However, if the representation of layout is to remain reasonably abstract, only a minimal amount of information can be maintained about each item. It is also important to keep in mind that nonattentional representations are not concerned with spatiotemporal coherence. Thus, even if a considerable amount of abstract information could be accumulated (e.g., Melcher, 2001), it would not be able to assist with the perception of *dynamic change*, although it might facilitate the detection of *difference* (Rensink, 2002a).

Preservation of attended information

The question of how much attended information is preserved across saccades is explored in an elegant way by Deubel et al. (2002, this volume), who examine how information from the presaccadic display interacts with information in the postsaccadic display. Their studies are based on the *blanking effect* (Deubel and Schneider, 1996), where the blindness to displacements made during saccades can be 'cured' by briefly blanking the saccade target after the eye has arrived at its new position. This effect suggests that more information may survive across saccades than would expected from change-blindness work. Deubel et al. carry out several interesting experiments that investigate this possibility.

The initial set of experiments investigates the preservation of position information. Deubel et al. present a nice summary of previous work showing that this kind of information is unlikely to be maintained across a saccade with a high degree of accuracy. They then propose that the position of any item in the vicinity of the estimated position will be taken as the reference location. Their experiments show evidence that an estimate of the postsaccadic position of the saccade target is also carried across the saccade, but that this is used only if no reference item is present.

This view of the transsaccadic preservation and integration of information is consistent with the framework described earlier, since given that a saccade target is an attended item, a certain amount of information about it will be held in stable form (including position information). The main addition here is a mechanism to cope with expected changes due to the saccade itself, namely, an anticipatory formation of a new link from the nexus to the estimated postsaccadic location.

An interesting issue that emerges from this proposal is the status of the blanked item. Deubel et al. argue that if the reference item is not found in the postsaccadic display, the assumption of stationarity is given up, and it is assumed that the item has moved elsewhere. However, it may also be that the blanked item is simply considered to be occluded (with its anticipated position left unchanged), and that its unblanking is interpreted as a shift to a new position where it is no longer occluded.

Deubel et al. also show that a similar kind of blanking causes a similar kind of increase in the ability to detect changes in other properties, such as shape. Owing to issues of projection, receptor density, etc., the representation of a given shape depends on its location on the retina, and it is certainly possible that a similar kind of anticipatory mechanism is used.

However, the experiments used to investigate this issue involved only a brief display of the presaccadic item, and so there may simply have been insufficient time for its consolidation in (attended) visual short-term memory. In other words, without the blank the consolidated representation might have been a combination of pre- and postsaccadic views, making detection of change unreliable. The insertion of the blank may have served simply to allow time to consolidate the (attended) presaccadic representation, or at least to mark it off as a distinct object. One test for this would be to repeat these experiments with a longer exposure of the stimulus (say, 300 ms) before the saccade is initiated. If blanking effects were still found, this would support the anticipation hypothesis; if not, it would support the consolidation hypothesis.

Access to detailed information

De Graef and Verfaillie (2002, this volume) provide a direct examination of the extent to which detailed information (i.e., the information in the array of detailed, volatile proto-objects) can be carried across a saccade and then accessed by various visual processes. Transsaccadic memory has often been presented as a limited-capacity system (often identified with visual short-term memory and attention); however, various studies indicate that other kinds of information are also preserved across saccades (see e.g., Tatler, 2002, this volume). De Graef and Verfaillie examine the possibility that the array of detailed information (in what they term a *visual analog*) can survive a saccade, and can be entered into subsequent descriptions of (coherent) objects.

The approach taken by De Graef and Verfaillie is an interesting variant of the technique used by Becker et al. (2000), namely, detecting change in a postsaccadic item that has been cued during the saccade. As in the case of Deubel et al. (2002, this volume), they find that a brief blanking creates some ability to detect change in the three-dimensional orientation of a saccade target, and that any blank of 50 ms or more is sufficient for this. However, if the item cued is a bystander object (i.e., not a saccade target), the observer remains unable to detect changes in its orientation. They argue from this that there is some ability to extract information from a visual analog, but that there remain some mysteries as to the details of its operation.

As De Graef and Verfaillie point out, the notion of a visual analog is similar to the idea of informational persistence (Irwin and Yeomans, 1986), and this in turn can be related to the memory trace of the array of proto-objects in early vision (Rensink, 2000b). All these descriptions concur in positing a dense array of items. Indeed, the proposal by De Graef and Verfaillie that the visual analog can represent in-depth (or three-dimensional) orientation is echoed in the findings of Enns and Rensink (1991) that early-level processes can form proto-objects that describe three-dimensional orientation.

There is less agreement, however, on the issue of whether proto-objects are moved during a saccade (resulting in a spatiotopic array) or whether they remain stationary (resulting in a retinotopic array). The work of Duhamel et al. (1992), for example, shows that receptive fields begin to anticipate saccade shifts, at least for fixation targets, and presumably all other attended items as well. However, it is an interesting question whether a similar translation takes place for the nonattended items.

The experiments of De Graef and Verfaillie are a good first step in addressing this question. However, their current design leaves open the possibility that no access to the proto-object array (or visual analog) is involved. To begin with, in the case where the cued item is the saccade target, the pattern is much the same as that found by Deubel et al. (2002, this volume), and an explanation of this can be given entirely in terms of the stabilization of the (attended) saccade target. (The lack of decay is exactly what would be expected of an attended item held in short-term memory.) Meanwhile, the failure to detect change in cued bystanders could be explained simply by a failure to access detailed information. Note that this failure does not imply that the volatile, detailed description has been completely destroyed by the saccade; rather, it may simply be that by the time attention has reached these items, they have simply decayed too much. (Indeed, the hint of improvement for the 50 ms blank may be due to the vestiges of this representation.) But as De Graef and Verfaillie suggest, a resolution of this issue can be obtained by further experiments that examine the effect of initial exposure, blank time, and cue time on performance.

Summary

As the chapters in this section show, change perception provides a powerful way to explore various aspects of vision, including implicit perception, the nature of visual attention, and the degree to which information is accumulated across saccades. Moreover, these results can be consolidated into a picture that casts light on the general architecture of the visual system. The picture that is emerging is one of a highly dynamic, 'just in time' system, in which the conscious perception of coherent structure is just one of several aspects of visual perception.

Thus, the study of change perception is changing many of our ideas about visual perception, as well as our ideas about change itself. Given that all things change, it is unlikely that we will ever arrive at a final picture of these matters. Nevertheless, it appears likely that we will continue to increase our understanding of how vision works, and it appears likely that much of this will be achieved by studying the perception of change.

Acknowledgements

The author would like to thank NSERC (Canada) for its support during the preparation of the manuscript.

References

Ballard, D.H., Hayhoe, M.M., Pook, P.K. and Rao, R.P.N. (1997) Deictic codes for the embodiment of cognition. *Behav. Brain Sci.*, 20: 723–767.

Becker, M.W., Pashler, H. and Anstis, S.M. (2000) The role of iconic memory in change-detection tasks. *Perception*, 29: 273–286.

Bridgeman, B., Hendry, D. and Stark, L. (1975) Failure to detect displacement of the visual world during saccadic eye movements. *Vision Res.*, 15: 719–722.

De Graef, P. and Verfaillie, K. (2002) Transsaccadic memory for visual object detail. In: J. Hyönä, D.P. Munoz, W. Heide and R. Radach (Eds.), *The Brain's Eye: Neurobiological and Clinical Aspects of Oculomotor Research*. Progress in Brain Research, Vol. 140, Elsevier, Amsterdam, pp. 181–196.

Dennett, D.C. (1991) *Consciousness Explained*. Little, Brown and Co, Boston, MA.

Deubel, H. and Schneider, W.X. (1996) Saccade target selection and object recognition: evidence for a common attentional mechanism. *Vision Res.*, 36: 1827–1837.

Deubel, H., Schneider, W.X. and Bridgeman, B. (2002) Transsaccadic memory of position and form. In: J. Hyönä, D.P. Munoz, W. Heide and R. Radach (Eds.), *The Brain's Eye: Neurobiological and Clinical Aspects of Oculomotor Research*. Progress in Brain Research, Vol. 140, Elsevier, Amsterdam, pp. 165–180.

DiLollo, V., Enns, J.T. and Rensink, R.A. (2000) Competition for consciousness among visual events: the psychophysics of reentrant visual processes. *J. Exp. Psychol. Gen.*, 129: 481–507.

Dornhöfer, S.M., Unema, P.J.A. and Velichkovsky, B.M. (2002) Blinks, blancs and saccades: how blind we really are for relevant visual events. In: J. Hyönä, D.P. Munoz, W. Heide and R. Radach (Eds.), *The Brain's Eye: Neurobiological and Clinical Aspects of Oculomotor Research*. Progress in Brain Research, Vol. 140, Elsevier, Amsterdam, pp. 119–131.

Duhamel, J.R., Colby, C. and Goldberg, M. (1992) The updating of the representation of visual space in parietal cortex by intended eye movements. *Science*, 225: 90–92.

Enns, J.T. and Rensink, R.A. (1991) Preattentive recovery of three-dimensional orientation from line drawings. *Psychol. Rev.*, 98: 335–351.

Irwin, D.E. and Yeomans, J.M. (1986) Sensory registration and informational persistence. *J. Exp. Psychol. Hum. Percept. Perform.*, 12: 343–360.

Kahneman, D., Treisman, A. and Gibbs, B. (1992) The reviewing of object files: object specific integration of information. *Cognit. Psychol.*, 24: 175–219.

Levin, D.T. and Simons, D.J. (1997) Failure to detect changes to attended objects in motion pictures. *Psychon. Bull. Rev.*, 4: 501–506.

Melcher, D. (2001) Persistence of visual memory for scenes: a medium-term memory may help us to keep track of objects during visual tasks. *Nature*, 412: 401–401.

Milner, A.D. and Goodale, M.A. (1995) *The Visual Brain in Action*. Oxford University Press, Oxford.

Pylyshyn, Z.W. and Storm, R. (1988) Tracking multiple independent targets: evidence for both serial and parallel stages. *Spat. Vis.*, 3: 179–197.

Redelmeier, D.A. and Tibshirani, R.J. (1997) Association between cellular-telephone calls and motor vehicle collisions. *N. Engl. J. Med.*, 336: 453–458.

Rensink, R.A. (2000a) When good observers go bad: change blindness, inattentional blindness, and visual experience. *Psyche*, 6, URL: http://psyche.cs.monash.edu.au/v6/psyche-6-09-rensink.html.

Rensink, R.A. (2000b) Seeing, sensing, and scrutinizing. *Vision Res.*, 40: 1469–1487.

Rensink, R.A. (2000c) The dynamic representation of scenes. *Vis. Cognit.*, 7: 17–42.

Rensink, R.A. (2001) Change blindness: implications for the nature of attention. In: M.R. Jenkin and L.R. Harris (Eds.), *Vision and Attention*. Springer, New York, pp. 169–188.

Rensink, R.A. (2002a) Change detection. *Annu. Rev. Psychol.*, 53: 245–277.

Rensink, R.A. (2002b) Visual attention. In: L. Nadel (Ed.), *Encyclopedia of Cognitive Science*. Nature Publishing Group, London, in press.

Rensink, R.A. and Enns, J.T. (1995) Preemption effects in visual search: evidence for low-level grouping. *Psychol. Rev.*, 102: 101–130.

Rensink, R.A., O'Regan, J.K. and Clark, J.J. (1997) To see or not to see: the need for attention to perceive changes in scenes. *Psychol. Sci.*, 8: 368–373.

Rensink, R.A., O'Regan, J.K. and Clark, J.J. (2000) On the failure to detect changes in scenes across brief interruptions. *Vis. Cognit.*, 7: 127–145.

Saiki, J. (2002) Multiple-object permanence tracking: limitation in maintenance and transformation of perceptual objects. In: J. Hyönä, D.P. Munoz, W. Heide and R. Radach (Eds.), *The Brain's Eye: Neurobiological and Clinical Aspects of Oculomotor Research*. Progress in Brain Research, Vol. 140, Elsevier, Amsterdam, pp. 133–148.

Scholl, B.J. and Pylyshyn, Z.W. (1998) Tracking multiple items through occlusion: clues to visual objecthood. *Cognit. Psychol.*, 38: 259–290.

Simons, D.J. (2000) Current approaches to change blindness. *Vis. Cognit.*, 7: 1–16.

Simons, D.J. and Levin, D.T. (1998) Failure to detect changes to people during a real-world interaction. *Psychon. Bull. Rev.*, 5: 644–649.

Stroud, J.M. (1955) The fine structure of psychological time. In: H. Quastler (Ed.), *Information Theory in Psychology: Problems and Methods*. Free Press, Glencoe, IL, pp. 174–207.

Tatler, B.W. (2002) What information survives saccades in the real world? In: J. Hyönä, D.P. Munoz, W. Heide and R. Radach (Eds.), *The Brain's Eye: Neurobiological and Clinical Aspects of Oculomotor Research*. Progress in Brain Research, Vol. 140, Elsevier, Amsterdam, pp. 149–163.

Thornton, I.M. and Fernandez-Duque, D. (2002) Converging evidence for the detection of change without awareness. In: J. Hyönä, D.P. Munoz, W. Heide and R. Radach (Eds.), *The Brain's Eye: Neurobiological and Clinical Aspects of Oculomotor Research*. Progress in Brain Research, Vol. 140, Elsevier, Amsterdam, pp. 99–118.

Wallis, G. and Bülthoff, H.H. (2000) What's in scene and not seen. *Vis. Cognit.*, 7: 175–190.

SECTION III

Smooth pursuit eye movements

Section Editors: W. Heide and D.P. Munoz

CHAPTER 14

Non-target influences on the initiation of smooth pursuit

Paul C. Knox * and Tarik Bekkour

Division of Orthoptics, University of Liverpool, Brownlow Hill, Liverpool L69 3BX, UK

Abstract: Smooth pursuit is usually regarded as a relatively stereotyped oculomotor response in which the early part of the response reflects primarily the properties of the visual stimulus and cortical motion processing. We have investigated pursuit initiation in human subjects using the gap paradigm to alter fixation conditions, and single *stationary* distractors to alter visual context. The results suggest that a number of processes, distinct from motion processing, are involved in pursuit initiation. The processes which are modified by gaps and distractors are closely related and interact with each other. They may be shared with the saccade system.

Introduction

Primates, including humans, have a wide repertoire of eye movements. There are two classes of eye movement which are important for achieving and maintaining foveation of visual targets: saccades and smooth pursuit (SP). It is clear that saccadic eye movements, an apparently simple behaviour, require multiple levels of neuronal processing involving areas throughout the neuraxis including the brainstem, cerebellum, midbrain and cortex. In contrast, in recent times, smooth pursuit has been regarded as a somewhat more simple, reflex-like, eye movement — a visuomotor reflex (Ferrera and Lisberger, 1995, 1997). According to this view, particularly in laboratory conditions in which a single moving target is tracked, the key stimulus determining the initiation of SP is raw retinal image motion and the key process requiring explanation is cortical motion processing and how this produces the drive signals required by the oculomotor system. However, many of the challenges that face the saccadic system must also face the pursuit system including target selection, breaking from stable fixation and filtering out distracting signals. Thus it seems likely that even in simplified laboratory conditions, multiple processes will be involved in the initiation of SP and that a number of these will be distinct from motion processing. One way of seeking to address this issue is to manipulate non-target aspects of SP tasks. If the visuomotor reflex view of SP is correct, such manipulations should have little or no effect on SP initiation while the stimulus target motion remains unaltered. However, systematic alterations of SP initiation by non-target aspects of stimuli would provide evidence of the involvement of multiple, perhaps largely independent, mechanisms in SP initiation.

The 'gap effect' on SP initiation is evidence of the importance of non-target influences on SP. When a temporal gap is introduced between the extinction of fixation target and the illumination of a moving target, SP latency is reduced (Knox, 1996, 1998; Krauzlis and Miles, 1996a,b; see Fig. 1). This effect is analogous to the gap effect on saccade latency (see Fischer and Weber, 1993 for review) and it has been suggested that a similar mechanism might account for both (Krauzlis and Miles, 1996a). Previously we found that when SP target contrast was reduced, SP latency increased, but the magnitude of the gap effect was unaffected (O'Mullane and Knox, 1999). This

---

* Correspondence to: P.C. Knox, Division of Orthoptics, University of Liverpool, Thompson Yates Building, Brownlow Hill, Liverpool L69 3BX, UK. Tel.: +44-0151-794-5736; Fax: +44-0151-794-5781;
E-mail: pcknox@liv.ac.uk

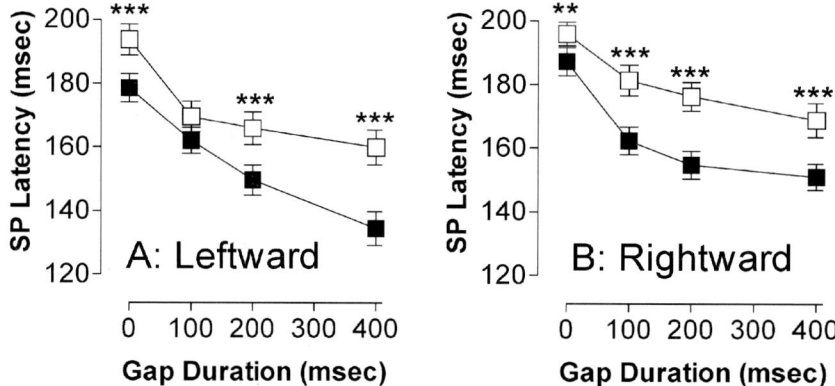

Fig. 1. Plots of mean (±95% confidence limits) SP latency against gap duration pooled for three subjects. Latencies for leftward (A) and rightward (B) smooth pursuit are plotted separately. In each plot, data from trials in which a single stationary distractor was present are plotted in open symbols. Data from trials in which no distractor was present are plotted in filled symbols. For each gap duration, means were compared using a Newman–Keuls test for multiple comparisons. Asterisks represent the level of statistical significance of differences between latencies with and without distractors: ** $p < 0.01$; *** $p < 0.001$.

was suggestive of the sort of separation of processes discussed above and supported the hypothesis of the involvement of multiple processes in SP initiation.

In the case of the gap effect on SP initiation it remains unclear which processes are being modified. Two general types of mechanism have been discussed with reference to gap effects, i.e. fixational and attentional. A number of neural structures have been tentatively identified as being part of a 'fixation system' for saccades (e.g. Munoz and Wurtz, 1992, 1993; Munoz et al., 1996; Petit et al., 1999; but see Gandhi and Keller, 1999). However it has yet to be shown that they play an identical role in fixation in relation to SP (see Krauzlis et al., 2000). The similarity in the gap effect for both saccades and SP, in addition to other evidence, indicates that a similar *break* from fixation precedes both classes of eye movement (Luebke and Robinson, 1988; Goldreich et al., 1992; Knox, 1996, 1998; Krauzlis and Miles, 1996b). Thus perhaps the gap effect on SP is a modulation of fixation mechanisms.

There is an alternative, though not mutually exclusive, hypothesis involving the modulation of attention which has not yet been ruled out. In the monkey cortical motion processing area MT, attentional signals can modify motion processing by altering single unit motion responses (Treue and Maunsell, 1996) and in human subjects attention can modify perceptual thresholds for motion (Raymond et al., 1998).

Presumably such signals might be involved in SP initiation and might be modified in gap conditions.

We decided to investigate other types of non-target stimulus manipulations in addition to temporal gaps. Again the parallels with experiments on saccades were instructive. Distractors have been used to probe the gap effect on saccades (Weber and Fischer, 1994) and it has been argued that the mechanisms modified by distractors are the same as those involved in the gap effect (Walker et al., 1997). Considerable use has been made of moving distractors in SP tasks in both monkeys (Ferrera and Lisberger, 1995, 1997; Lisberger and Ferrera, 1997) and humans (Krauzlis et al., 1999). In this situation there are two competing motion signals which initially influence SP. At some point after the initiation of SP an explicit choice must be made between the two moving targets as only one can be tracked (Ferrera and Lisberger, 1995). However, in the experiments we describe below, we have investigated the effect of presenting a single *stationary* distractor with the SP target. There is only ever one moving target, no competition between motion signals and no choice to be made between competing moving targets. This is a useful way of investigating the visuomotor reflex view of SP. A single stationary distractor, appearing some distance from the SP target should, presumably, have little effect on SP latency on this view. Where the SP stimulus (i.e. the motion signal generated by the SP target) always remains the same, there is no reason to believe that the properties of a single stationary distractor will have any systematic effect on SP latency. We have now tested the effects of a single stationary distractor on the initiation of SP and have found a number of interesting interactions.

Materials and methods

With local ethical approval and informed consent all experiments were conducted in adult human subjects with normal or corrected-to-normal visual acuity. They viewed a visual display with their left eye from 57 cm; the right eye was occluded. Visual stimuli were generated by a Visual Stimulus Generator 2/5 (Cambridge Research Systems, Rochester, UK); the fixation and SP targets and distractor were all $0.3° \times 0.3°$ dark squares presented on a light background. The fixation target was presented in the centre of the display for a variable period (0.5 s to 1.5 s). In all experiments the SP target appeared randomly 5° to the right or left of fixation, and moved back through the centre of the display at 14°/s. Fixation and pursuit targets, and the stationary distractor all had the same contrast. Subjects were presented with runs of 52 or 96 trials consisting of sets of four or eight tasks, in which leftward and rightward tasks and distractor condition were balanced and presented in random order. The randomisation of fixation time and target direction is important to prevent the build up of either predictive or anticipatory responses. Subjects were instructed to keep looking at the centre of the display until they saw a moving target which they were to track. In *Experiment 1*, we investigated the effects of a single stationary distractor appearing in the mirror image position to, and simultaneously with, the moving SP target in both gap and non-gap conditions. In sets of four interleaved tasks, one task had no gap, the other three had gaps of 100, 200 or 400 ms and in 50% of trials the distractor appeared. In all trials in which a distractor appeared it remained visible throughout the trial. Three subjects were exposed to 1248 trials in this configuration, providing up to 72 trials per subject per condition for analysis. In *Experiment 2*, we investigated the effect of introducing a delay between target appearance and target motion. Three subjects (one of whom was naive) were presented with runs of non-gap tasks in which after the fixation target was extinguished, either one target appeared 5° to either left or right of fixation or two targets appeared one 5° to the left and the other 5° to the right of fixation. There was then a delay of 200 ms before one of the targets moved at 14°/s back through the centre of the display. Three subjects (one naive) participated in *Experiment 3* in which we examined whether doing the tasks against a structured stationary background modified the distractor effect. The background consisted of vertical high contrast (92%) bars. Each bar was $0.3° \times 6°$, with 4.5° between bars. Nine bars were displayed above and nine below a 4.5° window in which the fixation and SP targets and distractors were presented. In *Experiment 4*, we investigated the effect of distractor eccentricity. Four subjects participated in variable eccentricity experiments, in which runs consisted of *either* normal or gap trials (gap = 200 ms). In each trial a distractor was presented at one of four eccentricities, 1°, 2°, 6° or 8° from fixation, on the opposite side to the SP target. We investigated whether the position of the distractor was important in *Experiment 5*. In runs consisting of sets of eight trials (six with and two without distractors), the distractor was presented either on the same horizontal axis as the SP target, or vertically above or below the position of the fixation target at one of two eccentricities, 2° or 4° from fixation. Three subjects (one naive) participated in these experiments.

Horizontal eye movement was recorded by means of an infra-red corneal reflection device (IRIS, Skalar Medical, Delft, Netherlands), and the eye position signal digitised with 12-bit precision at 1 kHz using a CED μ1401 (Cambridge Electronic Design, Cambridge, UK). The eye position and a time marker of the appearance of the pursuit target were displayed on the computer screen; data from 100 ms before to 500 ms after the appearance of the target were stored on disc for analysis off-line. Eye position traces were differentiated to yield traces of eye velocity. For each trial the two traces were displayed together. SP latency was measured from the velocity traces using a regression technique (see Krauzlis and Miles, 1996b; Morrow and Lamb, 1996). A linear regression of velocity against time was first fitted through the data from approximately 50 ms before to 50 ms after the time of target appearance. A second regression was calculated over the initial, acceleration, phase of the pursuit response. The calculated intersection between the two functions was taken to estimate the time of SP initiation. Only responses which were preceded by stable fixation, and were not contaminated by blinks or early saccades were analysed.

Experiment 1: the effect of synchronous mirror image distractors

Three subjects participated in the initial experiments with synchronous mirror image distractors. In all three, in the control condition in which only the SP target appeared, there was a gap effect on SP latency; when a gap was introduced between the extinction of the fixation target and the illumination of the pursuit target, SP latency was reduced (Fig. 1). Note that control trials were interleaved with distractor trials. Analysis of variance (ANOVA) was carried out for individual subjects, for each direction of pursuit separately, with the statistical significance of particular gap durations measured using the Newman–Keuls multiple comparison test. In all subjects, the overall effect of gaps was statistically significant ($p < 0.0001$). Compared with the normal condition (gap = 0 ms), the shortest gap duration used (100 ms) caused a statistically significant ($p < 0.05$ or better) reduction in SP latency in all three subjects, whether the target stepped left and moved right or stepped right and moved left. For pooled data, there was a statistically significant effect of gap duration on SP latency for both leftward ($F_{3,771} = 60.77$, $p < 0.0001$) and rightward ($F_{3,793} = 56.13$, $p < 0.0001$) SP. The shortest gap duration (100 ms) significantly reduced SP latency (left: $p < 0.001$; right: $p < 0.001$) and there were further statistically significant reductions comparing the 100 ms and 400 ms gaps (left: $p < 0.001$; right $p < 0.01$).

A single stationary distractor presented at the mirror image position to the SP target (5° from fixation, 10° from the SP target), increased SP latency in all subjects (see Fig. 1). In normal, non-gap, conditions there was some variability across subjects in the effect of the distractor. In one subject the distractor did not alter latency in a statistically significant manner in the normal (non-gap) condition, in a second there was no effect for targets moving to the right, and a statistically significant increase in SP latency to the left (16 ms, $p < 0.05$). In the third subject, SP latency was significantly increased for both leftward (17 ms, $p < 0.01$) and rightward (33 ms, $p < 0.001$) pursuit. However, distractors produced robust increases in latency in all the subjects in gap conditions. And indeed the largest increase in absolute terms was observed with a gap duration of 400 ms (an increase of 42 ms or 27% from the non-gap condition, $p < 0.001$). Because of this larger and more robust increase in latency in gap conditions, the effect of distractors could be viewed as being a reduction in the magnitude of the gap effect. The normal gap-induced reduction in latency was of smaller magnitude when a distractor was presented with the target. For example, in one subject when no distractor was present latency for leftward pursuit was reduced by 20%, from 175 ± 39 ms in the normal condition to 140 ± 34 ms with a gap of 400 ms. With a distractor, SP latency was reduced by 13 ms or 7% from 182 ± 36 ms to 169 ± 41 ms.

The pooled data reflected the pattern of latency changes in the individual subjects (Fig. 1). As Fig. 1 illustrates, the increases in latency tended to be greater in gap conditions, compared to the normal (non-gap) condition. The net result was that the gap effect was reduced in size. Latency was reduced by 44 ms without and 34 ms with a distractor for SP to the left, and by 36 ms without and 27 ms with for SP to the right, comparing the normal and gap = 400 ms conditions. Thus there was an interaction between the effect of distractors and the effect of gaps.

For each subject and each condition, frequency distribution histograms were plotted. Fig. 2A–D shows typical distributions of SP latency for leftward SP without distractors in a single subject. Note that even at the longer gap durations, there was little evidence of anticipatory pursuit. There was little evidence of a switch in the distributions between non-gap and gap conditions from a unimodal to a bimodal distribution (as has been reported for saccades; see Fischer and Weber, 1993). The addition of a single distractor, while increasing mean latency, also did not alter the shape of the latency distribution (Fig. 2E–H). For all subjects in all conditions distributions were tested for the assumption that they were gaussian; no evidence was found that violated this assumption.

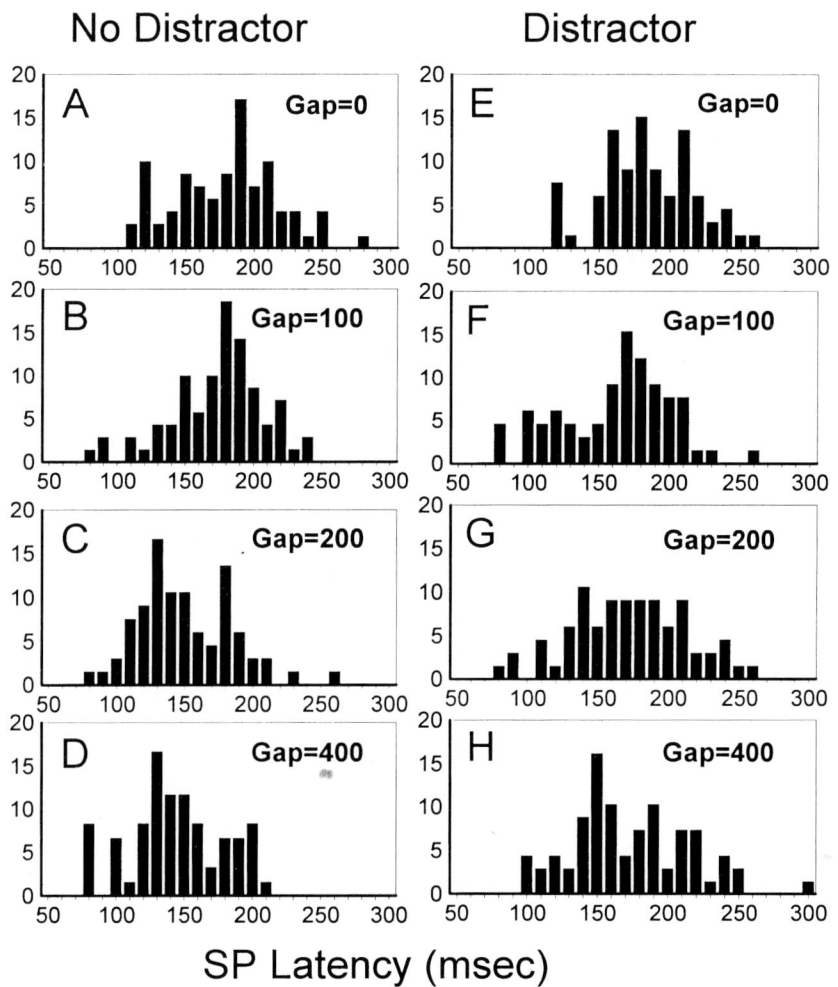

Fig. 2. Frequency distribution histograms of pursuit latency for a single typical subject (GOM) for leftward pursuit in the absence (A–D) and in the presence of (E–H) a single stationary distractor across the four gap durations (0–400 ms) used in this study.

Experiment 2: do distractors act by altering motion processing?

As discussed above, the visuomotor reflex view of SP stresses the importance of motion processing mechanisms in the initiation of SP, particularly in the conditions used in our experiments in which only one moving target was present. A single stationary distractor might exert its effects by interfering with motion processing. MT cells are known to respond to stationary objects falling in their receptive fields (Maunsell and van Essen, 1983). It is conceivable that a transient response in some cells to the stationary distractor might alter the population response of MT/V5 cells, and thus modify SP initiation. To test this possibility we compared latency when only one object (the target) appeared and was displayed for 200 ms with latency when two objects (target and distractor) appeared for 200 ms, 5° either side of fixation. After the 200 ms delay the target moved at 14°/s back through the centre of the display as in the other tasks. We reasoned that the 200 ms delay would allow sufficient time for onset transients to decline. The instruction to the subjects was to continue to look at the centre of the display until the moving target appeared.

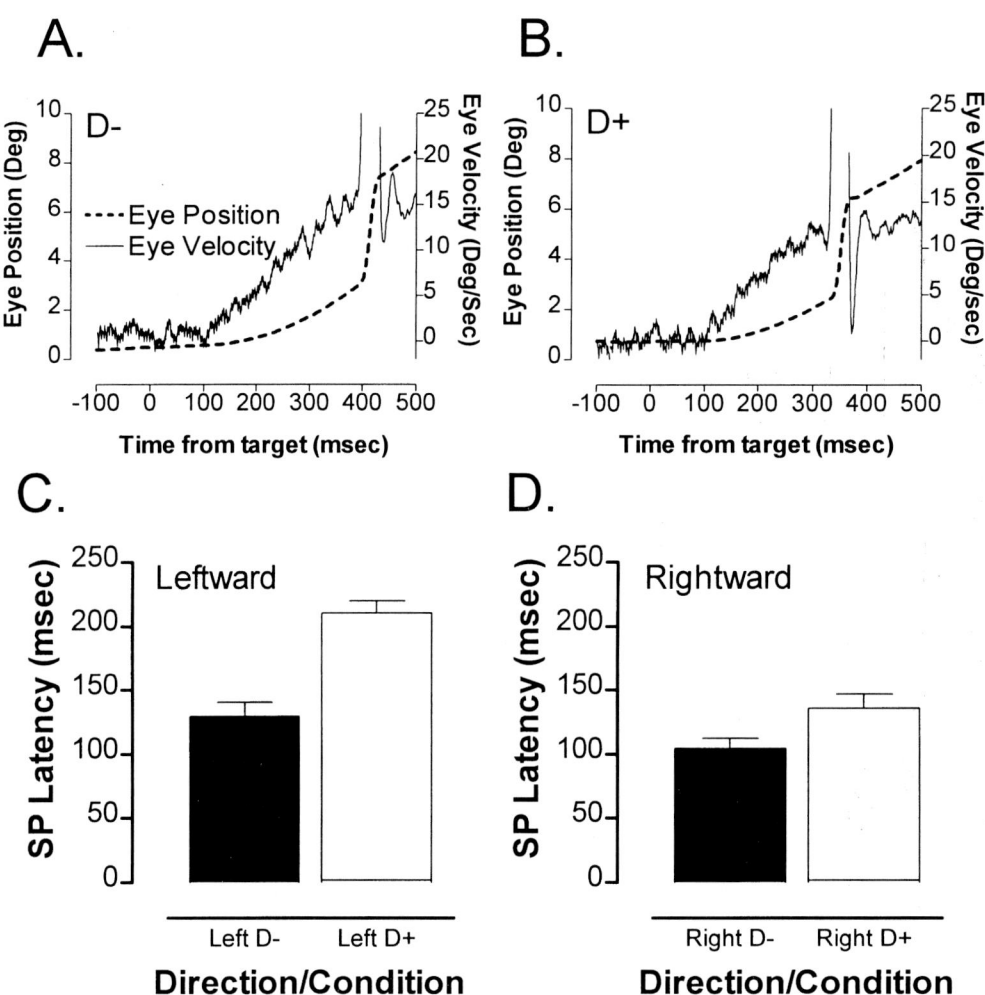

Fig. 3. The effect of introducing a 200 ms delay between target or target and distractor appearance and target motion. (A) Eye position (dotted trace) and eye velocity (solid trace) from one trial in which only the target appeared (no distractor, D−), 5° to the left of fixation. Time = 0 ms indicates time at which target moved at 14°/s to the right, back through the centre of the display. (B) Traces from trial in which both the target and distractor appeared (D+). Other conventions as for A. (C) Mean (with 95% confidence limits) latency for tasks in which target stepped right and moved to left. D− target only trials; D+ target and distractor trials. (D) Mean (with 95% confidence limits) latency for tasks in which target stepped left and moved to right. D− target only trials; D+ target and distractor trials. Data pooled across three subjects.

We found that in single object tasks subjects were able to continue viewing the centre of the display until the SP target appeared; they did not, in general, execute an early saccade which obscured SP initiation (see Fig. 3A). There were no qualitative differences between responses in single object trials and in trials in which two objects (target and distractor) appeared (Fig. 3B). For both leftward and rightward pursuit, there was a statistically significant increase in latency in the presence of the distractor (leftward 80 ms, $t = 11.09$, $p < 0.0001$; rightward 32 ms, $t = 4.531$, $p < 0.0001$; Fig. 3C,D). As might be expected, allowing the subjects a 200 ms 'preview' did cause a marked decrease in latency in most conditions compared to the non-delay condition (e.g. rightward SP without distractor: no delay 187 ± 32 ms, with delay 104 ± 37 ms). However, there remained little evidence of anticipatory SP, probably because the fixation period and target direction were randomised from task-to-task within runs (see section Materials and methods). Clearly the distractor effect persisted in these conditions.

Experiment 3: the effect of a stationary structured background

When pursuit is executed against a stationary structured background, steady state gain is reduced (Collewijn and Tamminga, 1984; Barnes and Crombie, 1985), and of more relevance to the present study, small increases in latency are observed (Keller and Khan, 1986). The question therefore arises as to whether distractors and stationary backgrounds might act through the same or similar mechanisms. We therefore exposed three subjects to mixed runs of distractor and non-distractor tasks, but with the addition of a structured background which remained visible throughout the run (see section Materials and methods). Only one gap duration (200 ms) was used in these experiments.

Typical data are illustrated in Fig. 4. As subject GOM participated in both these (Fig. 4A,B) and the earlier experiments without a structured background, appropriate data from Fig. 1 were re-plotted in Fig. 4C,D for comparison. The effect of the background was to increase latency across all conditions by a small amount. However, in the presence of a structured background, both gap and distractor effects persisted (e.g. GOM leftward $F_{3,180} = 13.15$, $p < 0.0001$; TB leftward $F_{3,175} = 10.69$, $p < 0.0001$). As might be expected from the results described above, in non-gap conditions distractor effects were small and not statistically significant (both GOM and TB: leftward $p > 0.05$; rightward $p > 0.05$, Newman–Keuls). However, with a 200 ms gap, the addition of a distractor once again caused a statistically significant increase in latency (GOM leftward $p < 0.001$, rightward $p < 0.01$; TB leftward $p < 0.01$, rightward $p < 0.001$).

Experiment 4: the effect of distractor eccentricity

The effect of distractor eccentricity was investigated in four subjects (including two naive subjects). In each of four tasks in these runs, a distractor appeared on the opposite side of the fixation target to the pursuit target, but randomly at one of four eccentricities (1°, 2°, 6° or 8°). Individual and pooled data are shown in Fig. 5. Distractor eccentricity influenced SP latency in all subjects. In one subject (Fig. 5, GOM) the effect of eccentricity was statistically significant for both directions and in both gap and non-gap conditions (one-way ANOVA; left normal $F_{3,144} = 11.37$, $p < 0.0001$; left gap $F_{3,144} = 12.98$, $p < 0.0001$; right normal $F_{3,145} = 5.94$, $p < 0.001$; right gap $F_{3,145} = 14.72$, $p < 0.001$). However, the gap effect was basically abolished. In another subject (Fig. 5, DN) there was no significant eccentricity effect in normal conditions (left $F_{3,98} = 6.2$, $p > 0.05$; right $F_{3,140} = 0.8$, $p > 0.05$) and a clear eccentricity effect in gap conditions (left $F_{3,96} = 2.7$, $p < 0.001$; right $F_{3,94} = 11.6$, $p < 0.0001$). There was now a clear gap effect when the distractor appeared 6° or 8° from fixation. The orientation of the effect of distractor eccentricity was clear; SP latency was longest when the distractor appeared near to the fixation target, and declined as the distractor was presented further from the fixation target.

In order to obtain an overall measurement of the eccentricity effect, data from the four subjects was pooled and subjected to linear regression analysis. As there was no significant difference between leftward and rightward pooled data, the data were collapsed across directions. Regression lines with 95% confidence limits are shown in Fig. 5E. Both regression lines significantly deviated from a line of zero slope (normal $F_{1,1002} = 23.7$, $p < 0.0001$; gap $F_{1,795} = 43.8$, $p < 0.0001$). There was also a significant difference between the slopes of the lines with the latency declining more steeply with eccentricity in gap compared to normal conditions (normal -2.3 ± 0.48; gap -4.0 ± 0.6; $p < 0.05$).

Experiment 5: horizontal versus vertical distractors

In all of the above experiments, the distractor and the target had the same vertical position and in the mirror image experiments, the horizontal distance of target and distractor from fixation was identical. It was therefore possible to argue that the distractor exerted its effects because it competed as a potential target, forcing a discrimination step not necessary when only a target was present. This might be conceived of as an

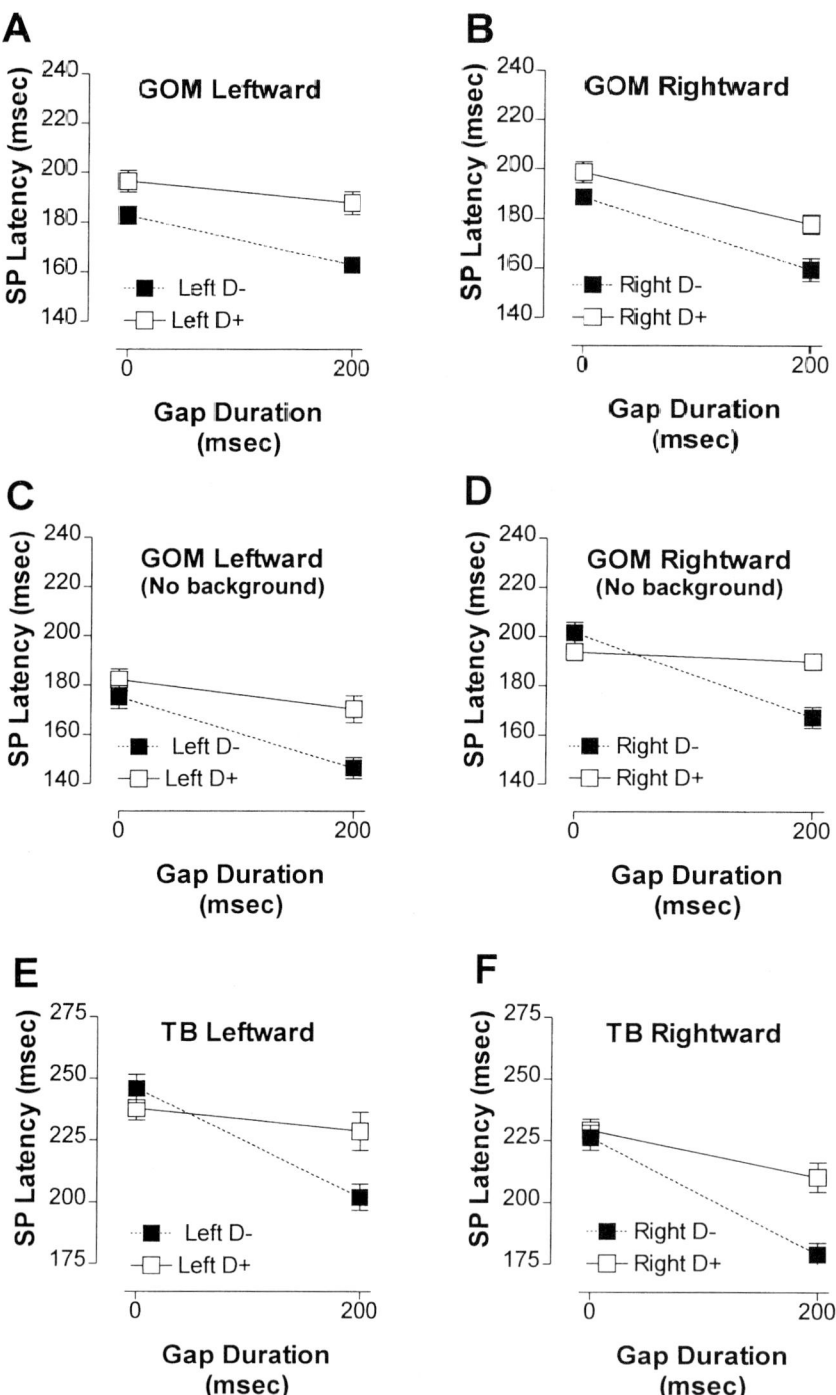

Fig. 4. Gap and distractor effects on SP latency when targets were presented against a structured background (see methods for details of the background). Mean ± SEM SP latency is plotted (in some case the error bars are smaller than the symbols). Data from two subjects (A–D: GOM; E,F: TB) are presented and leftward (A,C,E) and rightward (B,D,F) latencies are plotted separately. Data from trials without distractors are plotted in filled symbols; data from trials with distractors are plotted in open symbols. Note that GOM participated in earlier experiments without a structured background; the data in C and D are replotted from Fig. 1 for comparison.

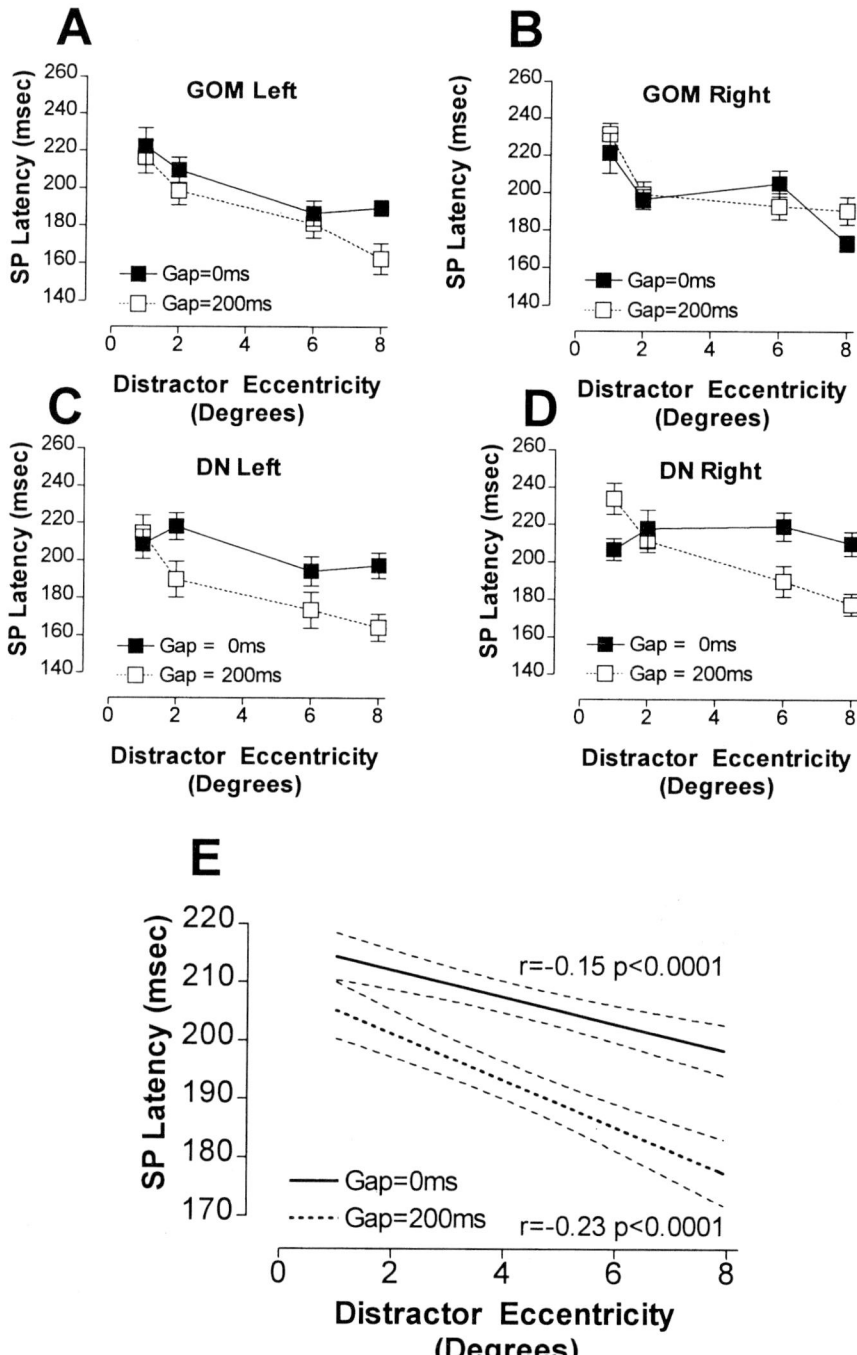

Fig. 5. Effect of distractor eccentricity on SP latency. Mean ± SEM latency is plotted for two individual subjects (A,B: GOM; C,D: DN). Filled symbols, non-gap conditions. Open symbols, 200 ms gap conditions. (E) Linear regression (with 95% confidence limits) of SP latency on distractor eccentricity; data pooled across four subjects collapsed across directions. Solid line, non-gap conditions. Regression parameters: slope -2.317 ± 0.48; intercept 216.70 ± 2.43; $r = -0.15$, $n = 1002$, $p < 0.0001$. Broken line, 200 ms gap conditions. Regression parameters: slope -4.001 ± 0.60; intercept 209.20 ± 2.94; $r = -0.23$, $n = 795$, $p < 0.0001$.

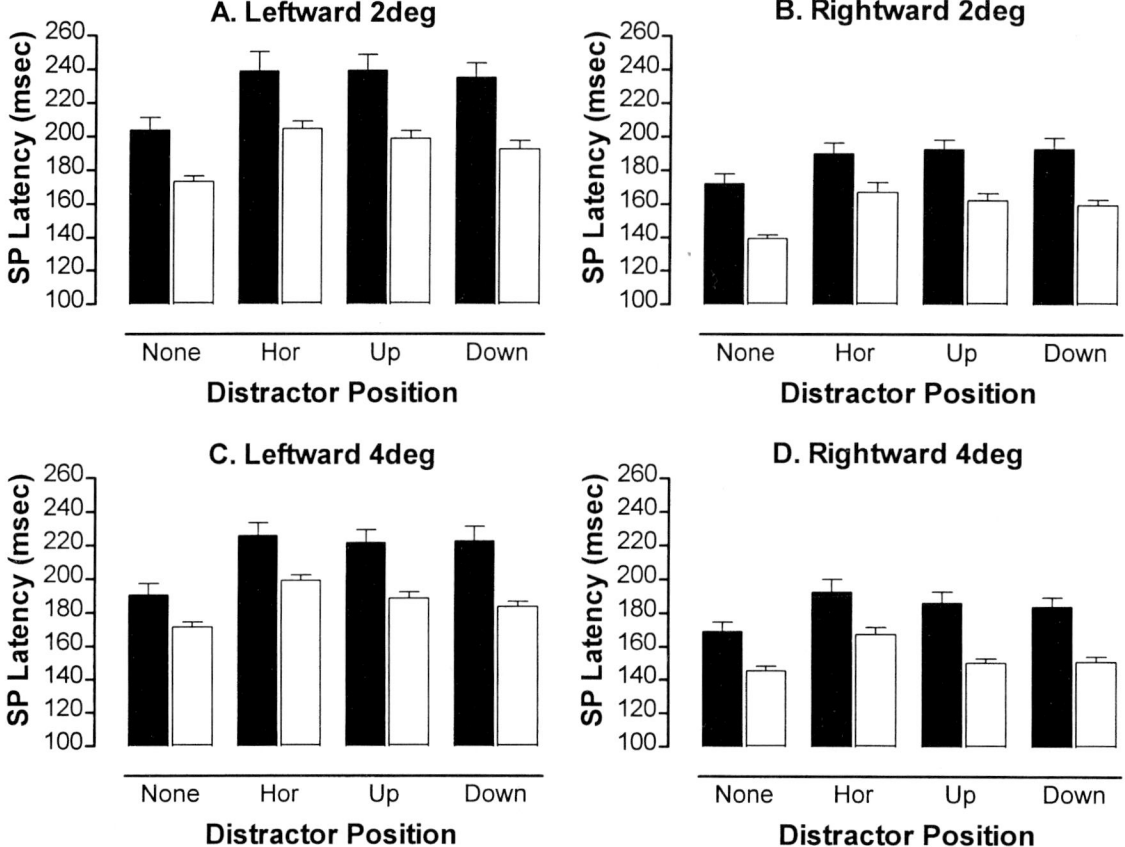

Fig. 6. Comparison of effect of single stationary distractor presented horizontally with distractor presented vertically above or below fixation. Bars show mean latency with 95% confidence limits. Filled bars, normal (non-gap) conditions. Open bars, gap 200 ms. Data pooled across three subjects. (A) Distractor eccentricity 2°. Target steps right, moves left. Leftward pursuit. None, only target presented; Hor, distractor appeared on same horizontal axis as the target, on opposite side of fixation; Up, distractor presented above fixation; Down, distractor presented below fixation. (B) Distractor eccentricity 2°. Rightward pursuit. (C) Distractor eccentricity 4°. Leftward pursuit. (D) Distractor eccentricity 4°. Rightward pursuit.

operation at a higher level, in the target selection system. In contrast, the distractor effect on saccades has been explained in terms of inhibitory fixation mechanisms, where the key factor is distractor eccentricity (Walker et al., 1997). We therefore investigated the effect of presenting distractors in positions where they could not be targets, vertically above and below the fixation target. Three subjects (one naive) were presented with runs of eight tasks in which the target motion was as described in the methods. In two tasks (one leftward, one rightward), no distractor appeared. In the other six, a distractor appeared at one of three positions (above, below or on the opposite side of fixation) at either 2° or 4° from fixation.

In the presence of a vertical distractor, SP latency was always increased as it was when a horizontal distractor appeared in the opposite hemifield to the target (Fig. 6). The magnitude of increase was very similar regardless of distractor position. The gap effect was robust across conditions, although there was some evidence that vertical distractors increased latency by less in gap conditions than horizontal distractors.

Discussion

In recent times smooth pursuit (SP) has been likened to a 'visuomotor reflex', a view which stresses the importance retinal image motion and cortical motion processing (e.g. Lisberger and Westbrook, 1985; Lisberger and Pavelko, 1989; see Lisberger et al., 1987 for review). According to this view, the initiation phase of pursuit (the open-loop period, comprising approximately the first 100 ms of the oculomotor response) is primarily a reflection of the visual inputs to the pursuit system. However, there is an older literature which tends to stress object perception and cognitive influences on pursuit (e.g. Steinbach, 1976; Kowler and Steinman, 1981; Kowler, 1989). This has been reinvigorated by recent experimental results and reviews (e.g. Beutter and Stone, 1998; Krauzlis and Stone, 1999; Stone et al., 2000). Our approach has been to investigate the initiation of SP by using the same target motion and changing other features of the stimulus. The results suggest that these non-target manipulations modify the initiation of SP by altering processes distinct from those involved in the transduction of retinal image motion.

In agreement with earlier studies (e.g. Knox, 1996, 1998; Krauzlis and Miles, 1996a,b), we found that the introduction of a temporal gap between the extinction of the fixation target and the illumination of the SP target caused a reduction in SP latency (Fig. 1). The magnitude of this reduction was monotonically related to the duration of the gap, and there was little evidence that latency began to increase again with the longest gap duration used in these experiments (400 ms). The reduction in mean latency was not due to an increase in low latency anticipatory responses. As the frequency distribution histograms illustrate, anticipatory responses were relatively rare; in the vast majority of trials, across all conditions, latency was consistent with visually guided SP. Although we have concentrated on latency here, a separate analysis of eye velocity in the 100 ms immediately after target appearance also suggests that predictive SP (Kowler, 1989) was not a feature of the subjects' responses in these experiments. This was probably because of the temporal uncertainty introduced by the variable fixation time, and the directional uncertainty stemming from the interleaving of tasks (Knox, 1998). Note that the gap paradigm is a non-target manipulation of the stimulus; the SP target moves from the same position, in the same direction and at the same speed in both gap and the appropriate non-gap task. Presumably the motion signals generated are the same. However, the time taken to initiate the behavioural response is significantly reduced in gap conditions.

In the distractor experiments, the motion stimulus is held constant once again. Now it is the addition of a single stationary distractor that increases SP latency. In initial experiments, the distractor was positioned 10° from the SP target and 5° from the fixation target, in the mirror image position to the target, on 50% of the trials. In the other 50% only the SP target appeared. In this configuration, when two objects appear after the fixation target is extinguished there are no clues as to which one is the SP target, until of course the motion from the SP target is detected. Interestingly, in this experiment there was evidence of an interaction between the gap and distractor effects. Because distractors increased latency more in gap than non-gap conditions, the magnitude of the gap effect was in effect reduced by distractors. This is different from the effect of other stimulus manipulations. We found that when target contrast was reduced, SP latency increased by the same amount across all conditions; the magnitude of the gap effect was unaltered (O'Mullane and Knox, 1999). This suggested a separation of motion processing and gap mechanisms. The evidence here is for linked or overlapping mechanisms for gap and distractor effects.

The distractor effect is not necessarily evidence for the involvement of mechanisms outwith the motion processing system. Because MT cells respond to stationary objects falling in their receptive fields, a stationary distractor as well as a moving target would evoke MT/V5 responses. However, MT responses to stationary stimuli are transient, while responses to moving stimuli are sustained. Therefore, introducing a delay between the appearance of either the target alone or the target and distractor together, and the target motion, should allow any transients to decay. We found that latency was still increased by the distractor compared to trials when only the target appeared. This provides evidence that the effect of stationary distractors should be explained in terms of mechanisms outwith the motion processing system.

Structured stationary backgrounds modify SP by generating an optokinetic signal which conflicts with the SP signal resulting in reductions in SP gain of the order of 10% (e.g. Collewijn and Tamminga,

1984; Kowler et al., 1984; Barnes and Crombie, 1985). There is also some evidence that SP latency is increased when target and background are present (Keller and Khan, 1986), presumably by making the visual context more complex and requiring object/background segregation. Could a single stationary distractor be operating in the same way as a structured background? If this were the case, then presenting the SP target and distractor against a structured background should have altered the distractor effect. Indeed, if the distractor acted as a background 'element' (perhaps along with other stationary objects in the subject's view like the edge of the stimulus monitor) then the presence of the larger, more salient background, would swamp any effects from the distractor itself. The addition of a (small) distractor should therefore no longer increase latency. The type of background used in the present experiments has been shown to be sufficient to alter SP gain (Worfolk and Barnes, 1992), and subjects reported that they were aware of the background moving in the opposite direction to the SP target during tracking. And we did observe small increases in latency across all conditions when the tasks were performed with the background. However, we also found that the pattern of effects observed with a distractor were essentially unaltered by the presence of a background; there were small and variable effects in non-gap conditions, and large increases in latency in gap conditions.

We also found that as distractor eccentricity increased, SP latency decreased; the longest latencies were observed when the distractor was closest to fixation. There were some differences between subjects in the effect of distractor eccentricity. In subject DN there was little sensitivity to eccentricity in non-gap conditions whereas in gap conditions there was a clear eccentricity effect. This meant that there was little evidence of a gap effect when the distractor was close to fixation, and a near normal latency advantage in gap conditions when the distractor appeared far from fixation. In subject GOM in both gap and non-gap conditions there was an eccentricity effect, but the gap-induced reduction in latency was all but abolished across all distractor eccentricities. In the analysis of the pooled data, these differences emerged as a significant difference between the slopes of gap and non-gap regression lines; the slope of the regression was significantly greater in gap conditions compared to non-gap conditions (Fig. 5E). Essentially, this finding implies that the magnitude of the gap effect (the difference in SP latency between gap and non-gap conditions) was dependent on distractor eccentricity. Thus the eccentricity results also suggest an interaction between gaps and distractors. They also suggest that a simple explanation for the eccentricity effect such as the cortical magnification factor, while probably playing some role, cannot be the whole story. There is no reason to suppose that there would then be any difference in the eccentricity relationship between gap and non-gap conditions.

The experiment in which we compared horizontal and vertical distractors demonstrated that the spatial position of the distractor was relatively unimportant. Subjects participating in experiments completed many trials and knew that the SP target always moved horizontally relative to the fixation target, although from trial to trial they did not know on which side of the fixation target the SP target would appear. It might be argued that the distractor exerted its effect because when presented along the target axis, it acted as a potential target forcing a target/distractor discrimination. Vertically located distractors, appeared outwith the target axis, and could not be confused with targets nor act as potential targets. They do have similar effects on SP latency. This supports the notion that distractors act not at a relatively high level, interfering with target selection, but at a relatively low level, on mechanisms distinct from motion processing.

Two types of mechanism have been invoked to explain alterations in oculomotor latencies produced by stimulus manipulations such as gaps and distractors, i.e. attentional and fixational. In attentional terms, the presence of a mirror image distractor in addition to the SP target would force the subject to monitor a larger portion of the visual world than when a target appeared alone. Limited attentional resources would thus be spread more thinly, increasing the time taken to detect target motion, leading to an increased SP latency. However, on this account a distractor near fixation would be expected to have less effect than a distractor far from fixation; SP latency would *increase* with distractor eccentricity. This contradicts the data we have presented. In fixational terms, it might be argued that the distractor, being a *stationary* object, would help to anchor fixation after the extinction of the nearby fixation target, thereby making the disengagement of fixation more difficult and therefore delaying the initiation of SP. This fixation effect would be strongest with the distractor near the current fixation position (i.e. near the position of the recently extinguished fixation target) and weakest when further away. SP latency would *decrease* with distractor eccentricity. This is consistent with our eccentricity data.

There is increasing evidence for the linkage of processes involved in saccades and SP. There are similar (though not identical) gap effects (Knox, 1996, 1998; Krauzlis and Miles, 1996b) and recent experiments have demonstrated saccade-linked enhancement of the motion signals used to drive SP (Gardner and Lisberger, 2001). It has been shown that distractors increase saccade latency, while having relatively little effect on saccade amplitude (Weber and Fischer, 1994). Moreover, this saccade distractor effect is also dependent on eccentricity; distractors near fixation have a larger effect than distractors far from fixation (Walker et al., 1997). One difference between the saccade and SP results is that whereas for saccades the eccentricity effect appears to be robust in both gap and non-gap conditions, for SP there is an enhancement of the effect of distractor eccentricity in gap conditions. One of the interesting features of the distractor effect on saccades is that it has a spatial structure. Distractors presented in the contralateral hemifield and in most of the ipsilateral hemifield relative to the target, modify saccade latency but do not affect saccade amplitude. However, distractors presented in the ipsilateral hemifield, within approximately 20° of the target axis do not affect saccade latency, but modify saccade amplitude. The results we have presented here (particularly the eccentricity results and the comparison of the effects of horizontal and vertical distractors) are broadly similar. We have presented preliminary spatial mapping evidence elsewhere that the distractor effect on SP initiation has a spatial structure that matches the saccade spatial structure closely (Bekkour and Knox, 2001). This similarity suggests once again a close relationship between the initiation of saccades and SP and perhaps the same underlying mechanisms.

So we have shown that a number of non-target stimulus manipulations modify the initiation of SP even when single target motion is relatively stereotyped. The two manipulations we have concentrated on here, temporal gaps and single stationary distractors, appear to operate through similar or linked mechanisms, perhaps related to fixation. These mechanisms are distinct from motion processing and are closely related to those involved in saccades. These findings, along with others showing that the pursuit system has at its disposal sophisticated velocity sampling and storage capabilities (Barnes et al., 2000, Chapter 16) and links between pursuit and perception (e.g. Beutter and Stone, 1998), suggest a sophisticated system that operates as much more than a motion reflex.

Acknowledgements

This work was supported by funding from the Wellcome Trust, the Royal Society and the Pace Fund.

References

Barnes, G.R. and Crombie, J.W. (1985) The interaction of conflicting retinal motion stimuli in oculomotor control. *Exp. Brain Res.*, 59: 548–558.
Barnes, G.R., Barnes, D.M. and Chakraborti, S.R. (2000) Ocular pursuit responses to repeated, single-cycle sinusoids reveal behaviour compatible with predictive pursuit. *J. Neurophysiol.*, 84: 2340–2355.
Bekkour, T. and Knox, P.C. (2001) Spatial mapping of distractor effect on smooth pursuit initiation. *Soc. Neurosci. Abstr.*, 784.9.
Beutter, B.R. and Stone, L.S. (1998) Human motion perception and smooth eye movements show similar directional biases for elongated apertures. *Vision Res.*, 38: 1273–1286.
Collewijn, H. and Tamminga, E. (1984) Human smooth and saccadic eye movements during voluntary pursuit of different target motions on different backgrounds. *J. Physiol.*, 351: 217–250.
Ferrera, V.P. and Lisberger, S.G. (1995) Attention and target selection for smooth pursuit eye movements. *J. Neurosci.*, 15: 7472–7484.
Ferrera, V.P. and Lisberger, S.G. (1997) The effect of a moving distractor on the initiation of smooth pursuit eye movements. *Vis. Neurosci.*, 14: 323–338.
Fischer, B. and Weber, H. (1993) Express saccades and visual attention. *Behav. Brain Sci.*, 16: 553–610.
Gandhi, N.J. and Keller, E.L. (1999) Comparison of saccades perturbed by stimulation of the rostral superior colliculus, the caudal superior colliculus and the omnipause neuron region. *J. Neurophysiol.*, 82: 3236–3253.

Gardner, J.L. and Lisberger, S.G. (2001) Linked target selection for saccadic and smooth pursuit eye movements. *J. Neurosci.*, 21: 2075–2084.

Goldreich, D., Krauzlis, R.J. and Lisberger, S.G. (1992) Effects of changing feedback delay on spontaneous oscillations in smooth pursuit eye movements of monkeys. *J. Neurophysiol.*, 67: 625–638.

Keller, E.L. and Khan, N.S. (1986) Smooth-pursuit initiation in the presence of a textured background in monkey. *Vision Res.*, 26: 943–955.

Knox, P.C. (1996) The effect of the gap paradigm on the latency of human smooth pursuit eye movement. *Neuroreport*, 7: 3027–3030.

Knox, P.C. (1998) Stimulus predictability and the gap effect on pre-saccadic smooth pursuit. *Neuroreport*, 9: 809–812.

Kowler, E. (1989) Cognitive expectations not habits control anticipatory smooth ocular pursuit. *Vision Res.*, 29: 1049–1057.

Kowler, E. and Steinman, R.M. (1981) The effect of expectations on slow oculomotor control. III. Guessing unpredictable target displacements. *Vision Res.*, 21: 191–203.

Kowler, E., van der Steen, J., Tamminga, E.P. and Collewijn, H. (1984) Voluntary selection of the target for smooth eye movement in the presence of superimposed full-field stationary and moving stimuli. *Vision Res.*, 24: 1789–1798.

Krauzlis, R.J. and Miles, F.A. (1996a) Decreases in the latency of smooth pursuit and saccadic eye movements produced by 'gap paradigm' in the monkey. *Vision Res.*, 36: 1973–1985.

Krauzlis, R.J. and Miles, F.A. (1996b) Release of fixation for pursuit and saccades in humans: evidence for shared inputs acting on different neural substrates. *J. Neurophysiol.*, 76: 2822–2833.

Krauzlis, R.J. and Stone, L.S. (1999) Tracking with the mind's eye. *TINS*, 22: 544–550.

Krauzlis, R.J., Zivotofsky, A.Z. and Miles, F.A. (1999) Target selection for pursuit and saccadic eye movements in humans. *J. Cogn. Neurosci.*, 11: 641–649.

Krauzlis, R.J., Basso, M.A. and Wurtz, R.H. (2000) Discharge properties of neurons in the rostral superior colliculus of the monkey during smooth pursuit eye movement. *J. Neurophysiol.*, 84: 876–891.

Lisberger, S. and Ferrera, V.P. (1997) Vector averaging for smooth pursuit eye movement initiated by two moving targets in monkeys. *J. Neurosci.*, 17: 7490–7502.

Lisberger, S. and Pavelko, T. (1989) Topographic and directional organization of visual motion inputs for the initiation of horizontal and vertical smooth-pursuit eye movements in monkeys. *J. Neurophysiol.*, 61: 173–185.

Lisberger, S.G. and Westbrook, L.E. (1985) Properties of visual inputs that initiate horizontal smooth pursuit eye movements in monkeys. *J. Neurosci.*, 5: 1662–1673.

Lisberger, S., Morris, E. and Tychsen, L. (1987) Visual motion processing and sensory–motor integration for smooth pursuit eye movements. *Annu. Rev. Neurosci.*, 10: 97–129.

Luebke, A.E. and Robinson, D.A. (1988) Transition dynamics between pursuit and fixation suggest different systems. *Vision Res.*, 28: 941–946.

Maunsell, J.H.R. and van Essen, D.C. (1983) Functional properties of neurons in middle temporal visual area of the macaque monkey I. Selectivity for stimulus direction, speed and orientation. *J. Neurophysiol.*, 49: 1127–1147.

Morrow, M.J. and Lamb, N.L. (1996) Effects of fixation target timing on smooth-pursuit initiation. *Exp. Brain Res.*, 111: 262–270.

Munoz, D.P. and Wurtz, R.H. (1992) Role of the rostral superior colliculus in active visual fixation and execution of express saccades. *J. Neurophysiol.*, 67: 1000–1002.

Munoz, D.P. and Wurtz, R.H. (1993) Fixation cells in monkey superior colliculus. I. Characteristics of cell discharge. *J. Neurophysiol.*, 70: 559–575.

Munoz, D.P., Waitzman, D.M. and Wurtz, R.H. (1996) Activity of neurons in monkey superior colliculus during interrupted saccades. *J. Neurophysiol.*, 75: 2562–2580.

O'Mullane, G. and Knox, P.C. (1999) Modification of smooth pursuit initiation by target contrast. *Vision Res.*, 39: 3459–3464.

Petit, L., Dubois, S., Tzourio, N., Dejardin, S., Crivello, F., Michel, C., Etard, O., Denise, P., Roucoux, A. and Mazoyer, B. (1999) PET study of the human foveal fixation system. *Hum. Brain Map.*, 8: 28–43.

Raymond, J.E., O'Donnell, H.L. and Tipper, S.P. (1998) Priming reveals attentional modulation of human motion sensitivity. *Vision Res.*, 38: 2863–2867.

Steinbach, M.J. (1976) Pursuing the perceptual rather than the visual stimulus. *Vision Res.*, 16: 1371–1376.

Stone, L.S., Beutter, B.R. and Lorenceau, J. (2000) Visual motion integration for perception and pursuit. *Perception*, 29: 771–787.

Treue, S. and Maunsell, J.H.R. (1996) Attentional modulation of visual motion processing in cortical areas MT and MST. *Nature*, 382: 539–541.

Walker, R., Deubel, H., Schneider, W.X. and Findlay, J.M. (1997) Effect of remote distractors on saccade programming: evidence for an extended fixation zone. *J. Neurophysiol.*, 78: 1108–1119.

Weber, H. and Fischer, B. (1994) Differential effects of non-target stimuli on the occurrence of express saccades in man. *Vision Res.*, 34: 1883–1891.

Worfolk, R. and Barnes, G. (1992) Interaction of active and passive slow eye movement systems. *Exp. Brain Res.*, 90: 589–598.

CHAPTER 15

Integration of motion cues for the initiation of smooth pursuit eye movements

Richard T. Born *, Christopher C. Pack and Ruilin Zhao

Department of Neurobiology, Harvard Medical School, 220 Longwood Avenue, Boston, MA 02115-5701, USA

Abstract: To clearly see a moving object, an observer must rotate his or her eyes with a velocity that matches that of the object. Such rotations are called smooth pursuit eye movements, and they depend critically on the ability of the primate brain to integrate information about object velocity from various local motion signals. When the local motion signals are in conflict, it is possible to use smooth pursuit eye movements as a continuous read-out of the motion integration process. This review discusses the results of recent behavioral experiments that have taken this approach, along with relevant neurophysiological and computational studies.

Introduction

Smooth pursuit is an important oculomotor behavior that allows a moving object to be held relatively stationary on the fovea so that it may be analyzed with high spatial acuity; see Eckmiller and Bauswein (1986), Lisberger et al. (1987), Keller and Heinen (1991) and Ilg (1997) for general reviews of smooth pursuit eye movements. The neural system that accomplishes this feat has been widely studied by both physiologists and psychologists because of the ease and precision with which its outputs (i.e. eye movements) can be measured, the ready manipulability of the inputs (i.e. visual stimuli), and, most significantly for this review, because of its intimate connection with visual motion processing. Because of this last fact, the behavior can serve as a convenient read-out of the algorithms at work on the sensory side. However, because the steady-state behavior of any closed-loop system, such as pursuit, is dominated by the very presence of negative feedback (Carpenter, 1988), it has mainly been the *initiation* of pursuit (or other 'open-loop' conditions) that has served this purpose.

The visual stimulus that drives the initiation of pursuit is target *motion* on the retina, or retinal slip (Rashbass, 1961). Such motion generates a number of visual 'error signals', including position, velocity and acceleration errors, all of which are involved in both the initiation and maintenance of the behavior, though retinal velocity error is the most important (Lisberger and Westbrook, 1985; Morris and Lisberger, 1987). Traditionally, these basic properties of pursuit have been studied in the laboratory by measuring the movements of the eyes in response to a single moving target, usually a small spot, presented against a dark, featureless background.

In the real world, however, the situation is more complicated. Often there are multiple possible targets present simultaneously, any given target may have an irregular shape — thus generating ambiguous and conflicting local motion signals — and target and eye motion usually occur against a richly textured background. All of these features present interesting problems that must be solved at the sensory end before useful motor signals can be generated.

---

* Correspondence to: R.T. Born, Department of Neurobiology, Harvard Medical School, 220 Longwood Avenue, Boston, MA 02115-5701, USA. Tel.: +1-617-432-1307; Fax: +1-617-734-7557; E-mail: rborn@hms.harvard.edu

How does the brain combine numerous local motion measurements to produce a veridical global direction of object motion that can be tracked by the eyes? Our review will focus on this question and what studies of pursuit eye movements have contributed to its answer.

Most of the results to be discussed below have been obtained in both monkeys (usually rhesus macaques) and humans. The chief advantage of the human preparation is that it allows one to compare, directly and relatively easily, the relationship between the *perception* of visual motion and a visually guided *behavior* that depends upon an internal representation of visual motion (Kowler and McKee, 1987; Watamaniuk and Heinen, 1999). While this has been an interesting and fruitful approach, for present purposes we will leave aside the question of whether these two brain 'functions' — perception and movement — make use of exactly the same representations or not. Suffice it to say that there appears to be a broad degree of overlap (Watamaniuk and Heinen, 1999; Beutter and Stone, 2000) but that the particular exigencies of each function would naturally lead to some differences depending on precisely how they are measured and compared; e.g. Mack et al. (1979).

Experiments in non-human primates, on the other hand, have the advantage of permitting comparisons between neuronal signals in motion processing regions of monkey visual cortex (most prominently, the middle temporal, MT, and the middle superior temporal, MST, visual areas, but in other parietal and frontal areas as well; see Keller and Heinen, 1991 for an overview) and the eye movements evoked by the same or similar stimuli. Virtually all studies of this nature have pointed to a very tight link between the neuronal properties in these two areas and the initiation of both smooth pursuit (Newsome et al., 1985; Dursteler and Wurtz, 1988; Komatsu and Wurtz, 1988, 1989; Movshon et al., 1990; Bremmer et al., 1997; Ferrera and Lisberger, 1997b; Groh et al., 1997; Lisberger and Movshon, 1999; Recanzone and Wurtz, 1999, 2000; Born et al., 2000; Pack and Born, 2001) and ocular following (Kawano et al., 1994; Kawano, 1999). Because of this relationship, we will also include a brief discussion of the relevant neuronal data.

Combining motion vectors: multiple targets

As noted above, in the majority of pursuit experiments, only a single, simple target is present in the field of view at any given time. One way to examine motion integration is to introduce a second simple target and to ask how the system treats the two associated motion vectors. This approach has been taken by two different labs (Ferrera and Lisberger, 1995, 1997a; Lisberger and Ferrera, 1997; Recanzone and Wurtz, 1999, 2000) with largely consistent results. If the two targets are presented nearby in both space and time and the animal has no prior knowledge to indicate which of the two targets is to be pursued, the read-out is a simple *vector average* of the two motion vectors (Ferrera and Lisberger, 1997a). If, however, the animal is supplied with prior knowledge concerning which target is to be pursued, it can use attention to suppress the motion vector from the irrelevant target (the 'distracter') thus producing a *winner-take-all* pursuit response (Ferrera and Lisberger, 1995).

Even with prior knowledge that ultimately allows for target selection, it appears that the earliest pursuit response is one of vector-averaging and that effects of attention appear only after some time (Recanzone and Wurtz, 1999). This was discovered by studying pursuit initiation (and the responses of neurons in MT and MST) during a task that required a monkey to track one of two possible visual stimuli: a 'target' and a 'distracter'. The animal had to identify which stimulus was the appropriate target (based on its shape) and then follow it. When both the target and the distracter moved simultaneously within the same region of retinal space (which was within the receptive field of the neuron under study), the authors were able to examine how these two visual motion signals were combined, both by the pursuit system, as indicated by the eye movements made by the monkey, and by the neurons. Interestingly, both measurements revealed that a vector average was used to combine the two signals when the two stimuli appeared within the receptive field for only a short time (a 'gap' of 150 ms) before the animal was instructed to make the eye movement (Fig. 1A). If the two stimuli appeared further apart and for a longer time (450 ms) before the animal was cued to make the eye movement, both the neurons and the pursuit 'behaved' as if the appropriate target was the

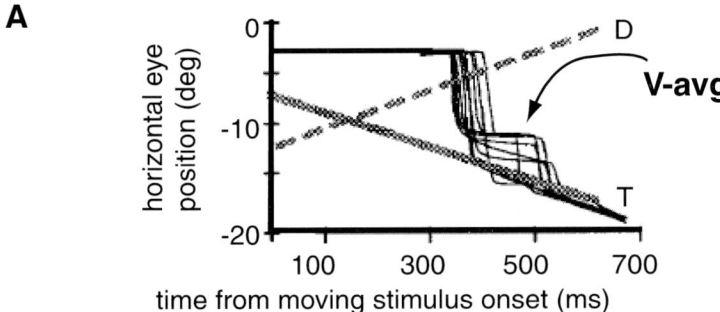

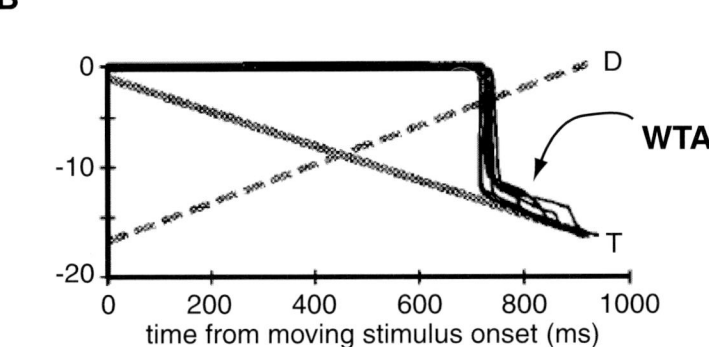

Fig. 1. Combining velocity vectors from two objects. (A) When a pursuit target (T) and a distracter (D) appear near each other in space and time, the resulting pursuit eye movement is a vector average (V-avg) of the two velocity vectors. (B) When the two objects appear well in advance of the cue to track and are separated by a greater distance, the distracter is effectively ignored and the pursuit shows a 'winter-take-all' (WTA) integration strategy, with the target winning. Modified from fig. 2 of Recanzone and Wurtz (1999).

only stimulus present (i.e. a winner-take-all method of combining the motion signals from the target and the distracter, with the target winning; Fig. 1B). It was as if, quite sensibly, the extra time had allowed the system to distinguish target from distracter and then suppress the response to the distracter's motion.

Very similar results were obtained when the two motion vectors were produced by a single visual target and a second 'virtual' target introduced by microstimulating direction columns in MT (Groh et al., 1997; Born et al., 2000; Fig. 2). In these experiments, the animal was required to pursue a single moving target that appeared within the receptive field of a given column of MT neurons. On half of the trials, the neurons at the site were activated for approximately 200 ms beginning at the onset of target motion. The interactions between the microstimulation and multiple different target velocities were studied at each site. Under these conditions, most comparable to those used by Lisberger and Ferrera in their 1997 paper and to the short-gap condition of Recanzone and Wurtz (1999), the pursuit response again proved to be a weighted average of the target velocity vector and an 'electrical' velocity vector introduced by the microstimulation. This computation appears to be quite widespread and robust, as the vector-averaging model best describes a large number of microstimulation experiments at different sites in MT (Groh et al., 1997; Born et al., 2000) and using a wide range of current amplitudes and

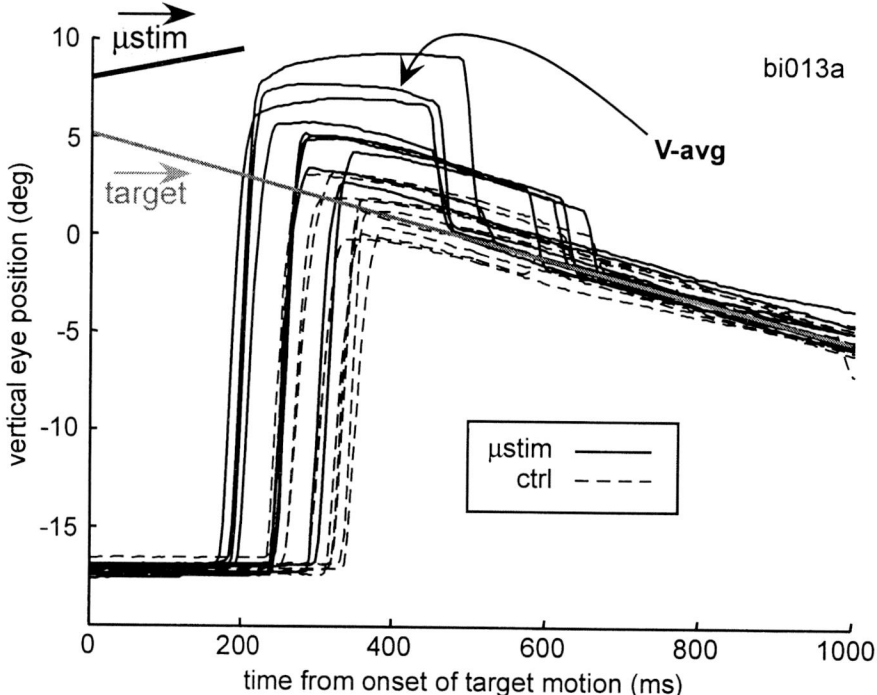

Fig. 2. Combining velocity vectors due to target motion and microstimulation of MT. On all trials the animal was required to track a small spot moving downwards at 10°/s. The resulting pursuit eye movement is a vector average (V-avg) of the two velocity vectors. In this case the 'electrical' vector introduced by microstimulation (biphasic current pulses of 40 μA at 200 Hz for ~200 ms) was upwards at approximately 8°/s. This vector was determined by a multivariate regression analysis of the interaction of microstimulation with 9 different target velocities ($p < 0.00001$), all of which were randomly interleaved with the trials shown.

pulse frequencies (R. Zhao and R.T. Born, unpubl. observations).

Additional support for vector-averaging comes from measurements of human pursuit initiation in response to random-dot cinematograms, i.e. large fields (10°) containing many (250) moving dots, each of whose direction was randomly chosen from a distribution of possible directions (Heinen and Watamaniuk, 1998; Watamaniuk and Heinen, 1999). For this type of stimulus no single dot provides consistent or veridical motion information, yet human observers are able to integrate over space and time and perceive smooth motion in the direction that corresponds to the *average* of the distribution (Williams and Sekuler, 1984). When humans are asked to track the motion in such displays with their eyes, they similarly pursue the statistical mean with great accuracy, exceeding that to a single target moving at the same velocity (Heinen and Watamaniuk, 1998; Watamaniuk and Heinen, 1999).

Combining motion vectors: complex shapes

Another approach to the problem of motion integration for pursuit eye movements is to use visual stimuli whose shape generates local motion vectors that differ from the velocity of the object ('global' motion). The reason that this generates an interesting problem for the pursuit system is that all of the available visual information is from neurons, such as retinal ganglion cells, with very small and discrete receptive fields. Thus the object's contours are effectively seen through many tiny apertures which make explicit only the component of motion perpendicular to the contour (Fig. 3). This 'aperture problem' must be solved by taking into account the motion of object features, called terminators, whose local motion is unambiguous. Furthermore, this information must be integrated in a way that ultimately allows terminator-based motion signals to prevail.

Inspired by the work of Lorençeau and colleagues

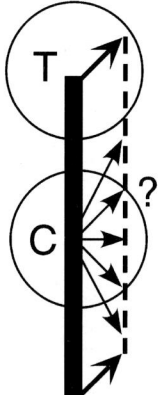

Fig. 3. Receptive field 'apertures' create ambiguous local motion signals. For a vertical bar moving upwards and to the right, a neuron with a small receptive field positioned along the contour (C) can measure only the rightward component of motion. This measurement is ambiguous, because it is consistent with many possible directions of actual bar motion. Only neurons whose receptive fields are positioned over the bar's terminators (T) can measure the direction of motion accurately.

(Lorençeau et al., 1993), who originally used such stimuli to study motion perception, a number of labs have recently used complex shapes to elicit both short-latency ocular following in humans (Masson et al., 2000) and smooth pursuit eye movements in monkeys (Pack and Born, 2001) and humans (Masson and Stone, 2000). The basic findings were similar in all cases: the initial direction of the pursuit (or ocular following) was strongly biased by the orientation of the contour, and the resulting eye movement looked like a weighted average of both terminator- and contour-based signals. Over time, the behavior evolved to follow the true direction of object motion, a situation that can be thought of as a winner-take-all computation, with the terminator motion winning.

A specific example of this 'contour effect' is shown in Fig. 4. In this case a macaque monkey, after a brief fixation period, was required to track the center of a moving bar that appeared at the fovea and could then move off in one of four different directions at a speed of 10°/s. The moving bar could assume one of three different orientations with respect to its direction of motion: perpendicular or tilted either backwards or forwards by 45°. For each different direction of target motion the eye movement data are represented as the component *parallel* to the direction of bar motion (Fig. 4, upper panel)

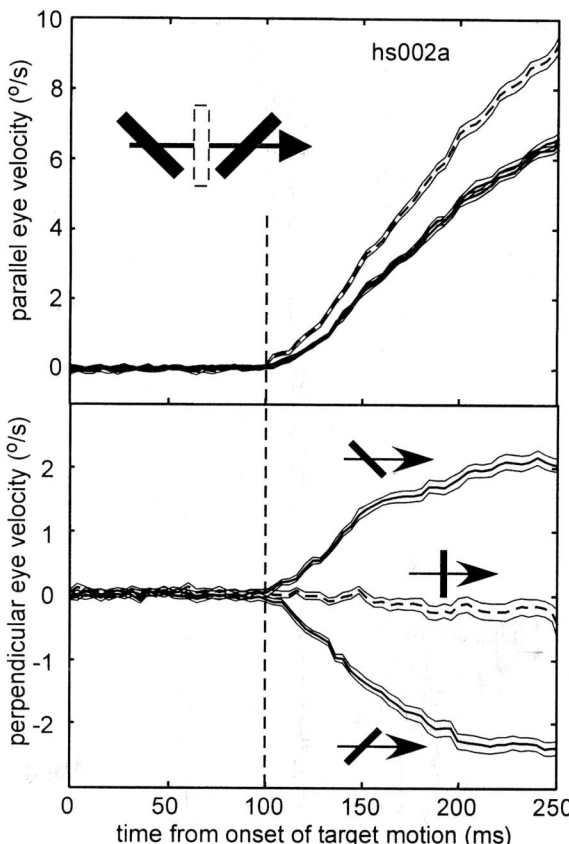

Fig. 4. Effect of contour orientation on the initiation of smooth pursuit. The animal was required to track the center of a long (25°) bar moving in one of four possible directions at 10°/s. When the bar's orientation was perpendicular to its direction of motion (dashed lines), pursuit was purely in the direction of bar motion with no perpendicular component. When the bar was tilted (solid lines), the initial pursuit eye movement deviated in a direction perpendicular to the orientation of the contour. Each thick line represents the mean; thin lines represent ±1 standard error of the mean.

and the component *perpendicular* to the direction of bar motion (Fig. 4, lower panel), thus allowing data from different directions of bar motion to be combined. (There was no systematic effect of target direction on the contour effect.) For simplicity, one can think of the data *as if* the direction of motion on all trials were purely rightward, so that any vertical eye movements represent a deviation from the true direction of target motion. Thus when the bar's orientation was vertical (control, dashed lines), the pursuit was only to the right with no vertical component as would be expected for any other simple moving target. If, however, the horizontally moving bar was tilted (solid lines), the initial pursuit deviated in a direction perpendicular to the contour orientation. This deviation is present in the very earliest phase of pursuit initiation (vertical dotted line), and it persists for approximately 150 ms, depending on a number of factors such as bar length (see below), speed and contrast. One additional point worth noting is that the initial *horizontal* pursuit is slower for the tilted bars than for the vertical bars and by exactly the amount predicted by the stimulus geometry and the aperture problem; i.e. the two curves superimpose if the vertical bar-pursuit values are multiplied by cosine (45°). This fact was not illustrated in our original publication (see fig. 3b of Pack and Born, 2001) due to the use of a small subset of eye movement trials from a single monkey.

If the initial response is simply a weighted average of contour- and terminator-related motion signals, then stimulus manipulations that change the relative amounts of the two signal types should produce predictable changes in the behavior. This has proven to be the case. For example, Masson et al. (2000) reduced the relative strength of the terminator signals by blurring the line endings and found a corresponding decrease in the amplitude of the terminator-driven component of ocular following. Conversely, Pack and Born, 2001 (Fig. 5) found that increasing the relative proportion of contour signals, by using longer bars, created a progressively larger contour-orientation bias in pursuit initiation. This latter experiment revealed that the pursuit system is capable of rapidly integrating along contours over very large regions of the visual field, extending to at least 35 degrees. This last result is also consistent with the aforementioned studies of human pursuit of random-dot cinematograms (Heinen and Watamaniuk, 1998), in which increasing the size of the dot field led to increases in the initial eye acceleration and decreases in pursuit latency.

In keeping with the close relationship between open-loop pursuit and signaling within visual motion cortex, Pack and Born (2001) found a neural correlate of this behavior in MT of the alert monkey. The earliest directional responses, beginning about 80 ms after the onset of stimulus motion, primarily encoded the component of motion *perpendicular* to

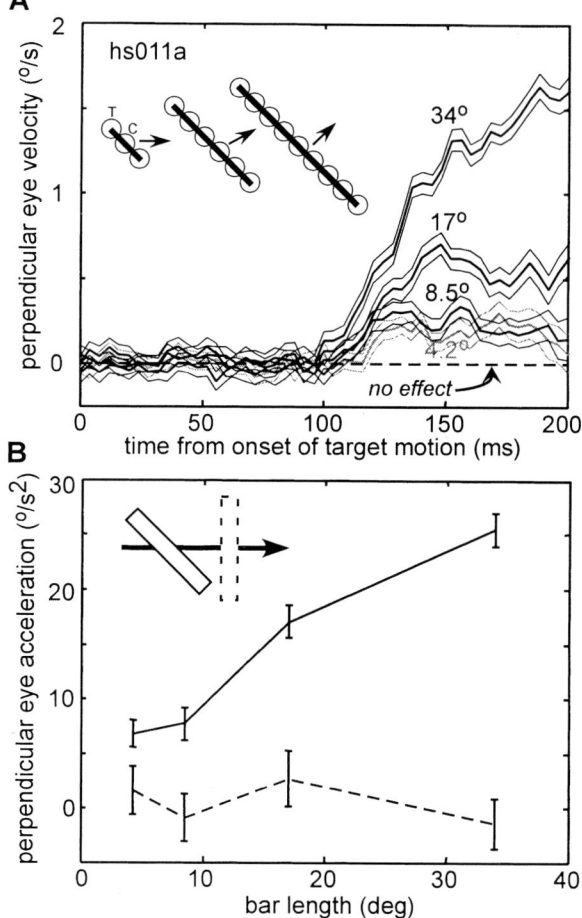

Fig. 5. Effect of bar length on the contour effect. (A) In this experiment, bars of different lengths and different relative orientations were randomly interleaved. For simplicity, only the component of the eye movement *perpendicular* to the direction of bar motion is plotted. Thus the control trials (bar moving perpendicularly with respect to its axis of orientation) show no velocity component in this direction (dotted line in A). The length of the bar has no effect on the latency of pursuit initiation, but has a clear effect on the initial slope (i.e. acceleration). Traces represent mean eye velocity ± the standard error of the mean. (B) The initial (0–40 ms) deviation in the eye acceleration is plotted as a function of bar length for both tilted bars (solid line; the 45° and 135° tilt data have been pooled) and for bars moving perpendicular to their axis of orientation (dashed line). Acceleration was calculated as the slope of a regression line fit to the first 40 ms of pursuit for each single trial. Error bars represent the standard error of the mean of the single-trial slope values.

the orientation of the contour (Fig. 6A). That is, they were strongly affected by the ambiguous contour signals. However, the later responses (>140 ms after

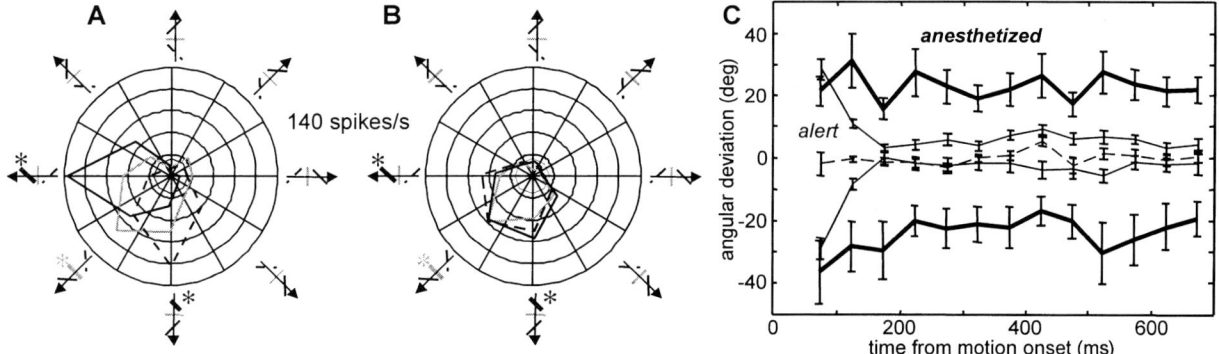

Fig. 6. MT and the aperture problem. (A) Over the first 20 ms of the directional response (65–85 ms after the onset of stimulus motion), the direction tuning reflects the component of motion perpendicular to the contour's orientation (*), whereas later responses, >140 ms after onset of target motion (B) are similar regardless of the orientation of the moving bars. (C) The population of MT neurons in the alert monkey ($n = 60$) converges to an orientation-invariant representation over about 60 ms; neurons recorded in the anesthetized animals never converge, even though their responses are equally vigorous and direction-selective. Modified from fig. 2 of Pack and Born (2001). Anesthesia data are from Pack et al. (2001).

motion onset) encoded the true direction of motion, regardless of contour orientation (Fig. 6B). Thus the responses of MT neurons reflect a similar solution of the aperture problem for motion over a period of about 60 ms. While this time-course is considerably faster than that found for pursuit, the bar-fields used to characterize the neurons contained many individual bars that were considerably shorter (3°) than the single bar used in the pursuit experiments, thus presenting a greater proportion of terminator signal. Indeed, preliminary data from our lab indicate that increasing the length of the bars prolongs the neural solution in the same way that it affects pursuit behavior (Fig. 5).

Interestingly, the same MT neurons, when studied in animals lightly *anesthetized* with isoflurane, completely failed to solve the aperture problem, even though they remained vigorously responsive and sharply tuned for direction of motion (Pack et al., 2001; Fig. 6C). Some have argued, based on contextual effects measured in primate V1 (Lamme et al., 1998a,b), that neural processes evolving over tens of milliseconds and highly susceptible to general anesthetics indicate a role for *feedback* from higher cortical areas. In the case of the neural and pursuit effects described above, this would implicate higher motion-processing areas such as the medial superior temporal (MST) or lateral intraparietal (LIP) areas. Both of these areas contain at least some neurons that have large direction-selective receptive fields (Saito et al., 1986; Komatsu and Wurtz, 1988; Blatt et al., 1990) and both have feedback connections to MT (Felleman and Van Essen, 1991). If the feedback hypothesis is correct, it should be possible to selectively impair the integration process by inactivating one or both of the regions. A second possibility, however, is that general anesthesia has a selective effect on a parallel stage of processing for terminator motion (Wilson et al., 1992). The second visual area, V2, is a good candidate for this so-called 'indirect' route to MT and the pursuit system with tantalizing, though inconclusive, findings regarding physiology (Levitt et al., 1994a; Mareschal and Baker, 1998), anatomy (Maunsell and Van Essen, 1983; DeYoe and Van Essen, 1985; Shipp and Zeki, 1989; Levitt et al., 1994b; Yabuta et al., 2001; see Born, 2001 for an overview) and function (Merigan et al., 1993). This hypothesis, too, should be testable with the appropriate inactivation experiments. Having both a robust neural and a behavioral correlate of this phenomenon should facilitate studies of its mechanism.

Combining motion vectors: complex motion

Yet another way to analyze motion integration for pursuit is to study initiation in response to more complicated moving stimuli, such as those combining 1st and 2nd order motion cues (Lindner and Ilg, 2000;

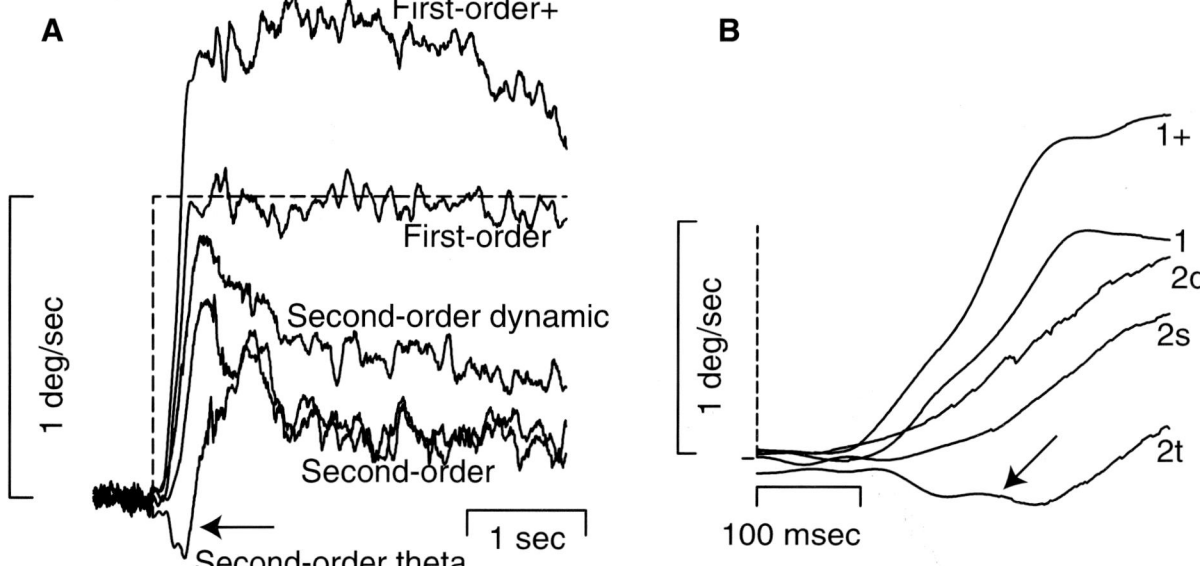

Fig. 7. Human pursuit initiation to targets defined by 1st or 2nd order motion stimuli. The gain of the initial phase of pursuit (B) is greatest for 1st order motion (1) and diminished for different varieties of 2nd order motion (2d, 2nd order dynamic; 2s, 2nd order static; 2t, 2nd order theta). Dashed lines show the target velocity profile. Note that for 2nd order theta motion, for which 1st and 2nd order motion directions are opposed, the initial eye movement is in the 'wrong' (1st order) direction (arrows). Adapted from fig. 5 of Hawken and Gegenfurtner (2001).

Hawken and Gegenfurtner, 2001). In these experiments, visual stimuli consisting of either 1st order motion (spatiotemporal changes in luminance) or 2nd order motion (spatiotemporal changes in, for example, texture or motion; see Chubb and Sperling, 1988; Cavanagh and Mather, 1989), or a combination of the two were used to create pursuit targets for human subjects. In both of these studies, pursuit initiation was better (i.e. higher gain) to 1st order than to 2nd order stimuli, though this difference was less marked at faster target speeds (Hawken and Gegenfurtner, 2001; Fig. 7). When the two types of motion were combined, 1st order motion dominated the earliest pursuit responses even though subjects were instructed to track the 'object' (i.e. 2nd order) motion, in some cases resulting in an initial eye movement in the wrong (1st order) direction (arrows in Fig. 7).

More recently, a similar approach has been used to study short-latency ocular following in humans (Masson and Castet, 2002). In this case the authors used 'uni-kinetic' plaids consisting of a drifting grating superimposed on a stationary grating tilted 45° with respect to the moving grating. This stimulus has the very useful property of producing conflicting motion signals: '1D' or contour motion signals in one direction (e.g. upwards in Fig. 8) and '2D' or pattern motion signals at a 45° angle (upwards and rightwards in Fig. 8). With these stimuli Masson and Castet (2002) observed that the earliest responses were completely dominated by the 1D direction, but, after a delay of about 25 ms, the eye movement direction deviated to reflect the influence of the pattern direction signals. Not only did they observe a clear latency difference for the 1D- versus 2D-related ocular responses, but they also found that the contrast response functions (CRFs) for the two components were completely different. The 1D CRF was steep and saturated at low contrast, similar to the contrast sensitivity function for magnocellular neurons in the lateral geniculate body (Derrington and Lennie, 1984), while that for the 2D response was much shallower and non-saturating, similar to the corresponding function for parvocellular neu-

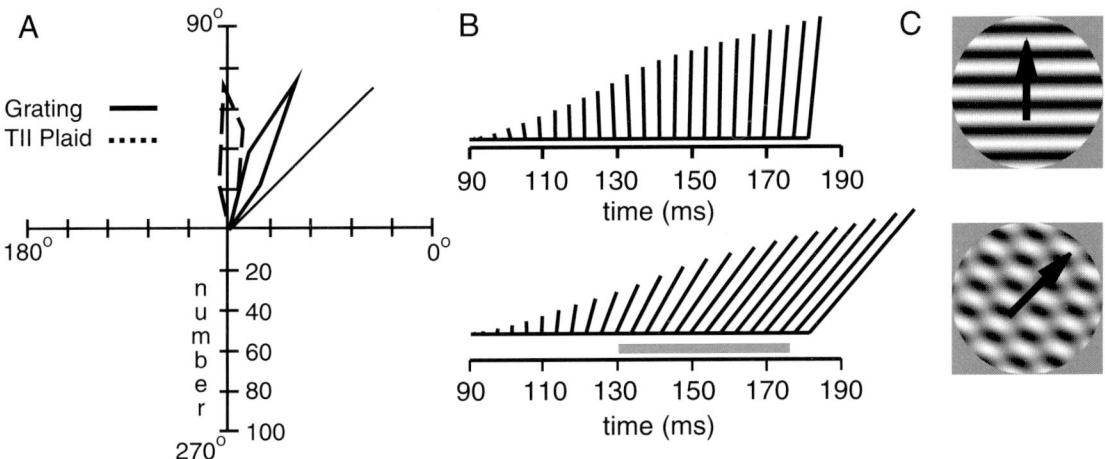

Fig. 8. Ocular following of 'uni-kinetic' plaids. The direction of the initial response is dominated by the 1D component (identical with that to a single grating drifting upwards, black arrow) but subsequently deviates towards the pattern (2D) direction, which contains a rightward component. (A) Polar histogram of the tracking directions (averaged over the time period indicated by the gray bar in B for either a single grating moving upwards or a plaid pattern moving upward and rightward. The solid line indicates the true direction of pattern motion (45°). (B) Instantaneous mean velocity vectors to the same two stimulus types (grating, top; uni-kinetic plaid, bottom). (C) Examples of the visual stimuli used in the experiments: grating (top) and uni-kinetic plaids (bottom). Modified from fig. 9 of Masson and Castet (2002).

rons. Taken together, these results constitute the best evidence to date for parallel motion channels driving smooth eye movements, and they mesh nicely with certain computational models of higher-order motion integration.

Models and the neural substrate

Because pursuit initiation is an open-loop behavior, it is convenient to analyze it as a succession of processing stages. Conceptually, pursuit initiation can be subdivided into three computational stages. The first stage represents local motion vectors of the kind that might be generated by a moving object. As shown in Fig. 3, these local motion vectors are not necessarily aligned with the direction of object motion. The second stage integrates the local motion signals into a global representation of object motion, and the third stage uses the global velocity signals to drive the eye velocity. For the most part, models of motion integration focus on the computations underlying stages one and two (Wilson and Kim, 1994; Simoncelli and Heeger, 1998; Lidén and Pack, 1999), while models of pursuit initiation are largely concerned with stages two and three (Robinson et al., 1986; Krauzlis and Lisberger, 1994). Because the second stage constitutes the output of motion integration and the input to pursuit initiation, it is of great theoretical interest in understanding the experimental findings discussed in this review.

Anatomically, the second stage is associated with MT in all of the models mentioned above. Indeed, there is compelling evidence that the responses of MT neurons are directly related to pursuit initiation (Newsome et al., 1985; Movshon et al., 1990; Groh et al., 1997) and motion integration (Movshon et al., 1986; Albright, 1991; Pack and Born, 2001). A controversial question concerns the nature of the computation by which MT neurons convert local motion signals into global representations of object motion. Recent physiological work has examined MT responses to a variety of motion stimuli, so it is now possible to place strong constraints on biological models of motion integration.

At a minimum, models of MT neurons must perform motion integration. A substantial proportion of the MT population in the alert animal responds to the global direction of object motion, rather than the local motion signals (Pack and Born, 2001; Pack et al., 2001). Furthermore, the motion integration process is not instantaneous: the early responses reflect the local motion signals, and the integrated motion signal is apparent only after 60–100 ms (Fig. 6). Given that the eye movement behavior exhibits a similar transition (Fig. 4), this property is crucial to any model of motion integration. Additionally, a motion integration system requires some type of segmentation system to prevent it from integrating motion signals from separate objects or from the background. The experiments of Recanzone and Wurtz (1999) have shown that MT neurons do indeed possess this property, and that it is at least partially under cognitive control. Similarly, other experiments (Duncan et al., 2000) suggest that MT neurons can switch between integration and segmentation depending on the surface layout of the stimulus. Finally, many MT neurons encode the direction of 2nd order motion (Albright, 1992; Churan and Ilg, 2001), consistent with the finding that 2nd order motion signals drive pursuit eye movements (Lindner and Ilg, 2000; Hawken and Gegenfurtner, 2001; Fig. 7). However, Churan and Ilg (2001) also showed that MT neurons do not respond to certain stimuli that drive pursuit eye movements, such as theta motion, indicating that MT is not the final or only integration stage in the pathway.

Existing models of motion integration cover a broad range of explanations, so it is useful to evaluate them in terms of the four properties outlined above: motion integration, temporal dynamics, motion segmentation, and response to 2nd order motion. Perhaps the simplest motion integration mechanism has been proposed by Simoncelli and Heeger (1998). Here motion integration is achieved by an appropriate feedforward weighting of local motion signals. The result is a vector representing the one velocity that is most consistent with the local motion signals (Adelson and Movshon, 1982). This approach can be expected to work very well for situations in which the pursuit target is a single moving object. However, this model lacks both temporal dynamics and a motion segmentation system, and does not respond to 2nd order motion, so it would need to be substantially extended to account for the pursuit eye movement phenomena described herein. A different feedforward approach, proposed by Nowlan and Sejnowski (1995), proposes that some MT cells integrate motion signals by according greater weight to parts of the stimulus that contain veridical motion information. This mechanism would measure the velocity at features such as endpoints, intersections, and corners, where the aperture problem shown in Fig. 3 does not apply. The same mechanism could be used to perform motion segmentation, but it is not clear how the model would generate temporal dynamics, or how it would respond to 2nd order motion. Another model that explicitly tracks object features was proposed by Lidén and Pack (1999). This model consists of separate motion integration and segmentation systems that are linked within MT by recurrent networks. The recurrent networks propagate motion signals across space, and in so doing provide a good qualitative fit to the temporal dynamics observed in MT (Pack and Born, 2001; Fig. 6C). This model has not been tested on 2nd order motion. The model of Wilson and Kim (1994) proposes an intermediate processing stage between V1 and MT that computes 2nd order motion. In model simulations, this additional route, identified with the second visual area (V2), adds a temporal delay and might account for that observed in MT. The model is also capable of motion integration and segmentation, and is therefore qualitatively capable of providing the four types of pursuit signals listed above. Finally, the model of Grossberg et al. (2001) accomplishes motion integration and segmentation, and simulates some of the phenomena that Wilson and Kim (1994) have attributed to the 2nd order pathway. This model relies on feedback connections to track image features in a manner similar to that of Lidén and Pack (1999) and with similar temporal dynamics. Each of the models predicts specific roles for the various visual areas in the primate brain, and each of these predictions is currently awaiting experimental validation.

Conclusions

A large number of experiments using a rich variety of visual stimuli have addressed the question of how the pursuit system integrates local motion cues into a veridical representation of object motion. The major consensus is that the earliest responses are not, in fact, veridical, but represent a quick-and-dirty vector-average that serves to get the eyes moving in approximately the right direction. This initial estimate is refined over time by taking into account higher-order properties of the stimulus, such as those attributable to terminators, or by limiting the pool of motion vectors averaged through, for example, selective attention. Although a wide variety of models offer solutions as to how this refinement might be accomplished, the specific physiological mechanisms at work remain unknown. Future experiments aimed at elucidating the mechanism of integration should focus on a functional dissection of the multiple anatomical pathways by which motion information reaches MT and other pursuit-related areas.

Acknowledgements

We thank Dr. Phillip Hendrickson for excellent technical assistance during the course of these experiments. This work was supported by NIH grants EY11379, EY12196 and RR00168 and a grant from the Whitehall Foundation.

References

Adelson, E.H. and Movshon, J.A. (1982) Phenomenal coherence of moving visual patterns. *Nature*, 300: 523–525.

Albright, T.D. (1991) Color and the integration of motion signals. *Trends Neurosci.*, 14: 266–269.

Albright, T.D. (1992) Form-cue invariant motion processing in primate visual cortex. *Science*, 255: 1141–1143.

Beutter, B.R. and Stone, L.S. (2000) Motion coherence affects human perception and pursuit similarly. *Vis. Neurosci.*, 17: 139–153.

Blatt, G.J., Andersen, R.A. and Stoner, G.R. (1990) Visual receptive field organization and cortico-cortical connections of the lateral intraparietal area (area LIP) in the macaque. *J. Comp. Neurol.*, 299: 421–445.

Born, R.T. (2001) Visual processing: parallel-er and parallel-er. *Curr. Biol.*, 11: R566–R568.

Born, R.T., Groh, J.M., Zhao, R. and Lukasewycz, S.J. (2000) Segregation of object and background motion in visual area MT: effects of microstimulation on eye movements. *Neuron*, 26: 725–734.

Bremmer, F., Ilg, U.J., Thiele, A., Distler, C. and Hoffmann, K.P. (1997) Eye position effects in monkey cortex. I. Visual and pursuit-related activity in extrastriate areas MT and MST. *J. Neurophysiol.*, 77: 944–961.

Carpenter, R.H.S. (1988) *Movements of the Eyes*. 2nd ed., Pion Ltd., London.

Cavanagh, P. and Mather, G. (1989) Motion: the long and short of it. *Spat. Vis.*, 4: 103–129.

Chubb, C. and Sperling, G. (1988) Drift-balanced random stimuli: a general basis for studying non-Fourier motion perception. *J. Opt. Soc. Am. A*, 5: 1986–2007.

Churan, J. and Ilg, U.J. (2001) Processing of second-order motion stimuli in primate middle temporal area and medial superior temporal area. *J. Opt. Soc. Am. A Opt. Image Sci. Vis.*, 18: 2297–2306.

Derrington, A.M. and Lennie, P. (1984) Spatial and temporal contrast sensitivities of neurones in lateral geniculate nucleus of macaque. *J. Physiol.*, 357: 219–240.

DeYoe, E.A. and Van Essen, D.C. (1985) Segregation of efferent connections and receptive field properties in visual area V2 of the macaque. *Nature*, 317: 58–61.

Duncan, R.O., Albright, T.D. and Stoner, G.R. (2000) Occlusion and the interpretation of visual motion: perceptual and neuronal effects of context. *J. Neurosci.*, 20: 5885–5897.

Dursteler, M.R. and Wurtz, R.H. (1988) Pursuit and optokinetic deficits following chemical lesions of cortical areas MT and MST. *J. Neurophysiol.*, 60: 940–965.

Eckmiller, R. and Bauswein, E. (1986) Smooth pursuit eye movements. *Prog. Brain Res.*, 64: 313–323.

Felleman, D.J. and Van Essen, D.C. (1991) Distributed hierarchical processing in the primate cerebral cortex. *Cereb. Cortex*, 1: 1–47.

Ferrera, V.P. and Lisberger, S.G. (1995) Attention and target selection for smooth pursuit eye movements. *J. Neurosci.*, 15: 7472–7484.

Ferrera, V.P. and Lisberger, S.G. (1997a) The effect of a moving distractor on the initiation of smooth-pursuit eye movements. *Vis. Neurosci.*, 14: 323–338.

Ferrera, V.P. and Lisberger, S.G. (1997b) Neuronal responses in visual areas MT and MST during smooth pursuit target selection. *J. Neurophysiol.*, 78: 1433–1446.

Groh, J.M., Born, R.T. and Newsome, W.T. (1997) How is a sensory map read out? Effects of microstimulation in visual area MT on saccades and smooth pursuit eye movements. *J. Neurosci.*, 17: 4312–4330.

Grossberg, S., Mingolla, E. and Viswanathan, L. (2001) Neural dynamics of motion integration and segmentation within and across apertures. *Vision Res.*, 41: 2521–2553.

Hawken, M.J. and Gegenfurtner, K.R. (2001) Pursuit eye movements to second-order motion targets. *J. Opt. Soc. Am. A Opt. Image Sci. Vis.*, 18: 2282–2296.

Heinen, S.J. and Watamaniuk, S.N. (1998) Spatial integration in human smooth pursuit. *Vision Res.*, 38: 3785–3794.

Ilg, U.J. (1997) Slow eye movements. *Prog. Neurobiol.*, 53: 293–329.

Kawano, K. (1999) Ocular tracking: behavior and neurophysiology. *Curr. Opin. Neurobiol.*, 9: 467–473.

Kawano, K., Shidara, M., Watanabe, Y. and Yamane, S. (1994) Neural activity in cortical area MST of alert monkey during ocular following responses. *J. Neurophysiol.*, 71: 2305–2324.

Keller, E.L. and Heinen, S.J. (1991) Generation of smooth-pursuit eye movements: neuronal mechanisms and pathways. *Neurosci. Res.*, 11: 79–107.

Komatsu, H. and Wurtz, R.H. (1988) Relation of cortical areas MT and MST to pursuit eye movements. I. Localization and visual properties of neurons. *J. Neurophysiol.*, 60: 580–603.

Komatsu, H. and Wurtz, R.H. (1989) Modulation of pursuit eye movements by stimulation of cortical areas MT and MST. *J. Neurophysiol.*, 62: 31–47.

Kowler, E. and McKee, S.P. (1987) Sensitivity of smooth eye movement to small differences in target velocity. *Vision Res.*, 27: 993–1015.

Krauzlis, R.J. and Lisberger, S.G. (1994) A model of visually guided smooth pursuit eye movements based on behavioral observations. *J. Comput. Neurosci.*, 1: 265–283.

Lamme, V.A., Super, H. and Spekreijse, H. (1998a) Feedforward, horizontal, and feedback processing in the visual cortex. *Curr. Opin. Neurobiol.*, 8: 529–535.

Lamme, V.A., Zipser, K. and Spekreijse, H. (1998b) Figure-ground activity in primary visual cortex is suppressed by anesthesia. *Proc. Natl. Acad. Sci. USA*, 95: 3263–3268.

Levitt, J.B., Kiper, D.C. and Movshon, J.A. (1994a) Receptive fields and functional architecture of macaque V2. *J. Neurophysiol.*, 71: 2517–2542.

Levitt, J.B., Yoshioka, T. and Lund, J.S. (1994b) Intrinsic cortical connections in macaque visual area V2: evidence for interaction between different functional streams. *J. Comp. Neurol.*, 342: 551–570.

Lidén, L. and Pack, C. (1999) The role of terminators and occlusion cues in motion integration and segmentation: a neural network model. *Vision Res.*, 39: 3301–3320.

Lindner, A. and Ilg, U.J. (2000) Initiation of smooth-pursuit eye movements to first-order and second-order motion stimuli. *Exp. Brain Res.*, 133: 450–456.

Lisberger, S.G. and Ferrera, V.P. (1997) Vector averaging for smooth pursuit eye movements initiated by two moving targets in monkeys. *J. Neurosci.*, 17: 7490–7502.

Lisberger, S.G. and Movshon, J.A. (1999) Visual motion analysis for pursuit eye movements in area MT of macaque monkeys. *J. Neurosci.*, 19: 2224–2246.

Lisberger, S.G. and Westbrook, L.E. (1985) Properties of visual inputs that initiate horizontal smooth pursuit eye movements in monkeys. *J. Neurosci.*, 5: 1662–1673.

Lisberger, S.G., Morris, E.J. and Tychsen, L. (1987) Visual motion processing and sensory–motor integration for smooth pursuit eye movements. *Annu. Rev. Neurosci.*, 10: 97–129.

Lorençeau, J., Shiffrar, M., Wells, N. and Castet, E. (1993) Different motion sensitive units are involved in recovering the direction of moving lines. *Vision Res.*, 33: 1207–1217.

Mack, A., Fendrich, R. and Pleune, J. (1979) Smooth pursuit eye movements: is perceived motion necessary? *Science*, 203: 1361–1363.

Mareschal, I. and Baker Jr., C.L. (1998) Temporal and spatial response to second-order stimuli in cat area 18. *J. Neurophysiol.*, 80: 2811–2823.

Masson, G.S. and Castet, E. (2002) Parallel motion processing for the initiation of short-latency ocular following in humans. *J. Neurosci.*, 22: 5149–5163.

Masson, G.S. and Stone, L.S. (2000) Initiation of smooth-pursuit eye movements to moving line-figure objects in humans. *Soc. Neurosci. Abstr.*, 26: 497.7.

Masson, G.S., Rybarczyk, Y., Castet, E. and Mestre, D.R. (2000) Temporal dynamics of motion integration for the initiation of tracking eye movements at ultra-short latencies. *Vis. Neurosci.*, 17: 753–767.

Maunsell, J.H. and Van Essen, D.C. (1983) The connections of the middle temporal visual area (MT) and their relationship to a cortical hierarchy in the macaque monkey. *J. Neurosci.*, 3: 2563–2586.

Merigan, W.H., Nealey, T.A. and Maunsell, J.H. (1993) Visual effects of lesions of cortical area V2 in macaques. *J. Neurosci.*, 13: 3180–3191.

Morris, E.J. and Lisberger, S.G. (1987) Different responses to small visual errors during initiation and maintenance of smooth-pursuit eye movements in monkeys. *J. Neurophysiol.*, 58: 1351–1369.

Movshon, J.A., Adelson, E.H., Gizzi, M.S. and Newsome, W.T. (1986) The analysis of moving visual patterns. In: C. Chagas, R. Gattass and C. Gross (Eds.), *Pattern Recognition Mechanisms*. Springer, New York, pp. 117–151.

Movshon, J.A., Lisberger, S.G. and Krauzlis, R.J. (1990) Visual cortical signals supporting smooth pursuit eye movements. *Cold Spring Harb. Symp. Quant. Biol.*, 55: 707–716.

Newsome, W.T., Wurtz, R.H., Dursteler, M.R. and Mikami, A. (1985) Deficits in visual motion processing following ibotenic acid lesions of the middle temporal visual area of the macaque monkey. *J. Neurosci.*, 5: 825–840.

Nowlan, S.J. and Sejnowski, T.J. (1995) A selection model for motion processing in area MT of primates. *J. Neurosci.*, 15: 1195–1214.

Pack, C.C. and Born, R.T. (2001) Temporal dynamics of a neural solution to the aperture problem in visual area MT of macaque brain. *Nature*, 409: 1040–1042.

Pack, C.C., Berezovskii, V.K. and Born, R.T. (2001) Dynamic properties of neurons in cortical area MT in alert and anaesthetized macaque monkeys. *Nature*, 414: 905–908.

Rashbass, C. (1961) The relationship between saccadic and smooth tracking eye movements. *J. Neurophysiol.*, 159: 326–338.

Recanzone, G.H. and Wurtz, R.H. (1999) Shift in smooth pursuit initiation and MT and MST neuronal activity under different stimulus conditions. *J. Neurophysiol.*, 82: 1710–1727.

Recanzone, G.H. and Wurtz, R.H. (2000) Effects of attention on MT and MST neuronal activity during pursuit initiation. *J. Neurophysiol.*, 83: 777–790.

Robinson, D.A., Gordon, J.L. and Gordon, S.E. (1986) A model of the smooth pursuit eye movement system. *Biol. Cybern.*, 55: 43–57.

Saito, H., Yukie, M., Tanaka, K., Hikosaka, K., Fukada, Y. and Iwai, E. (1986) Integration of direction signals of image motion in the superior temporal sulcus of the macaque monkey. *J. Neurosci.*, 6: 145–157.

Shipp, S. and Zeki, S. (1989) The organization of connections between areas V5 and V2 in macaque monkey visual cortex. *Eur. J. Neurosci.*, 1: 333–354.

Simoncelli, E.P. and Heeger, D.J. (1998) A model of neuronal responses in visual area MT. *Vision Res.*, 38: 743–761.

Watamaniuk, S.N. and Heinen, S.J. (1999) Human smooth pursuit direction discrimination. *Vision Res.*, 39: 59–70.

Williams, D.W. and Sekuler, R. (1984) Coherent global motion percepts from stochastic local motions. *Vision Res.*, 24: 55–62.

Wilson, H.R. and Kim, J. (1994) A model for motion coherence and transparency. *Vis. Neurosci.*, 11: 1205–1220.

Wilson, H.R., Ferrera, V.P. and Yo, C. (1992) A psychophysically motivated model for two-dimensional motion perception. *Vis. Neurosci.*, 9: 79–97.

Yabuta, N.H., Sawatari, A. and Callaway, E.M. (2001) Two functional channels from primary visual cortex to dorsal visual cortical areas. *Science*, 292: 297–300.

CHAPTER 16

The role of expectancy and volition in smooth pursuit eye movements

G.R. Barnes [1,*], A.M. Schmid [2] and C.B. Jarrett [1]

[1] *Department of Optometry and Neuroscience, UMIST, Manchester M60 1QD, UK*
[2] *NMR Center at the Mass. General Hospital, Charlestown, MA 02129, USA*

Abstract: The most important factor allowing the generation of pursuit eye movements prior to target onset is confidence in the likelihood of imminent target appearance. We show how these anticipatory pursuit responses are essentially ballistic motor primitives and how the signal that drives them is normally defined by stored information concerning target speed, duration and direction. But we also show how static cues may be used to grade the level of these motor primitives 'on-line'. We further demonstrate that, when concatenated, these graded motor primitives can be rapidly combined to form predictive smooth movement trajectories in response to complex multi-ramp sequences.

Introduction

Ocular pursuit serves to maintain the image of a moving visual target on or close to the high acuity foveal region of the retina. It is accomplished by a combination of smooth eye movements that attempt to match the velocity of the eye to that of the target, and saccadic corrections that realign the image on the fovea when necessary. The smooth component relies predominantly on velocity error (Rashbass, 1961), whereas saccadic control relies more on position error (Robinson, 1964), but both control types utilize both sources of feedback to some degree (Pola and Wyatt, 1980; de Brouwer et al., 2002). Pursuit is normally thought of as a voluntary process and, certainly, volition plays an important part in the initial process of selecting which target to pursue. However, there is also evidence that smooth eye movements can be induced reflexively by the visual feedback that results from the motion of even very small targets, if no other visual stimuli are present (Barnes and Hill, 1984; Pola and Wyatt, 1985). Indeed, volition may simply serve to selectively enhance the visual feedback for a chosen target and thus increase the gain of pursuit. On the other hand, the ability to use volitional control to actually initiate smooth movement appears to be limited. Early observations (von Noorden and Mackensen, 1962) showed that it was not possible to generate smooth eye movements of significant velocity in the absence of a moving visual target. Instead, attempts to do so led to a series of saccades interspersed with very low velocity (generally not more than 2°/s) smooth movements.

Whilst this apparent dependence of pursuit on visual feedback was clearly demonstrated, it was also acknowledged that other mechanisms could take over the pursuit response in circumstances where the target motion was highly predictable. The continuation of smooth eye movement that may be observed when the visual target is unexpectedly removed during pursuit of a constant-velocity target (von Noorden and Mackensen, 1962; Becker and Fuchs, 1985) has often been cited as one such example of this. In this case, though, it is difficult to dissociate the effects

---

* Correspondence to: G.R. Barnes, Department of Optometry and Neuroscience, UMIST, P.O. Box 88, Manchester M60 1QD, UK. Tel.: +44-161-200-3839; Fax: +44-161-200-3887; E-mail: g.r.barnes@umist.ac.uk

of prediction from the simple temporal decay of the oculomotor response, and therefore more robust evidence for the role of prediction is arguably needed. In fact, smooth eye movements should ideally be shown to begin prior to target motion — but this brings us full circle, because as already described, this feat appears almost impossible. To solve this apparent impasse, early investigators focused on the low velocity anticipatory smooth movements that do occur prior to target onset. Kowler and Steinman (1979a,b), for example, examined a number of important aspects of these movements, including the question of volitional involvement in their generation (Kowler, 1989), but unfortunately their relevance to normal ocular pursuit has always been questionable because eye velocities were always very low ($<2°/s$). So a major challenge followed, to demonstrate that much higher velocities of anticipatory eye movement can be generated prior to target onset, and to show that these movements might serve an important function in predictive control. Evidence for this has since been found, first in the experiments of Becker and Fuchs (1985) and later in studies by Barnes and Asselman (1991) and Kao and Morrow (1994).

This article will discuss more recent insights into the control of smooth pursuit eye movements, which have emphasized the important role of volition and expectancy. In particular we will draw upon the results of a number of recent experiments to explore three major issues: (a) what are the conditions that allow volitional anticipatory eye movements to be released, (b) what are the factors that allow those movements to be appropriately scaled so as to form an effective prediction of future target movement, and (c) how might these anticipatory movements be used to control a continuous predictive response to a periodic waveform such as a sinusoid. These issues will then be discussed in relation to the available neurophysiological evidence indicating areas of the brain likely to be involved in these processes.

General methods

Although a number of experiments will be described here, the methods had much in common, so that a general description can be given for all. The experiments were conducted with local ethics committee approval and all subjects participated with informed consent. All subjects had normal or corrected-to-normal vision, were healthy and had no relevant medical or psychiatric history.

Subjects were seated at the center of a circular screen (radius 1.5 m) with the head supported on a chin-rest and fixed by clamps to the side of the head. A visual target was presented on the screen and was made to move in the horizontal axis under the control of a motor-driven mirror. The target was composed of a circle with superimposed cross hairs, subtending 50 min of arc at the eye. Illumination of the target was controlled by an electromechanical shutter, allowing it to be switched on and off rapidly. Eye movements were recorded by an infrared limbus tracking technique (Skalar IRIS, Delft, Holland). All stimuli were presented in balanced, randomized combinations.

All stimuli presented here involved the intermittent presentation of the target whilst it was in motion. Repetition of identical target motion stimuli in this way has been found to be a reliable way of evoking a controlled anticipatory smooth pursuit eye movement (Barnes and Asselman, 1991). The stimuli were either presented at regular intervals or, in more recent studies, irregular timing of stimuli was combined with a timing cue that was given at a fixed time before the onset of the target (the Remembered Pursuit task, Barnes and Donelan, 1999).

Eye movements were analyzed by first identifying and removing the fast phase components of the response using a technique based on a combination of acceleration and velocity threshold criteria. A linear interpolation routine was used to bridge the gaps produced by removal of saccades from the eye velocity trajectory. Where measured variables are referred to as *steady-state* (SS) values these have been derived by averaging velocity trajectories for the third and subsequent presentations of the repeated stimulus. Two specific measures of eye movement were derived from each response to characterize predictive behavior, i.e. eye velocity at onset of the stimulus presentation ($V0$) and eye velocity 100 ms after onset ($V100$). Values at 100 ms were examined because this corresponds to the last time at which the response is likely to be uninfluenced by visual feedback on the basis of most estimates of pursuit reaction time (Rashbass, 1961; Tychsen and Lisberger, 1986; Carl and Gellman, 1987).

Evidence for a short-term store in ocular pursuit

One of the most important aspects of pursuit behavior suggested by early experiments (Barnes et al., 1987; Barnes and Asselman, 1991) was the notion of a short-term store for prediction. In these early experiments, the underlying stimulus was a triangular waveform. The target was not visible for the whole of the waveform, only for short periods as the target passed through the center point of the screen, as shown in Fig. 1. Subjects were simply instructed to follow the target as well as possible. In the example shown in Fig. 1, the target velocity was 36°/s, the exposure duration was only 120 ms and the interval between presentations was 1.26 s. During the first presentation, the subject was only able to make a reactive response. As a consequence, the first smooth movement did not start until after the target had gone out and the peak velocity was, not surprisingly, very low. But in the second and subsequent presentations the subject started to make anticipatory smooth movements, which built up to a steady state within 3–4 presentations. This build up of the response led to the hypothesis that the visual motion feedback available in the initial presentation might be used to build up an internal store of pre-motor drive that could then be released as a predictive estimate of the required eye velocity. In this way, it was thought that the release of relatively high velocity anticipatory smooth movements was facilitated, when in normal circumstances this would not be possible. This idea was supported by the observation that when the tar-

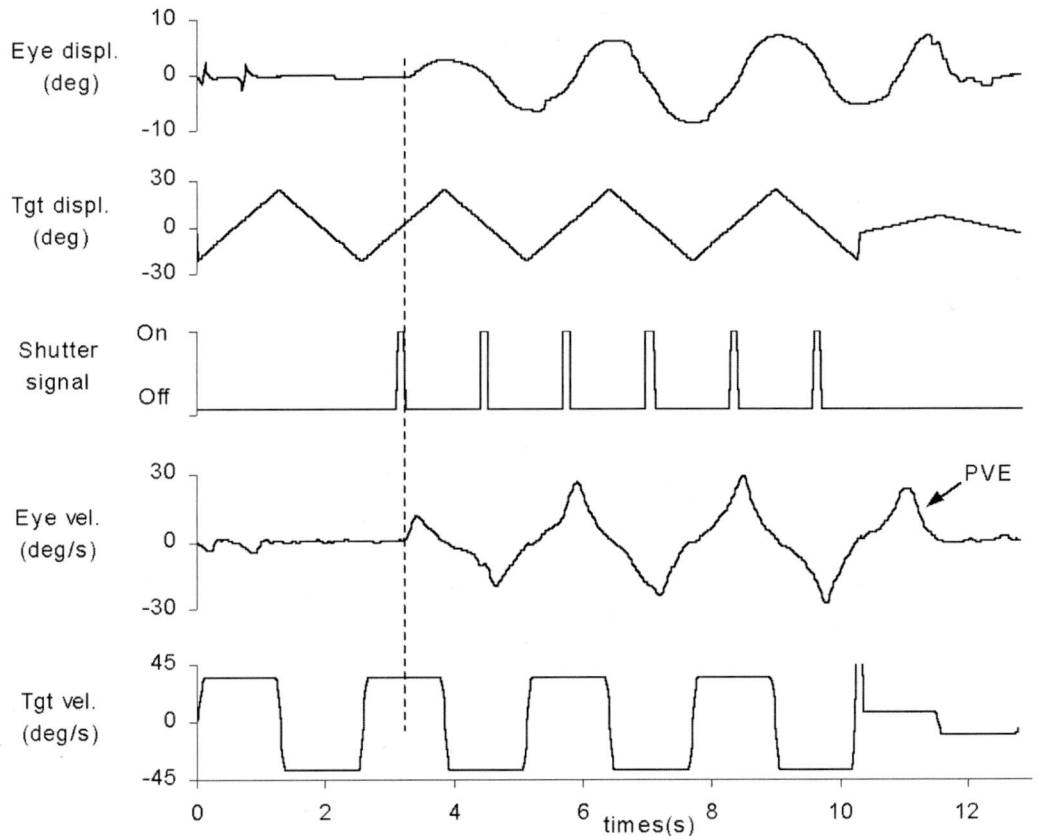

Fig. 1. Eye movements evoked by intermittent presentation of a target moving alternately to left and right at constant velocity (±36°/s). The underlying target motion stimulus was a triangular waveform of frequency 0.39 Hz. The target was exposed for a duration of 120 ms (indicated by the shutter signal) every half-cycle as it passed through center. Fast phase components have been removed from the eye velocity signal. PVE, predictive velocity estimate made when expected target failed to appear. (From Barnes et al., 1997, with permission.)

get unexpectedly failed to appear, a predictive velocity estimate (PVE, Fig. 1) was initiated, with appropriate timing, in the complete absence of a moving target. This PVE could not be sustained for very long, however, and generally started to decay around 100–150 ms after the target would have been expected to appear. Any further attempts by the subject to generate more smooth movements were normally unsuccessful, thus reinforcing previous findings that smooth movements cannot be sustained in the absence of a moving target. An important feature of the anticipatory movements was that their magnitude increased as target velocity increased, thus indicating that they could be used as a predictive estimate of required target velocity.

The role of expectancy and timing

The foregoing results suggested that the existence of stored pre-motor drive might be necessary to generate the anticipatory response and that, once it had been released in the absence of the target, the store might discharge, thus making further attempts impossible. However, in a subsequent experiment (Barnes et al., 1997) it was shown that this was not the case. In this experiment, the timing of target appearance was reinforced by giving audio cues 760 ms prior to each target appearance. When, at a particular point, the target failed to appear, subjects had been instructed to expect three blank presentations in succession (with timing cues continuing as normal) followed by target reappearance. In response to the first blank, subjects initiated one predictive velocity estimate (as in Fig. 1), but were unable to generate further anticipatory responses of significant velocity for the next two blanks even though the timing cues remained. This suggested that the store had been discharged. However, when the target reappeared after the third blank presentation — as the subjects *expected* — they were once again able to initiate a high velocity anticipatory response, even though this had not been possible in the intermediate phase. These results indicate that the store had not been discharged, but rather, that its output had been inhibited by the knowledge that the target would not be appearing for a certain interval. In subsequent experiments it has been possible to demonstrate that, provided the subject knows how many time cues are to be expected in the gap, there is often no reduction in the level of anticipatory response even for blank gaps as long as 14.4 s (Chakraborti et al., 2002).

Volitional control versus visual feedback

The concept of a short-term store for prediction was given further support by other experiments designed to investigate the volitional contribution to smooth pursuit (Barnes et al., 1995). It had been known for many years that when subjects were presented with a stabilized image on the retina they could initiate smooth movements by attempting to chase the eccentric image (Kommerell and Taumer, 1972). We hypothesized that subjects might be able to use stored information about the required eye velocity to control the velocity of smooth eye movement in this stabilized mode. Fig. 2 shows examples of the stimulus and responses generated.

In the initial part of each trial the subject was given a regular intermittent presentation of the moving target. After a number of cycles, the image was stabilized on the fovea. This stabilization was carried out in a dark period between presentations so that the subject was not able to observe the change when it occurred. In the initial 'closed-loop' period the subject built up anticipatory movements. When the stimulus was suddenly switched to stabilized mode the subject had already initiated another anticipatory movement, so that the eye was in motion at the time that the target appeared. Because it was then stabilized on the retina, the target was carried along by the movement of the eye. The subject was able to sustain this smooth movement for the duration of target exposure. Moreover, the subject was able to continue to volitionally generate smooth eye movements repeatedly every time that the target reappeared, alternating the movements from left to right. Since no retinal velocity error information was available to the subject during the stabilized image mode, these continued movements must have been carried out from a central source. The movements were dependent on voluntary activity; they could not be sustained without active involvement. In fact, accompanying experiments (Barnes et al., 1995) verified that subjects could control the direction of smooth eye movement simply by shifting attention to one or other side of the foveally stabilized image.

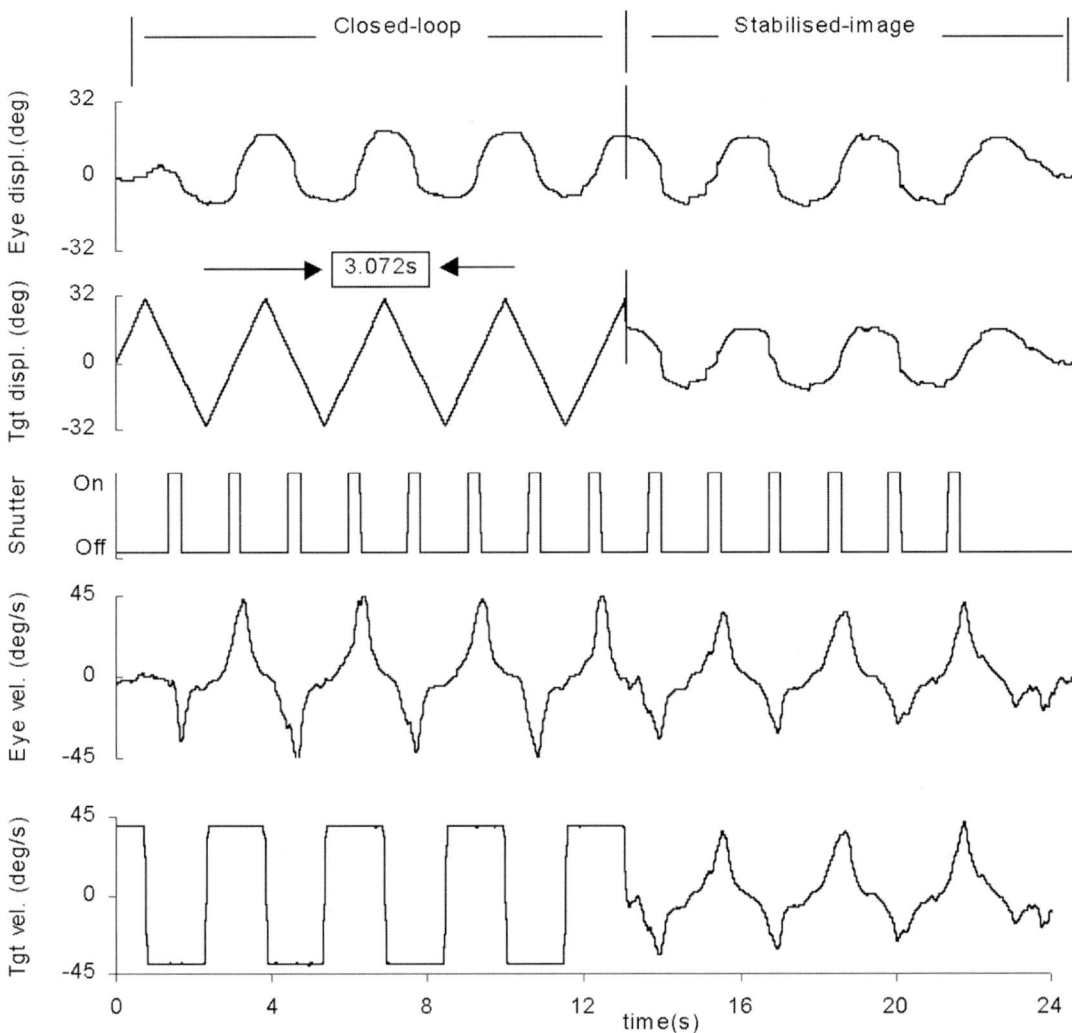

Fig. 2. Eye movements generated during intermittent presentation of a target moving with a triangular waveform (frequency 0.325 Hz; peak velocity 40°/s) under closed-loop and stabilized-image conditions. Pulses (second trace) indicate times at which the target was illuminated (pulse duration PD = 320 ms). Saccadic components have been removed from the eye velocity trajectory.

Examination of the velocity profiles of the individual responses to each target presentation showed that there was a close similarity between the responses in the stabilized and closed-loop modes up to 100 ms after the onset of the target as shown in Fig. 3A. After this, the presence of velocity error feedback led to an increase in the acceleration of the eye in the closed-loop mode, which resulted in an earlier attainment of peak velocity. The peak velocity attained in the stabilized mode ranged from 57 to 95% of that in the closed-loop phase, depending on closed-loop target velocity. This proportion is similar to that found by van den Berg (1988) using a rather different approach. It suggests that in pursuit of a predictable waveform, such as a sinusoid, a high proportion of the response is achieved through central drive, leaving visual feedback to make up only the remaining difference. Another feature common to stabilized and closed-loop responses was that the velocity often started to decline before the target actually disappeared (Fig. 3A). In the closed-loop mode this anticipatory slowing of the eye movement

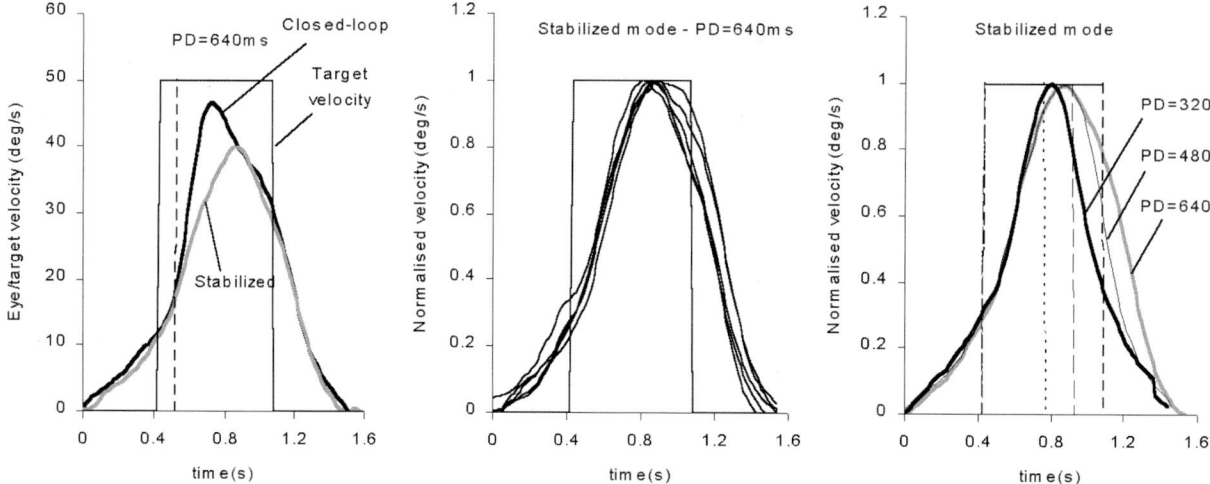

Fig. 3. (A) Averaged smooth component eye velocity trajectories obtained in stabilized-image and closed-loop conditions from means of three cycles in eight subjects. Target velocity was 50°/s. The target was illuminated for a duration (PD) of 640 ms as indicated by the pulse. Note the sudden increase in eye acceleration 100 ms after the start of the pulse (broken vertical line) in the closed-loop mode. (B) Normalized responses obtained by dividing stabilized trajectories by their peak velocity. Target velocity of prior closed-loop phase ranged from 10 to 50°/s. (C). Normalized eye velocity trajectories averaged across target velocities for target exposure durations (PD) of 320, 480 and 640 ms.

prior to the end of the target motion has been noted before (Robinson et al., 1986; Boman and Hotson, 1988; Wells and Barnes, 1999), but these results show that the underlying central component had also been programmed in a similar way.

An important feature of the stabilized responses was that peak velocity increased monotonically with the target velocity of the prior closed-loop phase, providing support for the idea that information stored in the closed-loop phase was being used to set the level of response in the stabilized phase. When the stabilized responses corresponding to different closed-loop target velocities were normalized by dividing each velocity profile by its own peak velocity, there was a considerable degree of similarity between them, even though actual peak eye velocity varied from 16.6 to 39.9°/s (Fig. 3B). In other words, the temporal development of the stabilized response was very similar, only the level changed. Moreover, as the duration of exposure increased, the initial part of the profile remained very similar, as shown in Fig. 3C, whereas the declining portion started later for longer exposure durations (PDs in Fig. 3). This trajectory thus had the hallmarks of being a ballistic response to an internal drive. The peak level of this predictive response is based on stored velocity information, whereas the onset and offset of the internal drive are controlled on the basis of stored timing information.

Learning sequences of movements

The experiments described so far have shown that subjects are able to generate predictive smooth movement trajectories to single ramp stimuli given the right expectancy. However, the major evidence for prediction in ocular pursuit comes from the examination of responses to continuous periodic motion stimuli, such as sinusoidal oscillation of the target. The next issue to consider then is how these predictive trajectories to short duration ramps might be related to prediction during continuous target motion. One possibility put forward previously (Barnes and Asselman, 1991) is that the sequential release of predictive trajectories in a serial order manner could lead to a composite response that is continuously predictive. Evidence to support this was provided by Boman and Hotson (1992), who showed that when the responses to single ramps are concatenated in this way the composite response mimics the response to a triangular wave target motion.

The predictive trajectory to a single ramp essentially forms a 'motor primitive' for smooth eye movements. It has been suggested that in other types of motor control such motor primitives form the basis of motor learning (Schmidt, 1988). If this could be applied to ocular pursuit then concatenation of the responses to a number of simple component trajectories of different speed and direction should allow a predictive response to quite complex trajectories to be built up. In order for this process to operate it would be necessary to demonstrate two attributes. First, there would have to be evidence of linear summation of the motor primitives and second, it would be necessary for subjects to be able to grade the magnitude and direction of successive motor primitives on the basis of expectancy. In a recent study (Barnes and Schmid, 2002) we have tested to see if this principle predicts the behaviorally observed tracking of a wide variety of complex target motion sequences.

The method employed was that of the 'remembered pursuit task'. The motion stimuli were presented at irregular intervals, but each presentation was preceded by an audio cue 600 ms prior to target appearance. Subjects were required to track target motion in the form of a sequence composed of two or four constant-velocity ramps.

Evidence for linear summation in double-ramp responses

The objective of the first experiment was to find evidence to support the hypothesis that the response to a sequence of two ramps is equivalent to the summation of responses to the individual ramps presented separately. Each double-ramp sequence consisted of two components, each of which could have a constant velocity (R1, R2) of $15°/s$ or $30°/s$ to the right (positive) or left (negative). A gap of 200 ms was left between ramps. During the gap the target either stopped ($G = 0°/s$) or continued moving at either the velocity of the first ($G = R1$) or second ($G = R2$) ramp. When G was zero, the target reappeared after the gap at the same location at which it had disappeared. When G was non-zero there was a positional shift ($3°$ for $G = 15°/s$; $6°$ for $G = 30°/s$) between the point at which it disappeared and the point at which it reappeared after the gap. In addition to the double-ramps, we also presented two further series in which the target was stationary during either the first or second component (referred to as single ramps; i.e. R1 or R2 = $0°/s$), thus effectively forming a 400 ms period of fixation.

Subjects, whether naïve or experienced, rapidly learned to produce anticipatory smooth pursuit responses to both single- and double-ramps, reaching a steady state (SS) after only 2–3 presentations of each new sequence. Even during the gap periods subjects were not truly aware of their anticipatory behavior; it appeared to be a natural consequence of their attempts to pursue as well as possible, as instructed. Examples of representative stimuli and responses are shown in Fig. 4. In these examples the two single-ramp stimuli (A and B) had component velocities (R1/G/R2) of 30/0/0 and 0/−15/−15 respectively. Summation of the velocities of these two single-ramp stimuli would result in the double-ramp stimulus shown in Fig. 4C, in which R1/G/R2 = 30/−15/−15. The hypothesis to be tested in this experiment was that the *composite response* obtained by the summation of the responses to the two single-ramp stimuli is equivalent to the actual response to the double-ramp stimulus.

When responses to the individual ramps of Fig. 4A,B were summated as indicated in Fig. 5A, the resulting composite response appears similar to the actual response to the double-ramp stimulus. (Note that for this summation process the smooth eye movement responses were time-locked to the audio warning cue.) A similar effect was also observed when the component ramps were in the same direction and had the same or different velocities (Fig. 5B,C), although there was more fluctuation in the recorded traces and, thus, less moment-by-moment correspondence.

To establish how well a linear summation model could be applied to these responses, two measures of eye velocity, V0 and V100, for the real and composite eye movements were compared at the beginning of the second ramp using linear regression analysis. Responses at these two times were chosen to be representative probes for the response throughout the critical period from 100 ms after the end of the 1st until 100 ms after the onset of the 2nd ramp, during which there is unlikely to be any influence of visual feedback (Carl and Gellman, 1987). There was a significant ($p < 0.001$) linear relationship between the double ramp and the summated single-ramp responses at these two probe points, the correlation

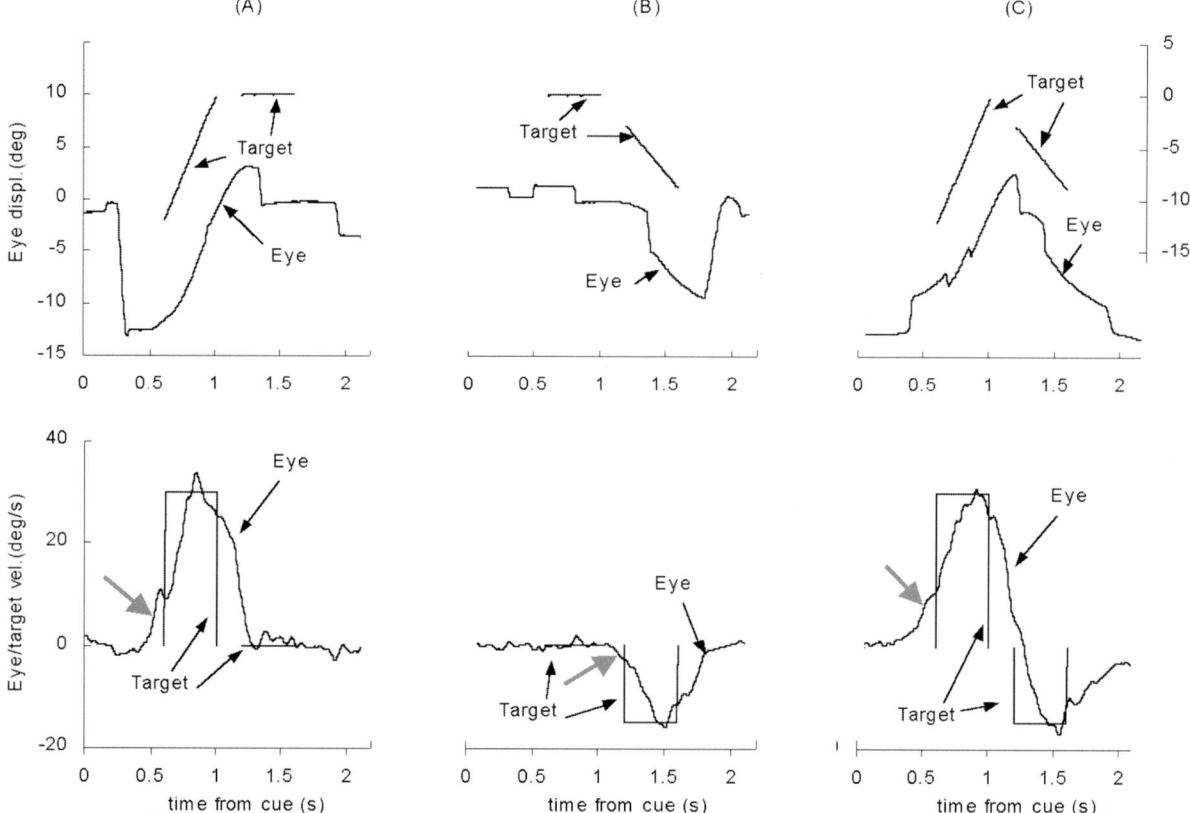

Fig. 4. Examples of eye displacement (upper plots) and the corresponding smooth component eye velocity (lower plots) evoked in response to regular repetition of single-ramp (A and B) and double-ramp (C) stimuli. These are single responses taken after steady-state conditions had been attained in a single subject. The target was visible only during the 400 ms periods for which it is indicated. Component velocities — R1/G/R2 — were (A) 30/0/0, (B) 0/−15/−15, and (C) 30/−15/−15 in degree per second. Large arrows indicate anticipatory eye movements. The abscissae indicate time after audio cue onset. Note that target displacement (right ordinate) is offset by 10° above eye displacement (left ordinate). (From Barnes and Schmid, 2002, with permission.)

coefficients being 0.969 for V0 and 0.987 for V100 ($n = 34$). The fact that the slope of these relationships was very close to unity (0.963 for V0; 1.039 for V100) also indicates that it was very close to a linear summation.

The technique used in this experiment is an extension of that previously used by Boman and Hotson (1992), who also showed an apparent linear summation of responses to low velocity ($<10°/s$) double ramps of opposing direction. Our results provide support for these earlier findings but, in addition, indicate that the summation principle (a) applies for higher velocity stimuli (up to $30°/s$), and (b) operates even when there is no change in direction between the first and second ramps.

Evidence for pre-programming in 4-ramp sequences: responses to catch presentations

In a second experiment, responses to 4-ramp sequences were examined (Barnes and Schmid, 2002). Successive ramps in a sequence were separated by 200 ms gaps and each ramp could have a velocity of $15°/s$ or $30°/s$ to left or right. In contrast to the previous experiment, gap velocity (G) was maintained at zero and there were no combinations in which any of the ramp components had zero velocity. The major objective of this experiment was to observe the responses that occurred in conditions where there was an unexpected change in the sequence. We therefore randomized the number of sequences within each

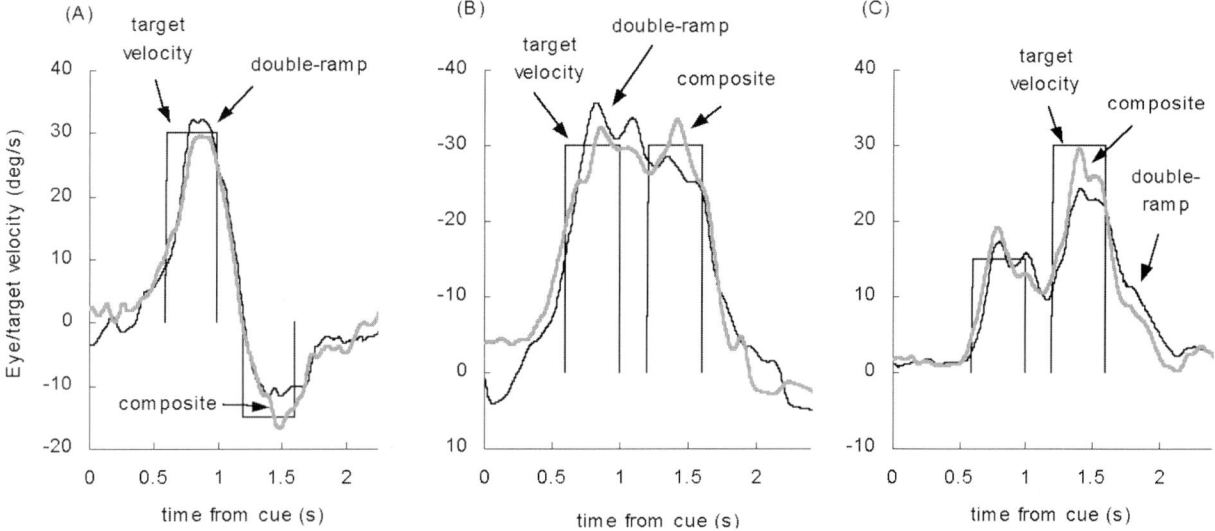

Fig. 5. Averaged double-ramp eye velocity responses (thin black) compared with composite responses (thick gray) derived by summation of constituent single-ramps of the type shown in Fig. 4A,B. Responses are SS averages from a single subject for the following combinations of R1/G/R2: (A) 30/−15/−15; (B) −30/−30/30; note inversion of ordinate; (C) 15/0/30. (From Barnes and Schmid, 2002, with permission.)

series (ranging from 5 to 8) and, between series, the speed and/or direction of one ramp component of the motion stimulus was changed in a way that could not be predicted by the subject. This is referred to as a *catch presentation*. The subject had no prior knowledge of when the change would occur, which ramp would change or what the new direction and speed would be.

Fig. 6 illustrates a part of the 4-ramp stimulus and the response of a single subject. The first two examples in this figure represent the last two presentations of one series, whereas the second pair represents the first two of a new series. The change that occurs represents the catch presentation. The first two responses, which represent the sixth and seventh presentations of this sequence, had similar velocity trajectories and represent part of the steady state (SS) that is normally attained after the first two presentations. As with the 2-ramp stimuli, even the naïve subjects were able to carry out this task quite naturally without prior training. Subjects were not specifically aware of whether they were making smooth or saccadic movements. Nor were they aware of the degree of anticipation that was taking place until the catch presentation occurred. When the catch presentation occurred in the opposite direction to the prior third ramp component (as in Fig. 6), the subject was well aware that a response had been initiated in the wrong direction for the current motion stimulus.

A wide variety of patterns of SS smooth eye velocity were generated in this experiment. Fig. 6 shows two such examples, but in total, 40 different patterns were generated and evidence was found that these complex patterns were the result of linear summation of the concatenated motor primitive responses to the single ramps shown earlier. To determine whether these patterns of response had been pre-programmed, we examined the eye movement characteristics at the time when unexpected changes were introduced into the 4-ramp stimulus.

Fig. 7 shows a detailed example of the velocity traces before and after such a change. This example corresponds to the eye movement data in the 3rd presentation shown in Fig. 6, in which the sequence was changed by modification of the direction, but not the speed, of the 3rd ramp. R3 changed from $+30°/s$ to $-30°/s$. As shown in Fig. 7A, the initial eye velocity of the *1st new* response to the modified part of the new sequence was similar to the steady-state response of the previous sequence (*SS prior*). Thus, in this specific example, the eye movement at the time of ramp 3 continued rightwards at a velocity

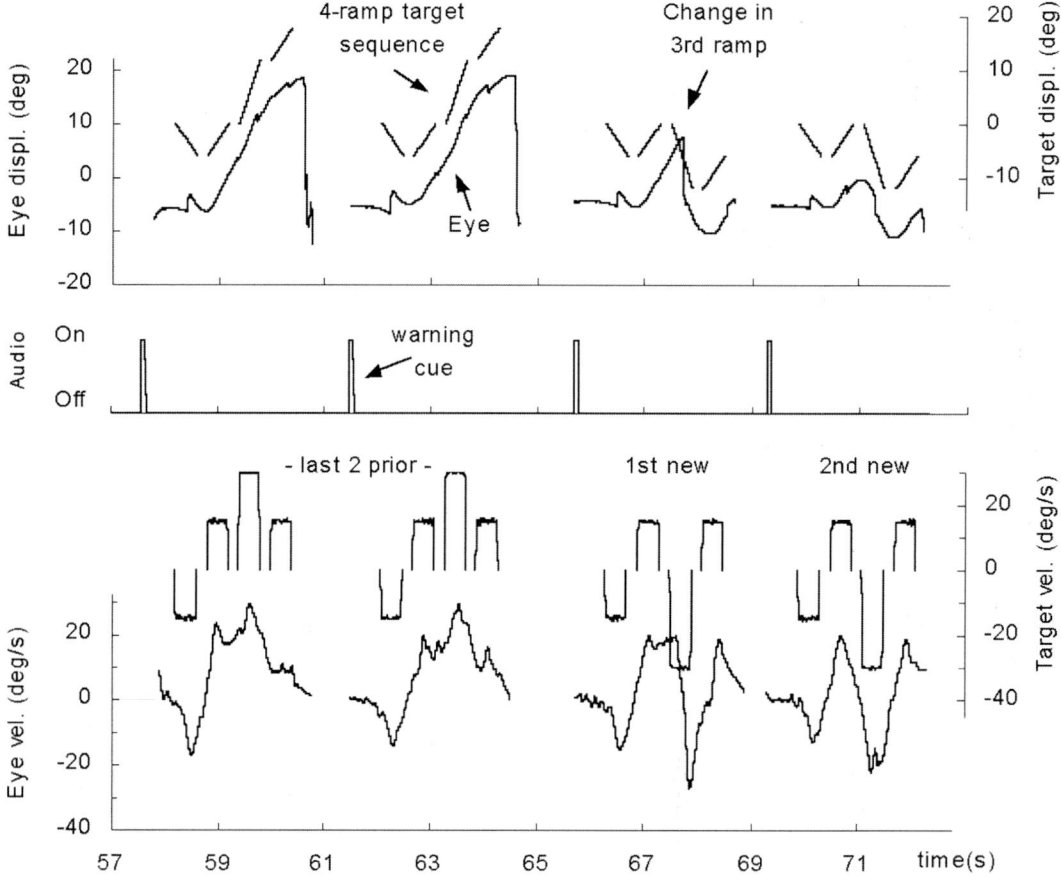

Fig. 6. An example of eye displacement and smooth component eye velocity in response to a 4-ramp target sequence. Each ramp was exposed for 400 ms with a blank gap of 200 ms between ramps. The example shows two presentations of one sequence followed by two of a new sequence, in which the velocity of the 3rd ramp component has changed from 30°/s to −30°/s. This change constitutes a *catch presentation*. Note that target displacement (right ordinate) is offset by 10° above eye displacement (left ordinate) and target velocity is offset by 40°/s above eye velocity. Each presentation was preceded by an audio cue 600 ms before onset of the first ramp component (center trace). (From Barnes and Schmid, 2002, with permission.)

appropriate for the recurrence of a +30°/s target movement for over 100 ms (shown by triangular marker), even though actual target movement was in the opposite direction. Referral to Fig. 6 indicates that eye displacement continued without any saccade during this initial period of the *1st new* presentation, but was then followed by a large corrective saccade that brought the eye position closer to target position. After this saccade, the eye velocity started to reverse in direction towards the new third ramp velocity. Comparison with the SS response to the new sequence (*SS new*, Fig. 7A) shows that the *1st new* response was delayed for the remainder of this presentation. However, in the second presentation of the new sequence the eye velocity trajectory (the *2nd new* response in Fig. 7B) was remarkably similar to the steady-state response for the new sequence (*SS new*), indicating that adjustment to the new sequence had occurred very rapidly.

V100 values for the response to the unexpectedly changed component of the sequence were compared with the SS V100 values for the corresponding component of the *prior* and *new* series by regression analyses. Comparison of V100 for the *1st new* response to the new sequence with the SS V100 of the *prior* sequence indicated a significant correlation

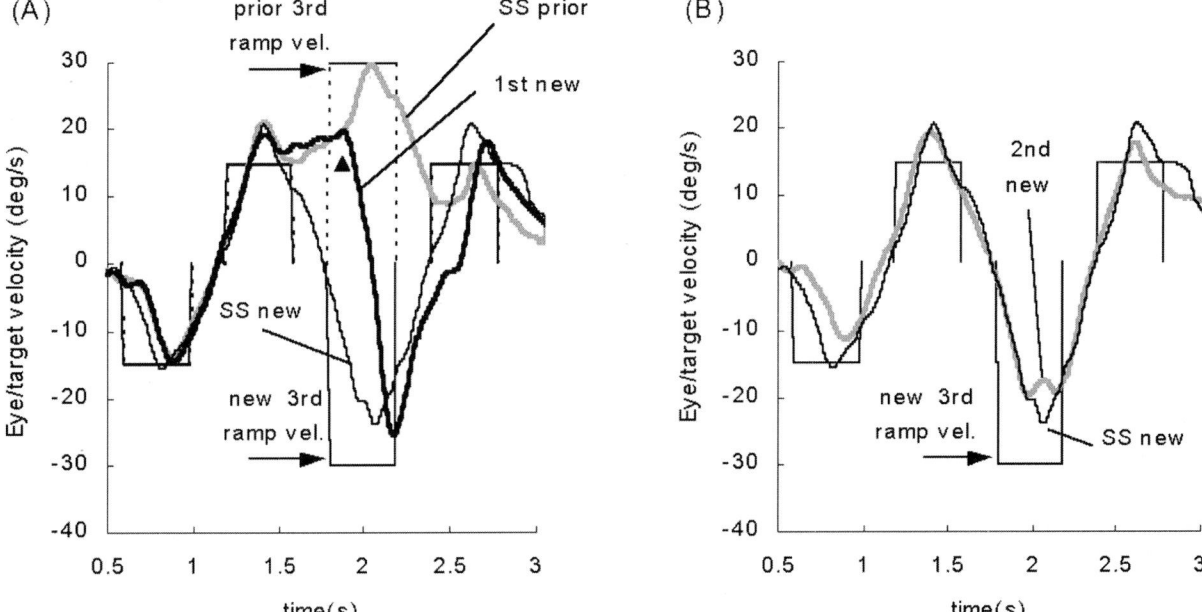

Fig. 7. Detail of changes in eye velocity that occurred before and after the catch presentation shown in Fig. 6, in which there was an unexpected change in the speed and direction of the 3rd ramp component of the 4-ramp sequence. R3 changed from +30°/s (R) to −30°/s (L). In (A), the *1st new* response (thick black) generated during the first presentation of the new sequence was initially very similar to the steady-state response (*SS prior*, thick gray) of the prior sequence. Apex of triangle marks 100 ms after target onset. In (B), the *2nd new* response (gray) generated in the second presentation of the new sequence was very similar to the steady-state response for the new sequence (*SS new*, black). (From Barnes and Schmid, 2002, with permission.)

($r = 0.98$; $n = 32$; $p < 0.001$) with a near-unity slope (0.99) of the best-fit line. In contrast, when V100 of the *1st new* response was compared with the SS V100 of the *new* sequence, no significant correlation was found. Conversely, comparison of V100 for the *2nd new* response to the new sequence with the SS V100 of the *prior* sequence revealed a very poor correlation whereas comparison of V100 for the *2nd new* response with the SS V100 of the *new* sequence indicated a significant correlation ($r = 0.95$; $n = 32$; slope = 0.92; $p < 0.001$).

These findings reveal crucial evidence of pre-programming. The results of the regression analyses show that the prediction of the future response is closely correlated with the response that occurred in the corresponding part of the prior sequence, even though this corresponding component occurred at a random time many seconds prior to the catch presentation. Since this effect was observed whichever of the four ramp components was modified, it indicates that the predictive response was based on the expected stimulus for each part of the sequence. This conclusion was given further support by the finding that for both 2- and 4-ramp sequences, the eye velocity at the onset of each ramp component in the steady state (V0) was predictively correlated with the velocity of the upcoming component of the sequence (Barnes and Schmid, 2002). When this information is taken in conjunction with the evidence presented earlier for the linear summation of successive anticipatory responses, it strongly suggests that the smooth eye movement response to the multiple ramps had been pre-programmed as a sequence of appropriately scaled anticipatory movements prior to each sequence presentation. Moreover, the evidence indicates that the pre-programming could be reset very quickly after there was an unexpected change in the stimulus since, by the time of the second presentation of the new sequence, V100 values were not significantly different to the SS for that new sequence.

Using static cues to grade the speed and direction of eye movement

The preceding studies have shown that subjects are able to store sequences of up to four velocity components and for every *expected* repetition of a sequence are able to use this information to anticipate each individual component within the sequence. This suggests that they can hold information about more than one speed and direction of movement in store simultaneously. This finding then led us to test whether subjects might be able to use such a store to generate anticipatory responses to targets of different direction and speed 'on the fly'. If their expectation of the nature of forthcoming targets was derived not from the memory of a pre-learned sequence but instead was derived 'on-line' from a symbolic cue, we hypothesized that it may be possible for them to volitionally scale the speed and direction of their anticipatory ocular pursuit in advance of each target, even when the speed and direction of successive targets is randomized.

The idea that expectations about forthcoming stimuli may be derived from cues has been examined before. Kowler (1989) used visual and auditory cues to provide information about the direction of forthcoming stimuli, and she reported that under these circumstances, anticipatory pursuit velocity was related more to cognitive expectations derived from the cues than to motor habit based on past history. We recently built on these findings, by showing that this principle holds for higher target velocities and responses (at $<2°/s$ the anticipatory movements in Kowler's study were too slow to be distinguishable from the kind of movements that most people are able to generate in the absence of a target anyway). Using a version of the 'remembered pursuit task', but this time with each random-direction target (leftward or rightward) of up to $40°/s$ preceded by a static, visual precue, we recorded velocity-scaled anticipatory responses in excess of $18°/s$ (Jarrett and Barnes, 2001). Furthermore, we showed that, given enough expectancy (in the form of an appropriate cue), subjects were able to transfer volitionally, anticipatory ocular pursuit responses to a novel direction, not previously traversed by target or eyes.

We next sought to test whether subjects were able to use static cues to exert volitional control over not only direction but also the speed of anticipatory pursuit. The plausibility of such an ability had been hinted at previously: Steinman et al. (1969) reported their own ability to track targets of varying velocities ($0.5°/s$, $1°/s$, $3°/s$, $6°/s$, and $11°/s$) at varying fractions of those velocities (1/4, 1/2, 3/4, but not double target velocity), at will. So, in a recent experiment (Jarrett and Barnes, 2002), again using the remembered pursuit paradigm, we tested the ability of eight normal subjects to scale volitionally, anticipatory smooth pursuit velocity. Subjects were presented with intermittently illuminated targets of random direction (left or right) and speed (10, 20, 30 and $40°/s$), preceded by static, symbolic cues (see legend, Fig. 8) which were predictive of *both* these random target parameters.

Following a single practice trial (also with randomized presentation) to allow an association to be made between cues and their respective targets, we found even naïve subjects *were* able to use static precues on-line to select both the direction of, and appropriately grade the speed of, anticipatory ocular pursuit responses in advance of targets of pseudorandom direction and speed. Raw data from this experiment (Fig. 8) show that this was possible from the very outset of the experiment, immediately following the practice trial. Crucially, observation of the V100 values (marked as lozenges) shows the appropriate scaling of this anticipatory activity before the possible influence of visual feedback. In line with previous observations V100 values increased significantly ($p < 0.05$) with increasing target speed. Moreover, there was no significant difference between the V100 values for randomized, cued presentations and for the control condition in which speed and direction remained constant in a given series.

These results indicate that, given enough expectancy (and in these experiments, consistently valid precues effectively served to maximize expectancy), subjects may exert relatively fine-tuned, volitional control 'on-line', over both the direction and speed of anticipatory ocular pursuit responses. Importantly, the demonstration of this ability opens up the possibility that subjects might also be able to use perceptual cues derived from ongoing target motion, such as perceived target deceleration, to forecast the future trajectory of a continuous target that is not regularly repetitive. However, the limitations of this

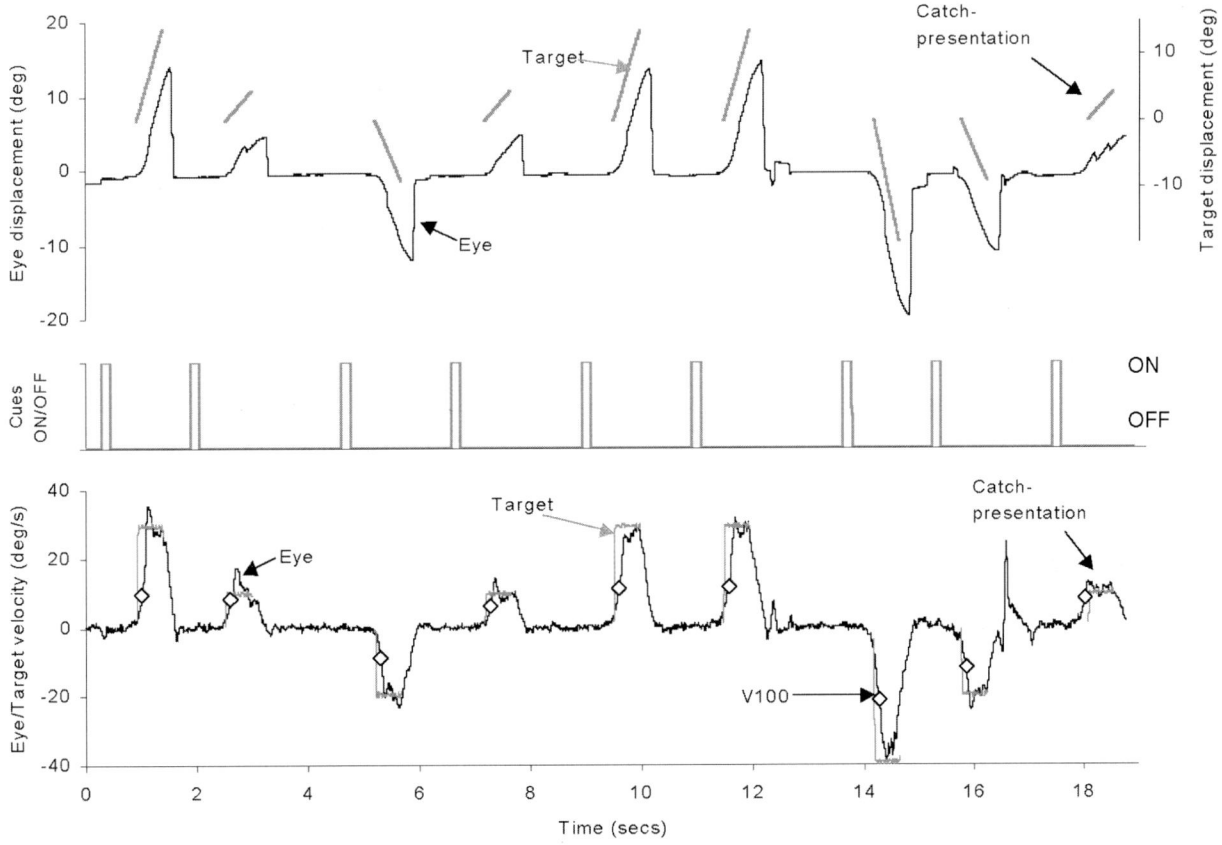

Fig. 8. Target and eye movements of one subject during presentation of static cues at center fixation point prior to each presentation of the impending target motion. Cues were composed of a number (1–4) indicating speed and an arrow indicating direction (e.g. 3>). The subject was able to scale anticipatory pursuit in advance of pseudo-randomized target velocities of 10, −20, −30, and 40°/s. Diamonds indicate eye velocity 100 ms after target onset (V100). (From Jarrett and Barnes (2002), with permission.)

top-down control remain to be elucidated. For example, velocity scaling may become saturated as the range of possible target velocities increases.

The neurophysiological substrate for motor learning in pursuit

Many of the characteristics associated with the type of extraretinal pursuit behavior reported here have already been identified in various neurophysiological studies. For example, the slowly increasing velocity profile of the anticipatory smooth movement, which we hypothesize forms the basis of the motor primitive for pursuit, has been observed by Gottlieb et al. (1993) and Tian and Lynch (1995) during microstimulation of the frontal eye field (FEF). In particular,

Gottlieb et al. found that when the image was stabilized on the retina the eye continued to accelerate for as long as stimulation continued and that the velocity increased with stimulus intensity. These are characteristics that would be required to control the timing and response level for the internal drive that forms the motor primitive for pursuit (Fig. 3). FEF is known to be in bi-directional communication with the site responsible for visual motion processing in the temporo-occipital junction (V5/V5A) and both areas exhibit activity related to extraretinal activity as well as retinal slip, as revealed by target blanking during pursuit (Komatsu and Wurtz, 1988; Tanaka et al., 1998). Timing of the release of activity from the FEF is probably controlled by the supplementary eye field (SEF) in the dorsomedial frontal cortex. Heinen and Liu (1997) have shown that in the macaque monkey the build up of activity in SEF is dependent on the predictability of the stimulus and that some cells in this area code for onset time whereas others code for offset time of the activity. There is evidence that the adjacent supplementary motor area (SMA) is particularly involved in controlling the release of volitional motor activity for other motor systems (Goldberg, 1985) and lesions in such dorsomedial frontal areas are known to give deficits in timing the release of voluntary movements (Halsband et al., 1993). Petit et al. (1996) found evidence of SEF participation in a PET study involving a pre-learned saccade sequence task and we have recently shown, with fMRI, that the associated preSMA and underlying anterior cingulate areas become progressively more activated during learning of a simple predictive pursuit task (Schmid et al., 2001).

Given that the response of the smooth pursuit system can be represented in terms of the short-term learning of a few motor primitive parameters, as suggested by our results, it implies the existence of a working memory for this information. This form of short-term storage has frequently been associated with the prefrontal cortex (PFC). In their saccade sequence task Petit et al. (1996) identified the superior frontal sulcus as a probable site for the storage of the spatial information necessary for this task in humans. There appears at present to be little information about a site for storing velocity-coded information other than a lesion study by Greenlee et al. (1995), implicating V5/V5A, but by its nature, this study could not identify whether frontal areas were also involved. It has been frequently observed that saccade and smooth pursuit areas are juxtaposed (e.g. in FEF, Tian and Lynch, 1996). So, by analogy, it might be suspected that storage for pursuit might be close to that for the saccadic system in the PFC. Dorsolateral PFC (DLPFC) is thought to be involved in the manipulation of information within working memory. Together with the intraparietal sulcus (IPS), it has been shown to be active in the early stages of sequence learning (Toni et al., 1998) and probably plays a vital role in comparing and validating internally generated motor output, based on stored information, with visual feedback (Goldberg, 1985). In accord with this, we have shown that DLPFC and IPS appear to play a similar role in a predictive pursuit task, being active in the initial presentations, but declining rapidly as anticipatory movements develop (Schmid et al., 2001).

Conclusions

Although smooth movements cannot normally be initiated volitionally in the absence of a moving target, the major reason for this appears to be the need to have a high expectancy of target motion. This expectancy is, to a certain extent, dependent on knowledge of the timing of the expected target movement, but the critical factor is confidence in the target's forthcoming appearance. When voluntary smooth movements are initiated they have a very characteristic velocity profile, with a slow build up of velocity that is quite different to the more rapid onset of the visually driven response. The evidence suggests that these anticipatory smooth movements are ballistic responses to an internal drive signal that forms a motor primitive. The parameters that define this drive signal are its amplitude, duration and direction. When motor primitives are issued in serial order fashion (concatenated) they can lead to the development of complex smooth movement trajectories as observed in the responses to 4-ramp sequences. Normally, the required amplitude level of the internal drive is based on information gleaned from past experience and held in a short-term store or buffer. This buffer appears to be capable of holding information about at least 4 levels of speed and direction. The stored information is rapidly acquired and this allows the system to be used to quickly build up a rudimentary motor program for predictive control. However, the stored information need not be tied to any particular sequence, since expectancy about future targets can be derived from static symbolic cues, thus allowing information contained in the store to be used to appropriately grade an ongoing response 'on-line'. The question of how many defining parameters for motor primitives can be held in store and whether more than one store is required for this process remains open.

Abbreviations

DLPFC   dorsolateral prefrontal cortex
FEF   frontal eye field

IPS   intraparietal sulcus
PFC   prefrontal cortex
PVE   predictive velocity estimate
SEF   supplementary eye field
SMA   supplementary motor area
SS   steady state

Acknowledgements

This work was supported by the Medical Research Council, UK and partly conducted in the former MRC Human Movement and Balance Unit, Queen Sq., London WC1N 3BG.

References

Barnes, G.R. and Asselman, P.T. (1991) The mechanism of prediction in human smooth pursuit eye movements. *J. Physiol. (Lond.)*, 439: 439–461.

Barnes, G.R. and Donelan, A.S. (1999) The remembered pursuit task: evidence for segregation of timing and velocity storage in predictive oculomotor control. *Exp. Brain Res.*, 129: 57–67.

Barnes, G.R. and Hill, T. (1984) The influence of display characteristics on active pursuit and passively induced eye movements. *Exp. Brain Res.*, 56: 438–447.

Barnes, G.R. and Schmid, A.M. (2002) Sequence learning in human ocular smooth pursuit. *Exp. Brain Res.*, 144: 322–335.

Barnes, G.R., Donnelly, S.F. and Eason, R.D. (1987) Predictive velocity estimation in the pursuit reflex response to pseudorandom and step displacement stimuli in man. *J. Physiol. (Lond.)*, 389: 111–136.

Barnes, G.R., Goodbody, S.J. and Collins, S. (1995) Volitional control of anticipatory ocular pursuit responses under stabilized image conditions in humans. *Exp. Brain Res.*, 106: 301–317.

Barnes, G.R., Grealy, M.A. and Collins, S. (1997) Volitional control of anticipatory ocular smooth pursuit after viewing, but not pursuing, a moving target: evidence for a re-afferent velocity store. *Exp. Brain Res.*, 116: 445–455.

Becker, W. and Fuchs, A.F. (1985) Prediction in the oculomotor system: smooth pursuit during transient disappearance of a visual target. *Exp. Brain Res.*, 57: 562–575.

Boman, D.K. and Hotson, J.R. (1988) Stimulus conditions that enhance anticipatory slow eye movements. *Vision Res.*, 28: 1157–1165.

Boman, D.K. and Hotson, J.R. (1992) Predictive smooth pursuit eye movements near abrupt changes in motion direction. *Vision Res.*, 32: 675–689.

Carl, J.R. and Gellman, R.S. (1987) Human smooth pursuit: stimulus-dependent responses. *J. Neurophysiol.*, 57: 1446–1463.

Chakraborti, S.R., Barnes, G.R. and Collins, C.J.S. (2002) Factors affecting the longevity of a short-term velocity store for predictive oculomotor tracking. *Exp. Brain Res.*, 144: 152–158.

De Brouwer, S., Missal, M., Barnes, G.R. and Lefevre, P. (2002) Quantitative analysis of catch-up saccades during sustained pursuit. *J. Neurophysiol.*, 87: 1772–1780.

Goldberg, G. (1985) Supplementary motor area structure and function: review and hypothesis. *Behav. Brain Sci.*, 8: 567–616.

Gottlieb, J.P., Bruce, C.J. and MacAvoy, M.G. (1993) Smooth eye movements elicited by microstimulation in the primate frontal eye field. *J. Neurophysiol.*, 69: 786–799.

Greenlee, M.W., Lang, H.J., Mergner, T. and Seeger, W. (1995) Visual short term memory of stimulus velocity in patients with unilateral posterior brain damage. *J. Neurosci.*, 15: 2287–2300.

Halsband, U., Ito, N., Tanji, J. and Freund, H.J. (1993) The role of premotor cortex and the supplementary motor area in the temporal control of movement in man. *Brain*, 116: 243–266.

Heinen, S.J. and Liu, M. (1997) Single-neuron activity in the dorsomedial frontal cortex during smooth-pursuit eye movements to predictable target motion. *Vis. Neurosci.*, 14: 853–865.

Jarrett, C.B. and Barnes, G.R. (2001) Volitional selection of direction in the generation of anticipatory smooth pursuit in humans. *Neurosci. Lett.*, 312: 25–28.

Jarrett, C.B. and Barnes, G.R. (2002) Volitional scaling of anticipatory ocular pursuit velocity using precues. *Cogn. Brain Res.*, in press.

Kao, G.W. and Morrow, M.J. (1994) The relationship of anticipatory smooth eye movement to smooth pursuit initiation. *Vision Res.*, 34: 3027–3036.

Komatsu, H. and Wurtz, R.H. (1988) Relation of cortical areas MT and MST to pursuit eye movements. I. Localization and visual properties of neurons. *J. Neurophysiol.*, 60: 580–603.

Kommerell, G. and Taumer, R. (1972) Investigations of the eye tracking system through stabilized retinal images. In: J. Dichgans and E. Bizzi (Eds.), *Cerebral Control of Eye Movements and Motion Perception*. Karger, Basel, pp. 288–297.

Kowler, E. (1989) Cognitive expectations, not habits, control anticipatory smooth oculomotor pursuit. *Vision Res.*, 29: 1049–1057.

Kowler, E. and Steinman, R.M. (1979a) The effect of expectations on slow oculomotor control, I. Periodic target steps. *Vision Res.*, 19: 619–632.

Kowler, E. and Steinman, R.M. (1979b) The effect of expectations on slow oculomotor control, II. Single target displacements. *Vision Res.*, 19: 633–646.

Petit, L., Orssaud, C., Tzourio, N., Crivello, F., Berthoz, A. and Mazoyer, B.M. (1996) Functional anatomy of a pre-learned sequence of horizontal saccades in humans. *J. Neurosci.*, 16: 3714–3726.

Pola, J. and Wyatt, H.J. (1980) Target position and velocity: the stimuli for smooth pursuit eye movements. *Vision Res.*, 20: 523–534.

Pola, J. and Wyatt, H.J. (1985) Active and passive smooth eye movements: effects of stimulus size and location. *Vision Res.*, 25: 1063–1076.

Rashbass, C. (1961) The relationship between saccadic and smooth tracking eye movements. *J. Physiol. (Lond.)*, 159: 326–338.

Robinson, D.A. (1964) The mechanics of human saccadic eye movement. *J. Physiol. (Lond.)*, 174: 245–264.

Robinson, D.A., Gordon, J.L. and Gordon, S.E. (1986) A model of the smooth pursuit eye movement system. *Biol. Cybern.*, 55: 43–57.

Schmid, A.M., Rees, G., Frith, C. and Barnes, G.R. (2001) A fMRI study of anticipation and learning of smooth pursuit eye movements in humans. *Neuroreport*, 12: 1409–1414.

Schmidt, R.A. (1988) *Motor Control and Motor Learning*. Human Kinetics, Champaign, IL.

Steinman, R.M., Skavenski, A.A. and Sansbury, R.V. (1969) Voluntary control of smooth pursuit velocity. *Vision Res.*, 9: 1167–1171.

Tanaka, M., Yoshida, T. and Fukushima, K. (1998) Latency of saccades during smooth-pursuit eye movement in man: directional asymmetries. *Exp. Brain Res.*, 121: 92–98.

Tian, J. and Lynch, J.C. (1995) Slow and saccadic eye movements evoked by microstimulation in the supplementary eye field of the cebus monkey. *J. Neurophysiol.*, 74: 2204–2210.

Tian, J. and Lynch, J.C. (1996) Functionally defined smooth and saccadic eye movement subregions in the frontal eye field of cebus monkeys. *J. Neurophysiol.*, 76: 2740–2753.

Toni, I., Krams, M., Turner, R. and Passingham, R.E. (1998) The time course of changes during motor sequence learning: a whole-brain fMRI study. *NeuroImage*, 8: 50–61.

Tychsen, L. and Lisberger, S.G. (1986) Visual motion processing for the initiation of smooth-pursuit eye movements in humans. *J. Neurophysiol.*, 56: 953–968.

Van den Berg, A.V. (1988) Human smooth pursuit during transient perturbations of predictable and unpredictable target movement. *Exp. Brain Res.*, 72: 95–108.

Von Noorden, G.K. and Mackensen, G. (1962) Pursuit movements of normal and amblyopic eyes. *Am. J. Ophthalmol.*, 53: 325–336.

Wells, S.G. and Barnes, G.R. (1999) Predictive smooth pursuit eye movements during identification of moving acuity targets. *Vision Res.*, 39: 2767–2775.

CHAPTER 17

Visual and cognitive control of attention in smooth pursuit

Yue Chen [1,*], Philip S. Holzman [1] and Ken Nakayama [2]

[1] *Department of Psychiatry, Harvard Medical School/McLean Hospital, Belmont, MA 02478, USA*
[2] *Department of Psychology, Harvard University, Cambridge, MA 02138, USA*

Abstract: In this chapter, we describe the role of attention in the control of smooth pursuit eye movements. As a voluntary and continuous eye movement, smooth pursuit is driven by both visual and cognitive signals. Here we show that whereas the entire process of smooth pursuit requires visual attention, the post-onset phase of the initiation and the maintenance smooth pursuit are under an additional sustained non-visual cognitive attention control. The temporal dynamics of these complementary controls of visual and non-visual cognitive attention support the continuous generation of smooth pursuit so that eye tracking of a moving target can be prompt and accurate.

Long-standing questions

Ever since smooth pursuit was classified as one of several types of eye movements, the role of attention has claimed a place in the understanding of the brain mechanisms underlying this oculomotor response. The issue is not whether attention is involved in the generation of smooth pursuit eye movements. As a voluntary eye movement, the smooth pursuit system inevitably uses visual attention when tracking a moving target of interest (e.g. Dodge and Fox, 1928). With visual attention engaged, continuous eye tracking appears to be remarkably adaptive and accurate (Westheimer, 1954). No theories or evidence have challenged the notion that visual attention is involved in smooth pursuit eye movements. One of the long-standing issues is, however, the role that attention plays in supporting the generation and the maintenance of this continuous eye tracking movement.

Smooth pursuit is a complex oculomotor response to a moving target; it involves sensory, cognitive and motor processes in the central nervous system. Several types of signals, visual and non-visual, can be used to drive various stages of smooth pursuit (Rashbass, 1961; Steinbach, 1976; Kowler, 1989). Two attention-related questions can be asked about the signals used in smooth pursuit:

(1) Is attention to each of these signals required for smooth pursuit?
(2) Is attention required for each of the different stages in smooth pursuit?

The empirical studies that address these questions are very recent, partly because our understanding about the nature of attention itself (e.g. Broadbent, 1958; Treisman and Gelade, 1980; Joseph et al., 1997; Nakayama and Joseph, 1997) as well as about the physiological control of smooth pursuit (Robinson, 1965; Lisberger et al., 1987; Newsome et al., 1988; Keller and Heinen, 1991; Chen et al., 1998; Heinen and Watamaniuk, 1998; Tanaka and Lisberger, 2001) have only recently been accumulated. Many theories and results acquired from studies on attention may be applied to address the two questions mentioned above, from which the attention control mechanisms of smooth pursuit can be putatively studied.

Of the signals used in smooth pursuit, visual detection of target movement is considered to be a

* Correspondence to: Y. Chen, Department of Psychiatry, Harvard Medical School/McLean Hospital, Belmont, MA 02478, USA. Tel.: +1-617-855-3615; Fax: +1-617-855-2778; E-mail: ychen@wjh.harvard.edu

necessary component as evidenced by the fact that continuous eye tracking can rarely occur or be sustained without the continuous presence of a moving target. Visual attention to a pursuit target was first appreciated based on phenomenological observations (Dodge and Fox, 1928), and has been explored in recent experimental studies (e.g. Khurana and Kowler, 1987; Ferrera and Lisberger, 1995). Based on the long history of research on this topic, a remaining question now is whether attention to visual signals is required for all stages of smooth pursuit. Moreover, the question about attention to non-visual signals, such as anticipation, in smooth pursuit has been rarely addressed.

Visual and non-visual attention

Everyone appears to know what attention is. But when it comes to the roles that attention plays in a specific behavioral process (such as smooth pursuit), the answer may become less clear to different people. According to William James (1890), attention can be described as "the taking possession of mind, in clear and vivid form, of one out of what seem several simultaneous possible objects or trains of thought." In this insightful remark, two types of attention are implicit, one visual and the other non-visual. The first type refers to the allocation of mind to one of 'several simultaneous possible objects'; this type of attention is what we now call visual attention. Control of visual attention is largely a bottom-up and stimulus-driven process. James' remark implies that visual attention is not an endless mental resource, i.e. one can pay attention only to one specific visual object at a time and has to withdraw attention from other visual objects at the same time, which was conceptualized later as limited capacity of attention (e.g. Moray, 1967). It is this type of conceptual thinking that guided many modern attention studies in the sensory, cognitive and motor domains.

For smooth pursuit eye movements, a common question that has been addressed in recent studies is how distraction of visual attention induced by a non-pursuit target affects the eye tracking responses. Khurana and Kowler (1987) showed that when observers tracked some moving letters with their eyes, the performance in a concurrent visual search for other letters was degraded, suggesting that the allocation of visual attention to smooth pursuit compromises the attention-demanding visual search task. Keller and Khan (1986) showed that initiation of smooth pursuit was adversely affected in monkeys when the pursuit target was presented in a textured background, results that have been confirmed later by other researchers (e.g. Kimmig et al., 1992; Mohrmann and Thier, 1995; Niemann and Hoffmann, 1997). Similarly, Ferrera and Lisberger (1995) showed that the initial smooth pursuit to a moving target in monkeys was compromised if a distractor moving in the opposite direction was presented at the same time. Recent brain imaging studies showed that when performing a smooth pursuit task, the activated brain areas, measured by regional cerebral blood flow, overlapped significantly with those when performing other attention-related tasks, implying that the same brain systems are recruited in these two types of tasks (Culham et al., 1998; Berman et al., 1999). These results support the notion that visual attention to selected targets is crucial for generating smooth pursuit eye movements.

It is natural to think that smooth pursuit requires visual attention because, after all, it is an eye tracking task to a selected visual target. It is not as apparent, however, to imagine that smooth pursuit also needs non-visual attention, such as keeping eye tracking in mind as a mental event or set that occurred previously or will occur soon in future. In James' remarks about attention, the second type (non-visual) refers to the allocation of the mind to one of 'trains of thought', which we call non-visual cognitive attention. In contrast to visual attention, non-visual cognitive attention is deployed to the physical and/or mental *events* that occur in the brain, but not necessarily to the physical *objects* in the visual world. Control of non-visual cognitive attention is a top-down and goal-directed process. Because of the roles of non-visual cognitive signals in smooth pursuit (Steinbach, 1976; Kowler, 1989), attention to visual signals may not be the only type of attentional resource that is used in controlling visual eye tracking.

Attentional controls for smooth pursuit

To control the dynamic and sustained oculomotor response involved in smooth pursuit, attentional resources must be continuously deployed. In order to study the role of visual and non-visual cognitive attention, one must control the attentional resources deployed at the different stages of smooth pursuit, because the signals that drive eye tracking differ from one stage to another.

One effective way to manipulate the allocation of attention is to introduce another behavioral task that is independent of smooth pursuit. In one experimental manipulation, we used a spatial frequency discrimination task for this purpose (Chen et al., 2000). Here, subjects are required to compare two static horizontal gratings, presented above and below the pursuit target, and judge which grating has a higher spatial frequency.

The rationale for this dual-task paradigm is based upon the limited capacity concept, that by engaging a secondary perceptual task that also requires attention, some amount of the attention used by smooth pursuit, the primary task, is taken away. This attentional redeployment from smooth pursuit to the secondary task should have an effect on the performance of the pursuit task. In principle, the effect of temporal transfer of attention between the pursuit task and the secondary task can be explained in terms of a psychological refractory period, a concept that is widely used to interpret the behavioral responses generated using dual-task paradigms (Smith, 1967; Pashler, 1994). The psychological refractory period refers to a time window within which a response to one signal has to be delayed or is impaired if a subject is already engaged in processing another previous signal. For a continuous process like smooth pursuit, the effect of a psychological refractory period takes place in the time period immediately after attention withdrawal by another (secondary) signal occurs (as depicted in Fig. 1).

Many behavioral responses, including saccadic eye movements, are discrete in nature, i.e. they are often non-continuous and abrupt events. Smooth pursuit eye movements, however, are gradual and continuous. One implication of these special temporal dynamics is that the design of experimental paradigms for smooth pursuit must take this temporal continuity characteristic into account. The dual-task paradigms are commonly used in studying discrete behavioral responses and must be modified in order to match the temporal dynamics of smooth pursuit. For assessment of the attention requirements in the whole process of smooth pursuit, one approach is to arrange the secondary task before (e.g. −200 ms), or at the same time as (0 ms), or after (e.g. +450 ms) the smooth pursuit task is presented (Fig. 2). The purpose of this time-locked attentional modulation is to determine the effects of attentional withdrawal on each of these different stages of smooth pursuit, allowing the roles of visual and non-visual cognitive attention to be examined.

Eye movements were recorded when subjects tracked a random dot pattern (Chen et al., 1998; Heinen and Watamaniuk, 1998). The pursuit target moved either to the left or to the right (randomized across trials) and at 10°/s. The apparatus for recording eye movements was a limbus eye tracker (Ober II EyeTrace System, Permobil Meditech AB, Sweden). Eye position signals were recorded in a computer and were aligned with target presentation for later off-line analysis. Eye velocities were derived by computing the first derivative of eye position signals after a low-pass filtering (Butterworth low pass filter, cut-off frequency 50 Hz). Eye accelerations were derived by computing the second derivative of eye position signals. Latencies of smooth pursuit were determined by inspection of eye movement records on a trial-by-trial basis.

From the single pursuit task to the pursuit/perceptual dual-task conditions, changes of eye track-

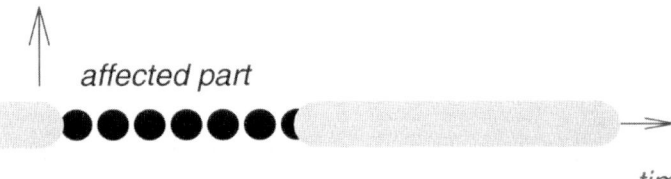

Fig. 1. Schematic illustration of the psychological refractory period during a continuous behavioral process. The black dots indicate the parts of the process (e.g. smooth pursuit) affected by attentional shift to another signal (e.g. spatial frequency discrimination) (the upward arrow), and are described as psychological refractory period.

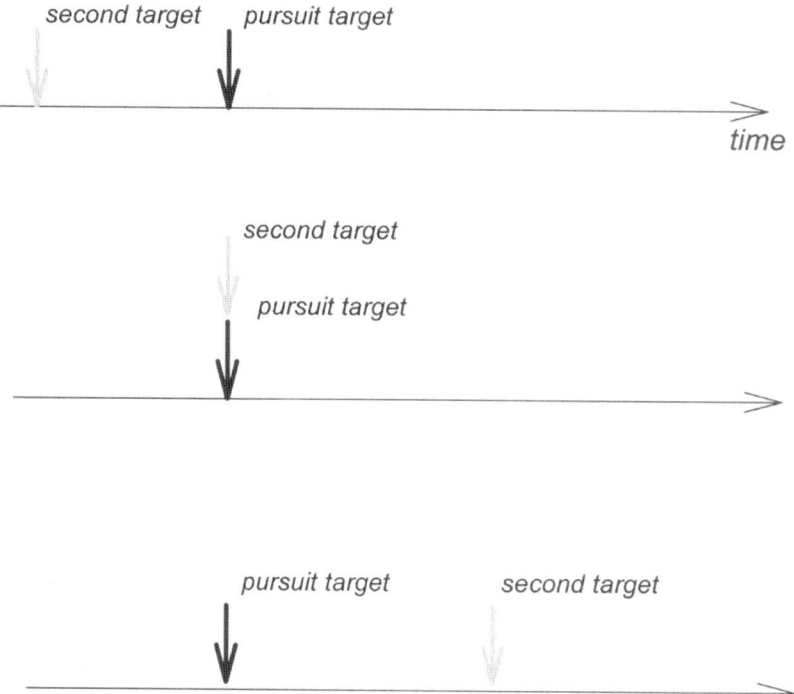

Fig. 2. Time-window locked attention withdrawal during smooth pursuit.

ing responses show a complex pattern (Chen et al., 2000), as shown in Fig. 3, and summarized in Fig. 4 and Table 1 below. In general, the eye movements under the dual-task conditions were less robust; that is, they showed delayed responding, sluggish accelerating and/or slow velocity compared with the single-task condition. A close examination of eye tracking in the three dual-task conditions reveals the following. (1) The triggering of smooth pursuit, measured by response latency, was affected only when the second task was present prior to or simultaneously with the pursuit task. (2) The initiation of smooth pursuit was affected no matter when the second task was presented. (3) The maintenance of smooth pursuit was affected primarily when the second task was present simultaneously with or after the pursuit task. The effects of the attentional withdrawal on smooth pursuit apparently depend on when the second task is introduced.

To understand how smooth pursuit is controlled by the attentional resources deployed at different stages, let us consider first the triggering stage of eye tracking in terms of the psychological refractory period. The delay of smooth pursuit occurs either

TABLE 1

Effects of attention withdrawal on smooth pursuit

Secondary task	Eye movement		
	Triggering (onset latency)	Initiating (initial acceleration)	Maintaining (sustained velocity)
Prior (−200 ms)	degraded	degraded	mildly degraded
Simultaneous (0 ms)	degraded	degraded	degraded
Delayed (+450 ms)	unaffected	degraded	degraded

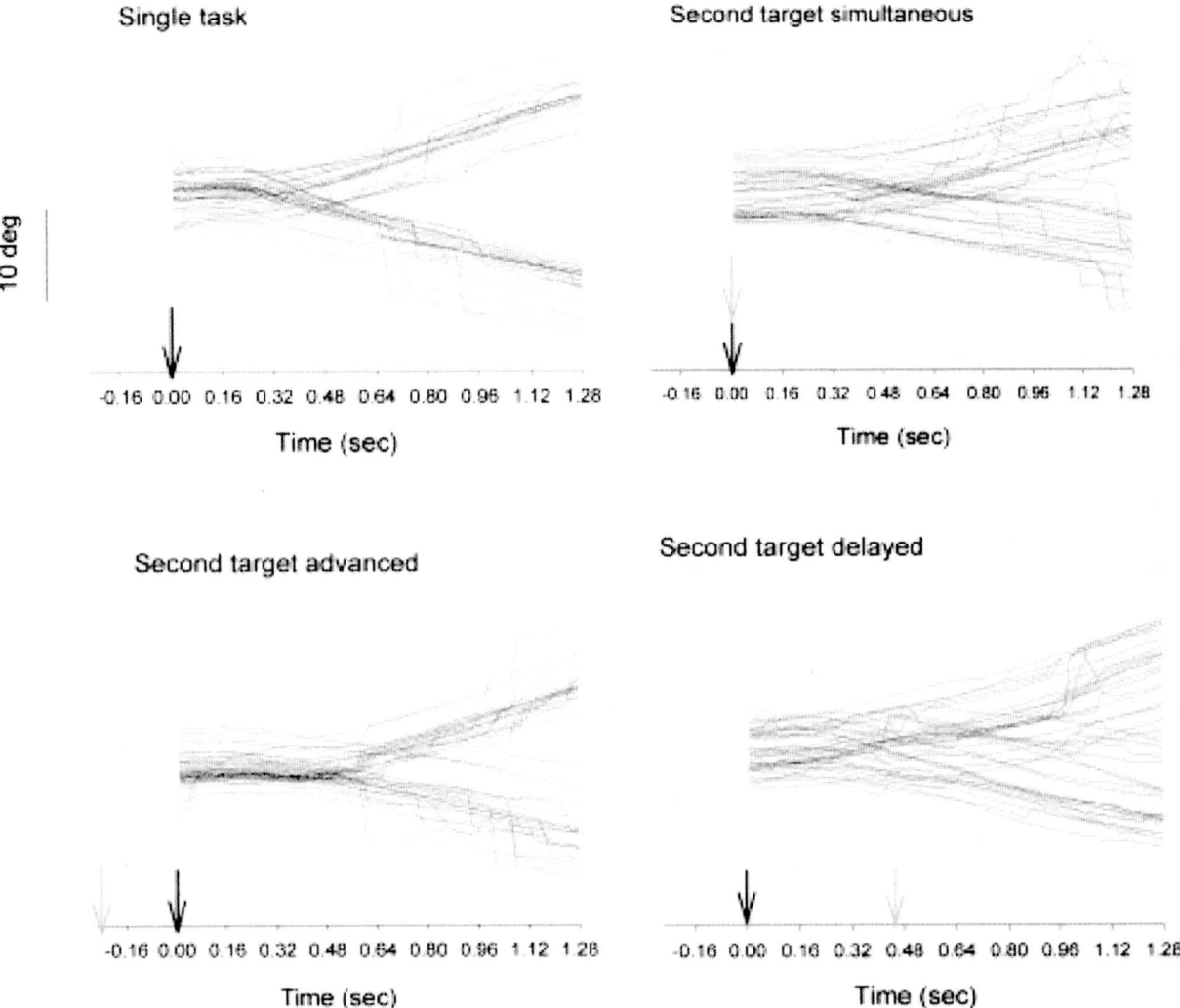

Fig. 3. Eye position traces under the single- and the three dual-task conditions (one subject).

when the second target is present before or when the pursuit and the second targets are presented at the same time. The psychological refractory period indicates that the deployment of visual attention to the perceptual target delays the triggering of smooth pursuit until after the signals from the non-pursuit target are completely processed. The concept also implies that if the non-pursuit target is presented later, the deployment of visual attention to the pursuit target should not be affected. Indeed, no delay of smooth pursuit under this dual-task condition indicates again the decisive roles of visual attention in triggering of smooth pursuit.

Visual attention alone, however, cannot explain the effects on initiating as well as on maintaining smooth pursuit. A slowing-down of smooth pursuit occurred when the non-pursuit target was present before, simultaneously with, and after the pursuit. According to the psychological refractory period, the slowing-down of smooth pursuit should not occur at the maintenance stage (starting at about 300 ms after the onset of pursuit target) if the non-pursuit target is presented before or at the same time with the pursuit target; this is so because the visual presentation of the non-pursuit target, which lasted only 100 ms, is long over when reaching this stage of eye movement.

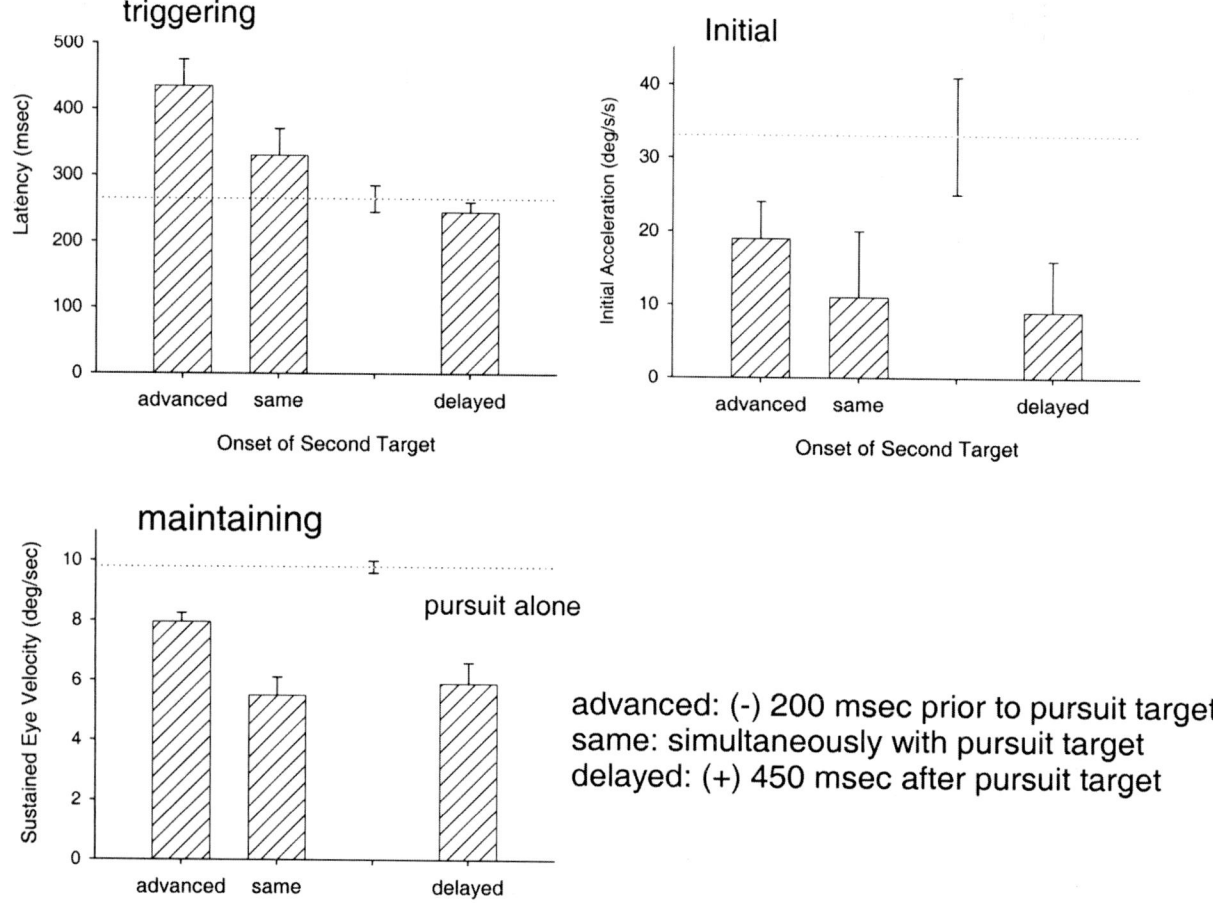

Fig. 4. Effects of attention withdrawal on the different stages of smooth pursuit. Data were averaged across three subjects. The error bars indicate ±1 standard error.

Thus, attention deployment to the second task, rather than to the visual presentation of the second target, appears to be responsible for slowing-down smooth pursuit. More telling is the sluggish initiation of smooth pursuit even before the non-pursuit target is present, because, under such a condition, visual attention to the later non-pursuit target has not yet been deployed and should not affect the initiating of smooth pursuit at all. The sluggish initiation of smooth pursuit must be attributed to the attentional deployment to non-visual aspects of the second task.

To better understand the nature of the non-visual attentional deployment, consider the second task as an event that begins as a trial starts, which happens before the visual presentation of the second target under this dual-task condition. When subjects performed the pursuit task first, they anticipated performing another impending task. Attention to the anticipated event, the second task, exacts a cost from the ongoing smooth pursuit, as expressed in a sluggish initiation of smooth pursuit. In this sense, the psychological refractory period means that attention deployment to the anticipation of the second task interferes with the initiating of smooth pursuit; the processing of the cognitive, not the visual, signals associated with the second task competes for attention with the pursuit task. This competition can occur long before the appearance of visual signals associated with the second task. Note that the deployment of the non-visual cognitive attention to the second task has no effect on the triggering of smooth pursuit (see the Table 1).

How can these diverse attentional resources be used to control smooth pursuit? Among the current models of attentional control of behavioral processes, the structural model (e.g. Broadbent, 1958) and the capacity model (Moray, 1967) appear to be useful in understanding the effects of attention withdrawal on smooth pursuit.

According to the structural model, attention is controlled within each domain, as depicted by the gray bands in Fig. 5. When two processes in one structure, e.g. domain 1, compete for attention, the attention controlling mechanisms modulate only the responses mediated within this structure (left panel in Fig. 5) and do not affect the responses mediated in other structures, e.g. domain 2, ... N. For example, in the instance of smooth pursuit, visual attention to a secondary visual signal (arrow) interferes only with visual attention to the pursuit signal (domain 1). Domain 2, ..., N here represent processes in non-visual domains and have minimal effects on smooth pursuit. Thus, the interference between the two responses is specific to the structure (domain) or mechanism that mediated these competing processes. In the capacity model, however, attention is controlled by an overall structure (domain). When two processes compete for attention, all responses are affected whether or not these processes are mediated in the same or different structures or mechanisms (right panel in Fig. 4). In this case, modulation of cognitive attention in non-visual domains affects smooth pursuit to visual signals. Thus, the interference between the two responses is not specific to one structure or mechanism. To understand attentional deployment between different tasks, both models may be needed because attentional modulation of actual behavioral responses is more flexible than is expected from the structure model; there the bottleneck for each structure controls only the response in that structure. On the other hand, attentional modulation of actual behavioral responses is more constrained than is expected from the capacity model, in which allocation of the attentional resources across different structures can be made without any restriction.

Our results show that the visual attention control mechanisms for smooth pursuit, from onset and initiation to maintenance, are more consistent with the structural model whereas the non-visual cognitive attentional control mechanisms for initiating as well as maintaining of smooth pursuit is more consistent with the capacity model. For the sake

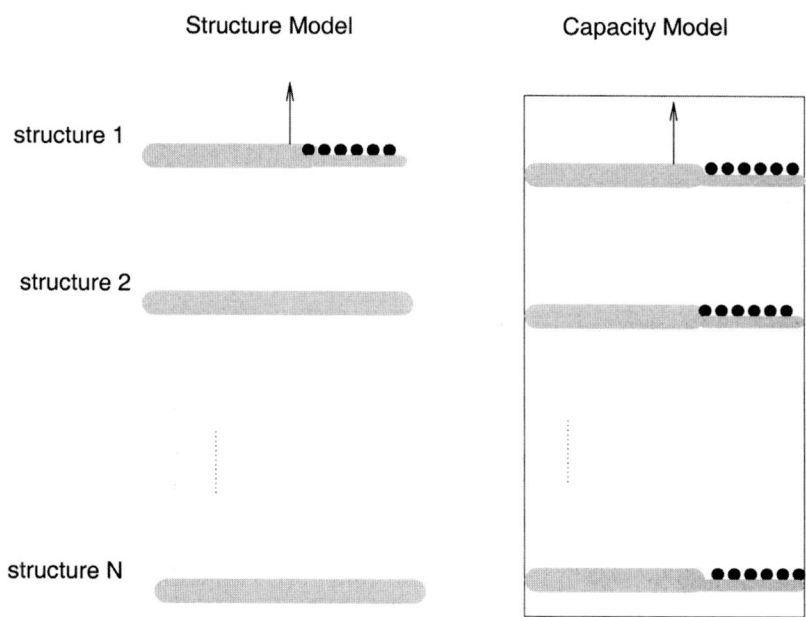

Fig. 5. Schematic illustration of the structural (left) and the capacity model of attention control.

of understanding the smooth pursuit results, let us consider visual processing as being in one structure and cognitive processing in another. In our experiments, the interfering smooth pursuit resulting from the competition for visual attention occurred only when the targets for the two tasks were presented together within a short time window. For example, the latency of smooth pursuit was prolonged when the target for the second task appeared shortly before (-200 ms) or simultaneously with the pursuit target, but not when the target for the second task was long delayed for 450 ms. That is to say, smooth pursuit in this triggering stage is influenced primarily by visual attention mechanisms. The structural model can characterize the visual attentional control better than the capacity model because *visual* eye tracking is affected mainly by the withdrawal of *visual* attention from another target. The non-visual cognitive attentional control mechanisms, such as the one for anticipating of the second task, play minor roles in this stage of smooth pursuit.

On the other hand, we can see that the interference resulting from the competition for non-visual cognitive attention occurs long before the target for the second task appears in the visual field. For example, the initial acceleration of smooth pursuit had already decreased when the target for the second task appeared 450 ms later, indicating that smooth pursuit in this initiating stage is also controlled by non-visual cognitive attentional mechanisms. The capacity model can characterize the non-visual cognitive attentional control better because *visual* eye tracking is affected not only by the visual aspect but also by *non-visual* cognitive attention, namely anticipation, to the secondary task. Unlike visual attentional control, the non-visual cognitive attentional control appears to embrace only the initiation and the maintenance of smooth pursuit, and affects eye tracking accuracy beyond the time period when visual attention withdrawal occurs.

The brain systems involved in smooth pursuit include occipital, parietal and frontal cortices. Damage to any of these brain areas can disrupt the process of eye tracking (e.g. Heide et al., 1996; Lekwuwa and Barnes, 1996). The parsing of attentional controls for smooth pursuit offers a theoretical basis on which the neural substrates of the complex oculomotor responses may be decomposed. In other words, this parsing may be carried out by identifying the role that different types of attention play in processing associated visual and cognitive signals. In this regard, a recent report on two types of attentional deficits, one on a transient task and the other on a sustained task, in patients with parietal damage is quite relevant (Battelli et al., 2001); the visual and non-visual cognitive attention mechanisms may show quite different temporal properties. And the brain systems for control of stimulus-driven and goal-directed attention are not the same; the bottom-up stimulus-driven system involves temporoparietal and inferiofrontal cortices whereas the top-down goal-directed system involves intraparietal and superior frontal cortices (Luo et al., 1998; Corbetta and Shulman, 2002).

Comparison with other types of behavioral processes

Compared with other behavioral processes, smooth pursuit eye movements have several distinct features with respect to attentional control. The most obvious one is the temporal continuity of the oculomotor tracking. Because of this temporal property, it is expected that allocation of attention for smooth pursuit is more distributed in the time domain than for non-continuous behavioral processes. For saccadic eye movements, the attentional requirements are modest and the attentional allocation is mainly around the time that the saccade target appears (Kowler et al., 1995). The temporally ballistic nature of attentional control of saccade eye movement is comparable to that of the visual attentional control for triggering smooth pursuit. In contrast, the non-visual cognitive attention controls for initiating and maintaining smooth pursuit are more temporally distributed. They do not have to be linked to a specific instant but rather to a whole event. The temporally distributed pattern of attentional allocation may reflect an optimal strategy for continuous recruitment and for continuous use of the limited capacity of attentional resources in smooth pursuit. At the same time, however, this continuous cognitive attentional requirement may allow smooth pursuit to be exposed to various disturbances over a longer period of time. This may be related to the fact that smooth pursuit, more than other types of eye movements, is susceptible to various central nervous system insults (Sharpe and Sylvester, 1978; Sibony et al., 1988; Thurston et al., 1988).

The visual and cognitive aspects of attentional control for smooth pursuit may also be understood by analogy to the visual and attentive tracking of flashed stimuli that evoke apparent motion perception. Visual detection of apparent motion is a highly transient process, as reflected by its high temporal resolution of about 50–60 Hz (Pantle, 1978). This temporal property of detecting apparent motion is analogous to that of visual attentional control in smooth pursuit, in which two visual targets compete for attention resources only when they are temporally adjacent. In contrast, attentive tracking — the application of non-visual mental effort to follow a visually ambiguous target (e.g. flashed stimuli) — is not a transient process and it has a low temporal resolution of about 7–8 Hz (Verstraten et al., 2000). This temporal property of attentive tracking is analogous to that of non-visual cognitive control in smooth pursuit, in which the competition between pursuit and another task for attention can be stretched over a relatively long time period.

The spatiotemporal distribution of attention should benefit not only smooth pursuit but also the task that is associated with smooth pursuit in real space–time, since attentional resources are presumably allocated with the attention-demanding pursuit task. Van Donkelaar (1999) compared the detection of a non-pursuit target that is close to the pursuit target with the detection of a non-pursuit target that is not close, and found that reaction time was shorter for the target that was closer, suggesting that smooth pursuit indeed grabs and holds attention as the eye tracks the target through space. This spatial aspect of visual attention control in smooth pursuit is similar to that in saccadic eye movements (McPeek et al., 1999) in that both processes require focal attention, rather than distributed attention.

The taking possession of attention is helpful for smooth pursuit and most, but not all, other behavioral processes. In the case of antisaccadic eye movements, less attention is more efficient in triggering the complex oculomotor response (Kristjansson et al., 2001). Since antisaccade eye movements are primarily driven by cognitive signals, it is not surprising that attentional control for the triggering stage of this eye movement differs from that of smooth pursuit.

Old paradox and new quest

This study suggests that two types of attention are used in the control of smooth pursuit. Visual attention is a determining factor for triggering the onset of smooth pursuit. Non-visual cognitive attention contributes to the high accuracy of eye tracking, which is achieved some time later after its onset. A distinct difference between the two types of attention is that the visual attention is much more transient than non-visual cognitive attention in the control of smooth pursuit.

Unlike other voluntary eye movements, namely, saccades, smooth pursuit cannot be initiated without the presence of a moving stimulus, and cannot be sustained very long after the disappearance of the pursuit target. This involuntary property is often taken as evidence for the role of visual stimulation in generating smooth pursuit. On the other hand, one can argue that visual attention cannot be deployed if the pursuit target to which one needs to attend is not available. Thus, the presence of a visual target and the deployment of visual attention appear to be the necessary dual-conditions for generating smooth pursuit. This visual attention comprises both voluntary and non-voluntary components (Holzman et al., 1976). In order to achieve and maintain accurate eye tracking, non-visual cognitive attention also needs to be engaged. A deep question is whether attention is just an effect or a cause of smooth pursuit. This dilemma of stimulus vs. attention may not be helpful if we view it only from a chicken–egg perspective. Instead, we regard the two processes as a competitive or complementary ones between sensory and attention components in the control of smooth pursuit eye movements. Attention is more critical when a visual stimulus is not salient than when it is salient. On the contrary, salience of a stimulus is more critical if attention to the stimulus is partly deployed somewhere else.

In most visual perception tasks, no one can possibly attend to the targets continuously; the focus has to drift among different targets. Smooth pursuit eye tracking represents one of the few conditions under which attention can be engaged on a target for a prolonged period of time. Therefore, eye tracking responses can be used to study the temporal dynamics of attention, either transient or sustained aspects.

Visual attention provides necessary control mechanisms for triggering smooth pursuit eye movements. After its onset, smooth pursuit also requires non-visual cognitive attention controls in order to achieve and maintain a high accuracy of eye tracking. The dynamics and continuous allocation of the two types of attention in smooth pursuit provide a model for understanding how a complex behavioral process applies the powerful, and yet limited, mental efforts supplied by the brain.

Acknowledgements

This work was supported in part by NIH, NARSAD and AFOSR grants. We thank Ms. Summer Sheremata for comments on an earlier version of this chapter.

References

Battelli, L., Cavanagh, P., Intriligator, J., Tramo, M., Henaff, M.A., Michel, F. and Barton, J. (2001) Unilateral right parietal damage leads to bilateral deficit for high-level motion. *Neuron*, 32: 985–995.

Berman, R.A., Colby, C.L., Genovese, C.R., Voyvodic, J.T., Luna, B., Thulborn, K.R. and Sweeney, J.A. (1999) Cortical networks subserving pursuit and saccadic eye movements in humans: an FMRI study. *Hum. Brain Mapp.*, 8(4): 209–225.

Broadbent, D. (1958) *Perception and Communication*. Pergamon, Oxford.

Chen, Y., McPeek, R., Intriligator, J., Holzman, P. and Nakayama, K. (1998) Smooth pursuit to a movement flow and associated perceptual judgments. In: (Eds.), *Current Oculomotor Research: Physiological and Psychological Perspectives*. Plenum, New York, pp. 125–128.

Chen, Y., McPeek, R., Intriligator, J., Kristjonssan, A., Mednick, S., Holzman, P., Nakayama., K. (2000) Attentional requirements for smooth pursuit. *Invest. Ophthalnol. Vis. Sci.*, V40: S381.

Corbetta, M. and Shulman, G.L. (2002) Control of goal-directed and stimulus-driven attention in the brain. *Nat. Rev. Neurosci.*, 3: 215–229.

Culham, J.C., Brandt, S.A., Cavanagh, P., Kanwisher, N.G., Dale, A.M. and Tootell, R.B. (1998) Cortical fMRI activation produced by attentive tracking of moving targets. *J. Neurophysiol.*, 80(5): 2657–2670.

Dodge, R. and Fox, J.C. (1928) Optic nystagmus. *Arch. Neurol. Psychiat.*, 24: 21–34.

Ferrera, V. and Lisberger, S.G. (1995) Attention and target selection for smooth pursuit eye movements. *J. Neurosci.*, 15: 7472–7484.

Heide, W., Kurzidim, K. and Kompf, D. (1996) Deficits of smooth pursuit eye movements after frontal and parietal lesions. *Brain*, 119(Pt 6): 1951–1969.

Heinen, S. and Watamaniuk, S. (1998) Spatial summation in smooth pursuit. *Vision Res.*, 38: 3785–3794.

Holzman, P.S., Levy, D.L. and Proctor, L.R. (1976) Smooth pursuit eye movements, attention, and schizophrenia. *Arch. Gen. Psychiatry*, 33: 1415–1420.

Joseph, J.S., Chun, M.M. and Nakayama, K. (1997) Attentional requirements in a 'preattentive' feature search task. *Nature*, 387: 805–807.

Keller, E.L. and Heinen, S.J. (1991) Generation of smooth-pursuit eye movements: neuronal mechanisms and pathways. *Neurosci. Res.*, 11(2): 79–107.

Keller, E. and Khan, E. (1986) Smooth-pursuit initiation in the presence of a textured background in monkey. *Vision Res.*, 36: 943–955.

Khurana, B. and Kowler, E. (1987) Shared attentional control of smooth pursuit eye movement and perception. *Vision Res.*, 27: 1603–1618.

Kimmig, H.G., Miles, F.A. and Schwarz, U. (1992) Effects of stationary textured backgrounds on the initiation of pursuit eye movements in monkeys. *J. Neurophysiol.*, 68(6): 2147–2164.

Kowler, E. (1989) Cognitive expectations, not habits, control anticipatory smooth oculomotor pursuit. *Vision Res.*, 29: 1049–1057.

Kowler, E., Anderson, E., Dosher, B. and Blaser, E. (1995) The roles of attention in the programming of saccades. *Vision Res.*, 35: 1897–1916.

Kristjansson, A., Chen, Y. and Nakayama, K. (2001) Less attention is more in the preparation of antisaccades, but not prosaccades. *Nat. Neurosci.*, 4(10): 1037–1042.

Lekwuwa, G.U. and Barnes, G.R. (1996) Cerebral control of eye movements I. The relationship between cerebral lesion sites and smooth pursuit deficits. *Brain*, 119: 473–490.

Lisberger, S.G., Morris, E.J. and Tychsen, L. (1987) Visual motion processing and sensory–motor integration for smooth pursuit eye movements. *Annu. Rev. Neurosci.*, 10: 97–129.

Luo, C.R., Anderson, J.M. and Caramazza, A. (1998) Impaired stimulus-driven orienting of attention and preserved goal-directed orienting of attention in unilateral visual neglect. *Am. J. Psychol.*, 11(4): 487–507.

McPeek, R.M., Maljkovic, V. and Nakayama, K. (1999) Saccades require focal attention and are facilitated by a short-term memory system. *Vision Res.*, 39(8): 1555–1566.

Mohrmann, H. and Thier, P. (1995) The influence of structured visual backgrounds on smooth-pursuit initiation, steady-state pursuit and smooth-pursuit termination. *Biol. Cybern.*, 73(1): 83–93.

Moray, N. (1967) Where is capacity limited? A survey and a model. *Acta Psychol.*, 27: 84–92.

Nakayama, K. and Joseph, J. (1997) Attention, pattern recognition and popout in visual search. In: R. Parasuraman (Ed.), *The Attentive Brain*. MIT Press, Cambridge, MA, pp. 279–298.

Newsome, W.T., Wurtz, R.H. and Komatsu, H. (1988) Relation of cortical areas MT and MST to pursuit eye movements. II. Differentiation of retinal from extraretinal inputs. *J. Neurophysiol.*, 60(2): 604–620.

Niemann, T. and Hoffmann, K.P. (1997) The influence of stationary and moving textured backgrounds on smooth-pursuit initiation and steady state pursuit in humans. *Exp. Brain Res.*, 115(3): 531–640.

Pantle, A.J. (1978) Temporal frequency response characteristic of motion channels measured with three different psychophysical techniques. *Percept. Psychophys.*, 24(3): 285–294.

Pashler, H. (1994) Graded capacity-sharing in dual-task interference? *J. Exp. Psychol. Hum. Percept. Perform.*, 20: 330–342.

Rashbass, C. (1961) The relationship between saccadic and smooth tracking eye movements. *J. Physiol. London*, 159: 326–338.

Robinson, D.A. (1965) The mechanics of human smooth pursuit eye movements. *J. Physiol.*, 159: 338–362.

Sharpe, J.A. and Sylvester, T.O. (1978) Effect of aging on horizontal smooth pursuit. *Invest. Ophthalmol. Vis. Sci.*, 17: 465–468.

Sibony, P.A., Evinger, C. and Manning, K.A. (1988) The effects of tobacco smoking on smooth pursuit eye movements. *Annu. Neurol.*, 23: 238–241.

Smith, M.C. (1967) Theories of the psychological refractory period *Psychol. Bull.*, 67: 202–213.

Steinbach, M.J. (1976) Pursuing the perceptual rather than the retinal stimulus. *Vision Res.*, 16: 1371–1376.

Tanaka, M. and Lisberger, S.G. (2001) Regulation of the gain of visually guided smooth-pursuit eye movements by frontal cortex. *Nature*, 409(6817): 191–194.

Thurston, S.E., Leigh, R.J., Crawford, T., Thompson, A. and Kennard, C. (1988) Two distinct deficits of visual tracking caused by unilateral lesions of cerebral cortex in humans. *Annu. Neurol.*, 23: 266–273.

Treisman, A. and Gelade, G. (1980) A feature-integration theory of attention. *Cognit. Psychol.*, 12: 97–136.

Van Donkelaar, P. (1999) Spatiotemporal modulation of attention during smooth pursuit eye movements. *Neuroreport*, 10(12): 2523–2526.

Verstraten, F.A., Cavanagh, P. and Labianca, A.T. (2000) Limits of attentive tracking reveal temporal properties of attention. *Vision Res.*, 40(26): 3651–3664.

Westheimer, G. (1954) Eye movement responses to a horizontally moving visual stimulus. *Arch. Ophthalmol.*, 52: 932–941.

CHAPTER 18

The allocation of attention during smooth pursuit eye movements

Paul Van Donkelaar* and Anthony S. Drew

Department of Exercise and Movement Science, Institute of Neuroscience, University of Oregon, Eugene, OR 97403-1240, USA

Abstract: The spatial–temporal allocation of attention during smooth pursuit eye movements is poorly understood. In this chapter we review evidence showing that attention contributes to both saccades and smooth pursuit. We then discuss results from our own recent studies using a dual-task paradigm in which subjects pursued a moving stimulus and pressed a button when targets appeared in the periphery. The results from these studies are consistent with the hypothesis that the allocation of attention is biased to a location just in front of the pursuit stimulus and that this bias can be altered by pursuit velocity.

Introduction

Attention allows us to detect and discriminate selected stimuli while effectively excluding most other stimuli impinging on sensory receptors. The benefits which accrue as a result of paying attention include decreased latencies in determining that a stimulus is present and increased sensitivity to subtle changes in the characteristics of the stimulus. In addition to these contributions to visual perception, attention also contributes to the accurate production of eye movements. While most of the work related to this issue has focussed on the contribution of attention to saccades, there is also evidence to suggest that attention contributes to smooth pursuit. We have recently undertaken a series of experiments that explicitly addresses the mechanisms underlying the spatio-temporal allocation of attention during pursuit. In what follows we will first review the evidence

---

* Correspondence to: P. Van Donkelaar, Department of Exercise and Movement Science, Institute of Neuroscience, 122C Esslinger Hall, University of Oregon, Eugene, OR 97403-1240, USA. Tel.: +1-541-346-2687; Fax: +1-541-346-2841; E-mail: paulvd@darkwing.uoregon.edu

demonstrating the role of attention during saccades. Next, we will discuss previous studies which suggest that a relationship between attention and smooth pursuit exists. Finally, we will review some of our own recent work that directly examines this relationship.

Attention and saccadic eye movements

Although visual attention is typically paid to the objects we are looking at, it can also be directed to locations away from the current fixation point of the eyes. Indeed, there is considerable evidence for the view that the spatial allocation of attention to selected objects is functionally linked to the generation of saccades to those targets (Fischer, 1999). This idea is supported by the fact that the areas of the brain that are activated during covert shifts of attention overlap to a substantial degree with those that are activated by saccadic eye movements (Corbetta, 1998). Further evidence for the influence of attention on saccadic eye movements comes from studies in which attention is directed to a different location than the saccade target. Kustov and Robinson (1996) examined this issue by comparing saccades evoked by stimulation of the superior colliculus during simple fixation and following attentional shifts to peripheral locations. During fixation stimulation at specific collicular sites elicits saccades of a fixed direction and amplitude. In contrast, stimulation at the same site following a shift of attention results in saccades that are deviated in the direction of the attentional shift. Analogous deviations in the trajectories of voluntarily generated saccades have been observed in human subjects when required to direct attention to locations that are dissociated from the saccade target (Sheliga et al., 1994, 1995). Saccades generated under these conditions also take longer to initiate and are less accurate than those produced when the locus of attention and the saccade target are coincident (Hoffman and Subramaniam, 1995; Kowler et al., 1995; Deubel and Schneider, 1996). Taken together, these results suggest that directing attention to a spatial location other than the saccade target has a direct impact on oculomotor programming.

Attention, visual motion processing, and smooth pursuit eye movements

Unlike the large body of research devoted to the role of attention in saccades, less is known about the mechanisms underlying the allocation of attention during smooth pursuit. There is, however, evidence which demonstrates that attention contributes to the processes underlying smooth pursuit output. First, to accurately pursue a visual stimulus the CNS must determine the velocity of the stimulus. Neurophysiological and functional imaging studies have demonstrated that neurons in the middle temporal (MT) and medial superior temporal (MST) areas are activated by visual motion stimulation (Zeki et al., 1991; Salzman and Newsome, 1994) and contribute to smooth pursuit output (Newsome et al., 1988; Barton et al., 1996). More recently, it has been demonstrated that the activity in these same areas is enhanced when the viewer is required to pay attention to a specific attribute of the visual motion (Treue and Maunsell, 1996; Beauchamp et al., 1997; Culham et al., 1998; Seidemann and Newsome, 1999; Treue and Martinez Trujillo, 1999). Thus, paying attention to visual motion influences the activity in CNS circuits involved in the initial transformation of sensory–perceptual information into subsequent smooth pursuit output. Moreover, the regions of the brain that functionally overlap for shifts of attention and saccade generation (see above) also contain cells that are involved in visual motion processing (Colby et al., 1993; Schaafsma and Duysens, 1996) and smooth pursuit output (MacAvoy et al., 1991; Petit et al., 1997; Shi et al., 1998).

Second, when a distractor target is present an attentionally modulated selection process occurs prior to pursuit initiation (Ferrera and Lisberger, 1995). The direction of motion of the distractor target systematically influences the initial pursuit response: latency is substantially increased when the distractor moves in the opposite direction to the pursuit target compared to when the two targets move in the same direction. Moreover, when the distractor target starts moving 100 ms prior to or after the onset of the pursuit target motion, the magnitude of this latency effect is markedly reduced (Ferrera and Lisberger, 1997a). Ferrera and Lisberger (1997b) have also demonstrated that a subset of cells in MT and MST display predictive modulatory activity during this task that may partially account for the behavioral observations. Taken together, these results are consistent with the notion that attention contributes during a finite window of time to the initiation of pursuit responses and that this contribution is partially mediated by the activity of motion processing cells in MT and MST.

Third, there is a correlation between attentional problems and visual motion processing and smooth pursuit deficits in individuals suffering from schizophrenia. These patients have difficulty covertly shifting attention to peripheral locations in space (Maruff et al., 1995; Moran et al., 1996; Sereno and Holzman, 1996). In addition, they display a reduced smooth pursuit gain (Friedman et al., 1995) and decreased visual motion processing abilities (Chen et al., 1999). Analogous attentional (McDonald et al., 1999) and smooth pursuit (Jacobsen et al., 1996) problems have been demonstrated in children suffering from attention deficit hyperactivity disorder (ADHD). The coexistence of these deficits in schizophrenic and ADHD individuals provides further evidence that attention may normally contribute to the processes underlying smooth pursuit.

Given that there appears to be a relation between attentional and pursuit processes, the next question that can be addressed is: what is the nature of this relation? Intuitively, the most obvious answer to this question is that attention helps us to pursue the target more effectively. The fact that we pay attention to the pursuit target is confirmed by the evidence that subjects can perform visual search tasks more quickly and accurately for target displays that are being pursued than for those that are not (Kowler and Zingale, 1985; Khurana and Kowler, 1987). Moreover, when subjects are required to allocate more attention than normal to the target that is being tracked, pursuit gain actually increases (Van Gelder et al., 1990).

The allocation of attention during pursuit

Although the research described above points to a tight relation between attention and smooth pursuit, it is not yet clear how attention is allocated either spatially or temporally during pursuit output. Some insight into this question can be gained by examining the characteristics of saccades directed at peripheral targets presented during ongoing pursuit. Such saccades have been shown to be initiated more quickly (Krauzlis and Miles, 1996; Tanaka et al., 1998) and completed more accurately (Gellman and Fletcher, 1992) for targets appearing ahead of the pursuit stimulus compared to those appearing in its wake. One interpretation of these effects is that more attention is allocated ahead of the pursuit target than behind it. This is based on the assumption that targets can be more quickly and accurately localized if attention is directed to the region of space in which they appear (Posner, 1980). However, these results may be partly confounded by differences in the orbital mechanics associated with making onward vs. backward saccades. In other words, biomechanically it may be simpler to generate the necessary changes in ocular muscle force required to produce a saccade to a target appearing beyond the pursuit stimulus than arresting eye motion and subsequently producing a saccade to a target appearing behind the pursuit stimulus. Although Tanaka and coworkers (1998) suggested that this is not likely to account for their observed latency effect because of the low velocities associated with pursuit responses (Robinson, 1965), it nevertheless is possible to test for this more directly. In particular, we have completed a series of recent experiments that made use of a new dual-task paradigm (Van Donkelaar, 1999; Drew and Van Donkelaar, 2002). Instead of making saccades

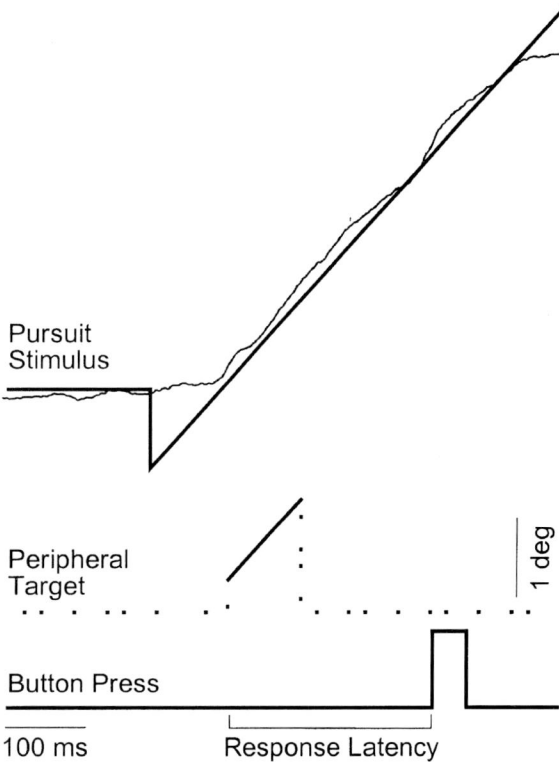

Fig. 1. Typical trial of the dual-task pursuit paradigm. Top part of figure shows step-ramp target motion (thick trace) and resulting pursuit eye movement (thin trace). Middle portion shows peripheral target. Dashed line, target not present; solid line, target present. Bottom portion shows output of response button with latency being defined as the time from the appearance of the peripheral target to the onset of the button press.

to targets appearing in the periphery during pursuit, subjects were required to react as quickly as possible to this event by pressing a button with the finger (Fig. 1). If more attention is directed to a particular portion of space around the pursuit stimulus then manual response latencies should be quicker for targets appearing in that location than in others. Thus, if more attention were directed ahead of the pursuit target, as the results from the saccadic studies cited above seem to suggest, then manual button pressing latencies should be shorter for peripheral targets appearing ahead of the pursuit stimulus than for those appearing behind it. In addition to examining attentional allocation across space, any variations in attention across time were assessed by presenting the peripheral targets during the onset, maintenance, or offset of the pursuit response. In this way it was possible to determine whether different pursuit epochs require more or less attentional resources.

Attention is not distributed evenly during pursuit

Fig. 2 displays the manual button pressing latencies for peripheral targets appearing 2.5° ahead of versus in the wake of the pursuit stimulus during the onset, maintenance, and offset of the pursuit response. Both the peripheral target and the pursuit stimulus moved rightwards at 10°/s. Clearly, latency varied as a function of both peripheral target location and pursuit epoch. Latencies were quicker for peripheral targets appearing ahead of the pursuit stimulus than for those appearing in its wake. In addition, latencies were quickest overall when the peripheral target appeared during pursuit maintenance. These results have several implications. First, they demonstrate that at each stage of the pursuit response, attention was directed ahead of the pursuit stimulus. Thus, when a peripheral target appeared there, reaction times were quicker than when the peripheral target appeared in the wake of the pursuit stimulus. Second,

these results imply that pursuit maintenance is less attention demanding overall than either the initiation or termination of pursuit. This makes sense when one considers the changes that occur during these epochs. During pursuit onset, for example, the subject must determine when pursuit motion begins and, depending upon the context, which direction and at what speed it is travelling. All of this information must then be transformed into the initial pursuit response. Presumably, these processes (as well as those required to terminate the response) are much more attention demanding than those required to maintain ongoing pursuit of a target moving at a constant velocity. Taken together, these results suggest that attention is not distributed evenly across either space or time during pursuit output.

Spatial extent of attention during pursuit

The first experiment used a single target appearing at a constant eccentricity (2.5°) in the periphery relative to the pursuit stimulus. Because of this limitation, it was impossible to determine the spatial extent to which attention was directed ahead of the pursuit stimulus. This issue was directly examined in a second experiment in which the pursuit stimulus was surrounded by 8 peripheral targets (4 ahead and 4 behind) each separated by 1°. During individual trials, one of these peripheral targets or the pursuit stimulus itself changed shape (from an 'x' to an 'o', or vice versa) and the subject was required to react to this event by pressing a button with the right index finger. Fig. 3A displays the manual button pressing latencies for each of these target locations for changes occurring during rightwards pursuit maintenance. This figure shows a tendency for subjects to have shorter latencies for target changes occurring up to 2° ahead of the pursuit stimulus, as well as at the pursuit stimulus itself compared to other target eccentricities. To quantify this trend in the data we computed the percent latency difference at each peripheral target eccentricity relative to the response latency when the pursuit stimulus changed shape. A graph of this measure reveals a dip for target changes occurring 1–2° ahead of the pursuit stimulus (Fig. 3B). This pattern of latencies suggests that attention is preferentially directed at, and just in front of, the pursuit stimulus.

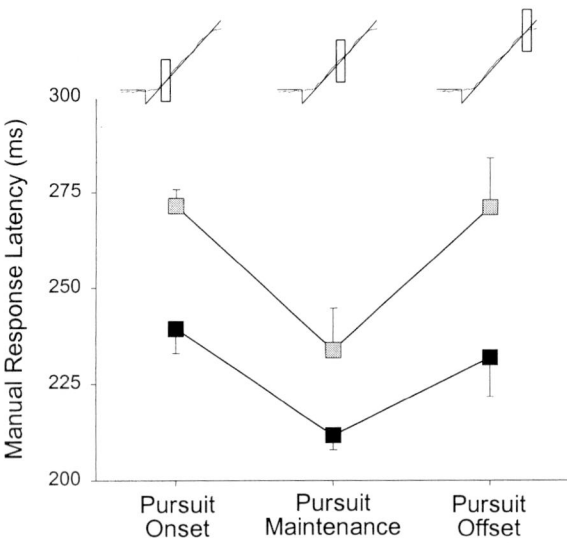

Fig. 2. Group medians for response latency when the peripheral target appeared ahead of (black squares) versus behind (gray squares) the pursuit stimulus during pursuit onset, maintenance, and offset. The images at the top of the figure show the period during which the peripheral target was present superimposed on a typical pursuit trajectory. Error bars, 1 SE.

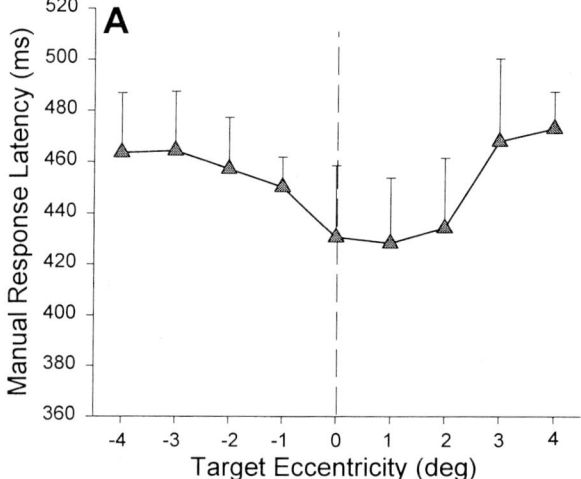
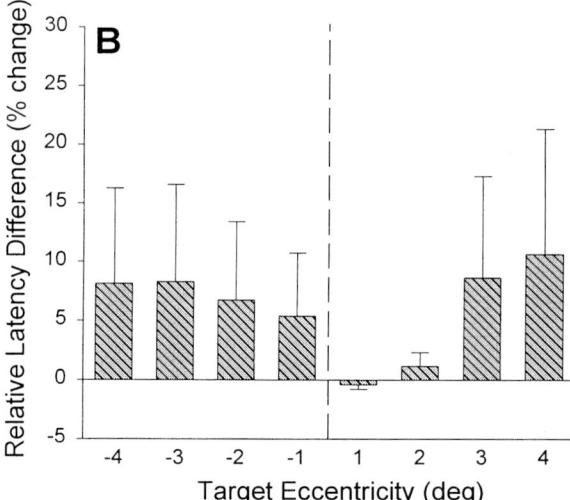

Fig. 3. (A) Group medians for response latency when the peripheral target (or pursuit stimulus) changed shape during pursuit maintenance. (B) Group means for the percentage change in response latency at each peripheral target location relative to that observed when the pursuit stimulus changed. Error bars, 1 SE.

Changes in the allocation of attention at different pursuit velocities

Having demonstrated that attention is directed at or just ahead of the pursuit stimulus, our next goal was to characterize how the attentional allocation may change with different pursuit velocities. In the previous experiments the pursuit stimulus moved at 10°/s. When pursuit velocities of 3, 5, and 15°/s were used, several noteworthy changes occurred in the pattern of response latencies (Fig. 4A). The first change is that there was an increase in the latency of the responses as pursuit velocity increased. This could be due to two factors. First, the changes in the targets may be more difficult to detect when the eye and the targets are moving at a faster velocity. Second, maintaining pursuit at higher velocities may be a more attention-demanding task. In particular, eye velocity is more likely to undershoot target velocity and result in a closer monitoring of any retinal slip. These two possibilities could be differentiated by using a probe reaction time task with nonspatial auditory cues rather than visual targets. If the increased latencies at higher pursuit velocities are due only to difficulty visually detecting the peripheral target, then reaction times to the auditory cues should not be influenced by increasing pursuit velocity. However, if the effect is due to increased attentional demands, then auditory reaction times should be affected by increasing pursuit velocity. The second change in the pattern of response latencies is that the position of the shortest latencies changes with increases in pursuit velocity. At 3 and 5°/s there is a dip in response latency only for changes occurring at the pursuit stimulus. At 10°/s, as mentioned above, the dip moves out to 1–2° ahead of the pursuit stimulus. Finally, at 15°/s, the dip appears 2–3° ahead of the pursuit stimulus. This trend in the data can be clearly observed in the figures depicting the relative latency difference at each peripheral target eccentricity compared to that obtained when the pursuit stimulus changed shape (Fig. 4B–E). Taken together, these data suggest that attention shifts away from the pursuit stimulus and moves further ahead into the periphery as target velocity increases.

Modeling the allocation of attention during pursuit

The results from these experiments confirmed that there is a latency benefit for manual responses made to targets appearing ahead of the pursuit stimulus. Further insight into the nature of this latency benefit was gained by applying Carpenter's model of latency to the data. This model (called LATER: linear approach to threshold with ergodic rate) has been used to explain the observed variability of re-

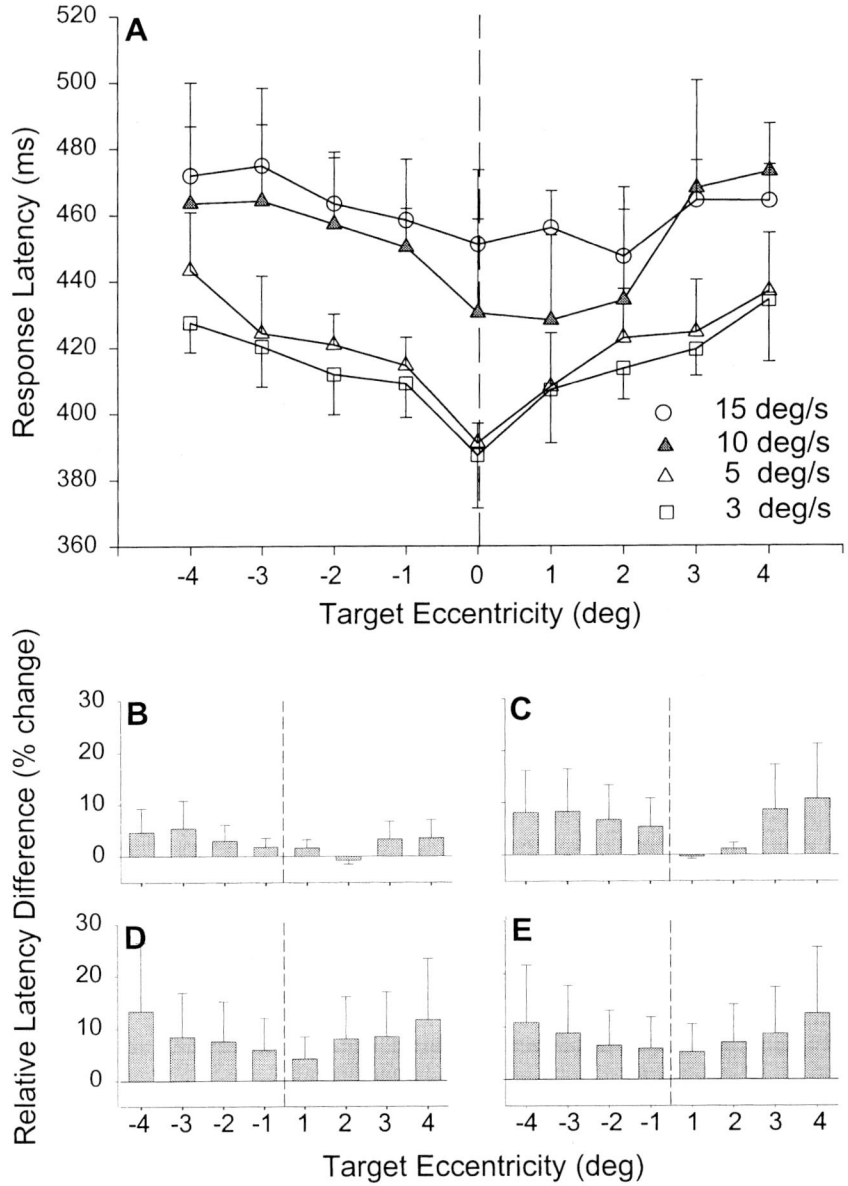

Fig. 4. (A) Group medians for response latency for different target changes when the pursuit display moved at 3, 5, 10, and 15°/s. Group means for the percentage change in response latency at each peripheral target location relative to that observed when the pursuit stimulus changed for target velocities of 15 (B), 10 (C), 5 (D), and 3°/s (E). Error bars, 1 SE.

action times and correctly predicts the effects on saccadic latency of altered expectations (Carpenter and Williams, 1995) and urgency (Reddi and Carpenter, 2000). It assumes that the latency on any particular trial is the result of a decision signal rising from a baseline level to a threshold with a certain rate of rise. Latency can therefore be defined mathematically with the following formula: $RT = (S_T - S_O)/r$, where RT = reaction time, S_T = threshold, S_O = baseline, and r = the rate of rise of the decision signal. The variability in response latency is assumed to be due to the stochastic nature of the rate of rise

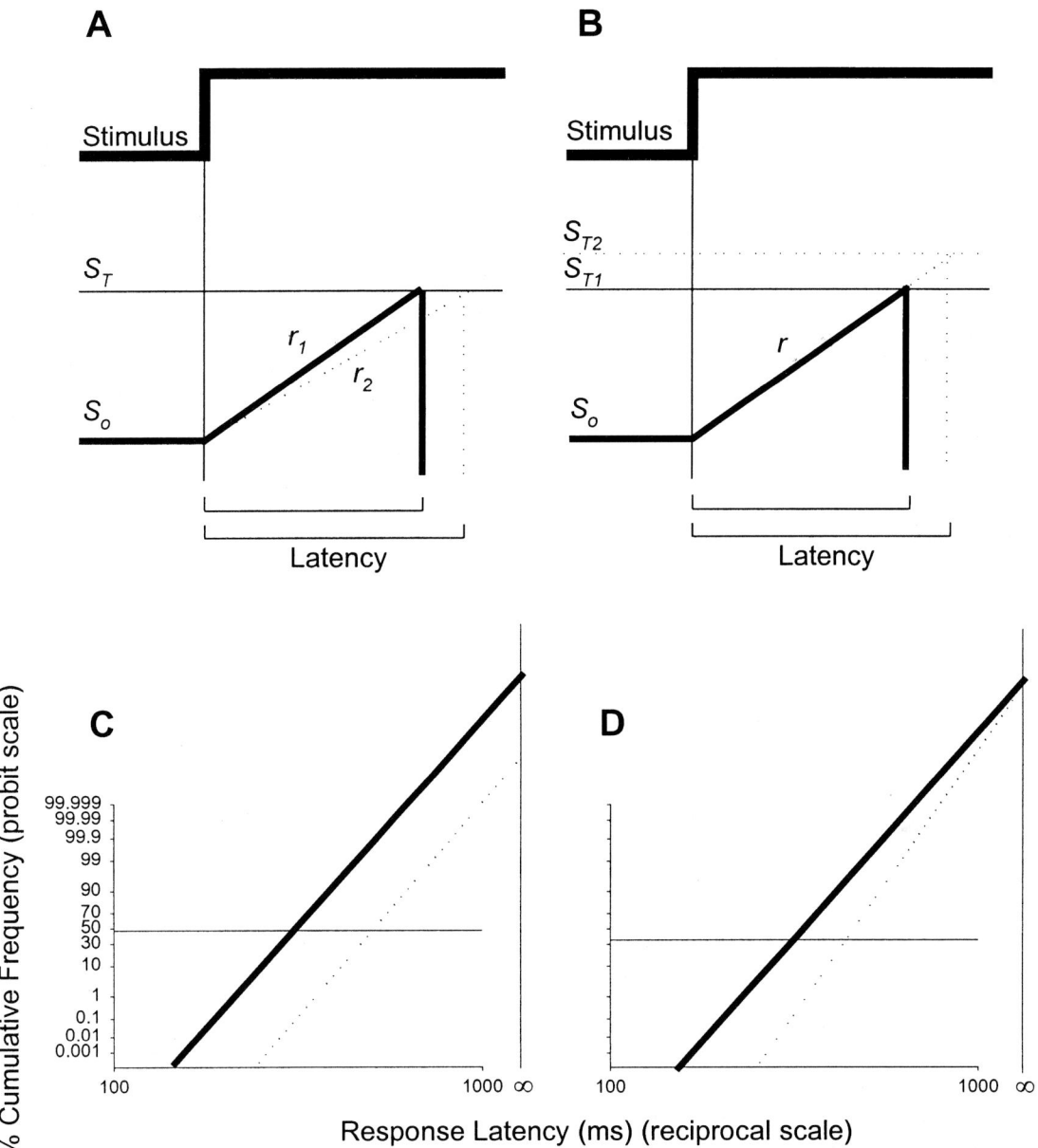

Fig. 5. Carpenter's LATER model. The model assumes that latency is the result of the time required for a decision signal to increase from a baseline level and cross a threshold. If the rate of rise of the decision signal is different in two conditions (A) it will result in two parallel regression lines in the reciprobit plot (C). By contrast, if the threshold is different in two conditions (B), the regression lines will swivel about the infinite latency intercept (D).

in the signal with r having some mean ($\mu_\bullet$) and variance (σ^2). Because of this stochastic nature, the reciprocal of latency will follow a Gaussian distribution. Replotting this distribution on a cumulative probability scale (a 'reciprobit' plot) will result in the data points falling along a relatively straight line. Performing a linear regression on this data gives a line of best fit with a median value of $(S_T - S_O)/\mu$ and an intercept at infinite time of $m = \mu/(\sigma\sqrt{2})$. Critically, this intercept is independent of S_T and S_O.

This implies that any changes in this value must be due to alterations in r. Thus, if the differences in latency from one condition to another are due solely to a change in the rate of rise of the decision signal (Fig. 5A), then the line of best fit in the reciprobit plot will shift in a parallel fashion (Fig. 5C). This will result in changes in the median value, but not the slope, of the lines of best fit. By contrast, if the differences in latency from one condition to another are due to a change in the distance between the baseline and threshold levels (Fig. 5B), then the line of best fit in the reciprobit plot will swivel about the infinite intercept point (Fig. 5D). This will result in changes in both the median value and slope of the lines of best fit.

We applied this model to data collected from another experiment in which most of the peripheral target changes occurred at 1° ahead (to the right of) or behind (to the left of) the pursuit stimulus with the display moving rightwards at 10°/s. These target locations and this speed were chosen because they resulted in the most consistent latency differences in the previous experiments. Changes in other peripheral targets occurred much less frequently and were used as catch trials. Fig. 6A shows the reciprobit plots for the latencies from a single subject when the peripheral target ahead of or behind the pursuit stimulus changed. Clearly, the line of best fit for 1° behind data is shifted in a parallel fashion to the right of the 1° ahead data. The slopes of the two lines are roughly the same, but the median latency in the 1° ahead condition is lower than that of the 1° behind condition. This trend in the data was confirmed for the group means for slope (Fig. 6B) and median latency (Fig. 6C). There was a significant effect for median latency but not for the slope values. Taken together, these data imply that the reduction in latency associated with paying attention ahead of the pursuit stimulus is due to an increase in the rate of rise of the decision signal related to determining whether a change occurred in the peripheral target.

Neurophysiological implementation of the LATER model

How is the decision signal suggested by Carpenter's LATER model implemented in the brain during our task? A number of recent observations made by other investigators are consistent with the idea that attention may modulate decision-making mechanisms by changing the rate of rise of a putative decision signal. First, it has been demonstrated that the responses of neurons in visual cortical areas are enhanced when the subject pays attention to the cells' preferred visual characteristic. Most relevantly, during both covert and overt orienting of attention to a specific spatial location the activity in the posterior visual areas of the brain is enhanced (Robinson et al., 1995; Luck et al., 1997). Second, integrating such an attentionally enhanced signal mathematically results in a signal that rises more quickly than a similarly integrated signal occurring during non-attentional trials. Thus, by paying attention to a relevant visual characteristic it is possible to affect the rate of rise of a signal. The fact that projections exist from the posterior visual areas involved the orienting of attention (e.g., posterior parietal cortex) to frontal areas involved in forming decisions about how to act (e.g., the dorsolateral prefrontal cortex) (Petrides and Pandya, 1984) suggests that there is a neuroanatomical substrate by which to carry out this integration process. Third, recordings from frontal eye field (FEF) cells during saccade generation demonstrate a steeper rate of rise in activity during saccades with quicker latencies (Hanes and Schall, 1996). As mentioned earlier, it has also been shown that saccades generated during pursuit are quicker when made to locations ahead of rather than behind the pursuit stimulus (Krauzlis and Miles, 1996; Tanaka et al., 1998). This difference in saccade latency during pursuit may be due in part to the rate of rise of activity in FEF cells being steeper for saccades made to locations ahead of the pursuit stimulus. Finally, to make the link to the present task it is necessary to show analogous changes in the build up of activity prior to the onset of limb movements. In fact, such a relationship has been found between the rate of growth of movement-related activity in the motor cortex and the time of movement initiation for a manual motor response (Lecas et al., 1986). Thus, when taken together these findings imply that Carpenter's model of latency can be used to explain how an attentionally enhanced signal is transformed into an increased rate of rise in a decision signal that subsequently affects response latency in the relevant effector. We speculate that a similar series of processing steps take place in our

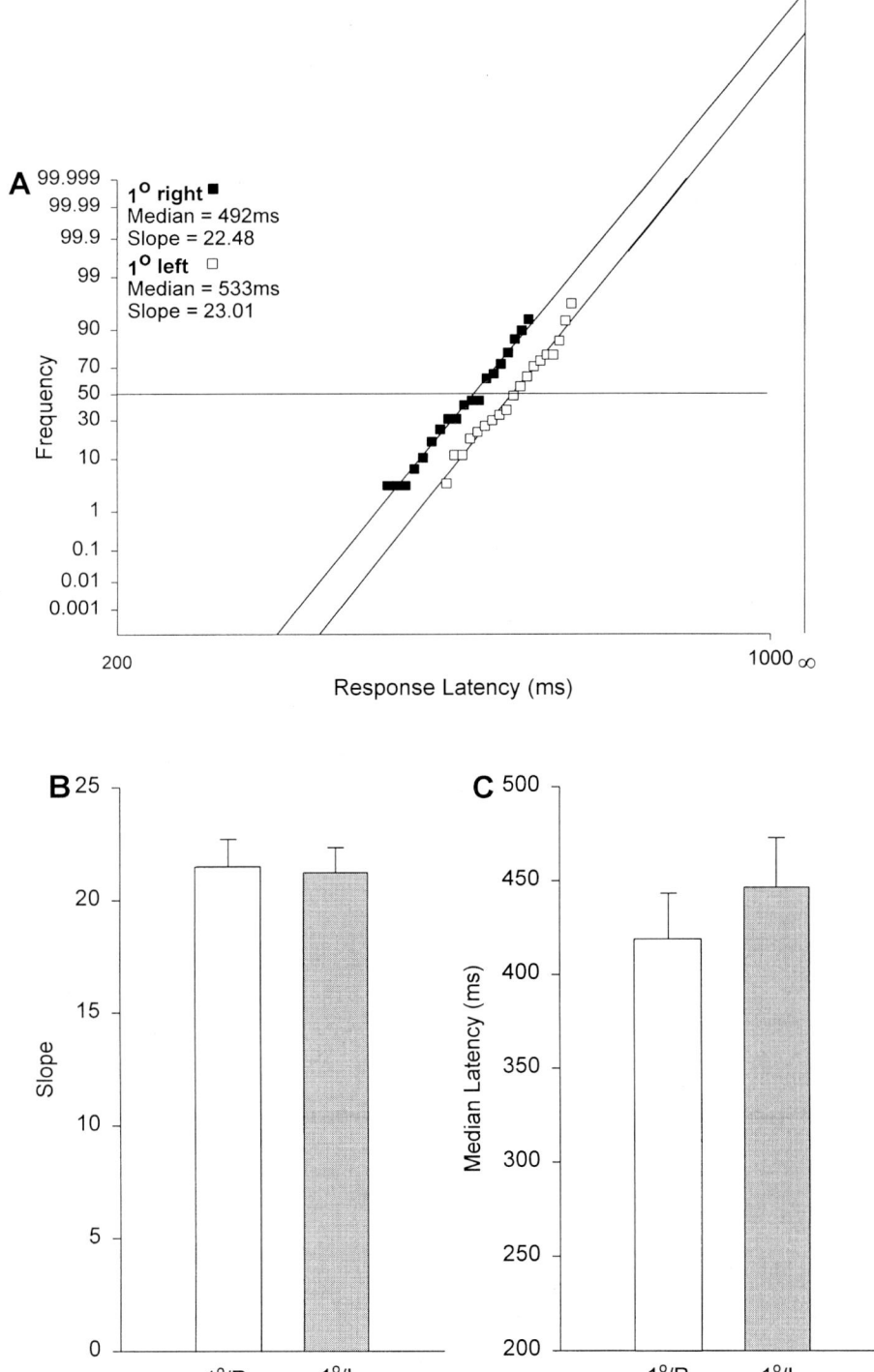

Fig. 6. (A) Typical reciprobit plot from a single subject for latencies to targets changing 1° ahead of or behind the pursuit stimulus. Group means for the slope of the two regression lines (B) and the median latency (C).

dual-task paradigm. In particular, implicit within the task of smoothly pursuing a visual target is the biased allocation of attention to an area of space just in front of the pursuit stimulus at the expense of areas in the wake of the pursuit stimulus. The visual processing signals associated with the appearance or change of a peripheral target ahead of the pursuit stimulus is thus enhanced by the biased allocation of attention. When these signals are integrated, they lead to a steeper rate of rise in a putative decision signal and consequently, a faster response latency.

Acknowledgements

This research was funded by National Science Foundation BCS-9982019 and the Medical Research Foundation of Oregon.

References

Barton, J.J., Sharpe, J.A. and Raymond, J.E. (1996) Directional defects in pursuit and motion perception in humans with unilateral cerebral lesions. *Brain*, 119: 1535–1550.

Beauchamp, M.S., Cox, R.W. and DeYoe, E.A. (1997) Graded effects of spatial and featural attention on human area MT and associated motion processing areas. *J. Neurophysiol.*, 78: 516–520.

Carpenter, R.H.S. and Williams, M.L.L. (1995) Neural computation of log likelihood in control of saccadic eye movements. *Nature*, 377: 59–62.

Chen, Y., Nakayama, K., Levy, D.L., Matthysse, S. and Holzman, P.S. (1999) Psychophysical isolation of a motion-processing deficit in schizophrenics and their relatives and its association with impaired smooth pursuit. *Proc. Natl. Acad. Sci. USA*, 96: 4724–4729.

Colby, C.L., Duhamel, J.R. and Goldberg, M.E. (1993) Ventral intraparietal area of the macaque: anatomic location and visual response properties. *J. Neurophysiol.*, 69: 902–914.

Corbetta, M. (1998) Frontoparietal cortical networks for directing attention and the eye to visual locations: identical, independent, or overlapping neural systems? *Proc. Natl. Acad. Sci. USA*, 95: 831–838.

Culham, J.C., Brandt, S.A., Cavanagh, P., Kanwisher, N.G., Dale, A.M. and Tootell, R.B. (1998) Cortical fMRI activation produced by attentive tracking of moving targets. *J. Neurophysiol.*, 80: 2657–2670.

Deubel, H. and Schneider, W.X. (1996) Saccade target selection and object recognition: evidence for a common attentional mechanism. *Vision Res.*, 36: 1827–1837.

Drew, A.S. and Van Donkelaar, P. (2002) The allocation of attention changes with increases in smooth pursuit velocity. *Vision Res.*, submitted.

Ferrera, V.P. and Lisberger, S.G. (1995) Attention and target selection for smooth pursuit eye movements. *J. Neurosci.*, 15: 7472–7484.

Ferrera, V.P. and Lisberger, S.G. (1997a) The effect of a moving distractor on the initiation of smooth-pursuit eye movements. *Vis. Neurosci.*, 14: 323–338.

Ferrera, V.P. and Lisberger, S.G. (1997b) Neuronal responses in visual areas MT and MST during smooth pursuit target selection. *J. Neurophysiol.*, 78: 1433–1446.

Fischer, M.H. (1999) An investigation of attention allocation during sequential eye movement tasks. *Q. J. Exp. Psychol.*, 52: 649–677.

Friedman, L., Jesberger, J.A., Siever, L.J., Thompson, P., Mohs, R. and Meltzer, H.Y. (1995) Smooth pursuit performance in patients with affective disorders or schizophrenia and normal controls: analysis with specific oculomotor measures. RMS error and qualitative ratings. *Psychol. Med.*, 25: 387–403.

Gellman, R.S. and Fletcher, W.A. (1992) Eye position signals in human saccadic processing. *Exp. Brain Res.*, 89: 425–434.

Hanes, D.P. and Schall, J.D. (1996) Neural control of voluntary movement initiation. *Science*, 274: 427–430.

Hoffman, J.E. and Subramaniam, B. (1995) The role of visual attention in saccadic eye movements. *Percept. Psychophys.*, 57: 787–795.

Jacobsen, L.K., Hong, W.L., Hommer, D.W., Hamburger, S.D., Castellanos, F.X., Frazier, J.A., Giedd, J.N., Gordon, C.T., Karp, B.I., McKenna, K. and Rapoport, J.L. (1996) Smooth pursuit eye movements in childhood-onset schizophrenia: comparison with attention-deficit hyperactivity disorder and normal controls. *Biol. Psychiatry*, 40: 1144–1154.

Khurana, B. and Kowler, E. (1987) Shared attentional control of smooth eye movement and perception. *Vision Res.*, 27: 1603–1618.

Kowler, E. and Zingale, C. (1985) Smooth eye movements as indicators of selective attention. In: M.I. Posner and O.S.M. Marin (Eds.), *Attention and Performance XI*. Lawrence Erlbaum, Hillsdale, NJ, pp. 285–300.

Kowler, E., Anderson, E., Dosher, B. and Blaser, E. (1995) The role of attention in the programming of saccades. *Vision Res.*, 35: 1897–1916.

Krauzlis, R.J. and Miles, F.A. (1996) Initiation of saccades during fixation or pursuit: evidence in humans for a single mechanism. *J. Neurophysiol.*, 76: 4175–4179.

Kustov, A.A. and Robinson, D.L. (1996) Shared neural control of attentional shifts and eye movements. *Nature*, 384: 74–77.

Lecas, J.-L., Requin, J., Anger, C. and Vitton, N. (1986) Changes in neuronal activity of the monkey precentral cortex during preparation for movement. *J. Neurophysiol.*, 56: 1680–1702.

Luck, S.J., Chelazzi, L., Hillyard, S.A. and Desimone, R. (1997) Neural mechanisms of spatial selective attention in areas V1, V2, and V4 of macaque visual cortex. *J. Neurophysiol.*, 77: 24–42.

MacAvoy, M.G., Gottlieb, J.P. and Bruce, C.J. (1991) Smooth-pursuit eye movement representation in the primate frontal eye field. *Cereb. Cortex*, 1: 95–102.

Maruff, P., Hay, D., Malone, V. and Currie, J. (1995) Asymmetries in the covert orienting of visual spatial attention in schizophrenia. *Neuropsychologia*, 33: 1205–1223.

McDonald, S., Bennett, K.M., Chambers, H. and Castiello, U. (1999) Covert orienting and focusing of attention in children with attention deficit hyperactivity disorder. *Neuropsychologia*, 37: 345–356.

Moran, M.J., Thaker, G.K., Laporte, D.J., Cassady, S.L. and Ross, D.E. (1996) Covert visual attention in schizophrenia spectrum personality disordered subjects: visuospatial cuing and alerting effects. *J. Psychiatr. Res.*, 30: 261–275.

Newsome, W.T., Wurtz, R.H. and Komatsu, H. (1988) Relation of cortical areas MT and MST to pursuit eye movements. II. Differentiation of retinal from extraretinal inputs. *J. Neurophysiol.*, 60: 604–620.

Petit, L., Clark, V.P., Ingeholm, J. and Haxby, J.V. (1997) Dissociation of saccade-related and pursuit-related activation in human frontal eye fields as revealed by fMRI. *J. Neurophysiol.*, 77: 3386–3390.

Petrides, M. and Pandya, D.N. (1984) Projections to the frontal cortex from the posterior parietal region in the rhesus monkey. *J. Comp. Neurol.*, 228(1): 105–116.

Posner, M.I. (1980) Orienting of attention. *Q. J. Exp. Psychol.*, 32: 3–25.

Reddi, B.A.J. and Carpenter, R.H.S. (2000) The influence of urgency on decision time. *Nat. Neurosci.*, 8: 827–830.

Robinson, D.A. (1965) The mechanics of human smooth pursuit eye movement. *J. Physiol.*, 180: 569–591.

Robinson, D.L., Bowman, E.M. and Kertzman, C. (1995) Covert orienting of attention in macaques. II. Contributions of parietal cortex. *J. Neurosci.*, 74(2): 698–712.

Salzman, C.D. and Newsome, W.T. (1994) Neural mechanisms for forming a perceptual decision. *Science*, 264: 231–237.

Schaafsma, S.J. and Duysens, J. (1996) Neurons in the ventral intraparietal area of awake macaque monkey closely resemble neurons in the dorsal part of the medial superior temporal area in their responses to optic flow patterns. *J. Neurophysiol.*, 76: 4056–4068.

Seidemann, E. and Newsome, W.T. (1999) Effect of spatial attention on the responses of area MT neurons. *J. Neurophysiol.*, 81: 1783–1794.

Sereno, A.B. and Holzman, P.S. (1996) Spatial selective attention in schizophrenic, affective disorder, and normal subjects. *Schizophr. Res.*, 20: 33–50.

Sheliga, B.M., Riggio, L. and Rizzolatti, G. (1994) Orienting of attention and eye movements. *Exp. Brain Res.*, 98: 507–522.

Sheliga, B.M., Riggio, L. and Rizzolatti, G. (1995) Spatial attention and eye movements. *Exp. Brain Res.*, 105: 261–275.

Shi, D., Friedman, H.R. and Bruce, C.J. (1998) Deficits in smooth-pursuit eye movements after muscimol inactivation within the primate's frontal eye field. *J. Neurophysiol.*, 80: 458–464.

Tanaka, M., Yoshida, T. and Fukushima, K. (1998) Latency of saccades during smooth-pursuit eye movement in man. Directional asymmetries. *Exp. Brain Res.*, 121: 92–98.

Treue, S. and Martinez Trujillo, J.C. (1999) Feature-based attention influences motion processing gain in macaque visual cortex. *Nature*, 399: 575–579.

Treue, S. and Maunsell, J.H. (1996) Attentional modulation of visual motion processing in cortical areas MT and MST. *Nature*, 382: 539–541.

Van Donkelaar, P. (1999) Spatiotemporal modulation of attention during smooth pursuit eye movements. *Neuroreport*, 10: 2523–2526.

Van Gelder, P., Anderson, S., Herman, E., Lebedev, S. and Tsui, W.H. (1990) Saccades in pursuit eye tracking reflect motor attention processes. *Compr. Psychiatry*, 31: 253–260.

Zeki, S., Watson, J.D., Lueck, C.J., Friston, K.J., Kennard, C. and Frackowiak, R.S. (1991) A direct demonstration of functional specialization in human visual cortex. *J. Neurosci.*, 11: 641–649.

CHAPTER 19

Commentary: Smooth pursuit eye movements: from low-level to high-level vision

Uwe J. Ilg *

Kognitive Neurologie, Neurologische Universitätsklinik, Hoppe-Seyler-Strasse 3, D-72076 Tübingen, Germany

Abstract: If an object of great interest moves in our environment, we are able to elicit smooth pursuit eye movements that keep the image of the moving object stationary on our fovea. The processing of visual motion underlying the execution of smooth pursuit eye movements is very similar to the processing underlying the perception of visual motion. During initiation of smooth pursuit, an averaging across all available motion information occurs. Cognitive factors including attention, prediction and learning are able to influence the execution of smooth pursuit. The pursuit target trajectory in space is represented in the discharge rates of neurons in the posterior parietal cortex of rhesus monkeys.

Introduction

Since the number of axons in our optic tract is limited, the spatial resolution of our visual system displays a marked anisotropy: only within the central visual field, the fovea centralis, we are able to discriminate up to 60 lines per degree of sight. The spatial resolution sharply decreases with eccentricity into the peripheral visual field. This anisotropy constitutes on the one hand an impressive example of data reduction. On the other hand, it imperatively asks for a very precise motor system which moves the retinal image of an object of interest into the fovea. If we are watching a stationary scene, this task is achieved by fast, ballistic eye movements called saccades. If the object of interest moves, we are able to move our eyes at an appropriate velocity yielding a stationary retinal image of the object on the fovea. These eye movements are called *s*mooth *p*ursuit *e*ye *m*ovements (SPEM) and constitute the subject of this chapter.

It seems to be trivial to generate slow or smooth eye movements voluntarily. If we ask a subject to move his hand slowly at a given velocity from point A to B, the subject does not have any difficulties in doing so. If a visual target moved on a computer monitor for instance, we were able to track the moving target precisely with our eyes. The eye velocity was perfectly matched to target velocity. Now we asked the subject to perform exactly the same eye movements without a target. We switched the computer monitor off and asked the subject to simply imagine the moving target and to track it. In this condition, the eye movements consisted in a sequence of saccades and fixation periods as illustrated in Fig. 1. Segments with smooth eye movements were completely absent in this condition. The fact that we are only able to perform SPEM in the presence of a moving target is the reason why these eye movements were frequently used as a biological probe for motion processing. If a subject performs SPEM, it can be taken as indication that successful processing of visual motion has taken place.

As the title of this chapter suggests, this tight link between visual motion processing and the execution of SPEM represents the start of the endeavor of this chapter. Based on the contributions by Richard Born,

---

* Kognitive Neurologie, Neurologische Universitätsklinik, Hoppe-Seyler-Strasse 3, D-72076 Tübingen, Germany.
Tel.: +49-7071-29-87602; Fax: +49-7071-29-5724;
E-mail: uwe.ilg@uni-tuebingen.de

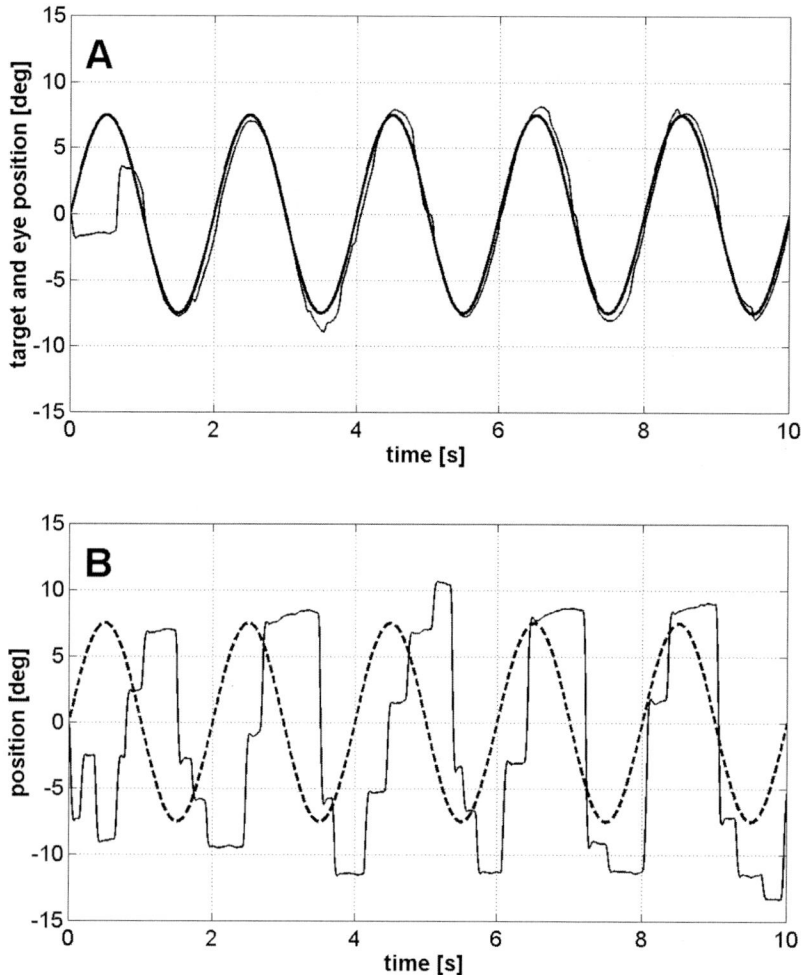

Fig. 1. The horizontal eye position of a human subject was measured by an infra-red eye tracker (IRIS from Skalar Medical). The moving target (pixel) was presented onto a 17' computer monitor 57 cm in front of the subject. In A, the target moved sinusoidally at 0.5 Hz with an amplitude of 7.5° shown by the solid line. In B, the monitor was switched off and the subject was instructed to perform the same eye movements as in A. The dotted line represents a possible imagined target position. Note the absence of smooth eye movements in B, only saccades and periods of fixation can be observed. Although the subject performed a series of saccades, he was able to reproduce the periodicity of the target movement.

Yue Chen, Paul Knox, Graham Barnes and Paul Van Donkelaar to this book, the role of cognitive factors such as attention, learning, and prediction on the execution of SPEM will be addressed. It will be discussed whether there are indications for common or separate mechanisms of visual motion processing underlying perception and execution of SPEM. Finally, the frame of reference of single neurons' responses during the execution of SPEM will be discussed.

Motion processing underlying perception and smooth pursuit eye movements

A very simple, but not trivial question asks for similarities or dissimilarities in the mechanisms of visual motion processing for perception and generation of SPEM. Is there a single mechanism that provides an input for perception and action systems, or act 'private' mechanisms in parallel for perception and action?

Influenced by the concept that the cortical visual system consists in two sub-systems, a ventral stream responsible for object identification (WHAT) and a dorsal stream underlying the localization of objects (WHERE) (Ungerleider and Mishkin, 1982), it was proposed that there are separate visual pathways for perception and action (Goodale and Milner, 1992). Initially, this proposal was supported by the observation in a patient who had difficulties in a manual matching task but could perform a manual grasping task correctly (Goodale et al., 1991). Further experiments addressing the question of separate systems for action and perception focused on the Ebbinghaus illusion. The perceived size of a central circle is influenced by the size of surrounding circles. However, if subjects were asked to grasp for the central circle, the grasping (i.e. the width between thumb and index finger) was not affected by the illusion (Aglioti et al., 1995). The strength of this argument for separate systems for action and perception was reduced by the findings of another laboratory showing similar effects on perception and grasping in the same condition (Franz et al., 2000). Recently, the question of separate systems for action and perception was also addressed by the analysis of the localization of a target flashed briefly before the execution of a saccade. Here, it was shown that manual pointing and verbal report gave different results: whereas the pointing towards a target was correct, the verbal report of the perceived target position reflected the earlier described compression of space (Burr et al., 2001). In summary, there are results from a broad range of experiments supporting the notion of separate systems for perception and action.

However, to specifically address the question whether separate systems with respect of processing visual motion are used for the perception and generation of SPEM, several experiments following a typical approach were performed in the past: on the one hand, the subjects' perception was examined using psychophysical techniques. On the other hand, the identical stimulus was used to elicit eye movements. A very typical stimulus in these studies consisted in a variable ratio of coherently moving dots superimposed onto randomly moving dots displayed within a stationary aperture (Newsome and Paré, 1988). If all dots were moving to the right, the subject clearly perceived rightward movement. If all dots were moving towards the left, the subject perceived leftward motion. If all dots were moving randomly, the perception of the subject was at chance level. The reports of the subjects constituted the *psychometric* function. At the same time, the elicited eye movements could be recorded and analyzed. To determine the *oculometric* function, the direction of the elicited eye movements was determined within a time window of 500 ms. To be able to only analyze the smooth eye movements, saccades were eliminated carefully. A first inspection of the *psychometric* and *oculometric* functions shown in Fig. 2 indicates that both functions are very similar (Krauzlis and Adler, 2001).

The fact that perception and oculomotor control involve the same mechanism was further supported by the observation that *psychometric* and *oculometric* functions could be similarly modified by prediction. Before the onset of the stimulus, the subjects saw a cue signaling the direction of the subsequent stimulus movement. If the cue predicted rightward movement, both functions were shifted to the left, i.e. a smaller amount of dots moving coherently to the right were necessary to elicit rightward perception as well as rightward eye movement (Krauzlis and Adler, 2001). A common mechanism of visual motion processing for perception and generation of eye movements was also suggested by the similarity of *oculometric* and *psychometric* function obtained when moving plaids were used (Krauzlis and Stone, 1999), in the case of the directional biases for elongated apertures (Beutter and Stone, 1998), when the effect of motion coherence (Beutter and Stone, 2000) and of motion integration (Stone et al., 2000) was examined.

Another attempt to reveal whether perception and oculomotor control share a common mechanism of visual motion processing consists in the use of paradoxical motion stimuli. These motion stimuli are called second-order motion to delineate them from first-order motion stimuli (Chubb and Sperling, 1988). Second-order motion cannot be decoded by an elementary motion detector (Reichardt, 1987) nor by the functionally equivalent energy model (Adelson and Bergen, 1985; Van Santen and Sperling, 1985). Four different types of motion stimuli are of interest to compare the perception of subjects and their power to elicit SPEM (see Fig. 3): luminance-

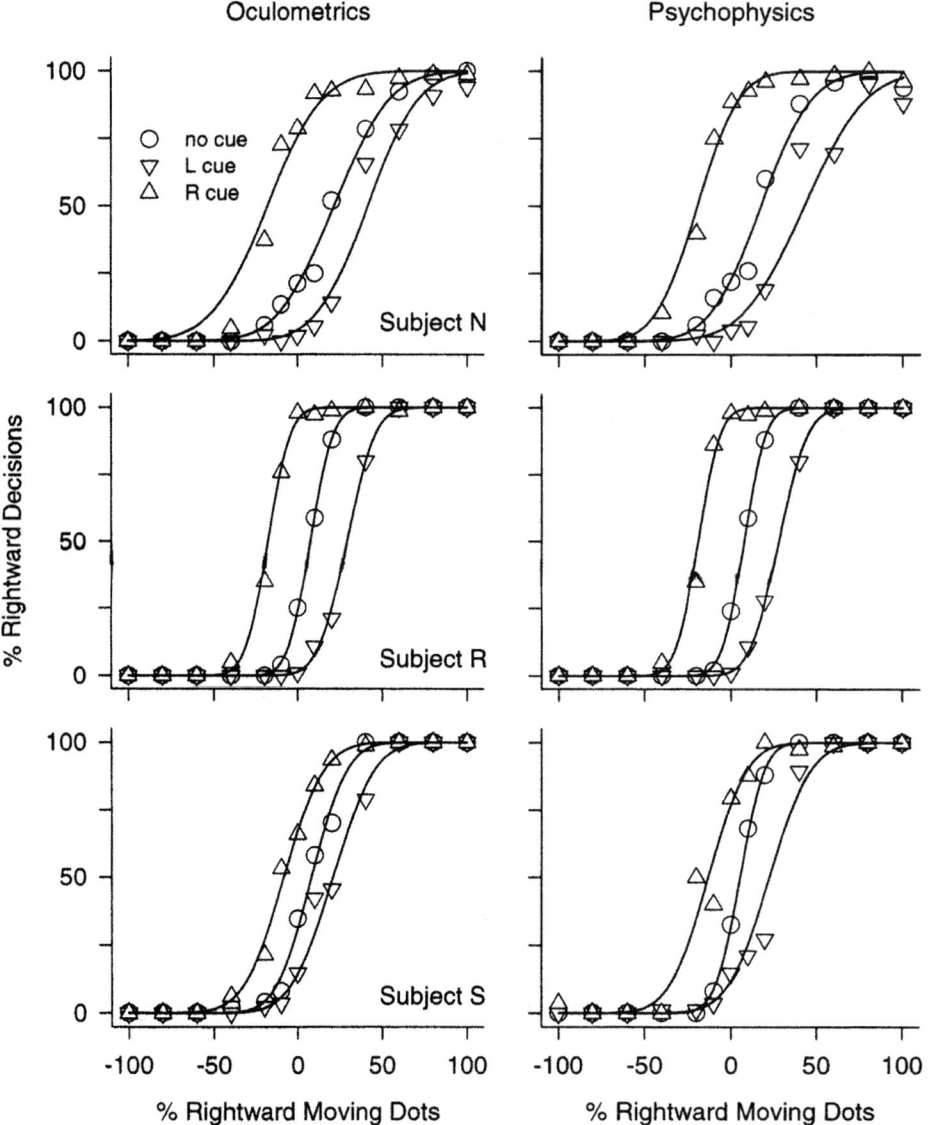

Fig. 2. Three subjects (N, R, and S) were exposed to a horizontal band of moving dots (width 45°, height 0.5°) displayed onto a computer monitor. They had to report the perceived motion within this band while their eye position was recorded. 100% on the x-axis indicates that all dots moved rightward, -100% indicates that all dots moved leftward. The *oculometric* functions were obtained from the analysis of eye movements within a 500 ms interval, the *psychometric* function resulted from the subjects' button presses. The *oculometric* and *psychometric* functions for three subjects are shown, when no prior information was given (circles), when a cue indicated rightward motion (upright triangles), or leftward motion (inverted triangles) (modified with permission from Krauzlis and Adler, 2001).

defined (LM), Fourier motion (FM), drift-balanced motion (DBM, Chubb and Sperling, 1988) and theta motion (TM, Zanker, 1993).

The psychophysical experiments revealed that human subjects (Chubb and Sperling, 1988; Zanker, 1993) and monkeys (Churan and Ilg, 2001) were able to perceive all these motion types correctly. As outlined above, the execution of SPEM is tightly connected to visual motion processing, so it is obvious to speculate whether the direction of pursuit

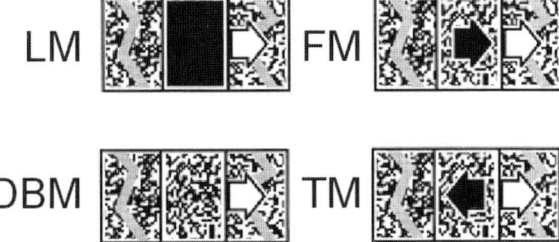

Fig. 3. A schematic representation of four motion stimuli is shown in space–time diagrams. In case of luminance-defined motion (LM), a rectangle with a different luminance than the background moved toward the right (indicated by the white arrow) across a dynamic random dot pattern (indicated by the gray zig-zag line). In case of Fourier motion (FM), a rectangular area of dots moved coherently. Here, object motion indicated by the white arrow and pixel motion illustrated by the black arrow was identical. In case of drift-balance motion (DBM), a rectangular aperture moved across the dynamic random dot pattern indicated by white arrow. No pixel motion occurred in this stimulus at all. Finally, in case of theta-motion (TM), the pixels within the rectangle moved towards the left (black arrow) while the rectangle itself moved to the right (white arrow).

was rather determined by the direction of the moving pixels or by the direction of the moving object. However, the smooth pursuit eye movements of subjects tracking objects defined by second-order motion followed the direction of the perceived object motion, not the direction of individual moving pixels (Butzer et al., 1997). There is no reason to assume different motion processing underlying the execution of SPEM and the perception of visual motion.

The latency of the initial saccade in the eye movement experiment revealed a strong dependency on the stimulus type: the first-order motion stimulus elicited initial saccades with a latency of 209 ms, the second-order motion stimuli resulted in a saccadic latency of 260 ms (Butzer et al., 1997). In psychophysical experiments, it was shown that second-order motion stimuli have to be presented for a longer period of time than first-order motion stimuli for successful discrimination of the subjects (Yo and Wilson, 1992; Derrington et al., 1993). This similarity in the dependence of latency and stimulus duration on the type of motion stimulus also indicates common visual motion processing for perception and action.

In summary, with respect to the processing of visual motion, there is multiple experimental evidence that the perception of motion and the generation of smooth pursuit eye movements share a common mechanism for motion analysis. The *psychometric* and *oculometric* functions obtained from various visual motion tasks are very similar and reveal a similar modification by expectation. In addition, the processing of second-order motion stimuli reveals similarities in perception and sensorimotor integration.

Initiation of smooth pursuit eye movements

An important question asks how SPEM are initiated. How is the transition from fixation to pursuit achieved? It is important to emphasize that only during pursuit initiation, before the onset of the eye movement itself, retinal image motion results exclusively from target motion in the environment. This period offers an ideal situation for studies addressing the question how visual motion signals are transformed into eye movement commands as discussed by Born et al. (2002, this volume). Since retinal image motion during initiation of SPEM is not yet influenced by a feedback signal, i.e. by the eye movement, this period is an *open-loop* phase in contrast to the *steady-state* phase occurring later during the maintenance of SPEM. During steady-state pursuit, target velocity in space has to be computed by adding the retinal image motion of the target and the executed eye velocity.

If we assume that the retinal image velocity of the target is determined during the open-loop period and transformed into an eye movement program, then eye position would lag target position forever. Obviously, this did not happen as the typical initiation of SPEM displayed in Fig. 4 shows. Approximately 150 ms after the onset of target movement, the eyes started to accelerate indicated by the increase in eye velocity. At about 300 ms following target onset, the subject performed an initial saccade compensating the lag of eye position. Immediately after the initial saccade, eye velocity was matched to target velocity. Studies on pursuit initiation usually determine the slope of increase in eye velocity (eye acceleration) and the latency of pursuit initiation in addition to the parameters of the initial saccade.

Closer examination of the initial saccade parameters revealed that the amplitude of this saccade was

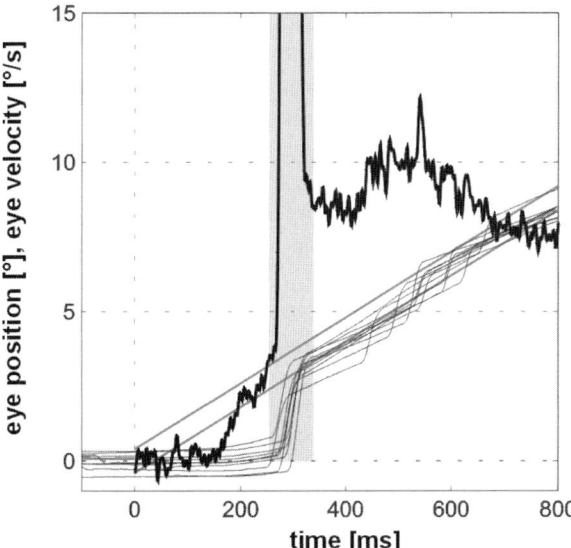

Fig. 4. Horizontal eye and target position (two parallel lines representing the left and right border of the target) together with the eye velocity of a human subject tracking a small moving target are displayed. Eye position traces of individual traces (thin lines) are shown together with the median eye velocity across all trials (bold line). The eye position was recorded by means of scleral search coils (Collewijn et al., 1975). As indicated, the target started to move at time zero. Note the stereotyped sequence of pre-saccadic eye acceleration followed by the initial saccade as well as the post-saccadic enhancement.

adjusted to the velocity of the target, i.e. the saccade ended where the target was after its execution, not at the position where the target was when the parameters of the saccade were computed (Gellman and Carl, 1991). The saccadic system does not only use retinal position error of the target to compute saccade amplitude, but also uses information about target velocity. A statistical analysis of the latency of pursuit and the initial saccade revealed that both values scattered independently (Merrison and Carpenter, 1994). This indicates that the generation of the initial saccade is an independent process from pursuit initiation. In addition, the latency of initial saccades during pursuit initiation was reported to be longer than the latency of saccades towards a stationary target with identical amplitude (Gellman and Carl, 1991).

Latencies and gap paradigm

With respect to the latency of an eye movement, it was shown that a brief (200 ms) temporal gap between the offset of the fixation target and the onset of the new saccade target reduced the saccadic reaction time (from Saslow, 1967 to Kalesnykas and Hallett, 2002). These saccades with short latency were called *express saccades* (Fischer and Boch, 1983). To understand why the saccadic reaction time is reduced in the gap paradigm, it is necessary to make the different steps involved in the generation of saccades clear. Obviously, the very first step in this sequence of events is the termination of fixation. If the fixation target is already switched off as in the gap paradigm, the saccade can be elicited earlier, since fixation is already released as a consequence of the gap.

Similar to the execution of saccades, the very first step in initiation of SPEM also consists in the termination of fixation. This leads to the question (see Knox and Bekkour, 2002, this volume) whether the gap paradigm also reduces the latency of SPEM onset. The outcome of the experiment was clear: a temporal gap between fixation target offset and pursuit target onset also reduced SPEM latency (Merrison and Carpenter, 1995; Knox, 1996; Krauzlis and Miles, 1996a,b). Interestingly, the contrast of fixation and pursuit targets affected the pursuit onset latency, but not the reduction in latency induced by the gap (O'Mullane and Knox, 1999). The similarity of the gap effect on saccadic and pursuit latencies can be traced back to a common neuronal substrate. It was shown that the activity of neurons in the superior colliculus represents a motor error signal for saccadic and pursuit eye movements (Krauzlis et al., 1997). These neurons increased their activity already during the gap period, before the target was presented. Since this was true for saccades as well as for SPEM (Krauzlis et al., 2002), it is very likely that the superior colliculus is involved in the preparation of saccades as well as SPEM.

In many studies on pursuit initiation, the investigators are interested in avoiding the disturbing initial saccade in order to describe precisely the mechanism of the slow build-up in eye velocity. This can easily be achieved if the target does not start to move from the point of fixation, but from a slightly changed position. This paradigm is called step-ramp paradigm.

If the size of the target step is equal to

step =

latency of the subject × target velocity × (−1),

eye position matches target position asymptotically without an initial saccade (Rashbass, 1961).

Post-saccadic enhancement

A prominent feature related to pursuit initiation consists in the huge difference in eye velocity immediately before and after the initial saccade (see Fig. 4) which is called post-saccadic enhancement (Lisberger, 1998). During execution of the saccade, there is no processing of visual motion. Vision is blocked during a saccade by a process called *saccadic suppression* (Bridgeman et al., 1975). So the initial saccade acts as a separator between the pre-saccadic acquisition of motion information and post-saccadic execution of pursuit. The exact reason for post-saccadic enhancement is unknown at present time. However, the post-saccadic enhancement documents that the sensitivity of motion processing during the preparation of SPEM is increased compared to fixation. These two stages of sensitivity can be symbolized by the two positions of a switch enabling or disabling visual motion processing (Lisberger, 1998). The analysis of small perturbations in target position during fixation and pursuit, respectively, yielded different results. During fixation, no modulation in eye velocity occurred as a consequence of a perturbation in target position. However, if the perturbation occurred during pursuit, a huge modulation in eye velocity was obtained (Schwartz and Lisberger, 1994). These findings strongly suggest that fixation is not pursuit of a target moving at zero velocity. Fixation and SPEM are two different types of eye movements and depend on two different control systems.

However, we can definitively exclude that post-saccadic enhancement can be explained by mechanical reasons such as inertia. If the step size of the target is much larger as explained above, the direction of the saccade is inverted to the direction of SPEM. Nonetheless, post-saccadic enhancement is observed in this condition excluding the possibility that mechanical inertia accounts for the observed enhancement.

Acquisition of motion signals

So far, the open-loop period of pursuit is characterized by sequential acquisition of all visual motion signals available, and subsequential transformation of the motion information into a motor command. Pre-saccadic eye acceleration is a function of the eccentricity of the target. Eye acceleration declined if the target started to move in the periphery compared to foveal vision (*man*: Tychsen and Lisberger, 1986; *monkey*: Lisberger and Westbrook, 1985). In addition, target movement towards the fovea resulted in higher eye acceleration than movement away from the fovea. To further characterize visual motion processing underlying the initiation of smooth pursuit eye movements, the use of second-order stimuli as explained in Chen et al. (2002, this volume) (see Fig. 2) turned out to be helpful. It has already been shown that during steady-state pursuit, the direction of SPEM was identical to the direction of perceived object motion (Butzer et al., 1997). Now, we asked whether the parameters of pursuit initiation (onset and acceleration) depended on the order of motion stimuli. As Fig. 5 shows, pre-saccadic pursuit initiation depended on the type of motion stimulus. The highest eye acceleration was elicited by Fourier motion. Drift-balanced motion resulted in a lower acceleration. In case of theta motion, the pre-saccadic pursuit was initiated into the direction of pixel motion, which was in contrast to steady-state SPEM (Lindner and Ilg, 2000). However, pursuit latency did not depend on the type of motion stimulus.

It is important to note that the first-order motion components in Fourier and theta motion were identical, the only difference was the relation between the first-order motion component and the direction of object motion. If the first-order component was the only source for pursuit initiation, the absolute value of eye acceleration should be identical for theta motion and Fourier motion. But there was a significant difference in the absolute values of eye acceleration, the theta motion stimulus elicited a significantly smaller acceleration than the Fourier stimulus. In addition, if the stimulus consisted in drift-balanced motion, i.e. without any moving pixels, pre-saccadic pursuit initiation was also observed. There are two conclusions from these results. Firstly, there are at least two systems for de-coding first- and second-

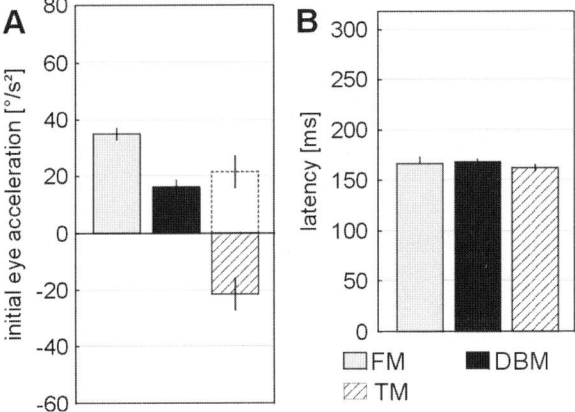

Fig. 5. Initiation of SPEM elicited by Fourier (FM), drift-balanced (DBM) and theta motion (TM). In A, the initial eye acceleration (mean and standard deviation for five subjects) elicited by the three different motion stimuli (4.6°/s) are shown. Note that in case of TM, the eyes started to move into the direction of pixel movement, i.e. opposite to the direction of object movement. However, there was a significant difference between the absolute value of acceleration obtained by TM (shown by the dashed rectangle) and by FM. In the absence of any pixel movements (DBM), the measured eye acceleration was significantly different from zero. B gives mean and standard deviation of pursuit onset latency. Note that the obtained latencies did not differ for the three types of motion (modified from Lindner and Ilg, 2000).

order motion, and secondly, these systems interact. Pursuit initiation cannot be described by a simple algebraic summation of the output of both systems.

It is important to note that luminance-defined stimuli elicited initial saccades with shorter latencies than all other motion-defined stimuli (Butzer et al., 1997). The luminance-defined stimulus could be perceived without further processing of visual motion information. In support, it was shown that increasing the saliency of the target by a different color compared to the background reduced the pursuit onset latency and increased the initial eye acceleration (Miura et al., 2001).

As perfectly described in Born et al. (2002, this volume), the middle temporal area (MT) in the brain of rhesus monkeys is essential for the visual motion processing underlying the initiation of SPEM (Pack and Born, 2001). If a moving line is viewed through a circular aperture, only motion perpendicular to line orientation can be observed. Individual neurons recorded from area MT of rhesus monkeys responded initially only to motion perpendicular to the moving line (first 20 ms of the response). Only the late response (>140 ms) signaled the true direction of line motion. Similarly, smooth pursuit eye movements of the monkeys tracking the moving bar changed their direction over time. Initial eye movements were perpendicular to the bar, irrespective of the direction of bar movement whereas steady-state pursuit was in the true direction of bar movement. Similar ocular behavior was reported from human subjects (Masson et al., 2000).

Effects of distracters

In studies on pursuit initiation discussed so far, only single objects moving across a homogeneous dark background were presented to the subjects. However, in a natural environment, many objects move at the same time across a structured background. Obviously, a selection process which requires selective attention is necessary in this natural condition. There is need to categorize the moving objects as possible targets and distracters. In this case, attention is fixed to the moving target and helps to extract only valid target information. However, selective attention is a necessary prerequisite for SPEM. We only perform these eye movements if we attend to a moving target, and we can only track one single target at a given time. So it was no surprise when it turned out that steady-state pursuit was not influenced by distracters. Obviously, the decision was already taken which moving object was the target for SPEM and selective attention helped to ignore the motion signals from the distracters. This is very similar to the finding that steady-state pursuit of a target moving across a structured background was only marginally influenced (see below, Collewijn and Tamminga, 1984). In contrast, the initiation of SPEM was massively affected by the presence of distracters. This sensitivity is quite similar to the sensitivity of pursuit initiation to the presence of a structured background (see below, Keller and Khan, 1986; Kimmig et al., 1992; Mohrmann and Thier, 1995). As described by Knox and Bekkour (2002, this volume), even stationary distracters were able to modify pursuit initiation, i.e. pursuit onset latency was increased in the presence of distracters. This increase in latency could be balanced by a temporal gap between fixation and pursuit targets as discussed above indicating that both mechanisms were separate and did not interact. However, the presentation of a stationary distracter yielded a reflexive or involuntary attraction of attention. So the increase in pursuit latency reported by Knox and Bekkour was quite similar to the results reported by Chen et al. in their chapter when the subject had to perform a spatial frequency discrimination task together with the execution of SPEM. In both situations, attention was withdrawn from the pursuit target resulting in an impairment of pursuit.

There are several studies addressing the effects of moving distracters on pursuit initiation and the underlying neuronal activity in the middle temporal (MT) and middle superior temporal (MST) areas. A common denominator in these studies is the question whether pursuit initiation as well as the recorded discharge rates in the presence of a distracter can be described by a winner-take-all, vector summation or vector average model.

If the target was cued by color (Ferrera and Lisberger, 1995), modifications of pursuit latency, but not of initial eye acceleration, were observed in the presence of a distracter. The pursuit onset latency was 100 ms in case of a single moving target. If the distracter moved in the same direction as the target, a reduction to 85 ms was observed. In contrast, if the distracter moved in opposite direction, the latency was increased to 150 ms (Ferrera and Lisberger, 1995). Subsequently, it was shown that the effects of the distracter depended on spatial and temporal proximity between target and distracter, and by the direction of motion (Ferrera and Lisberger, 1997). Recanzone and Wurtz (1999) also examined the effects of temporal and spatial separation of target and distracter. They used different shapes (rectangle and circle) to identify target and distracter. If the distance between target and distracter was small, pursuit initiation was best described by a vector-averaging model. If the distance was large, a winner-take-all model yielded best results. A similar shift from vector-averaging to winner-take-all mechanism was observed in the discharge rates of neurons recorded from areas MT and MST (Recanzone and Wurtz, 1999). If two targets moving perpendicularly were presented, the initial acceleration of SPEM could be described by a weighed vector averaging (Lisberger and Ferrera, 1997). In this study, there was no difference between target and distracter, the distracter simply disappeared 150 ms after motion onset. A vector averaging mechanism was also suggested by the results of *intra*cortical *m*icrostimulation (ICMS) in area MT during initiation of pursuit (Groh et al., 1997). Here, averaging occurred between visual motion signals related to the moving target and the artificially injected activity related to the ICMS. At the time of the initial saccade, obviously a decision was performed which target had to be pursued. Post-saccadic eye movements were best explained by a winner-take-all mechanism (Gardner and Lisberger, 2001).

In summary, the initiation of SPEM is characterized by a stereotyped sequence of pre-saccadic eye acceleration followed by an initial saccade. The huge increase in eye velocity immediately before and after the initial saccade is achieved by a process called post-saccadic enhancement which documents the increased sensitivity of motion processing during execution of SPEM compared to fixation. The open-loop period (i.e. before the onset of eye movement) is characterized by the acquisition of all available motion information. If more than a single target is presented, vector averaging between the motion signals dominates pre-saccadic eye acceleration. Subsequently, steady-state pursuit is characterized by a winner-take-all mechanism.

Cancellation of self-induced retinal image motion

It is a typical but artificial situation in the laboratory when subjects were asked to track a single target moving in front of a dark, homogeneous background. Under natural conditions, objects move in front of a structured background. The presence of a structured background during the execution of SPEM causes two peculiarities. Firstly, we do not perceive the self-induced retinal image shift under normal conditions. One might speculate that this might be due to a suppression of motion perception similar to saccadic suppression (Bridgeman et al., 1975). However, saccades are very brief, fast eye movements. The costs of visual impairment during saccades are quite small. For SPEM a similar suppression of vision is not possible since the execution of SPEM lasts much longer and critically depends on the processing of visual motion. With respect to the perception during execution of SPEM, it must be noted, that the perception of the stationary surround is not perfect. If you move a pencil across this text and you track the tip of the pencil, you will not be able to read the text, but you will perceive the characters moving in the opposite direction to the moving pencil. This apparent background movement is called Filehne illusion (Filehne, 1922). A successful attempt to explain why there is only a small misperception of self-induced retinal image motion consists in the *re-afference principle* (Von Holst and Mittelstaedt, 1950). According to this principle, our perception of motion does not only depend on retinal image motion, but is also influenced by the executed eye movements via an *efference copy signal*. In case of a stationary background, the size of the *efference copy* signal is identical to the self-induced retinal image motion, but with different polarity. Therefore, both signals cancel each other and perception signals a stationary background. In the course of elegant experiments, it was convincingly shown that the gain of the *efference copy* signal can be modified by artificial retinal image motion during execution of SPEM (Haarmeier and Thier, 1996).

The second peculiarity related to the presence of a structured background during the execution of SPEM consists in the fact that the execution of SPEM is only mildly affected by the background. The self-induced retinal image motion constitutes a perfect input signal for gaze-stabilization reflexes such as the optokinetic nystagmus. The effects of a structured background are different during initiation and steady-state pursuit. During pursuit initiation, and before the onset of the eye movement, retinal image motion is only caused by the movement of the target, not yet by an eye movement. Nevertheless, pursuit initiation is quite consistently affected by the presence of a structured background compared to pursuit initiation across a dark, homogeneous background: initial eye acceleration was reduced and pursuit latency was increased (Keller and Khan, 1986; Kimmig et al., 1992; Mohrmann and Thier, 1995). In contrast, during steady-state pursuit there are only marginal influences of the presence of a structured background on pursuit parameters. Pursuit gain was reduced mildly and compensated by an increase in the number of saccades (Yee et al., 1983; Collewijn and Tamminga, 1984; Ilg and Thier, 1996).

Some years ago, Urs Schwarz had the idea to address the puzzling problem of the insensitivity of the pursuit system to self-induced retinal image motion by the use of brief injections (200 ms) of global motion during various phases of the execution of SPEM. The short duration excluded motion adaptation, which is always present in motion processing. This approach turned out to be very successful for our understanding of the processing of self-induced retinal image motion. Immediately, a clear asymmetry in the obtained eye velocity profiles became evident (see Fig. 6): only if the background moved in same direction as the pursuit target, the eye velocity profile was briefly disturbed. If the background moved in opposite direction, no modulation of eye velocity was observed. Note that in natural conditions, i.e. if a target moves in front of a structured background, the direction of self-induced retinal image motion is always opposite to target motion. Obviously, the here described mechanism explains why the self-induced retinal image motion does not affect the ongoing eye movement (Schwarz and Ilg, 1999; Suehiro et al., 1999; Lindner et al., 2001).

In the meantime, we discovered that the asymmetry was due to a reduction in sensitivity for global motion in the direction opposite to the executed SPEM, i.e. in the direction of self-induced retinal image motion (see Fig. 6B). Furthermore, the asymmetry was bound to a retinal frame of reference: if the background moved in same direction as the target but at slower velocity, no modulation in eye speed occurred indicating that the processing was performed within a retinal coordinate system (see Fig. 6C). Recent experiments revealed that the asymmetric modulation in eye velocity also occurred if the target was removed briefly during background motion. This finding excluded the possibility that the asymmetry was due to the processing of relative retinal image motion. Note that relative motion is a very strong signal which is able to induce the perception of moving object simply by a moving background (*induced motion*, see Duncker, 1929). At the present time, it seems likely that the internal signal coding for the ongoing eye movement is essential to explain this asymmetry. It was already emphasized that the onset of SPEM can be understood as switching the motion processing to a higher sensitivity (Lisberger, 1998). In support of this notion, the injection of global image motion during fixation did not elicit

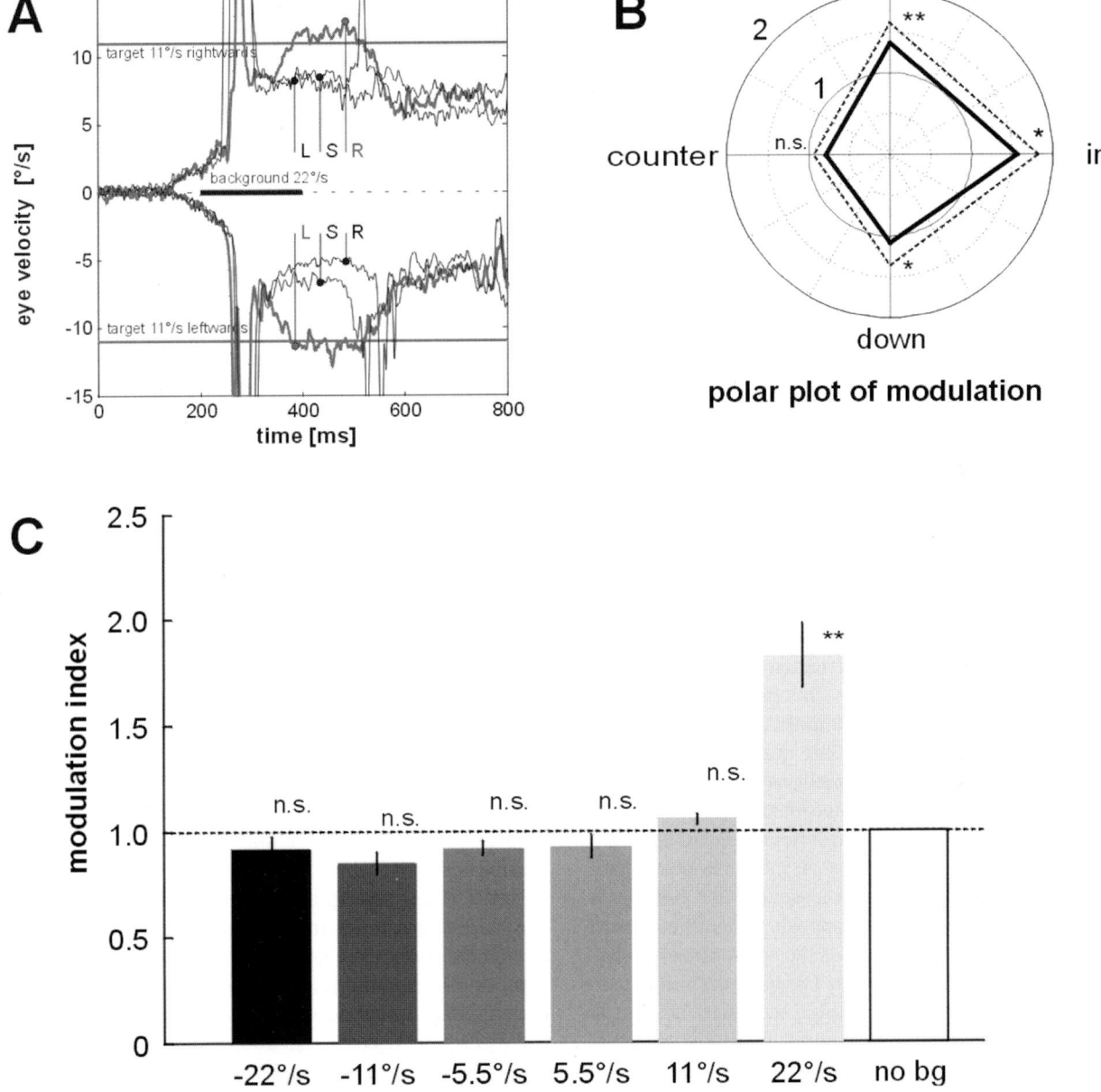

Fig. 6. (A) Smooth pursuit eye velocity profiles of a typical subject during various injections of background motion (22°/s) as indicated by the thick horizontal line during tracking of a small moving target (11°/s). The eye velocity profile obtained in the presence of a stationary background is labeled 'S', background movement towards the left is labeled with 'L', rightward movement with 'R'. Note that only in the condition when background and target moved in the same direction, a modulation in eye velocity was present. No difference between stationary background and background movement in opposite direction to target velocity was observed (modified from Schwarz and Ilg, 1999). (B) The amount of this modulation in eye velocity (mean and standard deviation across five subjects) was quantified as modulation index and plotted in polar coordinates with respect to the direction of target movement to emphasize the lack of modulation if the background moved in opposite direction to the target. (C) Shows the modulation index for various background velocities in same (positive) or opposite (negative values) direction as target movement. Note that only if background velocity was larger than target velocity a significant modulation in eye velocity occurred (modified from Lindner et al., 2001).

comparable eye movements, the sensitivity was reduced in all directions during fixation.

Our data resulting from brief injections of global motion nicely parallel the results from Richard Born and colleagues (2000) who used the earlier described *intra*cortical *m*icrostimulation (ICMS) in area MT to modulate the ongoing SPEM. It was shown earlier that area MT can be divided into regions with wide-field detector characteristics and regions with local-motion characteristics (Born and Tootell, 1992). In case of a wide-field detector, the visual response to a moving stimulus increased monotonically with stimulus size. In case of a local-motion detector, the response displayed a maximal value for a specific stimulus size, the response decreased for smaller and bigger stimuli (Born, 2000). Born and colleagues examined what happened if ICMS was applied at local-motion sites or wide-field sites (Born et al., 2000). They analyzed eye velocity just immediately following the initial saccade (20 to 60 ms after saccade) and obtained antagonistic results for both types of motion detectors. ICMS at a local-motion detector site resulted in a shift of eye position in the preferred direction of neurons at the stimulated site. In contrast, ICMS at a wide-field detector site resulted in a shift of eye position in the direction opposite to the preferred direction at the stimulated site. This effect of ICMS at a wide-field site was identical to the effects of global motion injection (Born et al., 2000).

Surprisingly, the presence of a structured background has only marginal effects on steady-state pursuit. Experimental evidence indicates that during the execution of SPEM, the sensitivity for global motion in the direction opposite to target movement (i.e. in the direction of the self-induced retinal image motion) is decreased. The cancellation of self-induced retinal image motion seems to be due to the involvement of extra-retinal factors such as an internal representation of the executed pursuit eye movement.

Role of anticipation, prediction, and attention

The tight linkage between visual motion processing and execution of SPEM might implicate that these eye movements exclusively depend on visual 'physical' factors such as retinal image motion. However, cognitive parameters have been shown to play an important role in the execution of SPEM as well as for the related perceptual processes. It was suggested that subjects pursue the perceptual rather than the retinal stimulus (Steinbach, 1976): subjects were able to track the hidden, invisible corner of a rectangle or the also invisible hub of a rolling wheel. Later it was demonstrated that humans as well as monkeys can track imaginary figures defined by parafoveal visual cues (*man*: Wyatt et al., 1994; *monkey*: Ilg and Thier, 1999).

The capability of anticipation or prediction to elicit SPEM has been known for a long time: expectation caused slow eye movements even before the appearance of a moving target. This observation was made for single target steps (Kowler and Steinman, 1979a) and for periodic target steps (Kowler and Steinman, 1979b). However, the velocity range of these eye movements was very low, below $1°/s$. To elicit higher smooth pursuit eye velocities, i.e. similar to the range of eye velocity during visual guided SPEM, Graham Barnes introduced the paradigm of the tachistoscopically illuminated target, which is explained in more detail in Barnes et al. (2002, this volume). Initially, the target moved on a triangular trajectory. After a few periods, the target was only briefly presented during its zero crossings (Barnes and Asselman, 1991). In this paradigm, subjects moved their eyes even before the target became visible.

To differentiate the various effects of prediction on eye movements, it turned out to be successful to separate mechanisms of short-term prediction from mechanisms of long-term prediction (Deno et al., 1995). Short-term prediction addresses the question where a target moving at constant velocity will be after a given time interval. The existence of this mechanism explains why the amplitude of the initial saccade is correctly adjusted to target velocity (Gellman and Carl, 1991). The mechanism of long-term prediction explains the zero-lag pursuit to periodically moving targets or the anticipatory eye movements during tachistoscopic target presentation.

Similar to the experiments conducted by Graham Barnes and colleagues (Barnes et al., 2002, this volume), we also used tachistoscopically illuminated target trajectories to elicit SPEM in the prospect of an upcoming target in man and monkey. The eye movements of a typical subject recorded in our laboratory are shown in Fig. 7.

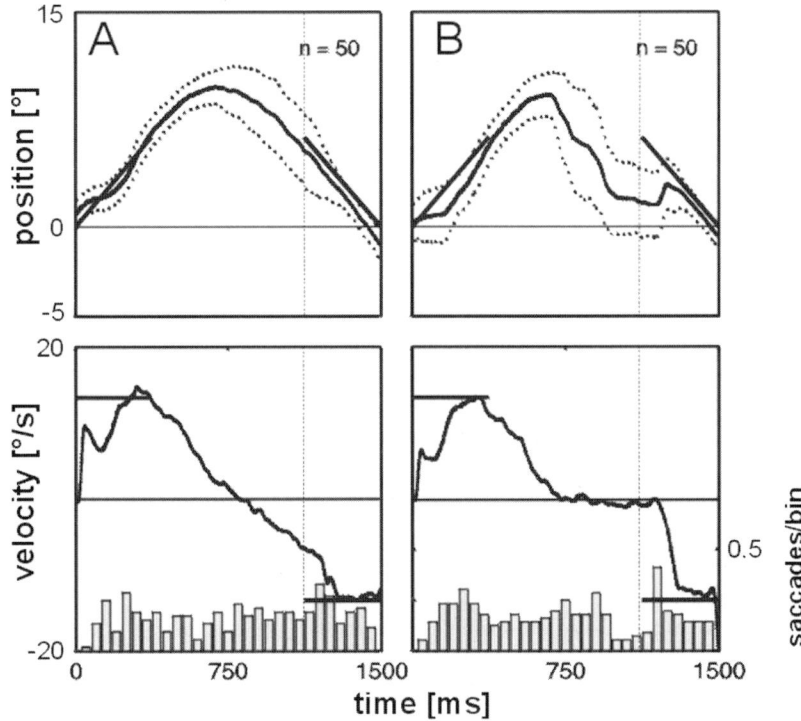

Fig. 7. Horizontal eye (mean and standard deviation) and target position and velocity as well as saccade histograms of a typical subject tracking a tachistoscopically illuminated target. Saccades were removed from the velocity records. For reasons of clarity, only the first half of the entire period is shown. Before these eye movements were recorded, the subject pursued at least for 10 periods the continuously presented moving target. In (A), the target trajectory was predictable. Note that eye velocity increased before the target (indicated by the horizontal bar) became visible (vertical dashed line). In (B), the target was not predictable since stimulus presentation was randomly intermixed with other trajectories. Note the absence of build-up in eye speed in this condition and the accumulation of saccades following the appearance of the target.

In order to examine SPEM driven by anticipation, we compared the eye movements obtained when the subject could predict the target trajectory with the eye movements obtained in a control paradigm. The control was physically identical to our test condition, but because these control trials were displayed together with other trial types, the subjects could not predict the target trajectory. In the control condition (see Fig. 7), the human subject did not move his eyes prior to target onset. The results from the experiments with rhesus monkeys failed to produce a significantly different eye movement pattern in the test and control conditions. Overall, our rhesus monkeys showed anticipatory pursuit to a much lesser extent than humans. The difference between man and monkey might reflect one out of two possibilities. Firstly, there might be an essential difference between the SPEM systems of man and monkey.

With respect to numerous reports in the literature, this does not seem to be very likely. Secondly, there might be differences in the instruction of human subjects and monkeys. Human subjects could be instructed verbally to generate anticipatory SPEM. It was proposed that the generation of anticipatory eye movements is due to an automatic process (Barnes and Asselman, 1991), accordingly the instruction should not play a crucial role. The differences in anticipatory eye movements between man and monkey might cast doubts on the hypothesis that the execution of anticipatory pursuit eye movements is driven by an automatic process.

The contributions in Born et al. (2002, this volume) show that the activity in extrastriate area MT was very closely related to the initiation of smooth pursuit eye movements. However, the processing of visual motion in this area was influenced by attention. If a monkey attended to a moving stimulus, the response was larger compared to a non-attended stimulation (Treue and Maunsell, 1996). Attention could not only be directed towards a specific location, but also to a specific feature of the stimulus. This feature-based attention also modulated the response of individual neurons (Treue and Martinez Trujillo, 1999). With these results in mind, it is obviously meaningful to examine the influence of directed or withdrawn attention on SPEM parameters.

As Chen et al. (2002, this volume) report, it is possible to combine a spatial frequency discrimination task with the execution of SPEM. The discrimination task was either presented before, simultaneously or subsequent to the onset of target movement. The pursuit onset latency was only increased if the second task was presented prior to the target. Initial eye acceleration was decreased in all cases and eye velocity of smooth pursuit maintenance was only decreased if the second task was presented simultaneously or subsequent to the pursuit target. These results could be explained by the limited capacity concept: if attention is withdrawn, less computational power is available and as a consequence, pursuit is degraded.

Another question is how the spotlight of attention moves when we perform SPEM, addressed by Van Donkelaar and Drew (2002, this volume). The task of the subject was to press a button as fast as possible in response to the appearance of a target. If the target was flashed ahead of the pursuit target, the manual reaction times were shorter compared to the target flash behind the pursuit target. This result indicates that the spotlight moves ahead of the target, examining the location where the pursuit target will be next.

Smooth pursuit eye movements and motor learning

Many eye movements are executed in response to a stimulus in the environment either as a reflex or at least in a reflex-like manner. Frequently, these stimulus–response loops are subject to adaptation or motor learning. Examples include the adaptation of the gain of the vestibulo-ocular-reflex (VOR, *man*: Collewijn et al., 1983; *monkey*: Miles and Fuller, 1974) or saccade amplitude (McLaughlin, 1967). In brief, adaptation or motor learning occurs if the stimulus–response loop generates consistently an error signal. Initially, the error is compensated using retinal information. Subsequently and after successful adaptation, the error is avoided by a modification of the primary response. With respect to SPEM, the amount of post-saccadic enhancement (see above) and the transformation of pre-saccadic visual motion information into an eye movement command could be subject to motor learning, as the following experiment shows. The basic paradigm was introduced more than 30 years ago (Barmack, 1970). If a target started to move at a given velocity and changed its velocity after a brief interval (100 ms), post-saccadic eye velocity was determined by the initial target velocity and not by its actual velocity. As a consequence, gaze position deviated from target position. If the paradigm was repeated (300 trials), post-saccadic eye velocity was adjusted to the new target velocity (Kahlon and Lisberger, 1996). It is possible to adapt to an acceleration or deceleration of the target.

The adaptation of initial eye acceleration offered a possibility to address the question whether vector averaging observed if two targets were presented simultaneously occurred rather early or late in the processing of visual motion. The obtained results clarified that the site of learning was located earlier in processing than the site of averaging (Kahlon and Lisberger, 1999). Despite this coarse localization, the exact site of learning is unknown at the present time. However, it is highly unlikely that neurons in area MT change their velocity tuning since area MT responds only to visual signals. Extra-retinal response properties related to the ongoing eye movement have not been found in this part of the brain. On the other hand, it is also not likely that the extraocular motoneurons or muscles change their properties during pursuit adaptation, since they are also involved in other types of eye movements. So the site of learning must be assumed somewhere in the pathway subserving SPEM, i.e. in neurons of area MST, of the frontal pursuit area (FPA), the dorsolateral pontine nuclei (DLPN) or the cerebellum (see Ilg, 1997 for overview).

Pursuit-related activity and its frame of reference

As mentioned earlier, the execution of SPEM is tightly connected to the processing of visual motion.

Elementary motion processing, either in case of correlation detectors (Reichardt, 1987) or in case of the energy model (Adelson and Bergen, 1985; Van Santen and Sperling, 1985), is achieved in a retinal frame of reference. This does not imply that motion processing takes place in the retina. Motion processing in primates is definitively a cortical feature, like the execution of SPEM itself. So it might be speculated that SPEM could also be generated within a simple retinal frame of reference. If this assumption was correct, SPEM could be explained as a simple feedback model with retinal image motion as input and eye movement as output (see Lisberger et al., 1987 for review).

However, there are qualms whether this statement is correct. Firstly, the perception of the moving target during pursuit is not confined to a retinal frame of reference. In case of perfectly adjusted SPEM, the image of the moving target remains stationary on the fovea. Despite the lack of retinal image motion, we perceive the target as moving which cannot result from processing within a retinal frame of reference. Secondly, pursuit is driven by perceptual rather than by retinal signals (Steinbach, 1976; Wyatt et al., 1994; Ilg and Thier, 1999). Pursuit can be executed in the expectation of an upcoming target, before the target is visible (see above). Finally, the strongest argument against the retinal frame of reference is elaborated below. The argument consists in the discharge rates of individual neurons in the posterior parietal cortex. The importance of areas MT and MST for the execution of SPEM was documented by single-unit responses (Newsome et al., 1988; Thier and Erickson, 1992; Lisberger and Movshon, 1999), by specific deficits following lesions (Dursteler et al., 1987; Dursteler and Wurtz, 1988; Yamasaki and Wurtz, 1991) and by ICMS in area MT (Groh et al., 1997; Born et al., 2000) and in area MST (Komatsu and Wurtz, 1989).

To answer the important question whether the observed pursuit-related activity can be explained by exclusively visual factors, the authors tried to exclude visual motion influences. A first step in the experiments was to avoid any background whose self-induced retinal image motion could be the source of pursuit-related activity. Subsequently, to avoid retinal target motion, the pursuit target was either switched off briefly or stabilized electronically on the retina. The pursuit-related activity recorded from area MT dropped as a consequence of this procedure indicating that area MT acts as a retinal image motion processor (Newsome et al., 1988; Lisberger and Movshon, 1999). In contrast, the activity recorded from area MST maintained unchanged (Newsome et al., 1988; Thier and Erickson, 1992). This robustness of discharge rates observed from area MST is taken as indication for the existence of extra-retinal signals affecting neurons in area MST. These extra-retinal signals most likely consisted in an eye movement signal. In contrast, neurons in area MT received only visual signals.

The extra-retinal properties were also demonstrated during pursuit of imaginary targets defined by parafoveal cues. As already noted, monkeys could be trained to perform SPEM towards an imaginary target (Ilg and Thier, 1999). In a study with three monkeys, we recorded from 85 neurons which responded identically during SPEM of real and imaginary targets (see Fig. 8). Note that during tracking of the imaginary target, there was no visual stimulation of the central visual field where the visual receptive field was located. We performed an important control experiment in which we moved the imaginary target while the monkey fixated a stationary target. Since the neurons did not respond in this condition, we were able to exclude the possibility that the similarity in responses was due to stimulation of the peripheral visual field, which was obviously identical in both stimulus conditions.

So there is multiple experimental evidence that the discharge rate of neurons in area MST is driven by visual and by extra-retinal signals. The possibility that neurons in area MST use a retinal frame of reference can therefore be excluded. However, the question remains whether the activity codes for eye-in-head, gaze or target velocity. In order to answer this question, we trained monkeys to execute either isolated eye or combined eye and head movements in response to a moving target. The color of the target signaled whether the monkey should use eye or head movements for tracking. Fig. 9 shows the response of a typical neuron recorded from area MST in the two different tracking conditions.

Although the eye-in-head movements differed substantially in the two tracking conditions, the discharge rates of the neuron were identical in both

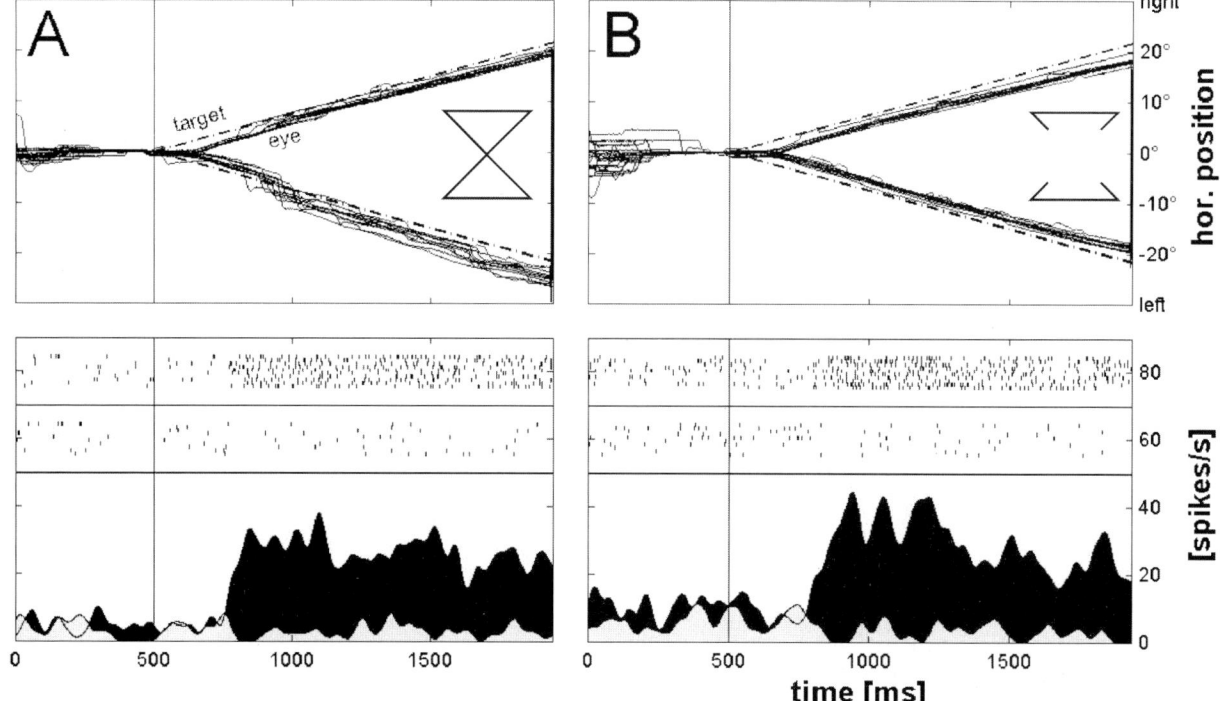

Fig. 8. Horizontal eye and target position together with the discharge rate of a typical neuron recorded from area MST of a rhesus monkey. The black spike density function and the upper raster display represents the response during pursuit in preferred direction, the gray density function and the lower raster display gives the response in non-preferred direction. The statistical analysis of the variance of the discharge rates (2-way ANOVA) revealed that the rate was significantly affected by the direction of target movement ($p < 0.0001$), but not by the type of target ($p = 0.28$, interaction of both factors: $p = 0.45$). The response during pursuit of the real target (A) was identical to the response during pursuit of the imaginary target (B). Both targets are shown in the right part of the figure, their height and width was 20°, the blanked area in the imaginary target was 12°.

cases. The gaze (eye-in-space) movements were also identical in both conditions. So the similarity in discharge rates might be explained as a consequence of identical gaze and resulting identical retinal image motion. However, as shown above, the activity of this neuron remained unchanged during brief removal of the target. In summary, we recorded 122 neurons from three rhesus monkeys in this paradigm. The activity of 51 neurons was not statistically significant different in the two tracking conditions, 45 of them showed extra-retinal response properties.

The similarity of responses during eye and head movements excluded the possibility that MST neurons code for eye-in-head movements. However, it is not clear whether the discharge rate coded for gaze or target velocity in space. To solve this question, we employed a combination of vestibular stimulation and a pursuit task. While the monkey was rotated sinusoidally around the yaw axis at 0.2 Hz, he tracked a target that moved horizontally at 0.33 Hz. The Fourier transformation of the neuronal response revealed that its power density function had a maximum at 0.33 Hz, the frequency of target movement in space. We tested 39 neurons out of the above-mentioned 51 neurons. Finally, linear regressions of the discharge rate versus gaze velocity and of the discharge rate versus target velocity revealed that the activity coded for target motion in space for 34 out of the 39 neurons tested. Our findings suggest that the activity in area MST codes for the trajectory of a target in an external frame of reference. Since the transformation from a retinal frame of reference towards an external reference frame is achieved at this level of cortical processing, this information can be

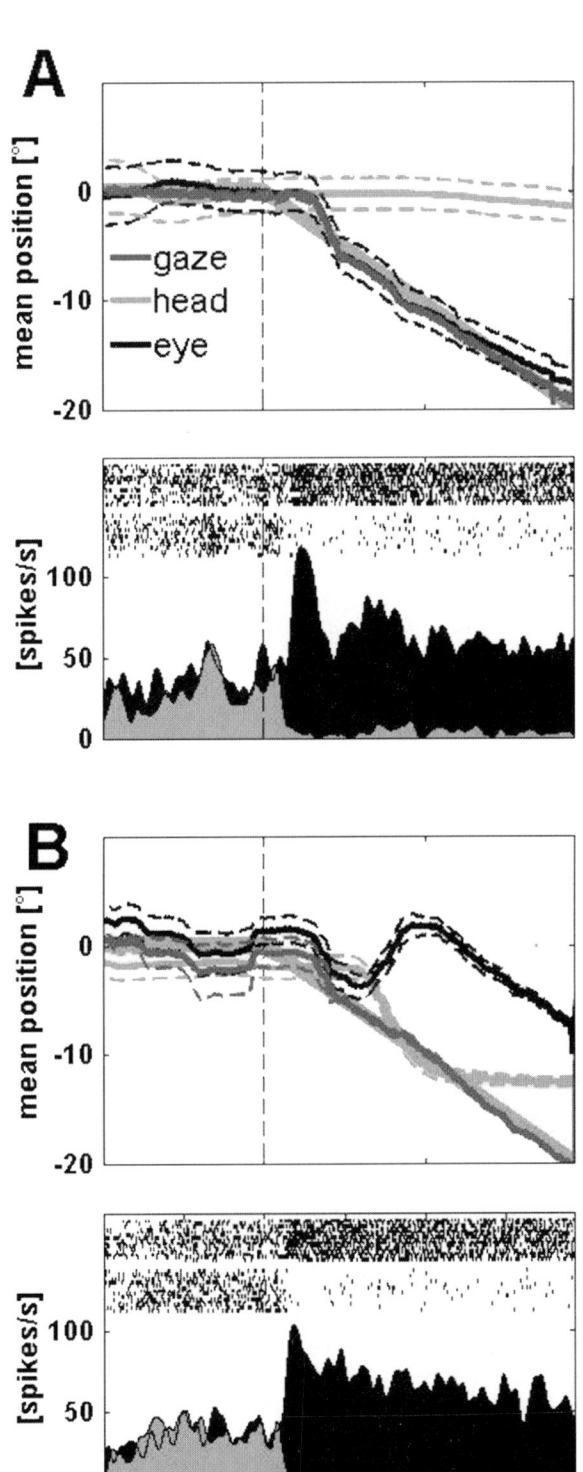

used for the generation of any general goal-directed behavior, not only for SPEM, but also for the perception of the moving target.

Conclusions

The execution of SPEM constitutes an ultimate link to visual motion processing as a typical example of low-level vision. However, as the examples in this chapter showed, the execution of SPEM is also massively influenced by high-level vision features such as the cognitive load of the paradigm, the structure of the background, or the predictability of target trajectory. Although the execution of SPEM is tightly related to visual motion processing which undoubtedly occurs within a retinal frame of reference, the neuronal activity recorded from the posterior parietal cortex during various tracking tasks codes for the target trajectory within an external reference frame.

Acknowledgements

I thank Urs Schwarz for more than a decade of stimulating collaboration. In addition, I would like to thank Axel Lindner, Stefan Schumann, Natalie Rüb and Jan Churan for performing many of the described experiments and critical discussions of the manuscript. I am grateful to Peter Thier for general support. Financial support from DFG and Hermann-and-Lilly-Schilling Foundation made this work possible.

Fig. 9. Gaze, eye, and head position of a rhesus monkey together with the discharge rate of a typical neuron recorded from area MST (black spike density function and upper raster display gives preferred direction, gray density function and lower raster display represents non-preferred direction). In (A), an eye movement trial was requested, the head remained stationary. In (B), the monkey had to execute a head movement trial. The statistical analysis (2-way ANOVA) revealed that the discharge rate was significantly affected by the direction of target movement ($p < 0.0001$), but not by the type of tracking ($p = 0.18$). So although the executed eye-in-head movements were quite different, the response of the neuron was identical in both conditions.

References

Adelson, E.H. and Bergen, J.R. (1985) Spatiotemporal energy models for the perception of motion. *J. Opt. Soc. Am. A*, 2: 284–299.

Aglioti, S., DeSouza, J.F. and Goodale, M.A. (1995) Size-contrast illusions deceive the eye but not the hand. *Curr. Biol.*, 5: 679–685.

Barmack, N.H. (1970) Modification of eye movements by instantaneous changes in the velocity of visual targets. *Vision Res.*, 10: 1431–1441.

Barnes, G.R. and Asselman, P.T. (1991) The mechanism of prediction in human smooth pursuit eye movements. *J. Physiol.*, 439: 439–461.

Barnes, G.R., Schmid, A.M. and Jarrett, C.B. (2002) The role of expectancy and volition in smooth pursuit eye movements. In: J. Hyönä, D.P. Munoz, W. Heide and R. Radach (Eds.), *The Brain's Eye: Neurobiological and Clinical Aspects of Oculomotor Research*. Progress in Brain Research, Vol. 140, Elsevier, Amsterdam, pp. 239–254.

Beutter, B.R. and Stone, L.S. (1998) Human motion perception and smooth eye movements show similar directional biases for elongated apertures. *Vision Res.*, 38: 1273–1286.

Beutter, B.R. and Stone, L.S. (2000) Motion coherence affects human perception and pursuit similarly. *Vis. Neurosci.*, 17: 139–153.

Born, R.T. (2000) Center–surround interactions in the middle temporal visual area of the owl monkey. *J. Neurophysiol.*, 84: 2658–2669.

Born, R.T. and Tootell, R.B. (1992) Segregation of global and local motion processing in primate middle temporal visual area. *Nature*, 357: 497–499.

Born, R.T., Groh, J.M., Zhao, R. and Lukasewycz, S.J. (2000) Segregation of object and background motion in visual area MT: effects of microstimulation on eye movements. *Neuron*, 26: 725–734.

Born, R.T., Pack, C.C. and Zhao, R. (2002) Integration of motion cues for the initiation of smooth pursuit eye movements. In: J. Hyönä, D.P. Munoz, W. Heide and R. Radach (Eds.), *The Brain's Eye: Neurobiological and Clinical Aspects of Oculomotor Research*. Progress in Brain Research, Vol. 140, Elsevier, Amsterdam, pp. 225–237.

Bridgeman, B., Hendry, D. and Stark, L. (1975) Failure to detect displacement of the visual world during saccadic eye movements. *Vision Res.*, 15: 719–722.

Burr, D.C., Morrone, M.C. and Ross, J. (2001) Separate visual representations for perception and action revealed by saccadic eye movements. *Curr. Biol.*, 11: 798–802.

Butzer, F., Ilg, U.J. and Zanker, J.M. (1997) Smooth-pursuit eye movements elicited by first-order and second-order motion. *Exp. Brain Res.*, 115: 61–70.

Chen, Y., Holzman, P.S. and Nakayama, K. (2002) Visual and cognitive control of attention in smooth pursuit. In: J. Hyönä, D.P. Munoz, W. Heide and R. Radach (Eds.), *The Brain's Eye: Neurobiological and Clinical Aspects of Oculomotor Research*. Progress in Brain Research, Vol. 140, Elsevier, Amsterdam, pp. 225–265.

Chubb, C. and Sperling, G. (1988) Drift-balanced random stimuli: a general basis for studying non-Fourier motion perception. *J. Opt. Soc. Am. A*, 5: 1986–2007.

Churan, J. and Ilg, U.J. (2001) Processing of second-order motion stimuli in primate middle temporal area and medial superior temporal area. *J. Opt. Soc. Am. A Opt. Image Sci. Vis.*, 18: 2297–2306.

Collewijn, H. and Tamminga, E.P. (1984) Human smooth and saccadic eye movements during voluntary pursuit of different target motions on different backgrounds. *J. Physiol.*, 351: 217–250.

Collewijn, H., van der Mark, F. and Jansen, T.C. (1975) Precise recording of human eye movements. *Vision Res.*, 15: 447–450.

Collewijn, H., Martins, A.J. and Steinman, R.M. (1983) Compensatory eye movements during active and passive head movements: fast adaptation to changes in visual magnification. *J. Physiol.*, 340: 259–286.

Deno, D.C., Crandall, W.F., Sherman, K. and Keller, E.L. (1995) Characterization of prediction in the primate visual smooth pursuit system. *Biosystems*, 34: 107–128.

Derrington, A.M., Badcock, D.R. and Henning, G.B. (1993) Discriminating the direction of second-order motion at short stimulus durations. *Vision Res.*, 33: 1785–1794.

Duncker, K. (1929) Ueber induzierte Bewegung. *Psychol. Forsch.*, 12: 180–259.

Dursteler, M.R. and Wurtz, R.H. (1988) Pursuit and optokinetic deficits following chemical lesions of cortical areas MT and MST. *J. Neurophysiol.*, 60: 940–965.

Dursteler, M.R., Wurtz, R.H. and Newsome, W.T. (1987) Directional pursuit deficits following lesions of the foveal representation within the superior temporal sulcus of the macaque monkey. *J. Neurophysiol.*, 57: 1262–1287.

Ferrera, V.P. and Lisberger, S.G. (1995) Attention and target selection for smooth pursuit eye movements. *J. Neurosci.*, 15: 7472–7484.

Ferrera, V.P. and Lisberger, S.G. (1997) The effect of a moving distracter on the initiation of smooth-pursuit eye movements. *Vis. Neurosci.*, 14: 323–338.

Filehne, W. (1922) Ueber das optische Wahrnehmen von Bewegungen. *Z. Sinnesphysiol.*, 53: 134–145.

Fischer, B. and Boch, R. (1983) Saccadic eye movements after extremely short reaction times in the monkey. *Brain Res.*, 260: 21–26.

Franz, V.H., Gegenfurtner, K.R., Bülthoff, H.H. and Fahle, M. (2000) Grasping visual illusions: no evidence for a dissociation between perception and action. *Psychol. Sci.*, 11: 20–25.

Gardner, J.L. and Lisberger, S.G. (2001) Linked target selection for saccadic and smooth pursuit eye movements. *J. Neurosci.*, 21: 2075–2084.

Gellman, R.S. and Carl, J.R. (1991) Motion processing for saccadic eye movements in humans. *Exp. Brain Res.*, 84: 660–667.

Goodale, M.A. and Milner, A.D. (1992) Separate visual pathways for perception and action. *Trends Neurosci.*, 15: 20–25.

Goodale, M.A., Milner, A.D., Jakobson, L.S. and Carey, D.P.

(1991) A neurological dissociation between perceiving objects and grasping them. *Nature*, 349: 154–156.

Groh, J.M., Born, R.T. and Newsome, W.T. (1997) How is a sensory map read out? Effects of microstimulation in visual area MT on saccades and smooth pursuit eye movements. *J. Neurosci.*, 17: 4312–4330.

Haarmeier, T. and Thier, P. (1996) Modification of the Filehne illusion by conditioning visual stimuli. *Vision Res.*, 36(5): 741–750.

Ilg, U.J. (1997) Slow eye movements. *Prog. Neurobiol.*, 53: 293–329.

Ilg, U.J. and Thier, P. (1996) Inability of rhesus monkey area V1 to discriminate between self-induced and externally induced retinal image slip. *Eur. J. Neurosci.*, 8: 1156–1166.

Ilg, U.J. and Thier, P. (1999) Eye movements of rhesus monkeys directed towards imaginary targets. *Vision Res.*, 39: 2143–2150.

Kahlon, M. and Lisberger, S.G. (1996) Coordinate system for learning in the smooth pursuit eye movements of monkeys. *J. Neurosci.*, 16: 7270–7283.

Kahlon, M. and Lisberger, S.G. (1999) Vector averaging occurs downstream from learning in smooth pursuit eye movements of monkeys. *J. Neurosci.*, 19: 9039–9053.

Kalesnykas, R.P. and Hallett, P.E. (2002) Saccadic latency effects of progressively deleting stimulus offsets and onsets. *Vision Res.*, 42: 637–652.

Keller, E.L. and Khan, N.S. (1986) Smooth-pursuit initiation in the presence of a textured background in monkey. *Vision Res.*, 26: 943–955.

Kimmig, H.G., Miles, F.A. and Schwarz, U. (1992) Effects of stationary textured backgrounds on the initiation of pursuit eye movements in monkeys. *J. Neurophysiol.*, 68: 2147–2164.

Knox, P.C. (1996) The effect of the gap paradigm on the latency of human smooth pursuit of eye movement. *Neuroreport*, 7: 3027–3030.

Knox, P.C. and Bekkour, T. (2002) Non-target influences on the initiation of smooth pursuit. In: J. Hyönä, D.P. Munoz, W. Heide and R. Radach (Eds.), *The Brain's Eye: Neurobiological and Clinical Aspects of Oculomotor Research*. Progress in Brain Research, Vol. 140, Elsevier, Amsterdam, pp. 211–224.

Komatsu, H. and Wurtz, R.H. (1989) Modulation of pursuit eye movements by stimulation of cortical areas MT and MST. *J. Neurophysiol.*, 62: 31–47.

Kowler, E. and Steinman, R.M. (1979a) The effect of expectations on slow oculomotor control. I. Periodic target steps. *Vision Res.*, 19: 619–632.

Kowler, E. and Steinman, R.M. (1979b) The effect of expectations on slow oculomotor control. II. Single target displacements. *Vision Res.*, 19: 633–646.

Krauzlis, R.J. and Adler, S.A. (2001) Effects of directional expectations on motion perception and pursuit eye movements. *Vis. Neurosci.*, 18: 365–376.

Krauzlis, R.J. and Miles, F.A. (1996a) Decreases in the latency of smooth pursuit and saccadic eye movements produced by the 'gap paradigm' in the monkey. *Vision Res.*, 36: 1973–1985.

Krauzlis, R.J. and Miles, F.A. (1996b) Release of fixation for pursuit and saccades in humans: evidence for shared inputs acting on different neural substrates. *J. Neurophysiol.*, 76: 2822–2833.

Krauzlis, R.J. and Stone, L.S. (1999) Tracking with the mind's eye. *Trends Neurosci.*, 22: 544–550.

Krauzlis, R.J., Basso, M.A. and Wurtz, R.H. (1997) Shared motor error for multiple eye movements. *Science*, 276: 1693–1695.

Krauzlis, R.J., Dill, N. and Kornylo, K. (2002) Activity in the primate rostral superior colliculus during the 'gap effect' for pursuit and saccades. *Ann. N.Y. Acad. Sci.*, 956: 409–413.

Lindner, A. and Ilg, U.J. (2000) Initiation of smooth-pursuit eye movements to first-order and second-order motion stimuli. *Exp. Brain Res.*, 133: 450–456.

Lindner, A., Schwarz, U. and Ilg, U.J. (2001) Cancellation of self-induced retinal image motion during smooth pursuit eye movements. *Vision Res.*, 41: 1685–1694.

Lisberger, S.G. (1998) Postsaccadic enhancement of initiation of smooth pursuit eye movements in monkeys. *J. Neurophysiol.*, 79: 1918–1930.

Lisberger, S.G. and Ferrera, V.P. (1997) Vector averaging for smooth pursuit eye movements initiated by two moving targets in monkeys. *J. Neurosci.*, 17: 7490–7502.

Lisberger, S.G. and Movshon, J.A. (1999) Visual motion analysis for pursuit eye movements in area MT of macaque monkeys. *J. Neurosci.*, 19: 2224–2246.

Lisberger, S.G. and Westbrook, L.E. (1985) Properties of visual inputs that initiate horizontal smooth pursuit eye movements in monkeys. *J. Neurosci.*, 5: 1662–1673.

Lisberger, S.G., Morris, E.J. and Tychsen, L. (1987) Visual motion processing and sensory–motor integration for smooth pursuit eye movements. *Annu. Rev. Neurosci.*, 10: 97–129.

Masson, G.S., Rybarczyk, Y., Castet, E. and Mestre, D.R. (2000) Temporal dynamics of motion integration for the initiation of tracking eye movements at ultra-short latencies. *Vis. Neurosci.*, 17: 753–767.

McLaughlin, S.C. (1967) Parametric adjustment in saccadic eye movements. *Percept. Psychophys.*, 2: 359–362.

Merrison, A.F. and Carpenter, R.H. (1994) Co-variability of smooth and saccadic latencies in oculomotor pursuit. *Ophthalmic Res.*, 26: 158–162.

Merrison, A.F. and Carpenter, R.H. (1995) 'Express' smooth pursuit. *Vision Res.*, 35: 1459–1462.

Miles, F.A. and Fuller, J.H. (1974) Adaptive plasticity in the vestibulo-ocular responses of the rhesus monkey. *Brain Res.*, 80: 512–516.

Miura, K., Suehiro, K., Yamamoto, M., Kodaka, Y. and Kawano, K. (2001) Initiation of smooth pursuit in humans: dependence on target saliency. *Exp. Brain Res.*, 141: 242–249.

Mohrmann, H. and Thier, P. (1995) The influence of structured visual backgrounds on smooth-pursuit initiation, steady-state pursuit and smooth-pursuit termination. *Biol. Cybern.*, 73: 83–93.

Newsome, W.T. and Paré, E.B. (1988) A selective impairment of motion perception following lesions of the middle temporal visual area (MT). *J. Neurosci.*, 8: 2201–2211.

Newsome, W.T., Wurtz, R.H. and Komatsu, H. (1988) Relation

of cortical areas MT and MST to pursuit eye movements. II. Differentiation of retinal from extraretinal inputs. *J. Neurophysiol.*, 60: 604–620.

O'Mullane, G. and Knox, P.C. (1999) Modification of smooth pursuit initiation by target contrast. *Vision Res.*, 39: 3459–3464.

Pack, C.C. and Born, R.T. (2001) Temporal dynamics of a neural solution to the aperture problem in visual area MT of macaque brain. *Nature*, 409: 1040–1042.

Rashbass, C. (1961) The relationship between saccadic and smooth tracking eye movements. *J. Physiol.*, 159: 326–338.

Recanzone, G.H. and Wurtz, R.H. (1999) Shift in smooth pursuit initiation and MT and MST neuronal activity under different stimulus conditions. *J. Neurophysiol.*, 82: 1710–1727.

Reichardt, W. (1987) Evaluation of optical motion information by movement detectors. *J. Comp. Physiol. A*, 161: 533–547.

Saslow, M.G. (1967) Effects of components of displacement-step stimuli upon latency for saccadic eye movement. *J. Opt. Soc. Am.*, 57: 1024–1029.

Schwartz, J.D. and Lisberger, S.G. (1994) Initial tracking conditions modulate the gain of visuo-motor transmission for smooth pursuit eye movements in monkeys. *Vis. Neurosci.*, 11: 411–424.

Schwarz, U. and Ilg, U.J. (1999) Asymmetry in visual motion processing. *Neuroreport*, 10: 2477–2480.

Steinbach, M.J. (1976) Pursuing the perceptual rather than the retinal stimulus. *Vision Res.*, 16: 1371–1376.

Stone, L.S., Beutter, B.R. and Lorenceau, J. (2000) Visual motion integration for perception and pursuit. *Perception*, 29: 771–787.

Suehiro, K., Miura, K., Kodaka, Y., Inoue, Y., Takemura, A. and Kawano, K. (1999) Effects of smooth pursuit eye movement on ocular responses to sudden background motion in humans. *Neurosci. Res.*, 35: 329–338.

Thier, P. and Erickson, R.G. (1992) Vestibular input to visual-tracking neurons in area MST of awake rhesus monkeys. *Ann. N.Y. Acad. Sci.*, 656: 960–963.

Treue, S. and Martinez Trujillo, J.C. (1999) Feature-based attention influences motion processing gain in macaque visual cortex. *Nature*, 399: 575–579.

Treue, S. and Maunsell, J.H. (1996) Attentional modulation of visual motion processing in cortical areas MT and MST. *Nature*, 382: 539–541.

Tychsen, L. and Lisberger, S.G. (1986) Visual motion processing for the initiation of smooth-pursuit eye movements in humans. *J. Neurophysiol.*, 56: 953–968.

Ungerleider, L.G. and Mishkin, M. (1982) Two cortical visual systems. In: D.J. Ingle (Ed.), *Analysis of Visual Behavior*. MIT Press, Cambridge, MA, pp. 549–586.

Van Donkelaar, P. and Drew, A.S. (2002) The allocation of attention during smooth pursuit eye movements. In: J. Hyönä, D.P. Munoz, W. Heide and R. Radach (Eds.), *The Brain's Eye: Neurobiological and Clinical Aspects of Oculomotor Research*. Progress in Brain Research, Vol. 140, Elsevier, Amsterdam, pp. 267–277.

Van Santen, J.P. and Sperling, G. (1985) Elaborated Reichardt detectors. *J. Opt. Soc. Am. A*, 2: 300–321.

Von Holst, E. and Mittelstaedt, H. (1950) Das Reafferenzprinzip. *Naturwissenschaften*, 37: 464–476.

Wyatt, H.J., Pola, J., Fortune, B. and Posner, M. (1994) Smooth pursuit eye movements with imaginary targets defined by extrafoveal cues. *Vision Res.*, 34: 803–820.

Yamasaki, D.S. and Wurtz, R.H. (1991) Recovery of function after lesions in the superior temporal sulcus in the monkey. *J. Neurophysiol.*, 66: 651–673.

Yee, R.D., Daniels, S.A., Jones, O.W., Baloh, R.W. and Honrubia, V. (1983) Effects of an optokinetic background on pursuit eye movements. *Invest. Ophthalmol. Vis. Sci.*, 24: 1115–1122.

Yo, C. and Wilson, H.R. (1992) Perceived direction of moving two-dimensional patterns depends on duration, contrast and eccentricity. *Vision Res.*, 32: 135–147.

Zanker, J.M. (1993) Theta motion: a paradoxical stimulus to explore higher order motion extraction. *Vision Res.*, 33: 553–569.

# SECTION IV

Eye-hand coordination

Section Editor: R. Radach

CHAPTER 20

Cortical frames of reference for eye–hand coordination

Paul Van Donkelaar *, Ji-Hang Lee and Anthony S. Drew

Department of Exercise and Movement Science, Institute of Neuroscience, University of Oregon, Eugene, OR 97403-1240, USA

Abstract: To reach for an object the brain must transform visual input from the eye into motor output of the arm. Recent neurophysiological experiments have shown that this transformation maps onto a network of brain areas including the posterior parietal (PPC) and premotor (PMC) cortices. In this chapter, we review evidence from our own experiments which demonstrate that this network can only partially complete the transformation when the eye and limb movement amplitudes are dissociated. We also discuss the effects of disrupting either the PPC or PMC using transcranial magnetic stimulation (TMS) on the ability to carry out the transformation successfully.

Introduction

The ease with which we perform the act of reaching out to point at or grasp an object belies the fact that this behavior requires a complex transformation of visual input into a coordinated motor response of the eyes and hand. How this process is carried out in the brain has been the focus of much recent investigation within neuroscience. At the heart of this issue is how the initial visual input coded with respect to the retina is transformed into appropriate oculomotor and manual motor output and how signals related to responses in each of these effectors interact with each other to produce the coordinated movements that are observed. A specific question that arises is how the oculomotor signals based in an eye-centered frame of reference influence the manual motor responses that are of necessity generated in a limb-centered frame of reference. We propose that if compensation for the eye-centered frame of reference is not complete by the time the manual response is generated, this should be apparent and quantifiable in the characteristics of the reaching movement. In a series of recent experiments we have examined this issue in relation to the conditions under which compensation occurs and the areas of the cortex that are responsible for it.

Neurophysiological studies

A growing body of literature from single unit neurophysiological studies in awake behaving non-human primates has demonstrated that parts of the posterior parietal cortex (PPC) code for oculomotor and manual motor output in an eye-centered frame of reference. Within the medial portion of the PPC there exists the parietal reach region (PRR) which contains arm movement-related cells that encode targets with respect to eye position (Batista et al., 1999). A large proportion of these reach-selective cells also fire around the time of saccade generation (Snyder et al., 2000). Such cells could play an important role in the coordination between eye and limb movements to visual targets. The PPC sends strong projections to the premotor cortex (PMC; Wise et al., 1997) and this latter area has also been shown to be involved in eye–hand interactions during reaching movements. The PMC is traditionally thought of as an area whose activity is strongly related to the coding of

---

* Correspondence to: P. Van Donkelaar, Department of Exercise and Movement Science, Institute of Neuroscience, University of Oregon, Eugene, OR 97403-1240, USA. Tel.: +1-541-346-2687; Fax: +1-541-346-2841; E-mail: paulvd@darkwing.uoregon.edu

arm movements (e.g., Fu et al., 1995; Riehle and Requin, 1995). Cells in this part of the brain typically display activity associated with the amplitude and direction of reaching responses; in other words, the goal of the output made with the arm. In this sense, this activity can be thought of as representing the target in an arm-centered frame of reference. More recent research has demonstrated that visual and oculomotor signals can influence the activity of reach-related cells in this part of the cortex (Mushiake et al., 1997; Boussaoud et al., 1998), and that visual responses can even vary with arm as opposed to eye position (Graziano, 1999). Taken together, this evidence implies that an arm-centered frame of reference predominates in the PMC.

Human eye–hand interactions

The available evidence from non-human primate studies indicates that neural activity related to coordinated eye and hand movements is transformed from an eye- to a hand-centered frame of reference as one moves from the PPC to the PMC. If this transformation is incomplete by the time the reach plan has been initiated, the information related to the eye-centered frame of reference should 'leak' into the pointing response. This leakage would not have any noticeable effect if the eye and hand both start at the same position. However, if the amplitude required of the eye movement is different from that required for the hand then any signals related to eye amplitude may have a quantifiable influence on the reach plan. We addressed this issue by having subjects make open-loop pointing movements from a central location to a peripherally presented target while simultaneously making saccadic eye movements from the same central starting position or from positions that required saccades 10–20° larger than the reaching response (Fig. 1; Van Donkelaar, 1997). In all cases, however, the reaching and saccadic movements were made to the same peripheral target location. In this way we were able to dissociate the eye and hand amplitudes and directly ask the question how the two systems may interact. If the saccadic signals do not influence reaching movements, then the amplitude of those movements should be uninfluenced by the fact that eye movements of different sizes accompany them. However, if there is an interaction, then the pointing amplitudes should increase with increases in saccadic amplitude. Fig. 2 shows the results of this manipulation on typical trials with each combination of hand and saccade amplitude as well as the group means for hand amplitude plotted as a function of saccade amplitude. It is clear that when the saccade started in the same position as the hand, there was a consistent undershooting of the target. As saccade size increased, however, the amplitude of the hand movement also increased. This occurred despite the fact that the eye and the hand were both directed at the same peripheral target. When visual feedback was available from the hand, the influence of saccade amplitude was not apparent. In addition, this effect does not appear to be due to a miscoding of space in the peripheral retina (see Henriques et al., 2002, this volume) since control experiments using visual fixation at the different eye target starting positions demonstrated a *constant* overshoot of the peripheral target with the hand. Taken together, these results are consistent with the idea that information related to saccade amplitude is integrated into the limb movement response.

In order to examine the time course of the interaction between eye and hand movements the initial acceleration of the arm was quantified as a function of the onset asynchrony between the beginning of the saccade and the beginning of the arm movement (Van Donkelaar, 1998). The idea is that the natural variation between saccade and hand movement onsets could provide some clues as to when in time saccadic signals started to influence the reach plan. Fig. 3 shows how the initial arm acceleration from a single subject varied as a function of the delay between the saccadic and hand movement onsets. The different symbols represent the three different saccade amplitudes used (10, 20, and 30°). As the saccade–hand delay increased, the magnitude of the initial hand acceleration decreased in a linear fashion. Indeed, for the group of subjects tested and different target amplitudes used, a positive linear correlation was obtained between these two variables in 87% of the cases. This result implies that the interactions between the saccadic and manual motor systems occur over a finite period of time around the onset of the saccade. Clearly, increasing the delay greatly reduces the impact the saccade has on the pointing response.

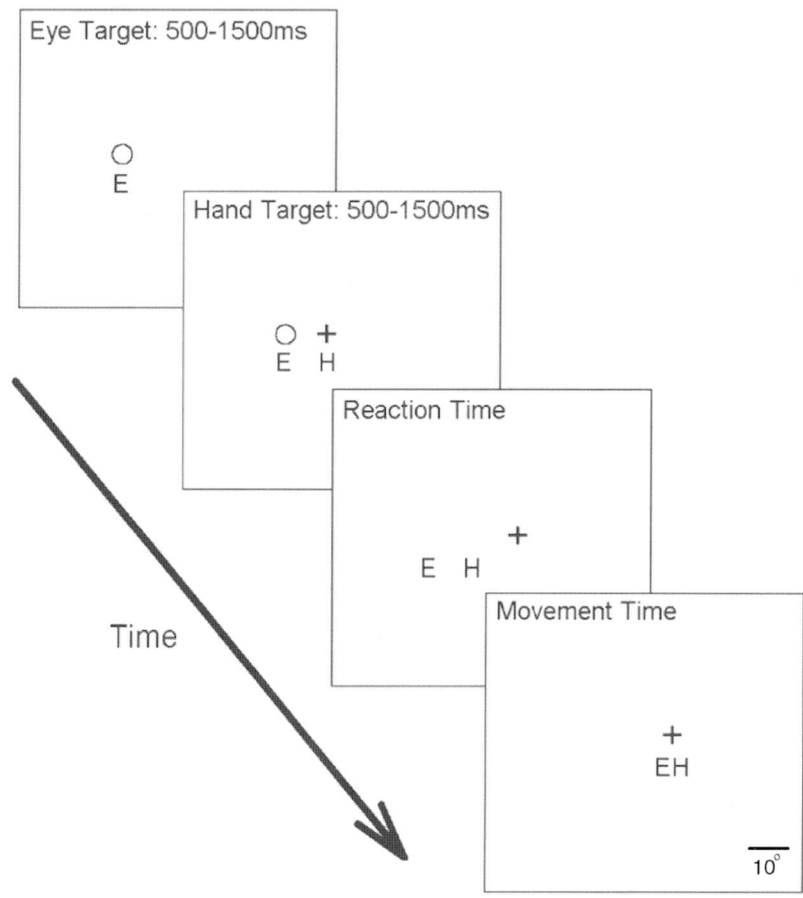

Fig. 1. Events occurring within a trial with a 10° hand movement and 20° eye movement. Initially, an eye target appears at one of three locations (centered, 10° to the left, 20° to the left) on the screen. After a variable delay a hand target appears directly in front of the subject. After a further variable delay both the eye and hand targets disappear and a peripheral target appears 10° to the right. The subject is required to make a combined eye and hand movement to this target in response. E and H represent the positions of the eye and hand, respectively. Target sizes are not to scale.

Taken together, these results demonstrate that eye and hand movement signals do interact in the human brain. More specifically they show that under certain circumstances saccadic signals generated in an eye-centered frame of reference are not completely compensated for during the planning of the reaching movement. Our goal in subsequent experiments was to examine how this transformation process maps onto the areas of the brain that are thought to play a key role in this process: the posterior parietal and premotor cortices. We addressed this question by using transcranial magnetic stimulation (TMS) to disrupt these areas during task performance.

Transcranial magnetic stimulation

One of the goals of systems neuroscience is to better understand the relationship between the activity in different brain regions and behavior. There are several approaches one can take in an attempt to address this issue in humans. One of the most powerful techniques is functional brain imaging. By measuring correlates of neural activity related to blood flow one is able to quantify the extent of the relation between brain activity and task performance. Before the advent of imaging techniques similar questions regarding brain–behavior relations were addressed

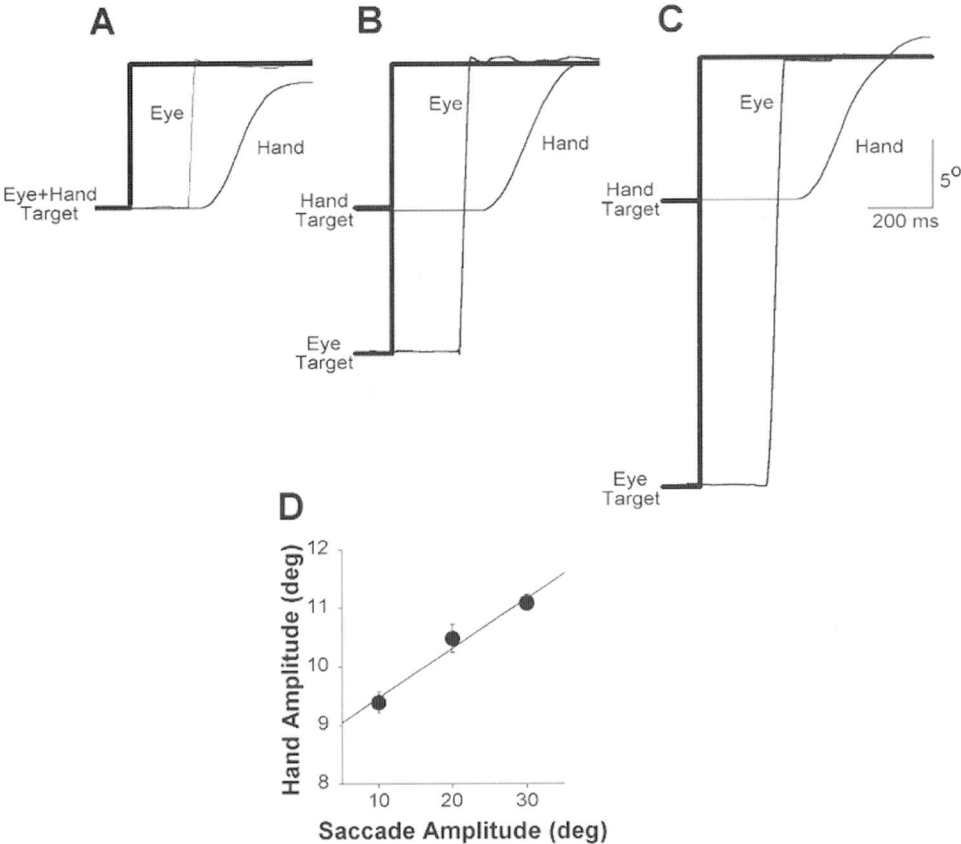

Fig. 2. Influence of saccades of different amplitudes on hand movements. Typical trials in which eye and hand start at same central position (A), or in which the saccade is 10° larger (B) or 20° larger than the hand movement. Notice that the hand amplitude increases with saccade amplitude. (D) Group means for hand amplitude plotted as a function of required saccade amplitude. Line of best fit is from a linear regression analysis. Error bars, 1 SE.

by quantifying the deficits that were observed when a particular area of the brain was damaged. The logic is that if a patient has difficulty with a certain behavior as a result of a lesion to a circumscribed brain region, then that region very likely contributes to that behavior in healthy humans. More recently, researchers have started using transcranial magnetic stimulation (TMS) in an analogous manner. TMS allows one to create a transient virtual functional lesion at a specific time relative to the processing of information related to the task of interest (Pascual-Leone et al., 1999). Of course no actual lesion occurs, rather the magnetic pulse appears to briefly disrupt the pattern of activity in the area being stimulated so that it is unable to contribute in a normal manner to the task being performed. By measuring the resulting performance deficits one can make strong inferences regarding the role played by the area being stimulated. TMS has at least two advantages over human functional imaging experiments. First, it can demonstrate that the activity in a particular area of the brain is necessary for, rather than simply correlated with, a specific behavior. Second, by delivering the disruptive stimulus at precise intervals it becomes possible to answer not only if but also when an area is involved in a task with a temporal resolution (tens of milliseconds; Walsh and Rushworth, 1999) that is greater than event-related fMRI (Josephs and Henson, 1999). TMS also has two advantages over human patient studies. First, the site at which the stimulation is delivered can be accurately controlled and relatively circumscribed from a functional point

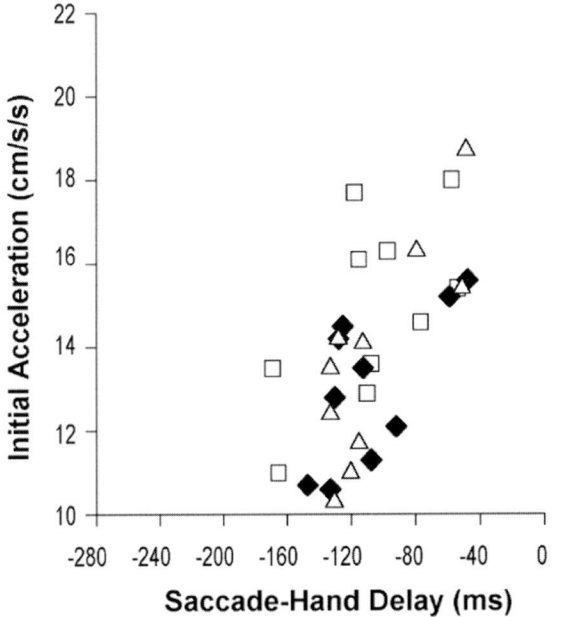

Fig. 3. Initial acceleration of the hand measured during the first 100 ms of hand movements plotted against the delay between saccade onset and hand movement onset for a single subject. Negative values indicate that the saccade started before the pointing movement. Different symbols represent different trial types with different saccade amplitudes (10°, diamonds; 20°, squares; 30°, triangles). Notice that as the delay between saccade and hand movement onset decreased the initial acceleration of the hand increased.

of view. For example, moving the stimulating coil by as little as 0.5 cm over the motor cortex can cause activation in different sets of hand muscles (Brasil-Neto et al., 1992). By contrast, lesions caused by a stroke can be quite extensive within an individual and quite variable from one patient to the next. Second, because of the short-term nature of the virtual functional lesion resulting from TMS, the subject is very likely unable to adapt to the deficit. The short-term nature of the effect is different from the situation with patient populations who sometimes may have months or even years to make behavioral (and neural) adjustments to accommodate for their lesions. Thus, TMS appears to be a very powerful additional tool that can be used to address the relation between the activity in a specific area of the brain and task performance.

Parietal TMS during eye–hand interactions

We have made use of TMS to examine the nature of the contribution of the PPC and PMC to eye–hand interactions. In an initial study we stimulated the PPC during the basic eye–hand task described above and quantified any changes that occurred in the oculomotor and manual motor output as a result (Van Donkelaar et al., 2000). The idea is that if the PPC is contributing to the coordination between these two motor systems then TMS delivered at the appropriate time should cause a significant reduction in the degree of coordination that is observed. We quantified this potential effect by measuring the slope of the relationship between hand movement amplitude and required saccade amplitude at different interleaved stimulation times. Fig. 4A shows the results for the group of five subjects for stimulation delivered over the PPC contralateral to the responding hand at 50, 100, 150, 200, or 250 ms after the presentation of the peripheral target. For comparison, the hand–saccade amplitude relationship is also shown when no stimulation was given. Clearly, the slope was modulated when TMS was applied 100–200 ms after target appearance. Fig. 4B displays the slope plotted as a function of the delay between the presentation of the target and delivery of TMS. The data from a control experiment with stimulation to the left occipital cortex are also included for comparison. In this figure the slopes have been normalized with respect to the baseline condition without stimulation. Statistical analysis revealed that the slope values were significantly smaller for PPC stimulation at intermediate times compared to earlier or later times or to occipital stimulation at any time. Further analysis revealed no significant changes for hand movement latency, saccadic latency, or saccadic amplitude.

To better understand how the changes in slope were related to the initiation of the saccade the data are replotted in Fig. 4C as a function of the 'TMS–saccade onset delay'. To obtain this value the time of TMS pulse application relative to the average saccade onset was calculated for each stimulation time and each subject. It is clear that pulses applied 0–100 ms prior to the onset of the saccade caused a substantial reduction in the slope. By contrast, pulses applied earlier or later had much less of an effect. These results are the first of their kind and are a

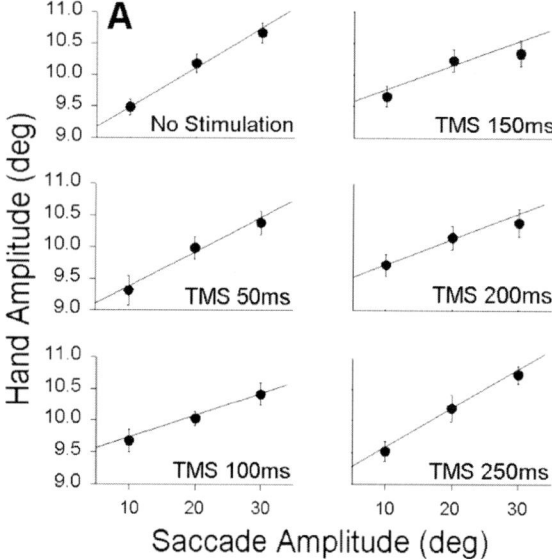
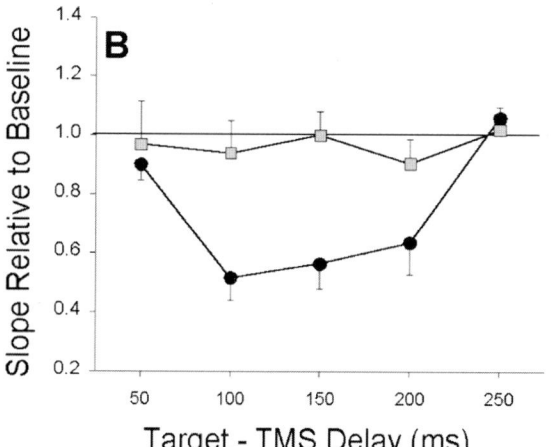
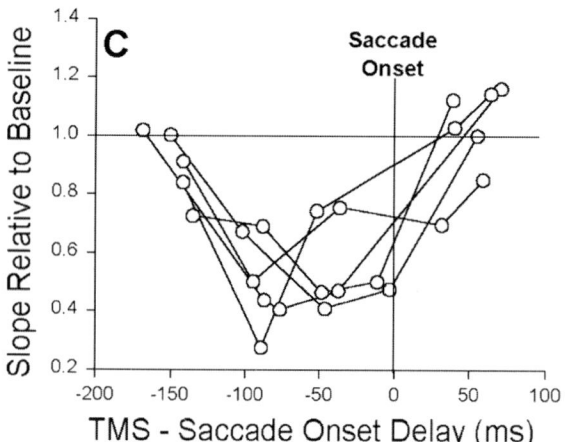

striking demonstration of how TMS combined with appropriate behavioral manipulations can yield valuable insight into the cortical information processing mechanisms underlying a specific task. In this case, they demonstrate that transiently disrupting the pattern of activation in the PPC 0–100 ms prior to the onset of a saccade causes a significant reduction in the effect the saccade has on a simultaneously produced limb movement. The reduced influence of the saccade occurred despite the fact that the saccade itself remained unaffected (see also Terao et al., 1999). We suggest that this was due to a disruption in the integration of saccade information into signals carrying limb movement related information within the PPC at this time. Stimulation at earlier or later times had no effect, demonstrating that the PPC contributes to eye–hand interactions during a finite period of time just prior to the saccade. Because the effects were observed during the presaccadic period, the signals must be part of an oculomotor efference copy rather than proprioceptive in origin. Similar inferences have been made previously by Duhamel and colleagues concerning the updating of the representation of visual space in the PPC across saccades (Duhamel et al., 1992a,b). The reduction in the effect of saccade amplitude during this period indicates that the subjects planned their reach response based upon the target goal with respect to the hand rather than the eye. In this sense, TMS appeared to disrupt the normal coding of the limb movement in eye-centered coordinates within the PPC. The fact that the largest effects were observed during the presaccadic period is also congruent with our finding that the saccadic influence on initial hand acceleration is larger when the saccade onset occurs 40–100 ms prior to the initiation of the hand movement (Fig. 3). Thus, these two different experiments provide converging evidence that the saccadic system influences the planning of

Fig. 4. Influence of TMS over the PPC on eye–hand coordination. (A) Plots of saccade–hand amplitude relation for stimulation at different times and no stimulation control. (B) Group mean for relative slope of saccade–hand amplitude relation at each stimulation time over the PPC (dots) and at a control site over the left occipital cortex (squares). (C) Relative slope plotted for each subject as a function of the average delay between stimulation and saccade onset. Error bars, 1 SE.

pointing movements and that this influence takes place, at least in part, within the PPC just prior to the saccade.

Premotor TMS during eye–hand interactions

In a more recent study, we have addressed whether the interactions between eye and hand movements are similar in the PMC to those observed in the PPC (Van Donkelaar et al., 2002). For this purpose the same procedures were used except that the stimulating coil was moved to a location overlying the PMC. Fig. 5 shows the results from this experiment. As with stimulation of the PPC, TMS over the PMC caused a systematic change in the saccade–hand movement amplitude relation. However, now instead of causing a decrease in the slope of this relation, it caused an increase when stimulation was given 100–200 ms after the presentation of the peripheral target. In other words, the saccade had a larger influence on the reaching response in these conditions than when TMS was not delivered or when it was delivered at the earlier (50 ms) or later (250 ms) delay intervals. This result implies that the compensation that normally occurs in the PMC for the eye-centered frame of reference imposed by the PPC occurs during a critical period of time just prior to the saccade so that the reaching response can be carried out in a limb-centered frame of reference.

Differing frames of reference in the human PPC and PMC

To capture the differences in the effects of TMS over the PPC and PMC we calculated a 'Compensation Index' (CI) for each stimulation site and time. The CI was computed by subtracting 1 from the slope of the line of best fit for the saccade–hand amplitude relation. With this index a value of zero would indicate that saccadic amplitude signals completely determine the amplitude of the reaching responses. This would result in pointing amplitudes that matched the saccade amplitude required for each trial (something that never happened). By contrast, a value of one would indicate total compensation for the eye-centered frame of reference derived from the PPC. This would result in pointing amplitudes that were appropriate for the distance from the starting position of the hand to the peripheral target and completely uninfluenced by saccadic signals. As is clear in Fig. 6, the CI values were closer to one than zero, ranging from 0.93 to 0.99. When no TMS was delivered the average CI value was ∼0.96. When processing occurring within the PMC was disrupted with TMS 100–200 ms after target presentation the CI values were significantly reduced. This indicates that the pointing responses were much more affected than normal by the eye-centered frame of reference arising from the PPC. By contrast, when processing occurring in the PPC was disrupted with TMS 100–200 ms after target presentation the CI values were significantly increased. This indicates that the pointing responses were much less affected than normal by the eye-centered frame of reference arising from the PPC. Thus, TMS appears to have opposite effects on eye–hand interactions when applied over the PPC and PMC.

Neurophysiological studies have demonstrated that the PPC contributes to reach planning in an eye-centered frame of reference (Batista et al., 1999; Snyder et al., 2000), whereas the PMC is more involved with the preparation of reaching movements in a limb-centered frame of reference (Fu et al., 1995; Riehle and Requin, 1995; Graziano, 1999). However, the fact that reaching movements ultimately reflect the distance from the hand to the target more so than that from the eye to the target (Van Donkelaar, 1997) implies that the limb-centered frame of reference encoded within the PMC compensates for the eye-centered frame of reference occurring within the PPC. Using TMS to disrupt the pattern of activation in the PMC and PPC provides an opportunity to examine the interaction between these two areas during tasks requiring eye–hand coordination. TMS over the PMC reduced the extent of compensation that was observed: the saccadic amplitude signals influenced the limb movements to a greater degree than normal. In contrast, TMS over the PPC increased the extent of compensation observed. In other words, the balance of influence that each area had on the task was disturbed by delivery of TMS.

Conclusions

We have demonstrated in a series of recent studies that the eye and hand motor systems interact in a sig-

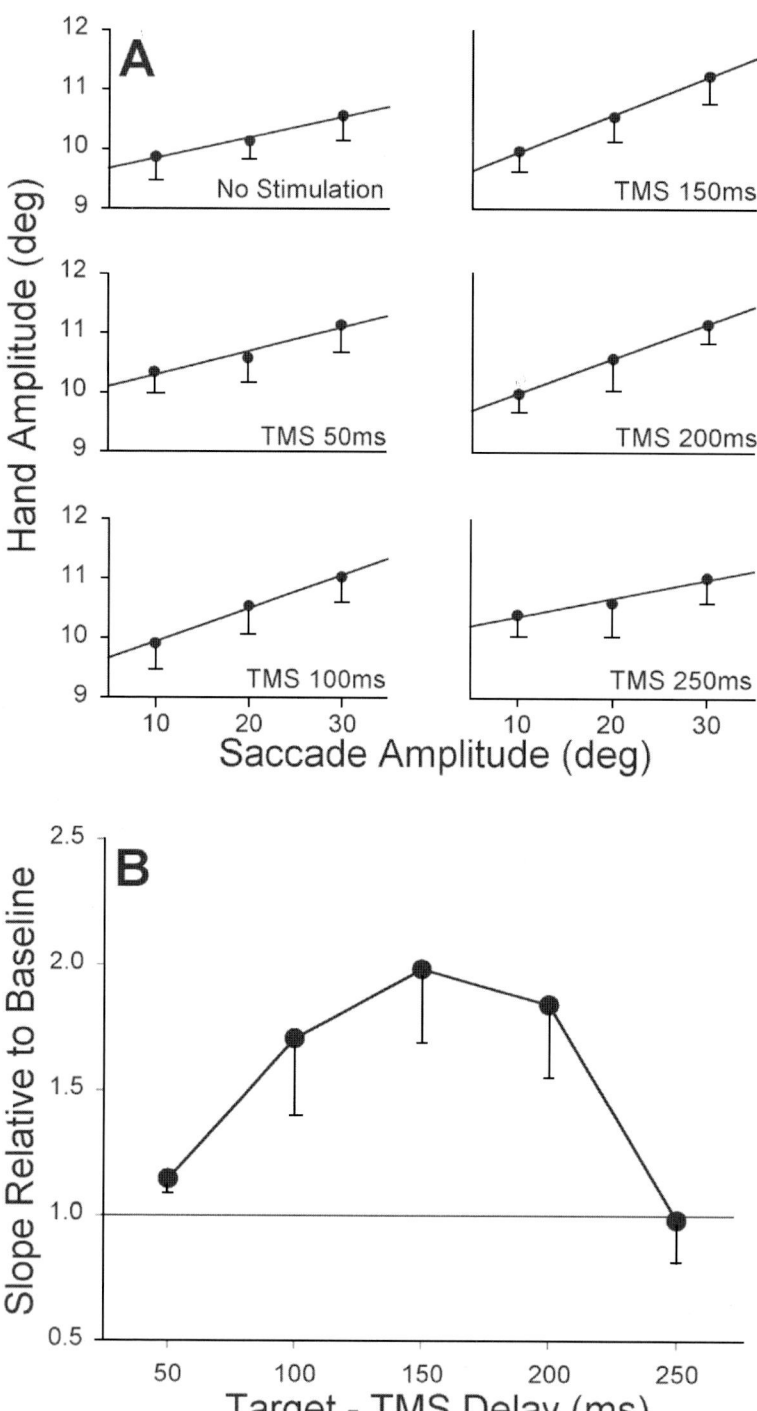

Fig. 5. Influence of TMS over the PMC on eye–hand coordination. (A) Group means for hand amplitude plotted as a function of required saccade amplitude. Condition appears in lower right hand corner of each graph. (B) Group means for relative slope of saccade–hand amplitude relation at each stimulation time. Error bars, 1 SE.

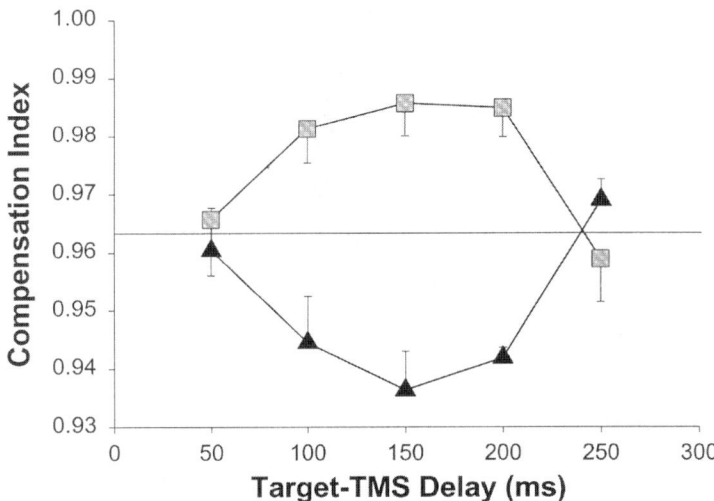

Fig. 6. Changes in the compensation index following PMC (triangles) and PPC (squares) stimulation. The increase in the compensation index during PPC stimulation indicates that the hand movements more strongly reflected a limb-centered frame of reference. The decrease during PMC stimulation reflects a stronger eye-centered frame of reference. Horizontal line represents compensation index value obtained when no TMS was delivered.

nificant and systematic manner during tasks that require coordination between oculomotor and manual motor output. Furthermore, by using TMS we have been able to demonstrate that these interactions reflect the transformation that occurs between an eye-centered frame of reference in the PPC and a limb-centered frame of reference in the PMC. While the research that has been reviewed examined the influence of saccadic eye movements on simple pointing responses, it is also clear that the interactions are bi-directional in that the presence of limb movements can affect saccade characteristics (Epelboim et al., 1997; Neggers and Bekkering, 2000). It will be important in the future to continue to address these issues in order to better understand how, when, and where within the brain these interactions occur.

References

Batista, A.P., Buneo, C.A., Snyder, L.H. and Andersen, R.A. (1999) Reach plans in eye-centered coordinates. *Science*, 285: 257–260.

Boussaoud, D., Jouffrais, C. and Bremmer, F. (1998) Eye position effects on the neuronal activity of dorsal premotor cortex in the macaque monkey. *J. Neurophysiol.*, 80: 1132–1150.

Brasil-Neto, J.P., McShane, L.M., Fuhr, P., Hallett, M. and Cohen, L.G. (1992) Topographic mapping of the human motor cortex with magnetic stimulation: factors affecting accuracy and reproducibility. *Electroencephalogr. Clin. Neurophysiol.*, 85: 9–16.

Duhamel, J.R., Colby, C.L. and Goldberg, M.E. (1992a) The updating of the representation of visual space in parietal cortex by intended eye movements. *Science*, 255: 90–92.

Duhamel, J.R., Goldberg, M.E., Fitzgibbon, E.J., Sirigu, A. and Grafman, J. (1992b) Saccadic dysmetria in a patient with a right frontoparietal lesion: the importance of corollary discharge for accurate spatial behaviour. *Brain*, 115: 1387–1402.

Epelboim, J., Steinman, R.M., Kowler, E., Pizlo, Z., Erkelens, C.J. and Collewijn, H. (1997) Gaze-shift dynamics in two kinds of sequential looking tasks. *Vision Res.*, 37: 2597–2607.

Fu, Q.G., Flament, D., Coltz, J.D. and Ebner, T.J. (1995) Temporal encoding of movement kinematics in the discharge of primate primary motor and premotor neurons. *J. Neurophysiol.*, 73: 836–854.

Graziano, M.S. (1999) Where is my arm? The relative role of vision and proprioception in the of limb position. *Proc. Natl. Acad. Sci. USA*, 96: 10,418–10,421.

Henriques, D.Y.P., Medendorp, W.P., Khan, A.Z. and Crawford, J.D. (2002) Visuomotor transformations for eye–hand coordination. In: J. Hyönä, D.P. Munoz, W. Heide and R. Radach (Eds.), *The Brain's Eye: Neurobiological and Clinical Aspects of Oculomotor Research*. Progress in Brain Research, Vol. 140, Elsevier, Amsterdam, pp. 329–340.

Josephs, O. and Henson, R.N. (1999) Event-related functional magnetic resonance imaging: modelling, inference and optimization. *Philos. Trans. R. Soc. Lond. B. Biol. Sci.*, 354: 1215–1228.

Mushiake, H., Tanatsugu, Y. and Tanji, J. (1997) Neuronal activity in the ventral part of premotor cortex during target–reach movement is modulated by direction of gaze. *J. Neurophysiol.*, 78: 567–571.

Neggers, S.F. and Bekkering, H. (2000) Ocular gaze is anchored to the target of an ongoing pointing movement. *J. Neurophysiol.*, 83: 639–651.

Pascual-Leone, A., Bartres-Faz, D. and Keenan, J.P. (1999) Transcranial magnetic stimulation: studying the brain–behaviour relationship by induction of 'virtual lesions'. *Philos. Trans. R. Soc. Lond. B. Biol. Sci.*, 354: 1229–1238.

Riehle, A. and Requin, J. (1995) Neuronal correlates of the specification of movement direction the monkey. *Behav. Brain Res.*, 70: 1–13.

Snyder, L.H., Batista, A.P. and Andersen, R.A. (2000) Saccade-related activity in the parietal reach region. *J. Neurophysiol.*, 83: 1099–1102.

Terao, Y., Fukuda, H., Ugawa, Y., Hikosaka, O., Hanajima, R., Furubayashi, T., Sakai, K., Miyauchi, S., Sasaki, Y. and Kanazawa, I. (1999) Visualization of the information flow through human oculomotor cortical regions by transcranial magnetic stimulation. *J. Neurophysiol.*, 80: 936–946.

Van Donkelaar, P. (1997) Eye–hand interactions during goal-directed pointing movements. *Neuroreport*, 8: 2139–2142.

Van Donkelaar, P. (1998) Saccade amplitude influences pointing movement kinematics. *Neuroreport*, 9: 2015–2018.

Van Donkelaar, P., Lee, J.H. and Drew, A.S. (2000) Transcranial magnetic stimulation disrupts eye–hand interactions in the posterior parietal cortex. *J. Neurophysiol.*, 84: 1677–1680.

Van Donkelaar, P., Lee, J.H. and Drew, A.S. (2002) Eye–hand interactions differ in the human premotor and parietal cortices. *Hum. Mov. Sci.*, in press.

Walsh, V. and Rushworth, M. (1999) A primer of magnetic stimulation as a tool for neuropsychology. *Neuropsychologia*, 37: 125–135.

Wise, S.P., Boussaoud, D., Johnson, P.B. and Caminiti, R. (1997) Premotor and parietal cortex: corticocortical connectivity and combinatorial computations. *Annu. Rev. Neurosci.*, 20: 25–42.

CHAPTER 21

Neuropsychological perspectives on eye–hand coordination in visually-guided reaching

David P. Carey *, Sergio Della Sala and Magdalena Ietswaart

Neuropsychology Research Group, Department of Psychology, University of Aberdeen, Old Aberdeen AB24 2UB, UK

Abstract: Substantial progress has been made in understanding the neural control of movement in the past 30 years. Lower cost technology for tracking movements of the eyes and the hands has increased our understanding of these two systems and their interactions in both neurologically intact individuals and non-human primates. Nevertheless the neuropsychology of eye–hand coordination during visually-guided tasks such as reaching and grasping remains relatively understudied. This chapter reviews some of the relevant neurophysiology and neuropsychology of eye–hand coordination during visually-guided reaching. Current models emphasising coordinate transformations are discussed in light of new patient data showing a particular type of failure of eye–hand coordination during reaching.

Movements of the eyes and the hands

Behavioural, physiological and psychological studies of eye movements have dominated primate motor control research. The amount of data on oculomotor control is vast, despite the fact that affordable, reliable and accurate technologies for recording high-speed activities like saccades are relatively new. Detailed studies of hand and arm movements have been made by many laboratories as well, and have benefited from many insights drawn from the earlier work on eye movements, as well as the development of similar technologies for motion recording and analysis. What is surprising is the lack of detailed neuropsychological work on how these two effector systems work together, in spite of several promising pointers provided by physiological and psychological investigations in neurologically intact participants (see Desmurget et al., 1998 for an excellent review). Brain systems that control reaching must process a number of sources of non-visual information, in addition to retinal location, in order to acquire visual targets successfully. Motor control theorists have always recognised that information about position of the target on the retinas must be integrated with information about position of the eyes in the head, the head on the trunk and the arm/hand/shoulder in order to prepare and execute successful reaches to visual targets. In this paper the relatively sparse data from neurological patients on eye–hand coordination in visually-guided reaching will be discussed, and contrasted with recent advances in the physiological studies of the same question.

A good starting point is a frequently cited paper by Fisk and Goodale (1985). This study was an early example of how simultaneous recordings of both eye and hand during reaching could provide important clues regarding their control. Using limbus tracking and high-speed video, eye and hand movements across the hemispace were recorded in eight neurologically intact participants. Fisk and Goodale (1985) took advantage of the facts that: (1) limb movements across the body midline (i.e. contralateral movements) tend to be slower than movements made into

---

* Correspondence to: D.P. Carey, Neuropsychology Research Group, Department of Psychology, University of Aberdeen, Old Aberdeen AB24 2UB, UK.

the space on the same side of the reaching limb (ipsilateral movements); and (2) eye movements tend to be initiated more quickly than arm movements to visual targets. As expected, they found slower reaction times for contralateral arm movements compared to ipsilateral arm movements. What was curious was that movements of the eyes that were 'identical' (i.e. to a target on the left side of the body midline) were initiated more slowly if a contralateral arm movement subsequently followed them. In other words, there was a temporal yoking of eye and hand movement reaction times: slower hand reaction times were coupled with slower eye movement reaction times, despite the fact that the eyes certainly *could* have arrived at the target earlier.

Several investigators have endorsed this kind of temporal coupling of eye and hand. For example, Prablanc and Martin (1992) have argued that the primary saccade is completed at a point near hand movement onset. More recent investigations of this issue by Helsen, Elliott and their colleagues suggest that the completion of the primary saccade occurs at or near the time when the hand is at peak acceleration (Helsen et al., 1998, 2000; Binstead et al., 2001). Others have argued that the particular type of eye–hand coupling found in any one study may depend upon the perceived or imposed accuracy and speed demands of a given aiming task (e.g. Fisk and Goodale, 1989; Carnahan and Marteniuk, 1991).

Experiments by Bekkering and Sailer (2002, this volume) elegantly demonstrated eye–hand symbiosis in a complementary and yet distinct way. Participants in their experiments were required to make rapid aiming movements to suddenly appearing visual targets. These authors also took advantage of the fact that saccadic eye movements to visual stimuli are usually completed while the moving hand is still approaching the target, and therefore could (in theory) be moved to a second visual target before the hand landed on the first. In a control condition, when the hand had landed on the visual target, a second target was illuminated ('static trigger' trials). The participants were required to look at the second target (as quickly as they could) while keeping their hand on the first. In the experimental condition ('dynamic trigger' trials), the second target was illuminated before the hand landed on the target but after the saccade to the first target was completed. As before, participants were to look at the second target as quickly as they could.

Remarkably, participants could not initiate saccades to the second target until the hand had reached the first target, as hard as they tried to do so. The saccade to the second target was severely delayed (relative to the onset of the second target) in the dynamic condition. Participants never initiated the second saccade until the arm movement was completed. Furthermore, there was no evidence that the second saccade could be planned (and just not initiated) during the terminal phase of the hand movement; no savings in reaction time for the second saccade were found once the hand had landed on the first target. These results have been subsequently replicated and extended, including movements made without vision of the reaching hand (Neggers and Bekkering, 2001). Other experiments have shown that the continuing presence of a visual target after the saccade has been completed facilitates endpoint accuracy of the hand, even when the hand is invisible (Prablanc et al., 1986).

Much like the Fisk and Goodale (1985) study described earlier, the Neggers and Bekkering (2000, 2001) experiments suggest that eye movements are temporally yoked to hand movements: there may be an optimal lead time for the eyes to arrive with respect to the hand (e.g. Fisk and Goodale, 1985) and there seems to be a requirement that the eyes remain fixed on a visual target until the hand movement is completed (Prablanc et al., 1986; Neggers and Bekkering, 2000, 2001). There is also some evidence for the reciprocal relationship — faster saccadic eye movement initiation may also lead to faster hand movement initiation (Bekkering et al., 1996; Lünenberger et al., 2000), although it is still unclear if the effects on hands depend on the faster reaction times of the eyes.

The evidence for spatial (in addition to temporal) coupling of eye and hand during reaching is less clear (cf. Sailer et al., 2000). Of course in most tasks eyes and hands are directed at the same target (although they have been dissociated in many other experiments such as extrafoveal pointing, or requiring saccades in one direction and arm movements in the other). Researchers have looked for evidence demonstrating the relation between terminal errors of the eyes and those of the hands (for example when the target is extinguished quickly and/or the reaching hand is invisible). Under some conditions the amplitude of the saccade was related to hand landing position (Van Donkelaar, 1997; Van Donkelaar et al., 2000; Johansson et al., 2001). In other conditions the landing position of the eye was predictive of hand landing position (Henriques et al., 1998). Using correlation coefficients the evidence is somewhat stronger for temporal rather than spatial coupling(s) of eye and hand. Nevertheless other methods have suggested better spatial rather than temporal coupling (Gielen et al., 1984; Rossetti et al., 1993; Bekkering et al., 1995).

Any temporal coupling of eye and hand should be dependent on sensorimotor areas of the brain such as subregions of parietal and premotor cortex (see Van Donkelaar et al., 2002, this volume). Alternatively, eye–hand coupling could depend on subcortical structures such as the superior colliculus (see Munoz, 2002, this volume; Munoz and Fecteau, 2002) and/or cerebellum (Glickstein, 1998). As of yet there is little direct evidence of temporal synchronies like those seen by Fisk and Goodale (1985) or by Neggers and Bekkering (2000, 2001) from single unit neurophysiology. However, several studies have implicated regions in the parietal (Andersen et al., 1998; Snyder, 2000; Snyder et al., 2000a,b; Ferraina et al., 2001) and/or frontal (Mushiake et al., 1996) lobes in eye–hand coordination. One laboratory has found arm-movement-related activity in the superior colliculus (Stuphorn et al., 2000), a structure more commonly associated with saccades and the neural control of fixation. Cerebellar contributions to both eye and hand movements have been documented; to date little of the evidence suggests a substantial role in eye–hand coordination during visually-guided reaching per se (although see Miall, 1998; the group discussion in Van Donkelaar and Lee, 1994; Glickstein, 1998).

Single unit investigations of eye–hand coordination

Much has been made in the past decade of gaze-related coding in several regions of monkey parietal and frontal cortex (several of these regions are depicted in Fig. 1). In its strongest form, an 'oculocentric' neuron would respond best to a visual target when the eyes of the animal are in a certain position in the orbit. A more common type of gaze signal in the cerebral cortex is found when a cell which is retinotopic (i.e. responds best when a target falls on a certain place on the retina) is 'modulated' by eye position. The retinotopic response grows or weakens

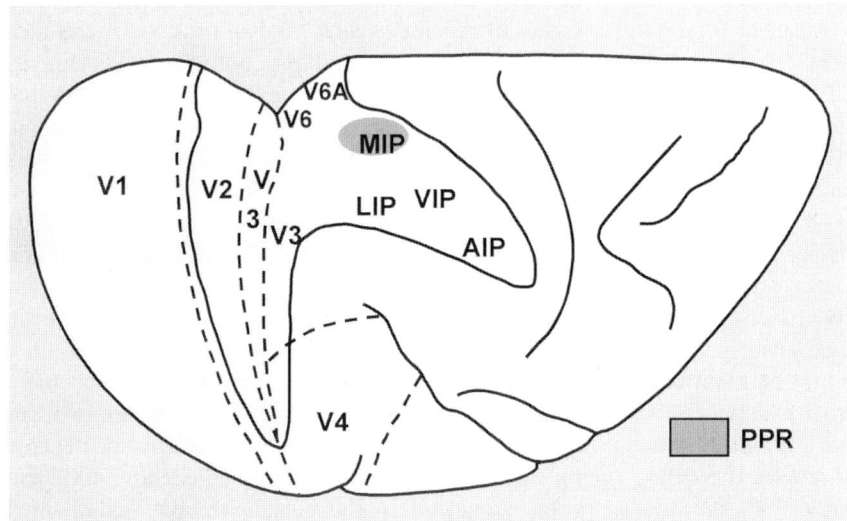

Fig. 1. Representation of the regions in Macaque parietal cortex implicated in eye and hand movement control. The lunate and intraparietal sulci have been opened to expose areas located in their depths. AIP, anterior intraparietal area; MIP, medial intraparietal area; PO, parieto-occipital area; LIP, lateral intraparietal area. The location of the parietal reach region is indicated in gray. Modified from Carey (2000).

depending on the position of the eyes within the head (even though the visual stimulus from a retinal point of view is kept constant). Gaze-modulation has been found in other types of single-cell activity, including in neurons with activity related to arm movements in a particular direction (e.g. Ferraina et al., 1997). Such neurons are obviously strong candidates for playing a major role in coordination of the eyes and hands. Their responses are easily incorporated into serial models of limb movement to visual targets, and have been bound up into models of coordinate transformations. For example, in structures closer to the retina such as the superior colliculus and V1, retinotopic coding of visual targets should be the norm. In intermediate regions such as subdivisions of the parietal cortex, gaze position coding should be more common than in regions further 'downstream', where head-centred and subsequently body-centred, hand-centred, and/or arm-centred codes should predominate. However, gaze modulation has now been discovered in a multitude of different cortical and subcortical brain regions, and is not easily categorised into early versus later stages of coordinate transformations (Desmurget et al., 1998; Boussaoud and Bremmer, 1999). Similarly although 'head-centred' coding has been found in downstream areas such as the supplementary eye field (SEF) of the medial frontal lobe (Tehovnik et al., 1998), it has also been found in earlier regions such as the ventral intraparietal area (VIP; Duhamel et al., 1997; Bremmer et al., 2001). Gaze modulation of human brain activity during finger movements — Baker et al., 1999; and pointing — DeSouza et al., 2000 has been demonstrated with neuroimaging but will not be reviewed in detail here.

From an eye–hand coordination perspective, the ubiquitous nature of gaze coding suggests a strong role for these signals, but their precise functional significance remains ambiguous. In any given neuron, a cell modulated by eye position might be receiving such a signal from an earlier unit in a network or might be the source of such signals for other units further downstream. For example, one of the cells described in Jouffrais and Boussaoud (1999) showed the greatest activation in a condition where the animal had to maintain fixation on a central location while reaching to an extrafoveal visual target. Such activity could be related to any one of a number of different processes, including specifying extrafoveal target location, or maintaining fixation and inhibiting the natural tendency to saccade to a target that is being reached towards, or even maintenance of instructional set.

Jouffrais and Boussaoud (1999) argue that if gaze modulation in dorsal premotor cortex is "used to build limb motor commands, limb-related activity should depend on whether or not the monkey made a saccade to the target prior to the reaching movement" (p. 205). However, from a computational point of view (so often embraced by the various coordinate transformation models) the presence or absence of a saccade to a visual target is largely irrelevant (see Xing and Andersen, 2000 for a review). Eye position (in head) coupled with retinotopic position of a non-foveated target is computationally no different than eye position (in head) coupled with a foveated target, unless an argument is made about receptor density fall-off in the retina. Such an argument is more appropriately targeted at acuity-related issues rather than localisation. In fact Goodale and Murphy (1997) suggested that visuomotor processing is relatively unaffected in the periphery relative to central vision compared with perceptual estimates of the same features.

Even if we assume that gaze-modulated cells are indeed playing an intermediate role in computing target position in (ultimately) an arm- or hand-centred frame of reference on a trial-to-trial basis, the data from physiological and psychological experiments suggest a more dynamic eye–hand synergy than that implied by a static signal providing eye position in the head. The Fisk and Goodale (1985) and Neggers and Bekkering (2000, 2001) studies suggest special linkages in time between *saccades* and moving hands during visually-guided reaching. A study by Honda (1984) demonstrated that acquiring targets by saccades produced more accurate hand movements in darkness than when pursuit eye movements acquired the same targets. These experiments as well as others suggest a special role in saccadic processes in accurate arm movements to visual targets. A special role for foveation in visually-guided reaching has also been suggested in the comprehensive two-channel model of feedback loops for error correction, suggested by Paillard and his colleagues (reviewed in Paillard, 1996. His arguments are discussed in more detail below).

Saccade and arm movement activity in the same neurons or groups of neurons?

Gaze modulation may play some role in eye–hand coordination in visually-guided reaching. A more direct link between eye and hand from single-unit neurophysiology is suggested by neurons which show both saccadic and arm-movement driven activity, and regions that are dominated by populations of cells which code for both saccades and arm movements. Several regions in the parietal lobe have been described which are active when monkeys make eye and hand movements (cf. Andersen et al., 1998; Battaglia-Mayer et al., 2001; Galletti et al., 2001; Marconi et al., 2001; Buneo et al., 2002). Andersen and colleagues have compared and contrasted single unit activity in areas dramatically specialised for the control of saccadic eye movements (e.g. the lateral intraparietal area, LIP) and control of arm movements (e.g. the parietal reach region, PRR. See also Shipp et al., 1998; Galletti et al., 1999). Although the early studies emphasised relatively independent coding of eye and hand movement properties between these two regions (and in single cells within the PRR and LIP), more recent accounts have uncovered the importance of eye movement- and eye position-related activity, even in 'reaching' cells in the PRR. For example, Batista et al. (1999) have found that the responses of reaching neurons were modulated by the initial position of eyes prior to the arm movement, whereas changes in the initial position of the arm had no effect on the subsequent arm-movement-related activity.

The same group has subsequently discovered that initial eye position is not the only eye-related property which influences the activity of cells supposedly restricted to coding arm movements. Snyder et al. (2000b) reported that despite a clear relationship between arm movements and firing patterns of PRR cells, 29% cells tested were influenced by saccadic eye movements in a task where no arm movement was required. The neurons were tuned for the same preferred directions for both delayed saccades made without reaches and delayed reaches made without saccades. A fascinating property of these single units is that the activity was not related to preparing a saccade per se. In their delayed saccade task, monkeys were required to make saccadic eye movements to targets after a delay period; therefore activity related to preparing the saccade should have been elicited during the delay. In fact, what Snyder et al. (2000b) found was that most PRR arm movement neurons increased firing during or immediately after the saccade and not during the delay period.

Snyder et al. (2000b) offered several different interpretations of their data. First, they favour the idea that the potential targets of reaching movements are represented in oculomotor rather than arm-centred coordinates. An oculomotor scheme used for several classes of target representation "may be a fairly general way of representing space and integrating different modalities within a particular spatial representation" (Andersen et al., 1998, p. 118).

A second, somewhat distinct explanation of the saccadic activity of PRR reach neurons is that whenever a saccade is executed to a visual target a "plan is formed in PRR that would carry the arm to the same target" (Snyder et al., 2000b, p. 1101). Of course, in fairly contrived laboratory conditions Macaque monkeys can be trained to dissociate eye and limb movements (as can university undergraduates), but in natural environments the two systems are often 'aimed' at the same target. It remains unknown whether both systems are driven by a common control mechanism or if one system in some control sense, 'drives' the other. Perhaps Snyder et al.'s heuristic (Snyder et al., 2000b) should be reversed to 'whenever a potential target for an arm movement appears, move the eyes to it first'.

In summary, gaze- and saccade-related effects on single-cell activity in the Macaque brain have rekindled interest in models of coordinate transformations. Recent neuropsychological work has also made use of these same types of model to help understand disorders of sensory-guided reaching seen in the clinic. Before discussing one particular example, the literature on deficits in reaching to visual targets will be reviewed.

Inputs rather than outputs in the parlance of reaching

In the previous century, the study of impaired performance in reaching after posterior brain damage has been concerned almost exclusively with the visual guidance of aiming. This bias is related to the popularisation of misreaching disorders in terms of Holmes–Balint syndrome, a triad of visuomotor/attentional disturbances which has been described in patients with bilateral parietal lobe dysfunction. These include gaze dysfunction (e.g. "psychic paralysis of gaze" as described by Balint — the patient had a great deal of difficulty in disengaging fixation (Husain and Stein, 1988; Harvey and Milner, 1995) and attentional disorders such as simultanagnosia (an inability to perceive more than one visual target at a time). The third component of Holmes–Balint syndrome is the symptom referred to as 'optic ataxia' (Harvey and Milner, 1995; De Renzi, 1996). Optic ataxia is a great difficulty in reaching to a visual target, in spite of being able to 'see' the target reasonably well. In some cases of Holmes–Balint syndrome, gaze dysfunction and attentional disorders largely disappear, whereas optic ataxia for targets in the periphery remains.

An important consideration for labelling such misreaching behaviour as optic ataxia is that the disorder should be restricted to the visual modality; that is, reaching to targets specified by other means *must* be reasonably intact. If the patient cannot reach accurately under other conditions (e.g. to named parts of his/her body) the disorder would be 'motoric' in nature and of less interest to the neuropsychologists who study sensory, perceptual and representational space in the brain. Clearly optic ataxia is an obvious candidate for neuropsychological explorations of eye–hand coordination.

Many of the same coordinate transformations discussed above will also be required when reaches are directed at non-visual targets. (Neggers and Bekkering (1999) have found even higher correlations between hand and eye movement latencies when participants reach to somatosensory targets than when they reach to visual targets). For example, sounds encoded in a head-centred frame may require conversion to gaze-centred and or arm/hand/shoulder-centred frames for looking and reaching towards such targets. And yet auditory localisation, with the exception of a few clinical reports (e.g. Tzavaras and Masure, 1975; Kase et al., 1977; De Renzi, 1988) is rarely assessed in any rigorous way in patients showing disordered reaching (De Renzi, 1982). In most reports where optic ataxia is claimed, intact reaching to proprioceptive targets is all that is usually reported (typically named body parts, e.g. Damasio and Benton, 1979, often just the nose as part of finger-to-nose assessment for cerebellar ataxia, cf. Kase et al., 1977, case 2). Sometimes, intact somatosensory function is merely mentioned (e.g. Pisella et al., 2000). The assessments are usually informal (i.e. as part of a bedside neurological examination) or just implied by the diagnostic labelling (cf. Hausser et al., 1980; Jakobson et al., 1991; Jeannerod et al., 1994; Milner et al., 1999, 2001). It is conceivable that a patient might be able to reach to a named body part such as his or her nose based on semantic knowledge, in spite of a profound disturbance in proprioception. For example, patients know that their nose is located just below the line of sight of the eyes. Indeed, there is some evidence that semantic information regarding body parts may enjoy a unique representation in the brain (e.g. De Renzi and Scotti, 1980; Suzuki et al., 1997). In some cases, proprioceptive guidance of movement has been assessed more rigorously by having the blindfolded subject's thumb or finger (positioned by the examiner) as the target of a grasping movement made with the other hand (Boller et al., 1975; Perenin and Vighetto, 1988). Unfortunately, the accuracy and efficiency of such movements have never been recorded and quantified (although see Levine et al., 1978 for an early attempt).

In spite of the above considerations, the theoretical focus in assessing patients with poor reaching has remained on visual input and analysis. For example, theorists debate whether or not deficits in the perception of space can account for the disordered reaching in patients with full Holmes–Balint's syndrome or optic ataxia (Holmes, 1918; Rondot et al., 1977; Perenin and Vighetto, 1988; Milner and Goodale, 1995; Baylis and Baylis, 2001). Other studies have addressed issues such as whether or not the disturbances in visual attention in such patients could account for their poor spatial behaviour in general (Hecaen and De Ajuriaguerra, 1954; Coslett and Saffran, 1991; Rizzo, 1993; Robertson et al., 1997; Kim and Robertson, 2001). Recently, scientists have documented disturbances in the visual guidance of grasping (Jakobson et al., 1991; Goodale et al., 1994; Jeannerod et al., 1994; Milner et al., 2001) in patients with full Holmes–Balint syndrome or optic ataxia. Other reports have been concerned with the time course of aiming movement responses to visual targets or changes in target position (Milner et al., 1999, 2001; Pisella et al., 2000).

Theory and metatheory of optic ataxia

This bias towards visual inputs may be ultimately responsible for the lack of definitive theories accounting for optic ataxia in its various guises. Some authors argue for a 'disconnection' syndrome account of the disorder, whereby motor systems are deafferented from the visual inputs which specify target position (Balint favoured such an interpretation, see Husain and Stein, 1988; Harvey and Milner, 1995; De Renzi, 1996). In their recent analysis of optic ataxia, Buxbaum and Coslett (1997, 1998) are critical of disconnection accounts (e.g. Rondot et al., 1977; see De Renzi, 1982 for a review of earlier arguments). They argue that disconnection of frontal lobe structures from visual cortex should result in 'complete' optic ataxia; therefore, demonstrations of 'subtotal' syndromes where patients only misreach to extrafoveal targets make such accounts untenable. Such a criticism makes sense when authors draw direct comparisons to the frontal lobe deafferentation experiments of Kuypers and his colleagues (Haaxma and Kuypers, 1975), because they are suggesting visual deafferentation of the neurons controlling arm movements as the mechanism behind misreaching. Those who do not make such comparisons could just as easily refer to disconnection phenomena at some intermediate level of control. For example, parietal lobe lesions could disconnect the visual cortices from the frontal eye fields (Bullier et al., 1996), or the cerebellum (Glickstein, 1998; Clower et al., 2001). Such lesions could also damage parietal lobe efferents to oculomotor control centres in the superior colliculus and/or brainstem (Baizer et al., 1993; Clower et al., 2001). These types of disconnection could disrupt eye movements to visual targets in some fashion, for example, which might contribute in some fashion to misreaching of the hand. Indeed, since many patients with optic ataxia have difficulties with oculomotor control, the relative impact of gaze disorders on misreaching has also been a major focus of the discussion (Rondot et al., 1977). However, such analyses rarely go beyond the demonstration that optic ataxia and gaze dysfunction *can* be dissociable (Rondot et al., 1977;

Perenin and Vighetto, 1988). In other words, optic ataxia can be seen in patients whose eye movements to visual targets are apparently spared. Rather less effort has been directed to understanding the complex interactions between position sense of eye, head and limb, efference copy of motor commands, etc. and how disruptions in these interactions can lead to different disturbances in visually-guided behaviour. (In fact, efference and eye proprioception may be used differently by perceptual systems which deal with maintaining a stable representation of the environment versus sensorimotor systems dealing with eye–hand coordination, recalibration etc. cf. Bahcall and Kohler, 1999).

The Buxbaum and Coslett (1997, 1998) transformational failure account

Buxbaum and Coslett (1997, 1998) suggest that the computational demands of visually-guided reaching provide an important framework for interpreting the deficits seen in optic ataxia and related syndromes. They argue that subtypes of optic ataxia may all be understood in terms of failures in the transformations of sensory inputs from retinal to oculocentric to hand or shoulder-centred codes required for successful reaching to visual targets. The proposal is that an important intermediate stage in such transformations turns head-centred codes into trunk-centred codes that have distinct left-body and right-body components, localised in the contralateral cerebral hemisphere. Buxbaum and Coslett (1997) suggest that lesions at different stages in their model can explain different varieties of optic ataxia, such as misreaching with either arm into the hemispace on the opposite side of the lesion or misreaching with only the contralateral arm into that space.

Buxbaum and Coslett (1997, 1998) argued that an important distinction in optic ataxia is that some patients fail to reach visual targets in spite of full foveal vision, while others will only fail if they are required to reach in extrafoveal vision (that is, reaching to a target which they are not looking directly at). They suggest that the pattern of behaviour presented by second type of patient is difficult to interpret as simple visuomotor disconnection. They state that "If OA [optic ataxia] is simply attributable to a disconnection of spatial and motor systems. . .

then conveying the limb to a target object should be equally inaccurate whether or not the object is foveated" (p. 160).

The deficits of these patients with 'extrafoveal optic ataxia' cannot be accounted for by visual field defects etc. An important consideration is that the errors in such patients are either randomly spread around the intended target, or, in some cases, are biased in the direction towards the side of the brain lesion (Ratcliff and Davies-Jones, 1972; Perenin, 1997). The patients described below showed errors that are fundamentally different than those seen in extrafoveal optic ataxia.

'Magnetic misreaching': a variant of extrafoveal optic ataxia?

In a report published in 1997 we (Carey et al., 1997) described a patient, Ms. D, probably affected by corticobasal degeneration, who presented with a slowly progressive bilateral ideomotor apraxia, coupled with apraxic gait and constructional disturbance. MRI scanning revealed severe bilateral parietal atrophy, particularly evident in the left superior parietal region. The most striking feature of Ms. D's case was a peculiar reaching disorder that we labelled as 'magnetic misreaching'. Magnetic misreaching refers to a pathological 'yoking' of the reaching hand to the direction of gaze, such that attempts to reach to extrafoveal targets inevitably fail, but *these failures are very specific*. Every time Ms. D. attempted to reach towards an extrafoveal target, she slavishly reached to the place where her eyes were pointing. Buxbaum and Coslett (1997) refer to what appears to be the same symptom in at least one (DP) of their two patients, although they limit their interpretation of DP's case by referring to his misreaching as yet another instance of extrafoveal optic ataxia (see also Buxbaum and Coslett, 1998). However, there is a key distinction between magnetic misreaching and extrafoveal optic ataxia: a patient with magnetic misreaching *must* reach to the place that she/he is looking at, while the errors of extrafoveal optic ataxics are randomly spread or simply biased towards the side of the brain lesion.

Magnetic misreaching may be related to vision of the reaching limb interacting in some complex way with eye position signals. For example, many models of saccadic eye movement control as well as arm movement control are based on 'error minimising'- reducing the size of the 'error' between target position (the desired endpoint of a movement) and the position of an effector on-line. Paillard has argued that foveation of a target provides a directional error signal for on-line control of the reaching limb, monitored by fast visual feedback loops of the extrafoveal retinae. These fast loops track the hand as it moves towards the foveated target (for review see Paillard, 1996). Use of motion cues in extrafoveal vision appears to be disrupted in the patient of Rizzo et al. (1992). This patient had severe deficits in the perception of visual motion, as well as difficulties reaching to visual targets. His misreaching deficit could be described as a variant of optic ataxia, since he could acquire a visual target more successfully when he reached *without a view of his hand in peripheral vision*.

If the sensorimotor systems controlling reaching operate in such a fashion, signals about target position might be compared to the *visual* position of the limb. Thus, once Ms. D initiated a ballistic movement under visual guidance towards a non-foveated target, her hand was 'captured' by an on-line *visual* control system which normally minimises target–hand distance. This perspective implies that Ms. D's misreaching might be conceptualised as a variant of optic ataxia, since the problem would be related to the visual guidance of movement. Such a view of optic ataxia is somewhat broader than the traditional interpretation, where the problem is thought to be with encoding the *position of the visual target*, or getting information about target position to the motor and premotor cortices (see Perenin and Vighetto, 1988 for review). Although Buxbaum and Coslett (1998) examined their patient DP's reaching when vision of his arm was eliminated, the visual guidance of aiming *once initiated* does not appear to feature in the transformational account (see their Fig. 3, for example).

An alternative account of magnetic misreaching

We favour a different interpretation of magnetic misreaching. Ms. D was not just *capable* of using eye position to specify targets, she was *compelled* to reach towards the place she was foveating. This pathological yoking of eye and hand in magnetic misreaching suggests that eye proprioception (or efference copy of oculomotor commands) was the only way that target position could be specified for the purposes of preparation and execution of a ballistic aiming movement. As noted above, typically, the eyes successfully acquire a target to be reached towards well before the hand reaches the target and the lead-time of the eyes seems to be controlled (Fisk and Goodale, 1985; Goodale, 1990).

Rather than failing at extrafoveal reaching, Ms. D's dysfunction should be interpreted in terms of her *only succeeding while foveating the target*. This view of magnetic misreaching underscores its distinctiveness from optic ataxia per se: non-visual means of specifying target position should result in failure, unless, for example, an auditory or somatosensory target could also be foveated. As we have reported previously, when we asked Ms. D to fixate a static target and reach to the 'opposite side of the table' she was unable to overcome the magnetic pull of her fixation. Even with such 'cognitive specification' of target direction, Ms. D. inevitably reached towards fixation (Carey et al., 1997). Buxbaum and Coslett (1997, 1998) did not provide any information about aiming at non-visual targets in DP, but, by labelling the syndrome as a variant of optic ataxia, they implied that the deficit was restricted to targets whose position was specified by vision. A second patient, AM, was also reported in the same papers, who apparently had to look at where his hand was moving, which caused all kinds of difficulty in reaching to foveal or extrafoveal targets. Again, as with DP, details of assessment of non-visual guidance of movement were not provided.

In order to evaluate the argument that non-visual aiming movement is impaired in magnetic misreaching, we have examined Ms. D's reaching behaviour to targets which were specified by other sensory modalities when she could not foveate the intended target. First, we wanted to examine and quantify her ability to point to her opposite limb, the position of which could only be specified by proprioceptive information. Secondly, we examined her ability to make pointing movements to auditory targets. In both of these conditions no visual information about target or limb was available, so any resulting disorder could not be labelled as optic ataxia.

Reaching to proprioceptive targets in magnetic misreaching

We asked Ms. D to point to one of her index fingers using the other, while blindfolded. Her arm was passively positioned by the examiner such that the 'target' finger was placed on one of 12 different positions across the tabletop (passive displacement minimises the amount of 'efference' from the target arm which could be used to specify target position). We tapped repeatedly on the target finger at the beginning of each trial, and asked her to confirm that she felt the taps and knew where the target finger was. Such a procedure should have provided tactile and proprioceptive information about the position of the fingertip, as well as drawing attention to the target's position in peripersonal space (Ms. D's verbal reports verified the attention-capturing features of the touches). She was then asked to reach quickly and accurately to the immobilised target finger with the index finger of her free hand. She was discouraged from moving once she had landed on the table top (or on her immobilised arm or on the arm of the examiner). We quantified her reaching accuracy by recording the movements at 60 Hz with a MacReflex motion analysis system (Qualisys, Inc.). We used each hand as a target for the other. We had Ms. D reach twice to each of 12 targets, six in each hemispace. Two infra-red reflective markers were attached to the dorsal surface of both of her index fingers. We calculated the two-dimensional distance between the two markers at her final resting position.

Ms. D made large errors when reaching to her own fingertip (see Fig. 2). In fact, her average error was 11 cm, outside the normal range for elderly control participants tested with the same procedure in our laboratory. The deficit was seen in movements made by either hand (while using the other hand as target). Her endpoint accuracy was substantially worse when moving her left hand to her right fingertip (mean error = 15.33 cm, SD = 6.56 cm) than when moving her right hand to her left fingertip (mean error = 6.55 cm, SD = 5.01 cm). Unfortunately, since the non-moving target was the other hand, this procedure makes it difficult to ascertain whether or not the deficit errors of proprioceptive guidance were related to the reaching hand, the target hand, or both hands. With either hand, she tended

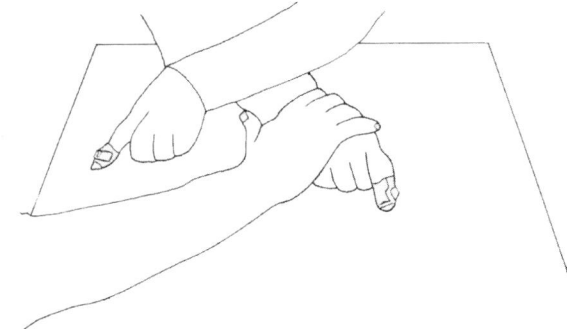

Fig. 2. Ms. D's right hand was held in place by the experimenter, and the final resting position of her reaching left limb is depicted (traced from a digitised image from videotape). In this trial, as in many others, Ms. D's reaching arm landed well to the right of the intended target.

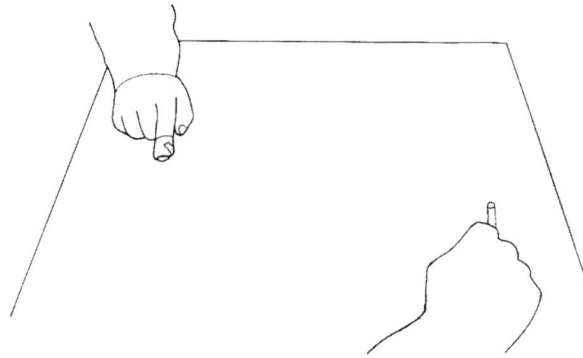

Fig. 3. The target for the reach was specified by the tapping of the pencil depicted in the lower portion of the figure (this was the upper left target from Ms. D's point of view). Her final reach endpoint for this trial appears well to the right of the target. We estimated an endpoint error of 39 cm for this particular trial.

to move in the direction of the target, but typically landed consistently right of the true target position. The mechanism underlying this bias is unclear, although it is in the direction which would be expected in a patient with dramatic 'ipsilesional bias' after right hemisphere damage. Ms. D's pathology was bilateral, and if anything was worse in the left parietal lobe (SPECT, MRI and neuropsychological data; see Carey et al., 1997 for further discussion), so her rightward bias remains unclear.

Reaching to auditory targets in magnetic misreaching

In a brief assessment, we examined Ms. D's reaches to targets defined by sound while she was blindfolded. Targets were defined by four corners of a sheet of A3 paper (42 × 29.7 cm), placed horizontally across the tabletop. The examiner tapped a corner of the A3 sheet and required Ms. D to initiate a ballistic reach to the sound of the tapping. Her errors were estimated from videotape. For some trials her actual endpoint was so far from the auditory target that it was no longer in the field of view of the videocamera. For these trials endpoint error was estimated given the final visible resting position of the reaching arm and wrist. As was the case in proprioceptive reaching, Ms. D made large errors with her left (33.8 cm, SD = 16.9 cm) and right hands (22.1 cm, SD = 13.2 cm). As before, she tended to land to the right of true target position (see Fig. 3).

Unlike in proprioceptive reaching, if anything, the left hand was slightly worse than the right hand.

As in proprioceptive reaching, Ms. D made large errors when attempting to point ballistically to the auditory targets. A schematic diagram of one of her attempts is depicted in Fig. 3.

Magnetic misreaching is multimodal

Our data suggest that Ms. D's reaching disorder was not restricted to targets specified visually, or to conditions when she was required to actively foveate some place other than the intended target. Additionally, her deficits did not seem to depend on vision of the reaching limb, as was the case with the patient of Rizzo et al. (1992). De Renzi (1988) and others (e.g. Levine and Rinn, 1986) have also reported cases of misreaching which are multimodal. In other cases, if intact reaching is not demonstrated in any modality, a very 'motoric' conceptualisation of the disorder could be suggested. Alternatively, a deficit of a non-modality-specific spatial representation would be another possibility.

In Ms. D's case, because she could reach to foveal targets her deficits cannot be understood in any simple model of disordered control of the limb per se. Additional, her ability to report spatial relationships for visual targets and the like was intact, so a very spatial conceptualisation of her disorder is just as unlikely. For this reason we excluded the possible diagnoses of optic ataxia, spatial disorientation or a 'parietal' ataxia in Ms. D (Carey et al., 1997).

Of course, our assessments of reaching to non-visual targets was only one feature of our testing sessions with her, and were, necessarily, brief. Additionally, Ms. D's auditory and somatosensory functions were not examined in any detail. (She was certainly capable of making eyes closed judgements of joint movement direction as part of a neurological examination, and her perception of speech and reaction to sounds in the environment appeared normal). Of course, other explanations of her poor misreaching behaviours that were independent of her magnetic misreaching were certainly possible, including higher level somatosensory deficits not immediately apparent to us. Nevertheless, her performance on non-visual reaching tasks did not reveal obviously intact guidance of movement by non-visual means, *except foveation*.

Can the coordinate transformation failure account explain magnetic misreaching?

Instead of visuomotor disconnection, Buxbaum and Coslett (1997, 1998) suggest that optic ataxia should be conceptualised as a failure in the necessary co-ordinate transformations which must intervene between visual input with respect to the retina and motor output with respect to the limbs. At first glance such a conceptualisation seems so broad that it includes every possible dysfunctional process in optic ataxia, since the transformational account encompasses all processes related to extracting target position from retinal input to a representation which is arm-, shoulder- or hand-centred (or even world-centred for that matter). Nevertheless, the model's emphasis on such coordinate transformations limits how well it could explain magnetic misreaching. In fact, neurophysiological studies of parietal lobe reflect a similar bias on the hierarchical models of transformations on the input side (i.e. extraction of target location relative to some body reference point) of these complex sensorimotor loops (see Battaglia-Mayer et al., 1998; Battaglia-Mayer and Caminiti, 2002, and Johnson et al., 1997 for critiques). The Buxbaum and Coslett (1997, 1998) model is about how target position in real space or space relative to an egocentric reference point is reconstructed in the brain. The model says little about how the eyes, head and arm get to that point once it has been specified.

The Buxbaum and Coslett (1997, 1998) model in its current form runs into difficulty in accounting for magnetic misreaching. Some type of deficit in oculocentric representation seems plausible, but both Ms. D and DP were perfectly able to direct their eyes to different visual targets, and were obviously able to use feedforward/feedback eye position signals to direct entirely successful reaching under those conditions. Another possibility (which the authors favour) is a break down in the hand-centred code which led DP to reach to the location specified by the oculocentric code. However, the series of processes which allow for pointing to non-foveated locations is not obviously specified in the transformational account, so it remains unclear why DP and Ms. D cannot combine the retinal signal of extrafoveal target location with eye position (which seems intact in this patients — they can point to foveal locations with different positions of the eyes in their orbits).

The performance of Buxbaum and Coslett's patients DP and AM are difficult to explain by dysfunctions in a single 'box' of their model. In both cases, a pathological yoking of hand and eye was postulated. Only in the case of AM could any claim be made for disordered oculocentric or retinocentric coding, since, in some instances, he could not direct his gaze to visual targets. Nevertheless, those instances are not specified in the model; AM failed to look at targets only when his eyes were 'captured' by his hand. Such capture is hard to understand as a failure in oculocentric coding per se or in mapping from oculocentric codes to head-centred or body-centred codes. Although the existence of single cells in the monkey which have 'arm centred' visual receptive fields have been described (Graziano et al., 1994), it is hard to see the place in the Buxbaum and Coslett model where such interactions occur.

Instead, we suggest that magnetic misreaching is a consequence of the disruption of several, probably parallel, sensorimotor loops which depend upon the integrity of the posterior parietal lobe. A second alternative hypothesis is based on the work of Andersen and colleagues (see below). In either case, these impairments disrupted sensory-guided movements for at least three modalities of target presentation. The only remaining 'sensory' route for target-directed reaching was via foveation, which, for extrafoveal targets, resulted in the pathological yoking of hand to eye of magnetic misreaching.

So how can we begin to understand the yoking of eye to hand (rather than hand to eye) which is described in patient AM? There is some evidence that attentional systems can be captured or biased towards hand actions, although the functional significance of such capture is puzzling. In fact, any sort of effortful visual monitoring of self-produced action seems completely contrary to models that emphasise efference copy or corollary discharge. In such schemes visual 'reafference' from self is ignored by the central nervous system, because processing resources are biased towards visual events consequent to the movements of external objects in the environment. Typically, such models emphasise a role of efference in perception of a stable world; nevertheless, clearly such signals could be used in a different way for sensorimotor control (see Colby (1999) for discussion, and Salinas and Thier (2000) for similar arguments about dual roles for gain modulation).

Can the coordinate transformation account explain extrafoveal optic ataxia?

In the Buxbaum and Coslett (1997, 1998) scheme, an oculocentric representation of the target is postulated, which is constructed by combining retinal target position with a feedforward or feedback signal of eye position. An oculocentric vector informs the system where the target is with respect to the head. This signal can then be combined with feedback from neck muscles to produce a body-centred representation of the target (usually conceived as relative to the torso or body midline).

If the model presupposes breakdown at these early stages, then patients with certain variants of optic ataxia would fail at reaching because for example, the retinocentric or oculocentric codes could not be constructed. Some of the oculomotor abnormalities seen in patients with full-blown Holmes–Balint syndrome could theoretically have disruptions of this sort. The consequence of such impairments would be poor reaching accuracy *because of* a failure to construct and/or utilise the retinocentric or oculocentric code. (Of course, as noted above, some patients with optic ataxia can make reasonably accurate eye movements to the very targets they cannot reach, so clearly some retinocentric and oculocentric processing is intact in such cases).

Foveation (or lack thereof) in such patients should be largely irrelevant, so a breakdown at this stage in the Buxbaum and Coslett model could explain foveal optic ataxia. The coordinate transformation account (or any particular model of how such transformations take place, e.g. Wise et al., 1997) emphasises how retinal information is combined with eye-in-head information. The position of any possible target on the retina is irrelevant as long as it can be specified in the retinocentric code. Therefore, it is not clear how the model accounts for non-foveal optic ataxia. To explain non-foveal optic ataxia, Buxbaum and Coslett (1997) speculate that "the actions of the eye and hand may be linked in a common system of spatio-motor coordinates" (p. 164). Such a system is difficult to place in their model.

A candidate for such a system in the parietal cortex is suggested by recent neurophysiological work. Andersen and his coworkers have found evidence that many of the cells in LIP which code for saccades to *auditory* targets utilise an oculocentric coordinate scheme (cells elsewhere in auditory cortex utilise head-centred coordinate frame, as would be expected for the purposes of auditory localisation). Moreover, the reach-related activity in PRR also represents targets in oculocentric coordinate frames. As noted above, Andersen and colleagues conclude that such a common scheme "may be a fairly general way of representing space and integrating different modalities within a particular spatial representation" (Andersen et al., 1998, p. 118). We favour a somewhat different interpretation: foveation is the 'default option' for primates. That is, orienting movements to auditory (and proprioceptive) targets allow primates to utilise the extremely well-adapted resolving power of the fovea. If there is any such common spatial coding, it makes perfect evolutionary sense for it to be centred on the eye. In fact, a recent report by Ben Hamed et al. (2002) showed that active fixation by an animal increases the proportion of neurons in LIP sensitive to central regions of the retina at the expense of the periphery (see also Ben Hamed and Duhamel, 2002). Whatever the functional interpretation of these intriguing neurophysiological data, our data suggest foveation signals provide the only remaining route for guiding hand movement in patients with magnetic misreaching.

Conclusions

The popularity of coordinate transformation schemes in single unit neurophysiology, physiology, motor control and neuropsychology has provided a tremendous stimulus for experimentation over the past 20 years. As neuropsychologists we agree with the critique of Buxbaum and Coslett (1997, 1998) of oversimplistic disconnection accounts of optic ataxia. We also appreciate that their model does note the potential contributions of non-visual sources of information to reaching to visual targets (e.g. arm and limb position) and that some computations may not take place in a completely serial, ordered way. The transformational account also acknowledges that target position should eventually be coded in some sort of egocentric code (either arm-, shoulder- or hand-centred). Nevertheless, it does not take into account any of the sensorimotor processes which happen after the target has appeared and the eyes begin to move. In this respect, the model, like much of experimental psychology in vision, is biased towards 'inputs' and not towards 'outputs' (Goodale, 1983). Other on-line processes largely ignored in coordinate transformation models are suggested by the fact that eye–hand localisation systems adapt extremely well to sudden shifts in target positions after the primary saccadic eye movement has been initiated. These transformations may depend on circuits of the posterior parietal cortex: Desmurget et al. (1999) found that transcranial magnetic stimulation (TMS) of posterior parietal cortex (PPC) disrupts error correction of hand movements, but only in conditions where the target jumped after the primary saccade.

Effectively, much controversy remains regarding what attributes of target position influence movement planning before eyes or hand begin to move. The data of Fisk and Goodale (1985) and others do suggest that arm movement direction is known to eye–hand coordinative structures before hand onset; e.g. given the 'slowing down' of eye movements to targets of contralateral hand movements. It may be that extent is also known in a similar fashion (Gribble and Everling, 2002), in which case hierarchical coordinate transformation accounts make more sense. In other words, if target position in direction *and distance* is known to sensorimotor control systems before movement onset, then effectively, serial transformations to an arm- or hand-centred frame have to have taken place. On-line computations in this view have evolved to deal with slight adjustments in hand and eye position due to noise in output specifications, or indeed possible changes in target position (insect and rodent prey of primates often move).

Clearly experiments of the sort described above, where eye and hand movements are simultaneously recorded, could contribute substantially to our understanding of dysfunctional mechanisms in Holmes–Balint syndrome, optic ataxia and magnetic misreaching. One difficulty in exploring more comprehensive models in individuals or groups of patients is that many recording systems require substantial control of eye movements, including making accurate saccades to and maintaining fixation on specified targets for calibration purposes. In some group studies of eye movements, patients with any fixation irregularities are excluded from the sample (e.g. Pitzalis and Di Russo, 2001). Head restraint, use of bite bars and other requirements can be very uncomfortable for elderly control participants, let alone for patients with eye movement dysfunction. In spite of these difficulties, several studies of eye movements have been made of patients with unilateral brain damage (Gaymard et al., 1998; Heide and Kömpf, 1998), suggesting that such difficulties are not insurmountable. Of course requiring arm movements in participants while eye movements are recorded adds an additional difficulty; the mechanical consequences of reaching and grasping are often transmitted to the torso, neck and head, adding artefacts to the eye movement recordings. As is often the case in science, technological advances such as more lightweight eye trackers, software which can account for head and arm movement artefact, and so on, will undoubtedly conquer the difficulties.

We believe that an understanding of processes from input to output is necessary for developing a comprehensive neuropsychological model of misreaching and the contributions of eye–hand coordination dysfunction in optic ataxia, Holmes–Balint syndrome and other sensorimotor disturbances. Magnetic misreaching is a good case in point: models of normal eye–head–hand control go some way in understanding the pathological yoking of hand to eye in Ms. D. and DP (see Jeannerod, 1988; Carey et al., 1997). Models of on-line error correction and coordination of multiple-effectors in space and time have been proposed which do not rely exclusively on coordinate transformations (cf. Johnson, 1993; Wolpert, 1997; Desmurget and Grafton, 2000), and may ultimately have greater explanatory power for case studies of misreaching, than models such as the transformational failure account.

Acknowledgements

The authors would like to thank Ms. D. for her courage and patience throughout testing. Grace Otto de Haart provided helpful comments on a previous draft of this manuscript. M.I. was supported by a Ph.D studentship from the Research Committee, University of Aberdeen. Claudio Galletti kindly advised us on Fig. 1. Some of this chapter was written while D.P.C. was supported by a Wellcome Trust Small Travel Grant.

References

Andersen, R.A., Snyder, L.H., Batista, A.P., Bueno, C.A. and Cohen, Y.E. (1998) Posterior parietal areas specialized for eye movements (LIP) and reach (PRR) using a common coordinate frame. In: G.R. Bock and J.A. Goode (Eds.), *The Sensory Guidance of Movement*. John Wiley and Sons, Chichester, pp. 109–122.

Bahcall, D.O. and Kohler, E. (1999) Illusory shifts in visual direction accompany adaptation of saccadic eye movements. *Nature*, 400: 864–867.

Baizer, J.S., Desimone, R. and Ungerleider, L.G. (1993) Comparison of subcortical connections of inferior temporal and posterior parietal cortex in monkeys. *Vis. Neurosci.*, 10: 59–72.

Baker, J.T., Donoghue, J.P. and Sanes, J.N. (1999) Gaze direction modulates finger movement activation patterns in human cerebral cortex. *J. Neurosci.*, 19: 10044–10052.

Batista, A.P., Buneo, C.A., Snyder, L.H. and Andersen, R.A. (1999) Reach plans in eye-centred coordinates. *Science*, 285: 257–260.

Battaglia-Mayer, A. and Caminiti, R. (2002) Optic ataxia as a result of the breakdown of the global tuning fields of parietal neurons. *Brain*, 125: 225–237.

Battaglia-Mayer, A., Ferraina, S., Marconi, B., Bullis, J.B., Lacquaniti, F., Burnod, Y., Baraduc, P. and Caminiti, R. (1998) Early motor influences on visuomotor transformations for reaching: a positive image of optic ataxia. *Exp. Brain Res.*, 123: 172–189.

Battaglia-Mayer, A., Ferraina, S., Genovesio, A., Marconi, B., Squatrio, S., Molinari, M., Lacquaniti, F. and Caminiti, R. (2001) Eye–hand coordination during reaching. II. An analysis of the relationships between visuomanual signals in parietal cortex and parieto-frontal association projections. *Cereb. Cortex*, 11: 528–544.

Baylis, G.C. and Baylis, L.L. (2001) Visually misguided reaching in Balint's syndrome. *Neuropsychologia*, 39: 865–875.

Bekkering, H., Abrams, R.A. and Pratt, J. (1995) Transfer of saccadic adaptation to the manual motor system. *Hum. Mov. Sci.*, 14: 155–164.

Bekkering, H. and Sailer, U. (2002) Commentary: Coordination of eye and hand in time and space. In: J. Hyönä, D.P. Munoz, W. Heide and R. Radach (Eds.), *The Brain's Eye: Neurobiological and Clinical Aspects of Oculomotor Research. Progress in Brain Research*, Vol. 140. Elsevier, Amsterdam, pp. 365–373.

Bekkering, H., Pratt, J. and Abrams, R.A. (1996) The gap effect for eye and hand movements. *Percept. Psychophys.*, 58: 628–635.

Ben Hamed, S. and Duhamel, J.-R. (2002) Ocular fixation and visual activity in the monkey lateral intraparietal area. *Exp. Brain Res.*, 142: 512–528.

Ben Hamed, S., Duhamel, J.-R., Bremmer, F. and Graf, W. (2002) Visual receptive field modulation in the lateral intraparietal area during attentive fixation and free gaze. *Cereb. Cortex*, 12: 234–245.

Binstead, G., Chua, R., Helsen, W. and Elliott, D. (2001) Eye–hand coordination in goal-directed aiming. *Hum. Mov. Sci.*, 20: 563–585.

Boller, F., Cole, M., Kim, Y., Mack, J.L. and Patawaran, C. (1975) Optic ataxia: clinical–radiological correlations with EMI scan. *J. Neurol. Neurosurg. Psychiatry*, 38: 954–958.

Boussaoud, D. and Bremmer, F. (1999) Gaze effects in the cerebral cortex: reference frames for space coding and action. *Exp. Brain Res.*, 128: 170–180.

Bremmer, F., Schlack, A., Duhamel, J.-R., Graf, W. and Fink, G.R. (2001) Space coding in primate posterior parietal cortex. *Neuroimage*, 14: S46–S51.

Bullier, J., Schall, J.D. and Morel, A. (1996) Functional streams in occipito-frontal connections in the monkey. *Behav. Brain Res.*, 76: 89–97.

Buneo, C.A., Jarvis, M.R., Batista, A.P. and Andersen, R.A. (2002) Direct visuomotor transformations for reaching. *Nature*, 416: 632–636.

Buxbaum, L.J. and Coslett, H.B. (1997) Subtypes of optic ataxia: reframing the disconnectionist account. *Neurocase*, 3: 159–166.

Buxbaum, L.J. and Coslett, H.B. (1998) Spatio-motor representations in reaching: evidence for subtypes of optic ataxia. *Cogn. Neuropsychol.*, 15: 279–312.

Carey, D.P. (2000) Eye–hand coordination: eye to hand or hand to eye? *Curr. Biol.*, 10(11): R416–R419.

Carey, D.P., Coleman, R.J. and Della Sala, S. (1997) Magnetic misreaching. *Cortex*, 33: 639–652.

Carnahan, H. and Marteniuk, R.G. (1991) The temporal organization of hand, eye and head movements during reaching and grasping. *J. Mot. Behav.*, 23: 109–119.

Clower, D.M., West, R.A., Lynch, J.C. and Strick, P.L. (2001) The inferior parietal lobule is the target of output from the superior colliculus, hippocampus and cerebellum. *J. Neurosci.*, 21: 6283–6291.

Colby, C. (1999) Parietal cortex constructs action-oriented spatial representations. In: N. Burgess, K.J. Jeffrey and J. O'Keefe (Eds.), *The Hippocampal and Parietal Foundations of Spatial Cognition*. Oxford University Press, Oxford, pp. 104–126.

Coslett, H.B. and Saffran, E. (1991) Simultanagnosia: to see but not two see. *Brain*, 114: 1523–1545.

Damasio, A.R. and Benton, A.L. (1979) Impairments of hand movements under visual guidance. *Neurology*, 29: 170–174.

De Renzi, E. (1982) *Disorders of Space Exploration and Cognition*. Wiley, Chichester.

De Renzi, E. (1988) Visuo-spatial disorders. In: C. Kennard and F. Clifford Rose (Eds.), *Physiological Aspects of Clinical Neuro-Ophthalmology*. Chapman and Hall, London, pp. 155–171.

De Renzi, E. (1996) Holmes–Balint syndrome. In: C. Code (Ed.), *Classic Cases in Neuropsychology*. Psychology Press, Hove, pp. 123–143.

De Renzi, E. and Scotti, G. (1980) Autopagnosia: fiction or reality? Report of a case. *Arch. Neurol.*, 23: 221–227.

Desmurget, M. and Grafton, S. (2000) Forward modelling allows feedback control for fast feedback loops. *Trends Cogn. Sci.*, 4: 423–431.

Desmurget, M., Péllisson, D., Rosetti, Y. and Prablance, C. (1998) From eye to hand: planning goal-directed movements. *Neurosci. Biobehav. Rev.*, 22: 761–788.

Desmurget, M., Epstein, C.M., Turner, R.S., Prablanc, C., Alexander, G.E. and Grafton, S.T. (1999) Role of the posterior parietal cortex in updating reaching movements to a visual target. *Nat. Neurosci.*, 2: 563–567.

DeSouza, J.F.X., Dukelow, S.P., Gati, J.S., Menon, R.S., Andersen, R.A. and Villis, T. (2000) Eye position signal modulates a human parietal pointing region during memory-guided movements. *J. Neurosci.*, 20: 5835–5840.

Duhamel, J.R., Bremmer, F., Ben Hamed, S. and Graf, W. (1997) Spatial invariance of visual receptive fields in parietal cortex neurons. *Nature*, 389: 845–848.

Ferraina, S., Garasto, M.R., Battaglia-Mayer, A., Ferraresi, P., Johnson, P.B., Lacquaniti, F. and Caminiti, R. (1997) Visual control of hand reaching movement: activity in parietal area 7m. *Eur. J. Neurosci.*, 9: 1090–1095.

Ferraina, S., Battaglia-Mayer, A., Genovesio, A., Marconi, B., Onorati, P. and Caminiti, R. (2001) Early coding of visuomanual coordination during reaching in parietal area PEc. *J. Neurphysiol.*, 85: 462–467.

Fisk, J.D. and Goodale, M.A. (1985) The organization of eye and limb movements during unrestricted reaching to targets in contralateral and ipsilateral space. *Exp. Brain Res.*, 60: 159–178.

Fisk, J.D. and Goodale, M.A. (1989) The effects of instructions to subjects on the programming of visually directed reaching movements. *J. Mot. Behav.*, 21: 5–19.

Galletti, C., Fattori, P., Kutz, D.F. and Gamberini, M. (1999) Brain location and visual topography of cortical area V6A in the macaque monkey. *Eur. J. Neurosci.*, 11: 575–582.

Galletti, C., Gamberini, M., Kutz, D.F., Fattori, P., Luppino, G. and Matelli, M. (2001) The cortical connections of area V6: an occipito-parietal network processing visual information. *Eur. J. Neurosci.*, 13: 1572–1588.

Gaymard, B., Pioner, C.J., Rivaud, S., Vermersch, A.I. and Pierrot-Deseilligny, C. (1998) Cortical control of saccades. *Exp. Brain Res.*, 123: 159–163.

Gielen, C.C.A.M., van den Heuvel, P.J.M. and van Gisbergen, J.A.M. (1984) Coordination of fast eye and arm movements in a tracking task. *Exp. Brain Res.*, 56: 154–161.

Glickstein, M. (1998) Cerebellum and the sensory guidance of movement. In: G.R. Bock and J.A. Goode (Eds.), *The Sensory Guidance of Movement*. John Wiley and Sons, Chichester, pp. 252–266.

Goodale, M.A. (1983) Vision as a sensorimotor system. In: T.E. Robinson (Ed.), *Behavioural Approaches to Brain Research*. Oxford University Press, Oxford, pp. 41–61.

Goodale, M.A. (1990) Brain asymmetries in the control of reaching. In: M.A. Goodale (Ed.), *Vision and Action: The Control of Grasping*. Ablex, Norwood, NJ, pp. 14–32.

Goodale, M.A. and Murphy, K.J. (1997) Action and perception in the visual periphery. In: P. Thier and H.-O. Karnath (Eds.), *Parietal Lobe Contributions to Orientation in 3D Space*. Springer-Verlag, Heidelberg, pp. 447–461.

Goodale, M.A., Meenan, J.P., Bülthoff, H.H., Nicolle, D.A., Murphy, K.J. and Racicot, C.I. (1994) Separate neural pathways for the visual analysis of object shape in perception and prehension. *Curr. Biol.*, 4: 604–610.

Graziano, M.S.A., Yap, G.S. and Gross, C.G. (1994) Coding of visual space by premotor neurons. *Science*, 266: 1054–1057.

Gribble, P.L., Everling, S., Ford, K. and Mattas, A. (2002) Hand–eye coordination for rapid pointing movements — arm movement direction and distance are specified prior to saccade onset. *Exp. Brain Res.*, 145: 372–382.

Haaxma, H. and Kuypers, H.G.J.M. (1975) Intrahemispheric cortical connections and visual guidance of hand and finger movements in the rhesus monkey. *Brain*, 98: 239–260.

Harvey, M. and Milner, A.D. (1995) Balints patient. *Cogn. Neuropsychol.*, 12: 261–264.

Hausser, C.O., Robert, F. and Giard, N. (1980) Balint's syndrome. *Can. J. Neurol. Sci.*, 7: 157–161.

Hecaen, H. and De Ajuriaguerra, J. (1954) Balint's syndrome (psychic paralysis of visual fixation) and its minor forms. *Brain*, 77: 373–400.

Heide, W. and Kömpf, D. (1998) Combined deficits of saccades and visuo-spatial orientation after cortical lesions. *Exp. Brain Res.*, 123: 164–171.

Helsen, W.F., Elliott, D., Starkes, J.L. and Ricker, K.L. (1998) Temporal and spatial coupling of point of gaze and hand movements in aiming. *J. Mot. Behav.*, 30: 249–259.

Helsen, W.F., Elliott, D., Starkes, J.L. and Ricker, K.L. (2000) Coupling of eye, finger, elbow and shoulder movements during manual aiming. *J. Mot. Behav.*, 32: 241–248.

Henriques, D.Y.P., Klier, E.M., Smith, M.A., Lowy, D. and Crawford, J.D. (1998) Gaze centered remapping of remembered visual space in an open-loop pointing task. *J. Neurosci.*, 18: 1583–1594.

Holmes, G. (1918) Disturbances of visual orientation. *Br. J. Ophthalmol.*, 2: 449–468; 506–516.

Honda, H. (1984) Functional between-hand differences in outflow eye position information. *Q. J. Exp. Psychol.*, 36A: 75–88.

Husain, M. and Stein, J. (1988) Rezso Balint and his most celebrated case. *Arch. Neurol.*, 45: 89–93.

Jakobson, L.S., Archibald, Y.M., Carey, D.P. and Goodale, M.A. (1991) A kinematic analysis of reaching and grasping movements in a patient recovering from optic ataxia. *Neuropsychologia*, 29: 803–809.

Jeannerod, M. (1988) *The Neural and Behavioral Organisation of Goal-Directed Movements*. Oxford University Press, Oxford.

Jeannerod, M., Decety, J. and Michel, F. (1994) Impairment of grasping movements following a bilateral posterior parietal lesion. *Neuropsychologia*, 32: 369–380.

Johansson, R.S., Westling, G.R., Backstrom, A. and Flanagan, J.R. (2001) Eye–hand coordination in object manipulation. *J. Neurosci.*, 21: 6917–6932.

Johnson, P.B. (1993) Towards an understanding of the cerebral cortex and reaching movements: a review of recent approaches. In: A. Berthoz (Ed.), *Multisensory Control of Movement*. Oxford University Press, Oxford, pp. 199–261.

Johnson, P.B., Ferraina, S., Garasto, M.R., Battaglia-Mayer, A., Ercolani, L., Burnod, Y. and Caminiti, R. (1997) From vision to movement: cortico-cortical connections and combinatorial properties of reaching-related neurons in parietal areas V6 and V6A. In: P. Thier and H.-O. Karnath (Eds.), *Parietal Lobe Contributions to Orientation in 3D Space*. Springer-Verlag, Heidelberg, pp. 221–236.

Jouffrais, C. and Boussaoud, D. (1999) Neuronal activity related to eye–hand coordination in the primate premotor cortex. *Exp. Brain Res.*, 128: 205–209.

Kase, C.S., Troncoso, J.F., Court, J.E., Tapia, J.F. and Mohr, J.P. (1977) Global spatial disorientation: clinico-pathologic correlations. *J. Neurol. Sci.*, 34: 267–278.

Kim, M.-S. and Robertson, L.C. (2001) Implicit representations of space after bilateral parietal lobe damage. *J. Cogn. Neurosci.*, 13: 1080–1087.

Levine, D.N. and Rinn, W.E. (1986) Opticosensory ataxia and alien hand syndrome after posterior cerebral artery territory infarction. *Neurology*, 36: 1094–1097.

Levine, D.N., Kaufman, K.J. and Mohr, J.P. (1978) Inaccurate reaching associated with a superior parietal lobe tumor. *Neurology*, 28: 556–561.

Lünenberger, L., Kutz, D.F. and Hoffman, K.-P. (2000) Influence of arm movements on saccades in humans. *Eur. J. Neurosci.*, 12: 4107–4116.

Marconi, B., Genovesio, A., Battaglia-Mayer, A., Ferraina, S., Squatrio, S., Molinari, M., Lacquaniti, F. and Caminiti, R. (2001) Eye–hand coordination during reaching. I. Anatomical relationships between parietal and frontal cortex. *Cereb. Cortex*, 11: 513–527.

Miall, R.C. (1998) The cerebellum, predictive control and motor coordination. In: G.R. Bock and J.A. Goode (Eds.), *The Sensory Guidance of Movement*. Chichester, John Wiley and Sons, pp. 272–290.

Milner, A.D. and Goodale, M.A. (1995) *The Visual Brain in Action*. Oxford University Press, Oxford.

Milner, A.D., Paulignan, Y., Dijkerman, H.C., Michel, F. and Jeannerod, M. (1999) A paradoxical improvement of misreaching in optic ataxia: new evidence for two separate neural systems for visual localization. *Proc. R. Soc. Lond. B.*, 266: 2225–2229.

Milner, A.D., Dijkerman, H.-C., Pisella, L., McIntosh, R.D., Tilikete, C., Vighetto, A. and Rossetti, Y. (2001) Grasping the past: delay can improve visuomotor performance. *Curr. Biol.*, 11: 1–20.

Munoz, D.P., Commentary: saccadic eye movements: overview of neural circuitry. In: J. Hyönä, D.P. Munoz, W. Heide and R. Radach (Eds.), *The Brain's Eye: Neurobiological and Clinical Aspects of Oculomotor Research. Progress in Brain Research*, Vol. 140. Elsevier, Amsterdam, pp. 89–96.

Mushiake, H., Fujii, N. and Tanji, J. (1996) Visually guided saccade versus eye–hand reach: contrasting neuronal activity in the cortical supplementary and frontal eye fields. *J. Neurophysiol.*, 75: 2187–2191.

Neggers, S.F.W. and Bekkering, H. (1999) Integration of visual and somatosensory target information in goal-directed eye and arm movements. *Exp. Brain Res.*, 125: 97–107.

Neggers, S.F.W. and Bekkering, H. (2000) Ocular gaze is anchored to the target of an ongoing pointing movement. *J. Neurophysiol.*, 83: 639–651.

Neggers, S.F.W. and Bekkering, H. (2001) Gaze anchoring to a pointing target is present during the entire movement and is driven by a non-visual signal. *J. Neurophysiol.*, 86: 961–970.

Paillard, J. (1996) Fast and slow feedback loops for the visual correction of spatial errors in a pointing task: a reappraisal. *Can. J. Physiol. Pharmacol.*, 74: 401–417.

Perenin, M.-T. (1997) Optic ataxia and unilateral neglect: clinical evidence for dissociable spatial functions in posterior parietal cortex. In: P. Thier and H.-O. Karnath (Eds.), *Parietal Lobe Contributions to Orientation in 3D Space*. Springer-Verlag, Heidelberg, pp. 289–308.

Perenin, M.T. and Vighetto, A. (1988) Optic ataxia: a specific disturbance in visuomotor mechanisms. *Brain*, 111: 643–674.

Pisella, L., Gréa, H., Tilikete, C., Vighetto, A., Desmurget, M., Rode, G., Boisoon, D. and Rosetti, Y. (2000) An 'automatic pilot' for the hand in the human posterior parietal cortex: towards a reinterpretation of optic ataxia. *Nat. Neurosci.*, 3: 729–736.

Pitzalis, S. and Di Russo, F. (2001) Spatial anisotropy of saccadic latency in normal subjects and brain-damaged patients. *Cortex*, 37: 475–492.

Prablanc, C. and Martin, O. (1992) Automatic control during hand reaching at undetected two-dimensional target displacements. *J. Neurophysiol.*, 67: 455–469.

Prablanc, C., Pélisson, D. and Goodale, M.A. (1986) Visual control of reaching movements without vision of the limb, I. Role of retinal feedback of target position in guiding the hand. *Exp. Brain Res.*, 62: 293–302.

Ratcliff, G. and Davies-Jones, G.A.B. (1972) Defective visual localization in focal brain wounds. *Brain*, 95: 49–60.

Rizzo, M. (1993) Balint syndrome and associated visuospatial disorders. *Bailleres Clin. Neurol.*, 2: 415–437.

Rizzo, M., Rotella, D. and Darling, W. (1992) Troubled reaching after right occipito-temporal damage. *Neuropsychologia*, 30: 711–722.

Robertson, I., Triesman, A., Freidman-Hill, S. and Grabowecky, M. (1997) The interaction of object and spatial pathways: evidence from Balints syndrome. *J. Cogn. Neurosci.*, 9: 295–317.

Rondot, P., DeRecondo, J. and Ribadeau Dumas, J.L. (1977) Visuomotor ataxia. *Brain*, 100: 355–376.

Rossetti, Y., Koga, K. and Mano, T. (1993) Prismatic displacement of vision induces transient changes in the timing of eye–hand coordination. *Percept. Psychophys.*, 54: 355–364.

Sailer, U., Eggert, T., Ditterich, T. and Straube, A. (2000) Spatial and temporal aspects of eye–hand coordination across different tasks. *Exp. Brain Res.*, 134: 163–173.

Salinas, E. and Thier, P. (2000) Gain modulation: a major computational principle of the central nervous system. *Neuron*, 27: 15–21.

Shipp, S., Blanton, M. and Zeki, S. (1998) A visuo-somatomotor pathway through superior parietal cortex in the macaque monkey: cortical connections of areas V6 and V6A. *Eur. J. Neurosci.*, 10: 3171–3193.

Snyder, L.H. (2000) Coordinate transformations for eye and arm movements in the brain. *Curr. Opin. Neurobiol.*, 10: 747–754.

Snyder, L.H., Batista, A.P. and Andersen, R.A. (2000a) Intention-related activity in the posterior parietal cortex: a review. *Vision Res.*, 40: 1433–1441.

Snyder, L.H., Batista, A.O. and Andersen, R.A. (2000b) Saccade-related activity in the parietal reach region. *J. Neurophysiol.*, 83: 1099–1102.

Stuphorn, V., Bauswein, E. and Hoffman, K.-P. (2000) Neurons in the primate superior colliculus coding for arm movements in gaze-related coordinates. *J. Neurophysiol.*, 83: 1283–1299.

Suzuki, K., Yamadori, A. and Fujii, T. (1997) Category-specific comprehension deficit restricted to body parts. *Neurocase*, 3: 193–200.

Tehovnik, E.J., Slocum, W.M., Tolias, A.S. and Schiller, P.H. (1998) Saccades induced electrically from the dorsomedial frontal cortex: evidence for a head-centered representation. *Brain Res.*, 795: 287–291.

Tzavaras, A. and Masure, M.C. (1975) Aspects différents de l'ataxie optique selon la latéralisation hémisphérique de la lésion. *Lyon Méd.*, 236: 673–683.

Wise, S.P., Boussaoud, D., Johnson, P.B. and Caminiti, R. (1997) Premotor and parietal cortex: corticocortical connectivity and combinatorial computations. *Annu. Rev. Neurosci.*, 20: 25–42.

Van Donkelaar, O., Lee, J.-H. and Drew, A.S. (2000) Transcranial magnetic stimulation disrupts eye–hand interactions in the posterior parietal cortex. *J. Neurophysiol.*, 84: 1677–1680.

Van Donkelaar, P. (1997) Eye–hand interactions during goal-directed pointing movements. *NeuroReport*, 8: 2139–2142.

Van Donkelaar, P. and Lee, R.G. (1994) Interactions between the eye and hand motor systems: disruptions due to cerebellar dysfunction. *J. Neurophysiol.*, 72: 1674–1685.

Van Donkelaar, P., Lee, J.-H., and Drew, A.S. (2002) Cortical frames of reference for eye–hand coordination. In: J. Hyönä, D.P. Munoz, W. Heide and R. Radach (Eds.), *The Brain's Eye: Neurobiological and Clinical Aspects of Oculomotor Research. Progress in Brain Research*, Vol. 140. Elsevier, Amsterdam, pp. 301–310.

Wolpert, D.M. (1997) Computational approaches to motor control. *Trends Cogn. Sci.*, 1: 209–216.

Xing, J. and Andersen, R.A. (2000) Models of the posterior parietal cortex which perform multimodal integration and represent space in several coordinate frames. *J. Cogn. Neurosci.*, 12: 601–614.

CHAPTER 22

Visuomotor transformations for eye–hand coordination

D.Y.P. Henriques, W.P. Medendorp, A.Z. Khan and J.D. Crawford *

York University, Centre for Visual Research, Departments of Psychology and Biology, 4700 Keele St., BSB, rm 291, Toronto, ON M3J 1P3, Canada

Abstract: In recent years the scientific community has come to appreciate that the early cortical representations for visually guided arm movements are probably coded in a visual frame, i.e. relative to retinal landmarks. While this scheme accounts for many behavioral and neurophysiological observations, it also poses certain problems for manual control. For example, how are these oculocentric representations updated across eye movements, and how are they then transformed into useful commands for accurate movements of the arm relative to the body? Also, since we have two eyes, which is used as the reference point in eye–hand alignment tasks like pointing? We show that patterns of errors in human pointing suggest that early oculocentric representations for arm movement are remapped relative to the gaze direction during each saccade. To then transform these oculocentric representations into useful commands for accurate movements of the arm relative to the body, the brain correctly incorporates the three-dimensional, rotary geometry of the eyes when interpreting retinal images. We also explore the possibility that the eye–hand coordination system uses a strategy like ocular dominance, but switches alignment between the left and right eye in order to maximize eye–hand coordination in the best field of view. Finally, we describe the influence of eye position on eye–hand alignment, and then consider how head orientation influences the linkage between oculocentric visual frames and bodycentric motor frames. These findings are framed in terms of our 'conversion-on-demand' model, which suggests a virtual representation of egocentric space, i.e. one in which only those representations selected for action are put through the complex visuomotor transformations required for interaction with actual objects in personal space.

Introduction

Eye–hand (or hand–eye) coordination is a topic that just about everyone can relate to. We need good eye–hand coordination to reach out and pick up a coffee cup, press a doorbell, or catch a ball. Indeed many of the skilled activities that distinguish humans from other species involve good eye–hand coordination. Most of these we take for granted — only in cases of extreme athletic prowess do we notice eye–hand coordination. But these more basic abilities become

* Correspondence to: J.D. Crawford, York University, Centre for Visual Research, Departments of Psychology and Biology, 4700 Keele St., BSB, rm 291, Toronto, ON M3J 1P3, Canada. Tel.: +1-416-736-2100 ext. 88641; Fax: +1-416-736-5814; E-mail: jdc@yorku.ca

all too significant when they are impaired, as in the neurological patients studied by Carey et al. (2002, this volume).

Given its centrality in our lives, it is not surprising that the study of this behavior has a long history (as early as Rene Descartes). Clearly this has remained a major topic of study, with various scientific contributions made in major laboratories of the 20th century. And yet at this time one will find no erudite 'Society for Eye–Hand Coordination', or 'Annual Meeting for Eye–hand Coordination'. However, as the contributions to this section of the current volume testify, it would seem that it is a topic which has reached its day, perhaps because we know just enough about these various sub-systems to now try putting them altogether.

Our particular interest is in the geometric aspects of the forward serial transformations within the brain that use vision to guide movement of the hand. Although many studies of eye–hand coordination look at the input (vision) and the output (hand movement), our focus is on the transformations that account for all of the linkages in between — from eye, to head, to body, to arm, to hand. Most of our studies are on pointing or 'touching', a pared-down version of eye–hand coordination minus the grasp element. Our goal is to build up a rigorous model — the kind that could actually control such a system if one were to build it from scratch. Our belief is that in building up such a model, we will gain a clearer understanding of the neural processes that one should look for in the brain. The following is not a general review of the topic: in the short space allowed here our aim is mainly to summarize some of our own work in this area, and to show how this work has motivated our thinking in this area.

Eyes on the prize

Many studies, including those described in the other contributions to this section and elsewhere (e.g. Gielen et al., 1984; Fisk and Goodale, 1985; Vercher et al., 1994; Engel et al., 2000) have demonstrated the intimate coupling between movements of the eyes and hand. But why do we need this? What is the advantage of coupling the eye and hand? One way to find out is to de-couple the system and see what happens, i.e. ask people to reach or point toward objects that they are not looking at. Under these conditions, Roland Johansson and colleagues have shown how reaching/manipulating movements that are normally precise become fumbling approximations. We wanted to quantify the effects of uncoupling on pointing performance (Henriques et al., 1998; Henriques and Crawford, 2000). This work followed from earlier observations by Bock (1986) and Enright (1995), showing that people point past remembered targets located in their visual periphery, which we confirmed and expanded on.

We found that when forced to point toward a central target in the absence of visual feedback, with the eyes deviated, subjects showed systematic misjudgments of target direction. Individual subjects showed different patterns of error, which varied rather anisotropically depending on the direction of the target relative to gaze. But overall, subjects showed a consistent pattern: a tendency to overestimate the distance of the target relative to gaze (Fig. 1A). When asked to direct their gaze 30°, 15°, and 5° both to the right and left of the pointing target, subjects' past-pointing increased with the amount of gaze deviation until saturating at about 2–4° error at 15° gaze deviation. Further controls — in which both the gaze target and pointing target were varied — confirmed Bock's finding that this effect was related to the amount of retinal deviation of the target, not eye position per se (Bock, 1986).

Why this degradation in performance? One obvious reason is that foveal vision has a much higher acuity. However this cannot be the full answer, because retinal acuity 5–15° from the fovea is still too good to explain the poor performance in our studies. Another possibility is that a 'gaze-guidance' system can use the line of sight as a special cue to guide the hand toward foveated targets. This might somehow account for the magnetic reaching behavior seen in Carey's patient (see Carey et al., 2002, this volume). But in another study where our subjects placed their finger onto a remembered target site (Henriques et al., 2001) they did not always look correctly onto the target, but these errors in fixation did not correlate with errors in reaching. For instance, when subjects looked slightly to the left of the target, they were no more likely to misreach to the left than to the right. Thus, contrary to what might be predicted by a gaze-guidance hypothesis, small, unconscious deviations in gaze do not drag the hand with them, though they do cause small non-specific degradations in performance. Instead, subjects may misreach more when their gaze misses the target site because the target falls outside the foveal part of vision. Thus, our favored explanation is that the system is simply better calibrated for foveated targets, and that conversely the neural outputs of other patches of retina are poorly calibrated for eye–hand coordination. This does not explain the specific overshooting pattern that we found, but that is a topic we will take up again in a later section.

Now you see it, now you don't

A visuomotor puzzle is how it is that we can look at a target, look away from it so that it is out of sight, and still know where the target is (Hallett and

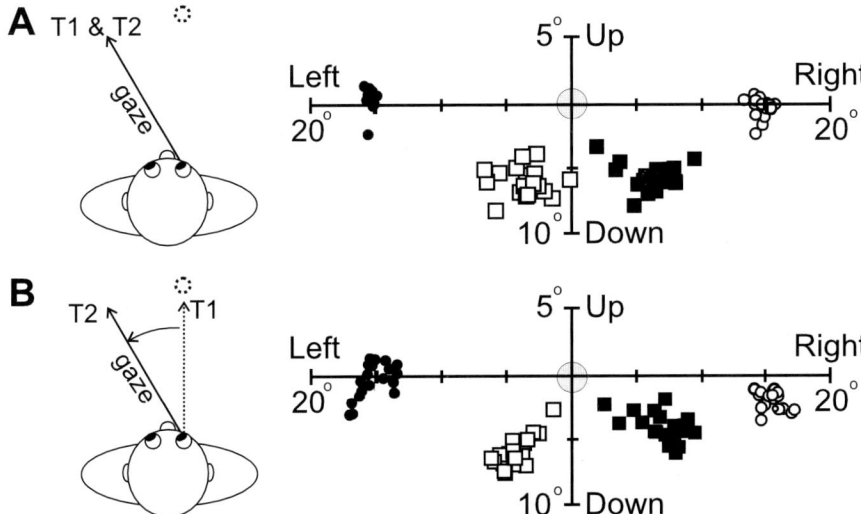

Fig. 1. Final 2-D pointing directions (squares) and gaze direction (circles) relative to central target for a head-fixed subject. Left column: the two tasks, where subjects either view the target peripherally (A) or foveate the target (T1) before looking also to the left (T2) (B). Right column: in the top task (A), the subject past-points in the direction opposite to gaze; this is due to an overestimation of the retinal eccentricity of the target. In the bottom task (B), the subject also past-points in the direction opposite to their final gaze direction, although they fixated the target first (this paradigm is further illustrated in Fig. 2, middle column). Open symbols indicate 15° rightward fixation trials; solid symbols indicate 15° leftward fixation trials. Modified from Henriques et al., 1998.

Lightstone, 1976; Mays and Sparks, 1980). Clearly, a fixed retinal impression of the target location would be insufficient and downright misleading, so the brain must be doing something more sophisticated.

One idea was that the brain builds up representations of space by comparing vision with eye position, head position, and so on (Flanders et al., 1992). Unfortunately, the neurophysiological evidence for this mechanism, at least in visuomotor transformations, remains somewhat sketchy, boiling down to some fairly subtle eye position signals (Andersen and Mountcastle, 1983; Schlag et al., 1992; Graziano et al., 1994; Bremmer et al., 1999; Jouffrais and Boussaoud, 1999) with no clear maps of head-centered or body-centered space. Perhaps these maps are distributed in some way (Bremmer et al., 1999). But a more recent suggestion, consistent with certain signals recorded in the visuomotor structures of the brain (Duhamel et al., 1992; Mazzoni et al., 1996), suggests that each time the eyes move, an internal copy of this movement is used to remap our internal on-line representations of visual space in a retinal frame.

The gaze-dependent pointing errors described in the previous section (Fig. 1A) provided the opportunity to test between these mechanisms in the eye–hand coordination system (Fig. 2). We reasoned that since subjects make pointing errors as a function of retinal eccentricity (as described above), then they should make these same errors when redirecting their gaze produces a similar 'retinal eccentricity' for the remembered fixated target site — as if their internal representations were remapped to the same retinal location during an eye movement (Fig. 2, right column), even if they looked at the target with the fovea (Henriques et al., 1998). For instance, if subjects point past a remembered target seen while they are looking 15° to its left, they should also past-point after they move their eyes to 15° left subsequent to fixating the flashed target. On the other hand, if subjects formed static, head- or body-centered representations of targets (Fig. 2, left column) then pointing based on an initially foveated target should not be affected by subsequent eye movements (that, indeed is the point of this model).

In summary, in the paradigm illustrated both in Figs. 1B and 2, where people redirect their gaze away from the fixated target before pointing to its remembered location, a head-centered model would

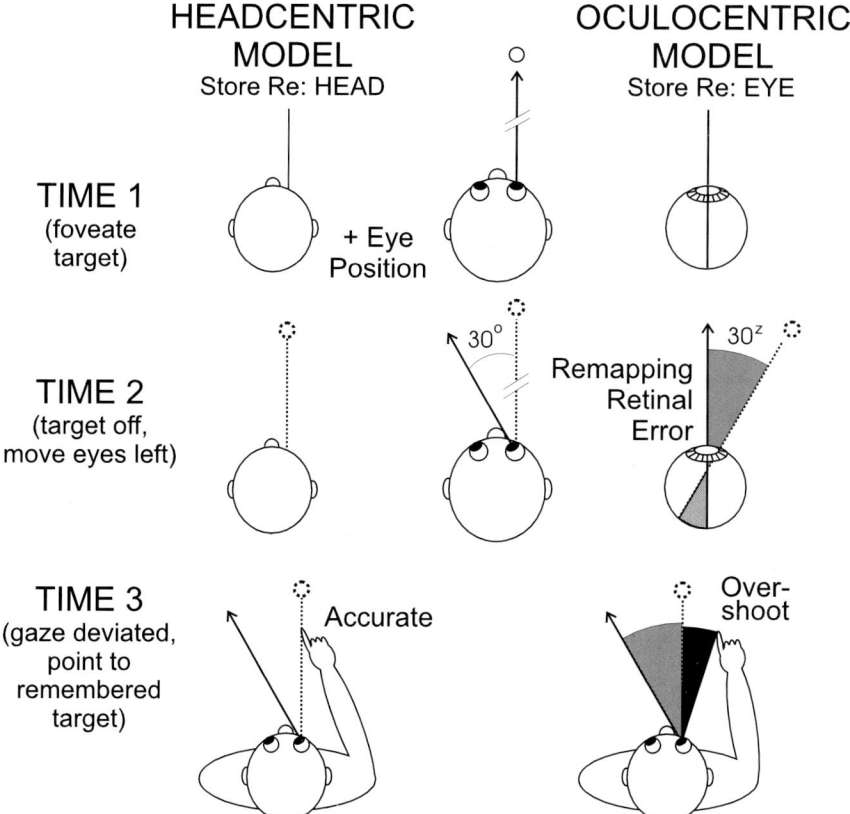

Fig. 2. Predictions of the headcentric (left) and oculocentric (right) models of visuospatial memory on subjects' pointing to a remembered target. The test paradigm (shown in the middle, as well as in Fig. 1B), has subjects look at the target (time 1) and then look 30° left after the target disappears (time 2) before pointing to its remembered location (time 3). The key feature of this test is that during the visuomotor transformation for pointing, subjects usually exaggerate the retinal eccentricity of the remembered direction of non-foveal targets (top row of Fig. 1, also Bock, 1986; Enright, 1995). The headcentric model holds that we compute target direction relative to the head (by combining retinal signals with eye position) as soon as we fixate the target (in time 1). Note that retinal eccentricity at time 1 is zero and therefore is not subject to the exaggeration effect. According to the headcentric model, this head-centered memory trace remains stable during the intervening eye movement at time 2, so that accurate pointing is predicted at time 3. The oculocentric model holds that the target is coded relative to current gaze direction and as a result the leftward eye movement at time 2 must be compensated for, by the counter-rotating of the retinotopic memory trace 30° to the right (time 2, right panel). Now the subject must point based on a peripherally shifted retinotopic memory trace, which is susceptible to the exaggeration effect. Therefore, the oculocentric model predicts that subjects will past-point in the direction opposite to the final gaze direction. Modified from Henriques et al., 1998.

predict accurate open-loop pointing (Fig. 2, bottom left), whereas an eye-centered remapping model would predict that subjects past-point in the direction opposite to gaze (Fig. 2, bottom right) like they do when they point to the remembered location of a peripherally viewed target (as shown by the data in Fig. 1A). Note that neither model explains past-pointing in the peripherally viewed target condition shown in Fig. 1A, but given this phenomena, the two models predict different pointing performance for the paradigm shown in Fig. 2. Thus, the results in Fig. 1A merely provides the necessary control for pointing based on peripheral retinotopic representations.

Our results clearly favored the eye-centered remapping model (Fig. 1B). When subjects foveated a briefly flashed target in complete darkness, and then deviated their eyes, they did not point accurately as they did when they maintained gaze on the remembered target site throughout the trial. Instead, they made the same errors in pointing as if they had viewed the target in the new retinally peripheral location (compare Fig. 1B to Fig. 1A). In other words, it looks like they were pointing based on a shifted, retinotopic representation. Based on this result, we concluded that the eye–hand coordination system uses this same mechanism (Henriques et al., 1998), which had previously been proposed and described for the oculomotor system. Shortly afterwards Andersen and colleagues (Batista et al., 1999) discovered that single-unit responses are consistent with such a mechanism in the parietal reach region (PRR) — an arm control center with retinotopically organized receptive fields.

Near vs. far

The previously described study by Henriques et al. (1998) was done exclusively with pointing targets that were well beyond reach, in so-called extrapersonal space. However, a number of neuropsychological studies have suggested that different neural mechanisms are used for coding near (peripersonal) space (for a review see Colby and Goldberg, 1999). This makes some sense for eye–hand coordination. Anything within reach is coded by preparatory activity in primary motor cortex (M1), whose signals are clearly not organized in eye-centered coordinates (Fu et al., 1993; Riehle and Requin, 1995; Mushiake et al., 1997; Crammond and Kalaska, 2000). Why not code for near targets using the stable, muscle-centered, eye-movement independent codes of M1?

To test which spatial mechanism dominates human reaching behavior, across eye movements, in near space, we repeated the paradigm in Henriques et al. (1998) (Fig. 2), but this time using three sets of arm pointing/reaching targets — one beyond reach, one at 42 cm, and one at 15 cm. According to the hypothesis that near and far space are coded differently, subjects should have shown the same result as before for the far target, but should have shown a more stable reaching response for the near targets, unaffected by the intervening eye movement. But this is not what happened (Medendorp and Crawford, 2002). Instead, subjects showed the same effect for all three-target sets: that predicted by the eye-centered remapping model. It would be a mistake to conclude that this means that the muscle/body centered representations are never used to code near space in M1 and other structures, but this result does suggest structures like PRR which do utilize remapping to override those responses, updating them after each eye movement. Perhaps, the near–far distinction may be more relevant for perception than for action. If so, our results support the notion that target locations are remembered by shifting retinotopic representations as a function of each eye movement, and suggest that this is a general spatial mechanism for near and far space.

Cyclops had it easy

When we speak of eye–hand coordination, we immediately propagate an implicit error: only a mythical one-armed Cyclops has eye–hand coordination. Most of us have to coordinate two eyes with two hands, but one generally chooses one hand in reaching, often the dominant hand. But which eye is chosen? Or is it some synthesis of the two?

This gets us into the sticky territory of ocular dominance and the cyclopean eye. Ocular dominance has many meanings. Here we consider just alignment of the hand with the eye. For example, in our monocular pointing studies, we have found that subjects tend to align the fingertip between the eye and the target, as if they were reaching out to touch it (as opposed to aligning the line of the arm to the target). So, which eye do they choose? In neurophysiological terms, which eye dominates the eye-centered representations in the brain described above?

One appealing idea, put forward in the 19th century by Wells and more recently championed by Ono (Wells, 1792; Ono and Barbeito, 1982), is that the inputs from the two eyes are synthesized and referenced to a virtual 'cyclopean eye' positioned between them. But, even this theory would require the fingertip to be positioned along the line of sight of one eye or the other to be perceived as dead ahead of the cyclopean eye (this may sound contradictory, but makes sense in terms of Wells' original experiments). Thus, the question arises again, which eye does the hand coordinate with?

A number of classical studies suggest that the hand prefers to align with a dominant eye (Miles, 1930; Crider, 1944; Coren and Kaplan, 1973; Porac and Coren, 1976). However, we noted that all

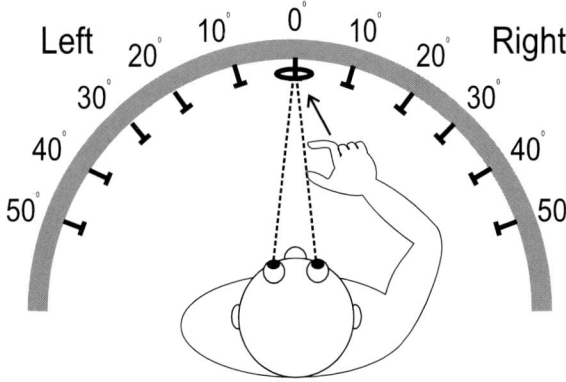

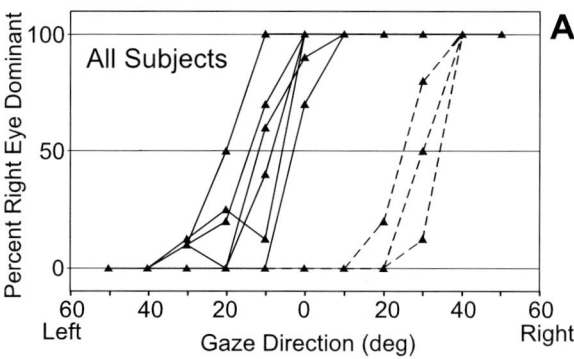

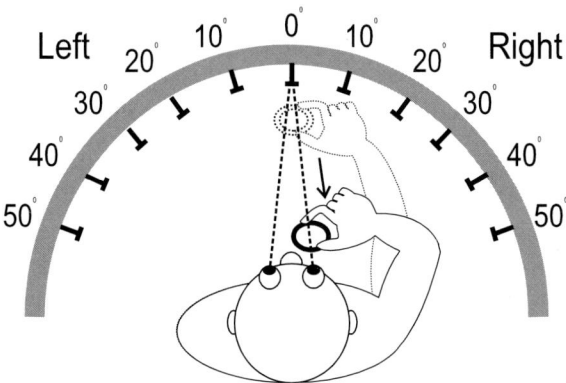

Fig. 3. Illustration of a reach–grasp task to test whether ocular dominance shifts between the eyes as a function of gaze direction. Method: subjects were instructed to fixate on one of 11 rings placed horizontally (50° left and right of center) in a semi-cylinder, and grasp the ring (top) and bring it all the way back to their face in a smooth fluid motion, without allowing it to cross either line of gaze (bottom). Modified from Khan and Crawford, 2001a.

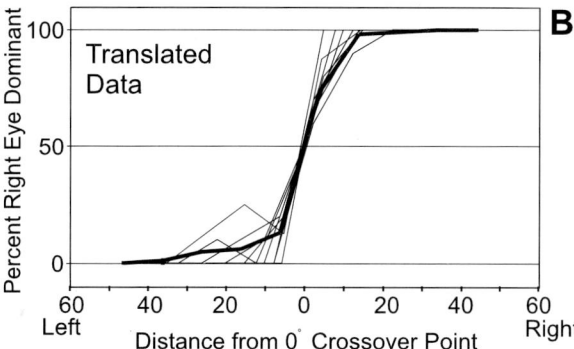

Fig. 4. Gaze position dependence of ocular dominance. (A) The percentage of trials where the right eye was dominant (0% indicates that the left eye was always dominant) is shown for each gaze/target direction for 10 subjects. Solid lines: right eye dominance at center. Dashed lines: left eye dominance at center. (B) Same data shifted so that the 50% crossover point aligns with zero on the abscissa. The thick line shows the average across all subjects. Modified from Khan and Crawford, 2001a.

of these studies were done with targets located straight ahead. But what about more peripheral targets? Would it not make sense for the system to be more flexible, and chose either eye, depending on which one had the better field of view?

To test this idea, we used a variation of an old paradigm (Crider, 1944) where we had subjects reach out and grasp a ring while visually fixating a target through that ring, and then bring the ring back to 'the eye' without allowing it to cross the line of sight (Fig. 3). Subjects are expected to choose the 'dominant' line of sight, and indicate this by bring-

ing the ring back to the corresponding eye. Their performance on this task proceeded as we had expected (Khan and Crawford, 2001a): subjects tended to choose the right eye for rightward (but still binocular) targets, and the left eye for leftward targets (Fig. 4). The switch in choice generally occurred surprisingly close to, but just off, center, so that if subjects had been tested only at the center target they would have appeared to be either left eye or right eye dominant. In a similar, more recent test of this hypothesis, we asked subjects to point toward targets at various horizontal eccentricities, and then examined the kinematics of their arm position to determine if the hand had been aligned with the left or right eye (Khan and Crawford, 2001b). Again, we found a clear tendency for subjects to choose the left eye for leftward targets and vice versa, although curiously this tendency was reduced by visual feedback. This may be a motor strategy that allows the hand to coordinate with either one eye or the other in way that optimizes vision, perhaps relying on eye position signals or some other cue.

The importance of knowing eye position

Speaking of eye position signals, how does the eye–hand coordination system transform eye-centered visual signals into useable commands for arm movement? At first glance, the eye-centered remapping mechanism described in the previous sections would seem to obviate the need to continuously take eye position into account. But that is only true with regard to the mechanism for coding and storing spatial memory described in those sections. Once one has to actually act on those representations, the eye position signals become vital.

Why is this so? Supposing that one always started off by looking and pointing in the same direction, one might think it a simple matter to drive the arm along the arc in parallel with the displacement of the target as coded on the retina, or the target's retinal displacement. To code the arm movement, the brain would map the retinal vector directly onto a motor vector. One obvious flaw with coding arm motor commands this way is that most of the time the arm does not start aligned with gaze. When we go from a resting position to reach for a target, we are generally accurate, even when we do not have visual feedback of the arm and target (e.g. Crawford et al., 2000; Henriques and Crawford, 2000). The only way to do this is by combining the visual signal with an internal sense of eye position (von Helmholtz, 1867; Mittelstaedt, 1983).

The recognition that the brain needs to take eye position into account when computing target direction has led some theories to suggest that the brain might approximate the required arm/eye rotation by a simple vector addition — merely adding all retinal vectors onto a vector coding initial eye direction (Hallett and Lightstone, 1976; Mays and Sparks, 1980; Flanders et al., 1992). But this vector-addition strategy would lead to marked errors in some situations because displacements in retinal coordinates are not the same as displacements in head or shoulder coordinates (Crawford and Guitton, 1997). For example, the way that straight lines project onto the retina depends on eye position in a complex manner. In Fig. 5, we have two earth-fixed, horizontal arcs centered on an eyeball. In Fig. 5A, the eye is fixating a diamond at eye-level, while in Fig. 5B, the eye is fixating a diamond 30° up. For each diamond, a square is placed 60° to its right, so that both objects lie on the same horizontal arc in space. The left and right columns show how the images of these objects project on the retinal for two different perspectives. When the eye fixates the eye-level diamond (Fig. 5A), the retinal image of the eye-level square falls on the retinal meridian (dashed line on the back of the transparent eye). But when the eye fixates the diamond 30° up (Fig. 5B), the retinal image of the square falls below the horizontal meridian of the eye — owing to the upward rotation of the eye. Thus, spatial displacements that might be visually horizontal (i.e. on the retina) at one eye position become oblique at other eye positions, whereas in head/shoulder coordinates they stay the same. If the brain tried to compute these objects' location relative to the head or the shoulder simply by using vector addition, it would misestimate the elevations of at least some objects, and would misaim resultant eye and arm movements.

To test the way that the eye–hand coordination system handles this problem, we had subjects point between various horizontally displaced targets, in the absence of visual feedback (Crawford et al., 2000). What we found was that: (1) the projections of these target displacements onto the retina varied strongly with eye position in a complex, non-linear fashion; and (2), despite this, pointing movements were essentially accurate. In other words, the visuomotor transformation for pointing did not just take the 'first-order' aspects of eye position into account (i.e. adding the visual vector to an eye position vector), it in effect accounted for 3-D eye rotation and performed the correct non-linear reference frame transformation.

Using your head

Similar arguments hold for taking head orientation into account. For example, if one were to purposefully keep the eyes centered while looking around,

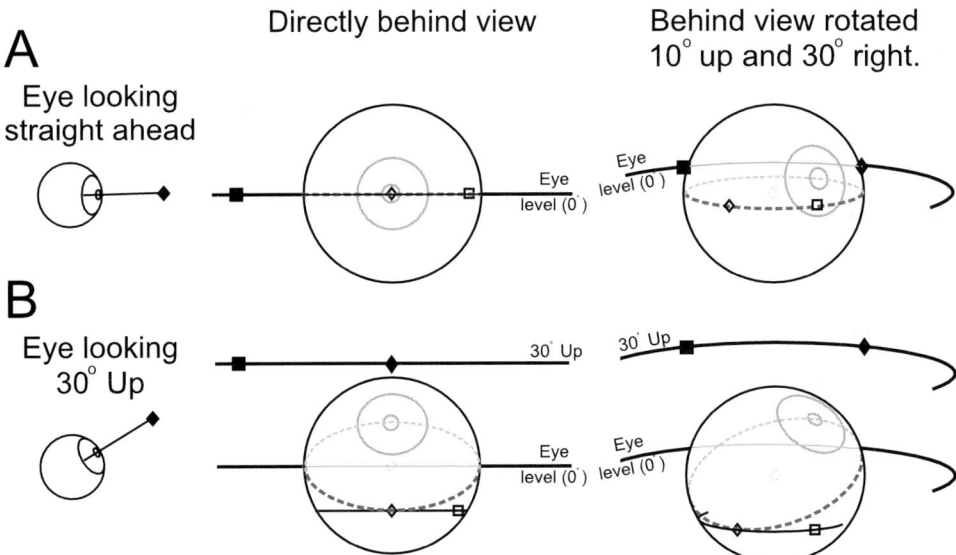

Fig. 5. Simulated eye position-dependent geometry of retinal stimulation. Two views of the eyeballs and targets are shown: one directly behind edge-on (left column) and one behind and slightly up and to the right (right column). The eyeball is transparent, so we can see its nodal point (small circle), its horizontal meridian (dashed sphere), the two external objects (closed symbols) and their retinal projections on the back of the eye (open symbols). For both eye positions (A, eye directed straight ahead; and B, eye rotated 30° upward), the eye is fixating a diamond target. A square is located 60° to the right of the diamond at the same elevation, on a horizontal arc (wrapped around the eye) at: eye level (A) and 30° up (B). When the eye looks at the eye-level diamond (A), the retinal image of the square lies on the horizontal meridian. But when the eye looks up at the diamond on the top arc (B), the image of the square no longer falls on the horizontal meridian.

the head moves pretty much like an eye (Ceylan et al., 2000) and at least for far targets, the geometry described in the previous section holds pretty much the same: one needs to take head orientation into account in a non-linear fashion.

But head movement has other, special implications for eye–hand coordination. This is because the centers of rotation of the eye, head and shoulder do not coincide. As a result, each time the head rotates, it causes the eyes to translate through space relative to the shoulder, which changes the angular direction of targets relative to the eye (but not the shoulder). One could rely on visual feedback of the hand — during pointing or reaching — to make up for any differences this might make, but we were interested to see if the system took this into account without such feedback.

To do this, we had subjects point toward distant targets with the head in different horizontal positions (Henriques and Crawford, 2002). This caused significant changes in the line from the eye to the target (recall that this is the line that subjects use for aligning pointing when looking straight ahead). Nevertheless, subjects were able to re-calculate this line, and accurately place the fingertip at the right location for any head position. In a related experiment (Henriques et al., 2001) we found that subjects were similarly able to account for head orientation and the resulting translation of eye location when computing the visual angle of near targets for reaching movements. These results show not only that head orientation is taken into account, but also, moreover, that the eye–hand coordination system possesses a sophisticated *representation* of body geometry that takes into account the differences in the centers of rotation of the eyes, head, and shoulder in the absence of on-line visual feedback. Such a representation is likely constructed or at least fine-tuned by learning.

Arms and the man

Eye–hand coordination must end in a movement of the hand. But at what point in the brain is the transition from mechanisms specific to eye–hand coordination to those purely associated with arm control? A reasonable dividing line would be the point where gaze and head signals no longer influence neural firing rates, where these are purely modulated by the kinematics and dynamics of the arm movement. Most of the current evidence suggests that this has not yet occurred at the level of premotor cortex (Mushiake et al., 1997), but is completed by or within M1 (Mushiake et al., 1997; Crammond and Kalaska, 2000).

By corollary, one might not expect eye–hand coordination to have much to do with the details of arm kinematics that are not related to aiming the hand or conforming grasp to the target. A prime example would be the neural constraints to determine redundant degrees of freedom in the arm control system (Bernstein, 1967). Nevertheless, (without going into detail) there are considerable similarities between some of the three-dimensional kinematics constraints observed in the upper arm and in the eye (Straumann et al., 1991; Theeuwen et al., 1993). Based on this, it was once suggested that these constraints were developed in unison in order to facilitate coordination of the eye and arm in the workspace (Straumann et al., 1991).

In order to test this, we dissociated gaze from arm movements and measured the three-dimensional constraints in the latter (Medendorp et al., 2000). In a similar situation, we had previously found that dissociating gaze from head movement disrupted the normal 3-D control of the head, demonstrating the intimate coupling of these two systems (Ceylan et al., 2000). However, the same did not occur: although dissociating gaze from the arm again led to a disruption in movement accuracy, it had no effect on the three-dimensional constraints on arm orientation (Medendorp et al., 2000). Based on these findings, we conclude that such constraints are organized in neural structures downstream from those which employ gaze signals to compute arm movement direction.

Synthesis and conclusion

As stated in the introduction, the first aim of this work is to create a model of eye–hand coordination that can help us to understand visually directed arm movements, and help guide our neurophysiological investigations. The working model that we have been using for the past few years is illustrated in Fig. 6. Admittedly it is cartoonish in several respects: in its reliance on forward serial transformations (we all know the brain is really heavily parallel and recurrent in organization), in its representation of signals (no one should expect such discrete, explicit representations in the brain), and in its simplicity (even many aspects of the work described here have been left out). And yet in outline, it agrees with much of the known physiology.

This model might also account for some symptoms observed in the neuropsychology literature. For example, Carey et al. (2000) report a patient who reaches 'magnetically' toward the direction of fixation. Our model would predict this if the extra-foveal portions of the early gaze-centered representation for arm movement (i.e. perhaps the parietal reach region) were lost (a condition not unlikely given the tendency to over-represent extra-foveal space). If only activity in the foveal zone were possible, the downstream transformations would automatically convert this into a reaching movement toward the fixation object (and conversely would be unable to reach toward non-foveal objects).

A key feature of this model is its use of early representations of attended target locations in a retinal frame, representations that must be updated with each eye movement. Only the target that is selected for action is put through the subsequent transformations: comparisons with eye and head orientations, computation of inverse kinematics and dynamics of the arm and so on. From a biological perspective, this is a space and energy saving feature: there would be an enormous cost to try to perform these operations on every point in space, and very little advantage. This goes a long way toward explaining why the early stages of arm control seem to be organized in eye-centered coordinates (Henriques et al., 1998). But it also has a surprising implication. Whereas introspection may suggest that we have a complete map of visuomotor space, this model suggests that this is an illusion — only the overall transformation provides such a map, and only on those representations we choose to act on. The catch is that every time we test our intuition by choosing to act on a representation, it confirms our intuition of a complete map. In this sense, this is a 'virtual' map of

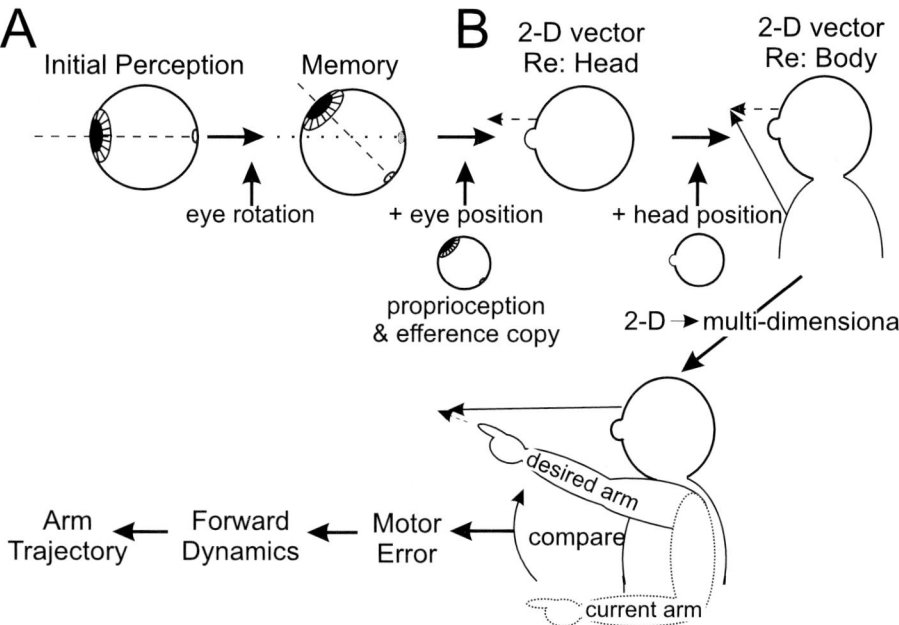

Fig. 6. Conversion-on-demand hypothesis of visuomotor representation and visuomotor control. Target representations are initially held in an eye-centered frame, and can be shifted in this frame to compensate for intervening eye movements through dynamic remapping (A). Once a target has been selected for action, its final retinal representation is put through a reference frame transformation (by comparing it with 3-D orientation of eyes and head) to generate an accurate 3-D motor signal in motor reference frame (B). Modified from Henriques et al., 1998.

space, similar to ideas that have been proposed for visual perception (Howard, 1982).

A less realistic aspect of the cartoon in Fig. 6 is the suggestion of explicit signals of desired target location relative to the head, etc. These are clearly not found in actual physiology, which tends to employ retinal codes (Gnadt and Andersen, 1988; Sparks, 1989; Duhamel et al., 1992). However, when one simulates the same transformations by training a neural net to transform a visual vector into a motor vector (Smith and Crawford, 2001a,b), one finds that the network learns to do so through fairly simple position modulations, resulting in an organization that captures the basic conceptual flow of Fig. 6, while using signals that resemble actual physiology. Thus, as originally suggested by Andersen and colleagues, reference frame transformations can be explicit (Zipser and Andersen, 1988), but in fact one can entirely get rid of the need for position maps for a more realistic model. Indeed, models that do not rely on explicit position codes turn out to be more flexible and powerful (Ceylan et al., 2000). Incorporating these ideas, and all of the findings described above in this article into a complete computational model following the outline provided in Fig. 6 will be a major goal of our future work.

Acknowledgements

This research is supported by CIHR group grant, Canadian NSERC and PREA. J.D.C is supported by the Canadian Research Chair program, D.Y.P.H is supported by an E.A Baker Foundation CIHR Research Doctorate Award, and W.P.M. is supported by the Human Frontiers Science Program.

References

Andersen, R.A. and Mountcastle, V.B. (1983) The influence of the angle of gaze upon the excitability of the light-sensitive neurons of the posterior parietal cortex. *J. Neurosci.*, 3: 532–548.

Batista, A.P., Buneo, C.A., Snyder, L.H. and Andersen, R.A. (1999) Reach plans in eye-centered coordinates. *Science*, 285: 257–260.

Bernstein, N. (1967) *The Coordination and Regulation of Movements*. Pergamon Press, Oxford.

Bock, O. (1986) Contribution of retinal versus extraretinal signals towards visual localization in goal-directed movements. *Exp. Brain Res.*, 64: 467–482.

Bremmer, F., Graf, W., Ben-Hamed, S. and Duhamel, J.R. (1999) Eye position encoding in the macaque ventral intraparietal area (VIP). *NeuroReport*, 10: 873–878.

Carey, D.P. (2000) Eye–hand coordination: eye to hand or hand to eye? *Curr. Biol.*, 10(11): R416–R419.

Carey, D.P., Della Sala, S. and Ietswart, M. (2002) Neuropsychological perspectives on eye–hand coordination in visually guided reaching. In: J. Hyönä, D.P. Munoz, W. Heide and R. Radach (Eds.), *The Brain's Eye: Neurobiological and Clinical Aspects of Oculomotor Research. Progress in Brain Research*, Vol. 140. Elsevier, Amsterdam, pp. 311–327.

Ceylan, M.Z., Henriques, D.Y.P., Tweed, D.B. and Crawford, J.D. (2000) Task-dependent constraints in motor control: pinhole goggles make the head move like an eye. *J. Neurosci.*, 20: 2719–2730.

Colby, C.L. and Goldberg, M.E. (1999) Space and attention in parietal cortex. *Annu. Rev. Neurosci.*, 22: 319–349.

Coren, S. and Kaplan, C.P. (1973) Patterns of ocular dominance. *Am. J. Optom. Arch. Am. Acad. Optom.*, 50: 283–292.

Crammond, D.J. and Kalaska, J.F. (2000) Prior information in motor and premotor cortex: activity during the delay period and effect on pre-movement activity. *J. Neurophysiol.*, 84: 986–1005.

Crawford, J.D. and Guitton, D. (1997) Visual-motor transformations required for accurate and kinematically correct saccades. *J. Neurophysiol.*, 78(3): 1447–1467.

Crawford, J.D., Henriques, D.Y.P. and Vilis, T. (2000) Curvature of visual space under vertical eye rotation: implications for spatial vision and visuomotor control. *J. Neurosci.*, 20: 2360–2368.

Crider, B.A. (1944) A battery of tests for the dominant eye. *J. Gen. Psychol.*, 31: 179–190.

Duhamel, J.-R., Colby, C.L. and Goldberg, M.E. (1992) The updating of the representation of visual space in parietal cortex by intended eye movements. *Science*, 255: 90–92.

Engel, K.C., Anderson, J.H. and Soechting, J.F. (2000) Similarity in the response of smooth pursuit and manual tracking to a change in the direction of target motion. *J. Neurophysiol.*, 84: 1149–1156.

Enright, J.P. (1995) The non-visual impact of eye orientation on eye–hand coordination. *Vision Res.*, 35: 1611–1618.

Fisk, J.D. and Goodale, M.A. (1985) The organization of eye and limb movements during unrestricted reaching to targets in contralateral and ipsilateral visual space. *Exp. Brain Res.*, 60: 159–178.

Flanders, M., Helms-Tillery, S.I. and Soechting, J.F. (1992) Early stages in a sensorimotor transformation. *Behav. Brain Sci.*, 15: 309–362.

Fu, Q.F., Suarez, J.I. and Ebner, T.J. (1993) Neuronal specification of direction and distance during reaching movements in the superior precentral premotor area and primary motor cortex of monkeys. *J. Neurophysiol.*, 70: 2097–2116.

Gielen, C.C., van den Heuvel, P.J. and van Gisbergen, J.A. (1984) Coordination of fast eye and arm movements in a tracking task. *Exp. Brain Res.*, 56: 154–161.

Gnadt, J.W. and Andersen, R.A. (1988) Memory related motor planning activity in posterior parietal cortex of macaque. *Exp. Brain Res.*, 70: 216–220.

Graziano, M.S., Yap, G.S. and Gross, C.G. (1994) Coding of visual space by premotor neurons. *Science*, 152: 1603–1608.

Hallett, P.E. and Lightstone, A.D. (1976) Saccadic eye movements to flashed targets. *Vision Res.*, 16: 107–114.

Henriques, D.Y.P. and Crawford, J.D. (2000) Direction dependent distortions of retinocentric space in the visuomotor transformation for pointing. *Exp. Brain Res.*, 132(2): 179–194.

Henriques, D.Y.P. and Crawford, J.D. (2002) Role of eye, head and shoulder geometry in the planning of accurate arm movements. *J. Neurophys.*, 87: 1677–1685.

Henriques, D.Y.P., Klier, E.M., Smith, M.A., Lowey, D. and Crawford, J.D. (1998) Gaze-centered re-mapping of remembered visual space in an open-loop pointing task. *J. Neurosci.*, 18: 1583–1594.

Henriques, D.Y.P., Crawford, J.D., Medendorp, W.P. and Gielen, C.C.A.M. (2001) The eye–hand coordination system accounts for head orientation and target depth during reaching toward near targets. *Abstr. Soc. Neurosci.*, 27(2).

Howard, I.P. (1982) *Human Visual Orientation*. Wiley, New York.

Jouffrais, C. and Boussaoud, D. (1999) Neuronal activity related to eye–hand coordination in the primate premotor cortex. *Exp. Brain Res.*, 128: 205–209.

Khan, A.Z. and Crawford, J.D. (2001a) Ocular dominance reverses as a function of gaze angle. *Vision Res.*, 41: 1743–1748.

Khan, A.Z. and Crawford, J.D. (2001b) Coordinating one hand with two eyes: gaze-dependent reversal of ocular dominance in a pointing task. *Abstr. Soc. Neurosci.*, 940.12.

Mays, L.E. and Sparks, D.L. (1980) Saccades are spatially, not retinotopically coded. *Science*, 208: 1163–1164.

Mazzoni, P., Bracewell, R.M., Barash, S. and Andersen, R.A. (1996) Spatially tuned auditory responses in area LIP of macaques performing delayed memory saccades to acoustic targets. *J. Neurophysiol.*, 75: 1233–1241.

Medendorp, W.P. and Crawford, J.D. (2002) Visuospatial updating of reaching target in near and far space. *NeuroReport*, 13: 633–636.

Medendorp, W.P., Crawford, J.D., Henriques, D.Y.P., Van Gisbergen, J.A.M. and Gielen, C.C.A.M. (2000) Kinematic strategies for upper arm — forearm coordination in three dimensions. *J. Neurophysiol.*, 84: 2302–2316.

Miles, W.R. (1930) Ocular dominance in human adults. *J. Gen. Psychol.*, 3: 412–420.

Mittelstaedt, H. (1983) A new solution to the problem of the subjective vertical. *Naturwissenschaften*, 70: 272–281.

Mushiake, H., Tanatsugu, Y. and Tanji, J. (1997) Neuronal activity in the ventral part of premotor cortex during target–reach movement is modulated by direction of gaze. *J. Neurophysiol.*, 78: 567–571.

Ono, H. and Barbeito, R. (1982) The cyclopean eye vs. the sighting-dominant eye as the center of visual direction. *Percept. Psychophys.*, 32(3): 201–210.

Porac, C. and Coren, S. (1976) The dominant eye. *Psychol. Bull.*, 83(5): 880–897.

Riehle, A. and Requin, J. (1995) Neuronal correlates of the specification of movement direction and force in four cortical areas of the monkey. *Brain Behav. Res.*, 70: 1–13.

Schlag, J., Schlag-Rey, M. and Pigarev, I. (1992) Supplementary eye field: influence of eye position on neural signals of fixation. *Exp. Brain Res.*, 90: 302–306.

Smith, M.A. and Crawford, J.D. (2001a) Network properties in a physiologically realistic model of the 2-D to 3-D visuomotor transformation for saccades. *Abstr. Soc. Neurosci.*, 27(1).

Smith, M.A. and Crawford, J.D. (2001b) Self-organizing task modules in explicit coordinate systems in a neural network model for 3-D saccades. *J. Comput. Neurosci.*, 10: 127–150.

Sparks, D.L. (1989) The neural encoding of the location of targets for saccadic eye movements. *J. Exp. Biol.*, 146: 195–207.

Straumann, D., Haslwanter, T., Hepp-Reymond, M.C. and Hepp, K. (1991) Listing's law for eye, head and arm movements and their synergistic control. *Exp. Brain Res.*, 86: 209–215.

Theeuwen, M., Miller, L.E. and Gielen, C.C.A.M. (1993) Is the orientation of head and arm coupled during pointing movements? *J. Motor Behav.*, 25: 242–250.

Vercher, J.-L., Magenes, G., Prablanc, C. and Gauthier, G.M. (1994) Eye–head–hand coordination in pointing at visual targets: spatial and temporal analysis. *Exp. Brain Res.*, 99: 507–523.

von Helmholtz, H. (1867) *Handbuch der Physiologischen Optik*, Bd. 3. Voss, Hamburg, Germany.

Wells, W.C. (1792) *An Essay Upon Single Vision with Two Eyes: Together with Experiments and Observations on Several Other Subjects in Optics*. Cadell, London.

Zipser, D. and Andersen, R.A. (1988) A back-propagation programmed network that simulates response properties of a subset of posterior parietal neurons. *Nature*, 331: 679–684.

CHAPTER 23

Implications of distracter effects for the organization of eye movements, hand movements, and perception

Uta Sailer *, Thomas Eggert and Andreas Straube

Klinikum Grosshadern, Department of Neurology, Center for Sensorimotor Research, Marchioninistr. 23, D-81377 Munich, Germany

Abstract: The end positions of eye and hand movements were both drawn towards a distracter that was presented nearby the target. They thus showed a so-called global effect. In contrast, perception was not influenced by the presence of a distracter. These results are discussed with regard to the question whether eye, hand, and perception are based on shared or separate target representations and readout triggers. We conclude that separate representations and readout triggers for eye and hand are the most likely case.

Introduction

The coordination of eye and hand movements is essential for manipulating objects in everyday life. This manipulation entails looking at the object, identifying and consciously perceiving the object, and reaching toward it. These different aspects may involve differences in visual processing for eye and hand.

We tested eye movements, hand movements, and perception by presenting targets together with an irrelevant nearby distracter, a paradigm known as the 'global effect' paradigm. By comparing the effect of the distracter on eye movements, hand movements, and perception we addressed the question of whether eye and hand movements have a common target representation in the brain.

Eye movements

The amplitude of visually triggered and guided saccades is influenced by the presence of a distracter in the proximity of the target. Under this condition, saccades are known to land at a position intermediate between the target and the distracter, i.e. at the 'center of gravity' of the configuration. Apparently, the individual targets are not completely resolved spatially by the saccadic system. This effect is referred to as spatial averaging or the global effect.

In the typical paradigm two stimuli are presented simultaneously. The task can be to fixate either one of them (Findlay, 1982) or to fixate the target, which may be defined by its form (Coeffé and O'Regan, 1987), color (Ottes et al., 1985), or both (Findlay and Gilchrist, 1997).

The global effect was found to be dependent on the latency of the saccade, because it is characteristic of visual saccades with short latencies (Findlay, 1982; Ottes et al., 1985). Saccades with longer latencies tend to land nearer the target. On the basis of these findings, it has been suggested that the global effect arises from the limited time available for processing information about target position prior to a saccade. Saccades with longer latencies do not show this averaging effect.

---

* Correspondence to: U. Sailer, Klinikum Grosshadern, Department of Neurology, Center for Sensorimotor Research, Marchioninistr. 23, D-81377 Munich, Germany. Tel.: +49-89-7095-4818; Fax: +49-89-7095-4801; E-mail: usailer@nefo.med.uni-muenchen.de

There are two explanations for the global effect and its disappearance with longer latencies. The first concerns the temporal course of visual information processing. Visual processing starts with a coarse spatial scale, which is refined with time (Coeffé and O'Regan, 1987; Watt, 1987). If saccades are triggered during such a coarse stage of visual processing, peripheral stimuli can only be resolved poorly. According to this view, saccadic accuracy improves with longer latencies, because detailed visual information about the configuration has become available over time.

The second explanation holds that the spatial resolution of the configuration is not the reason for the global effect, because it improves too fast to be a problem. In contrast, the process of target selection is thought to require more time. It is thus assumed that the global effect results from the saccade being initiated before the target has been discriminated from the distracter (Ottes et al., 1985; Coeffé and O'Regan, 1987; Aitsebaomo and Bedell, 2000). Contrary to an incomplete resolution process (the explanation above), this discrimination process would be subject to higher level input, such as information about the identity of target and distracter. This explanation assumes that saccadic accuracy is better with longer latencies, because target selection has been completed.

The results of two recent studies favor the second interpretation. The first study used flashed targets, thus restricting the degree of available visual target information. This study also observed the global effect for short-latency saccades, but not for long-latency saccades (Eggert et al., 2000). Because the target was present for only a short time (50 ms), visual target information could not be further accumulated during the additional latency period. Therefore, it seems likely that the latency dependence of the global effect is due to an unfinished target selection process.

Similarly, a second study investigated this possibility by varying target duration and the time available for target selection while employing a mask (Aitsebaomo and Bedell, 2000). It showed that the extent of saccadic averaging was reduced both by prior auditory cues that indicated which target represented the goal and by longer target duration. The authors concluded that saccadic averaging is mostly due to the ambiguity of which of two targets represents the goal of the saccade and to a lesser extent, to the brief processing time of target location prior to the saccade.

Hand movements

Recently, more and more evidence is indicating that there is a global effect for hand movements as well. A first hint in this direction was a study that presented a distracter before the target (Lee, 1999). While short-latency hand movements (below 200 ms) were mostly directed toward the distracter, higher-latency movements (above 300 ms) were mostly directed toward the target. Movements with an intermediate latency were often directed between the distracter and the target. This effect is similar to that typically observed for eye movements.

More direct evidence comes from a study from our group (Sailer et al., 2002), in which the global effect paradigm was applied to hand movements. Two different target configurations were employed. Using a distracter less eccentric than the target, one experiment showed that the amplitude was smaller in the presence of a distracter for both eye and hand movements (see Fig. 1). However, while eye movements landed in between the target and the dis-

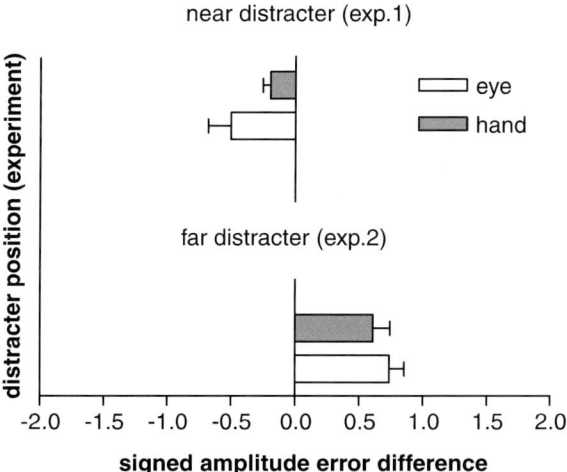

Fig. 1. Global effect of eye and hand, defined as the difference in signed amplitude error between trials with and without distracter, for two different distracter positions (blocked presentation). The mean of single- and dual-task conditions is shown.

tracter, hand movements essentially showed reduced overshoot and actually landed closer to the target. As the distracter effect on hand movements was not very large and manual latencies were also somewhat increased, a second experiment was conducted to establish whether there really was a global effect for hand movements or whether hand movements simply became more accurate. Both alternatives would result in the observed reduced overshoot. The second experiment involved the same task, but used a distracter that was more eccentric than the target. Increased accuracy would have resulted in reduced overshoot, whereas a distracter effect would have resulted in an increased overshoot. Indeed, hand movements showed a global effect, i.e. increased overshoot with a distracter. This effect was confirmed in two further experiments, one of which randomized the relative positions of distracter and target.

In all experiments, the global effect for hand movements was independent of whether hand movements were accompanied by eye movements (dual-task) or not (single-task). Thus, subjects did not simply point to where they were looking. This suggests that the global effect is not an effect specific to the eye that just transferred to the hand motor system. Instead, the hand seems to have its own global effect.

Perception

The distracter obviously affects both eye and hand movements. However, humans also consciously perceive the configuration. Current explanations of the global effect do not clarify if it is a purely motor phenomenon or if it is also encountered in perception. To this aim, Eggert et al. (2000) compared a saccade task with a perceptual localization task. The same briefly flashed stimuli were used in both tasks. A distracter was presented together with the target but closer to the center. In the perceptual task, a single reference stimulus was presented before this configuration appeared. The position of the reference stimulus was varied by $1°$ from trial to trial. The position of the target with regard to the reference stimulus was also varied in an adaptive procedure from trial to trial, starting from $5°$ until $1.5°$. Subjects had to indicate by responding with a joystick whether the target was more peripheral or more central than the reference stimulus. A global effect would have been shown by subjects perceiving the target at a more central location with the distracter than without. More specifically, if there is a global effect in perception, a larger number of 'central' judgments should occur in the presence of a distracter.

The results showed a classic global effect for primary saccades, but not for secondary saccades and perceptual localization. This finding demonstrated that correct information about the target is available at a later point in time and that this information is used both by secondary saccades and perceptual localization.

Comparison of the global effect for eye, hand and perception

So far we have discussed the global effect for eye movements, hand movements, and perception separately. However, what does it tell us about how the three are combined? We will first discuss the implications on spatial coupling of eye and hand before addressing the relationship of movement and perception.

As the global effect occurs during target selection, a similar global effect for both eye and hand would mean that they are coupled at the level of target selection. Thus, the level at which eye and hand are coupled or are not coupled can clearly be determined. To this aim, we directly compared the behavior of eye and hand movements in the presence of a distracter in one common analysis (Sailer et al., 2002). This procedure allowed us to determine if the global effect was similar for eye and hand.

In two experiments with blocked presentation of the near or far distracter (experiments 1 and 2), the global effect was similar in direction and magnitude for eye and hand movements. Both eye and hand movements were drawn toward the distracter (see Fig. 1). However, in an experiment with randomized presentation of the near and far distracter, only eye movements showed a global effect in the presence of the near distracter, whereas hand movements did not (see Fig. 2). Manual latencies did not differ for the near and the far distracter.

To discuss these results with respect to eye–hand coordination, we have to specify the kind of information to be shared. It is thus necessary to differentiate between the representation of the configuration, i.e. target and distracter, and the point in time when this

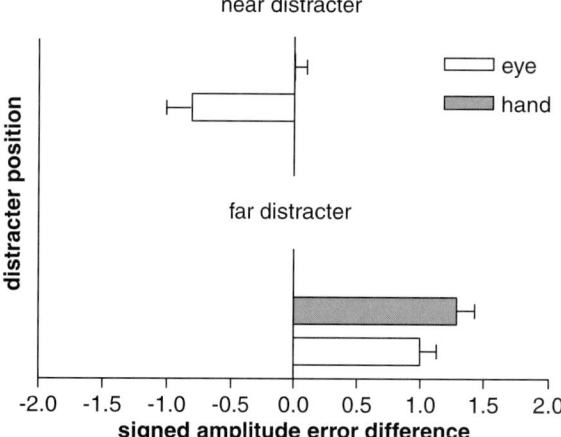

Fig. 2. Global effect of eye and hand for two different distracter positions (randomized presentation). The mean of single- and dual-task conditions is shown.

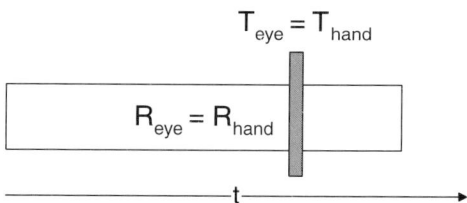

Fig. 3. Schematic illustration of case 1 with regard to possible combinations of common and separate configuration representations and readout triggers (see Table 1). Horizontal bars named 'R' show the representation of target and distracter during the stage of target selection, i.e., before the target has been separated from the distracter. Vertical bars named 'T' show the point in time when the target information within this representation is accessed, i.e., the readout trigger mechanisms.

information is read out (accessed). For reasons of simplicity, the mechanism determining the timing of this readout will be called the readout trigger. Such a discrete decision about the direction of a saccade occurring before the beginning of the movement was suggested by Becker and Jürgens (1979). For open loop hand movements, i.e. when target information cannot be continuously updated, target information also has to be read out at a particular point in time. In this context, it is important to note that the moment that target information is read out (readout trigger) differs from the moment that movement is initialized (latency).

Both the representation of target and distracter and the readout trigger could either be the same for eye and hand or not, as shown in Table 1.

According to this scheme, eye and hand can only be said to be based on a common target representation in case 1. 'Common target representation' designates the target information that is read out, i.e. the target information that determines the movement. Cases 2–4 would all result in separate target representations.

The results will first be discussed with regard to evidence against case 1 (see Fig. 3). There was a remarkable similarity of the global effect for eye and hand movements with blocked presentation of the near or far distracter, but not with randomized presentation. With randomized presentation, the global effect induced by the near distracter was different for eye and hand. This finding cannot be reconciled with case 1, i.e. one common configuration representation and one common readout trigger, because then the global effect should always be the same for eye and hand.

This conclusion may come as a surprise because the results of other authors indeed suggest a combination of eye and hand as in case 1. For example, in a double-step paradigm, the cluster of data points (Gielen et al., 1984) as well as the changes in trajectory (Van Sonderen et al., 1988) were similar for eye and hand. The authors interpreted their data as indicating a common target representation in the sense of case 1 for eye and hand. The difference between the interpretation of their results and our present results may be due to the different paradigms used. In a double-step paradigm, there is no competition between stimuli and thus, no selection is required. One may speculate that a difference in eye and hand responses only occurs under conditions of selection, depending perhaps on the degree of interference or

TABLE 1

Combination of relationships between eye and hand

Readout trigger	Configuration representation	
	One in common	Two separate ones
One in common	Case 1	Case 2
Two separate ones	Case 3	Case 4

2.) one common representation (R), two separate readout triggers (T)

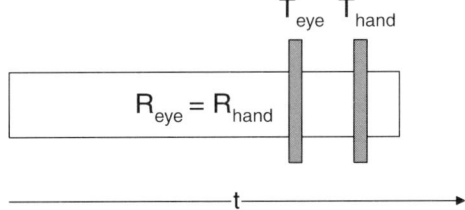

Fig. 4. Schematic illustration of case 2 (for explanation of labels see Fig. 3).

3.) two separate representations (R), one common readout trigger (T)

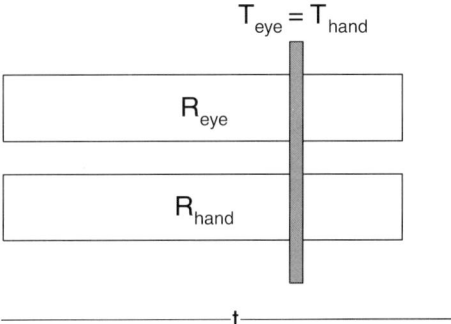

Fig. 5. Schematic illustration of case 3 (for explanation of labels see Fig. 3).

competition between the stimuli. In the present experiment, the competition between responses was possibly greater with randomized presentation of the near and far distracter.

Case 2 (Fig. 4) assumes that information of the same configuration representation is read out at two separate points in time for eye and hand. If this point occurs earlier for eye movements, then the global effect should always be larger for eye movements than for hand movements. If this point occurs earlier for hand movements, the global effect should always be larger for hand movements. In the present experiment, the global effect was mostly the same for hand and eye movements, and under one condition (randomized presentation of the near distracter, see Fig. 2), it was larger for eye movements. This would mean a high variability of the readout triggers, i.e. under some conditions target information would be read out at about the same time for eye and hand, and under different conditions target information would be read out earlier for the hand. However, such variability and, even more, an earlier readout of target information for hand movements do not seem plausible. A further argument against case 2 is that a smaller global effect for the hand with the randomized near distracter means that in this case the target information readout has taken place at a later point in time. A later readout trigger, in turn, would automatically increase the movement's latency. However, hand movement latency was not increased. Thus, the assumptions of case 2 seem improbable.

Case 3 (Fig. 5) assumes that the configuration is represented separately for eye and hand, but that the information is read out from this representation at the same time for eye and hand. This case also seems unlikely given that during randomized presentation of the near distracter hand movements showed a much smaller global effect than eye movements (see Fig. 2), although hand movement latencies were much higher. Common explanations of the global effect imply that it only occurs if the separation between target and distracter is incomplete. As this separation is believed to improve with time, the global effect should be reduced with increasing latencies. Therefore, if one common readout trigger is assumed, the smaller global effect of the hand compared to the eye can only be explained with the target distracter separation being completed earlier for the hand than for the eye. However, there is no obvious reason why this should happen with the near distracter in the randomized condition. Thus, the hypothesis of a common readout trigger seems implausible.

Under natural conditions, accurate hand movements require much more information about the target than eye movements. To grasp an object, information about its size, weight, texture, etc. has to be taken into account. This information, which is irrelevant for making an eye movement toward the same object, has to be incorporated in the target representation for the hand. Therefore, it seems reasonable to assume that the target or configuration representation for hand movements is separate and that it lasts longer and can be read out at a later point in time than that for eye movements (as case 4 suggests). In the light of the present results, this

4.) two separate representations (R), two separate readout triggers (T)

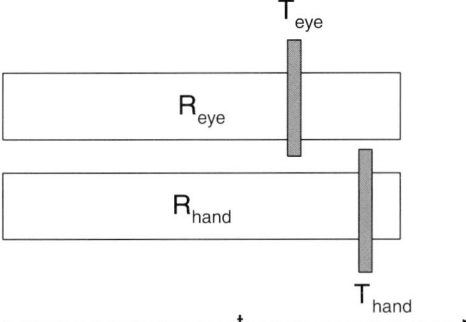

Fig. 6. Schematic illustration of case 4 (for explanation of labels see Fig. 3).

case seems the most convincing. It assumes that eye and hand movements are based on two separate representations of the configuration and on two separate readout triggers (see Fig. 6). This combination can easily explain why under some conditions the global effect is the same for eye and hand and why under other conditions it is different. The similarity of the global effect for both eye and hand could be due to the exchange of information between eye and hand, i.e. either between the two separate representations of the configuration or between the two separate readout triggers. If the two readout triggers were synchronized, then under some conditions case 4 would be difficult to distinguish from case 3.

A combination of eye and hand as in case 4 can provide maximal flexibility, which may be necessary to satisfy the different 'needs' of eye and hand reactions. For eye movements, quick arrival at the target may be most important, not the acquisition of a maximally detailed target representation. In contrast, for the hand, accuracy may be more crucial than speed. Although numerous studies indicate that the representation of the target is updated while the movement is going on, it is possible that the hand requires more information than the eye already at the point of initial readout of target information. It would be interesting to know if the global effect for the hand would change if the instruction were to emphasize on accuracy, not speed.

A further advantage of an organization as in case 4 is that it allows for two representations of different targets for eye and hand at the same time. This means the eye could already start to represent a new target while the hand is still acting on the basis of information about the old target. Such a strategy would be helpful when planning sequential movements in advance. For instance, when picking up an object, the eyes went on to a new area before the fingers touched the object (Pelz et al., 2001, see also Hayhoe et al., 2002, this volume). This indicates that the saccade to the new target is planned during the ongoing hand movement. In other words, while the hand is performing a movement on the basis of the representation of one target, the representation of the new eye target is already built. However, such a behavior may only occur under conditions of predictable target locations as is the case in real-life situations. Neggers and Bekkering, 2000 (also discussed in Carey et al., 2002, this volume) found in a laboratory experiment that no second eye movement could be initiated until the hand movement towards the first target was completed. Nevertheless, this effect is also compatible with a structure as suggested in case 4. Possibly the system makes less use of a flexible handling of target representations under the restricted conditions of a laboratory experiment. In summary, to our mind, case 4, i.e. two separate configuration representations and readout triggers, seems to be the most plausible combination of eye and hand spatial coupling.

The question arises as to the place of perception with regard to eye and hand? If case 4 for eye and hand is assumed, another separate configuration representation and selection mechanism could be used for perception. Such a combination would allow the eye to continue planning a saccade to a new target while perception was still working on the old representation. However, it is also possible that perception does not use a separate configuration representation, but simply results from a readout of later refined eye or hand representations.

Putting it all together: inhibition- and enhancement-based explanations of the global effect

Distracter effects on the trajectories of eye and hand movements have been explained by the programming and subsequent inhibition of a response toward the distracter (Howard and Tipper, 1997; Tipper et al., 1997). Such an explanation could also apply to the global effect. When programming a response toward the distracter, a group of neurons is activated. This activity is reduced by inhibition that is thought to mainly come from low-level mechanisms such as lateral inhibition. The resulting response is based on the combined activity of a group of neurons. Therefore the movement's trajectory — or end position — is changed by the selective inhibition of the subset of neurons activated by the distracter.

Others have favored a more top-down approach to explain such selection processes. Instead of the irrelevant stimulus being inhibited, they suggest that the relevant stimulus is boosted (e.g. Duncan, 1998; Chelazzi et al., 2001). They argue that stimuli in the visual field compete for representation, and that this competition is biased toward the behaviorally relevant stimulus.

Inhibition of the irrelevant distracter could occur within the superior colliculus (SC). Cells in the SC gave a larger response to a receptive field stimulus when it was the target than when it was the distracter (Goldberg and Wurtz, 1972). This effect seems to be specific for eye movements. It led Desimone and Duncan (1995) to conclude that competition takes place independently within the oculomotor system, but has yet to be coordinated with competition within visual processing areas. Competition for the hand motor system may also take place independently, the SC being a likely candidate, as it is also active during hand movements (Werner et al., 1997). Because the neurons coding eye and arm movements lie close to each other and because motor areas project to the SC, its role in hand movement control or in the coordination of eye and hand has been discussed (e.g. Stuphorn et al., 2000). Mediation of activity in the SC via higher areas could arise from the connections of the SC to the parietal cortex and the frontal eye field (Schall, 1995).

Regardless of the explanation preferred, our results suggest that the inhibition or enhancement effect acts differently on eye and hand. Our finding that the responses of eye and hand were quite similar under certain conditions suggests that the competition may be resolved separately for eye and hand, but that the separate competition or attentional processes for eye and hand are integrated. This is in accordance with the idea that competition is not resolved within specific parts of the sensorimotor network, but reflects distributed states of the network as a whole (Duncan, 1998).

In conclusion, the global effect paradigm is a promising approach for analyzing how eye movements are coupled both with hand movements and perception. We suggest that this coupling can best be achieved by separate configuration representations and separate readout triggers. However, future research combining the three activities in one experiment is necessary to confirm this interpretation.

Acknowledgements

This work was supported by the Deutsche Forschungsgemeinschaft, SFB 462 'Sensomotorik' and Klinische Forschergruppe BR 639. The authors thank Marc Hassenzahl and Iain Gilchrist for inspiring remarks and Judy Benson for copy-editing the manuscript.

References

Aitsebaomo, A.P. and Bedell, H.E. (2000) Saccadic and psychophysical discrimination of double targets. *Optom. Vis. Sci.*, 77: 321–330.

Becker, W. and Jürgens, R. (1979) An analysis of the saccadic system by means of double step stimuli. *Vision Res.*, 19: 967–983.

Carey, D.P., Della Sala, S. and Ietswart, M. (2002) Neuropsychological perspectives on eye–hand coordination in visually guided reaching. In: J. Hyönä, D.P. Munoz, W. Heide and R. Radach (Eds.), *The Brain's Eye: Neurobiological and Clinical Aspects of Oculomotor Research. Progress in Brain Research*, Vol. 140. Elsevier, Amsterdam, pp. 311–327.

Chelazzi, L., Miller, E.K., Duncan, J. and Desimone, R. (2001) Responses of neurons in macaque area V4 during memory-guided visual search. *Cereb. Cortex*, 8: 761–772.

Coëffé, C. and O'Regan, J.K. (1987) Reducing the influence of non-target stimuli on saccade accuracy: predictability and latency effects. *Vision Res.*, 27: 227–240.

Desimone, R. and Duncan, J. (1995) Neural mechanisms of selective visual attention. *Annu. Rev. Neurosci.*, 18: 193–222.

Duncan, J. (1998) Converging levels of analysis in the cognitive neuroscience of visual attention. *Philos. Trans. R. Soc. Lond. B. Biol. Sci.*, 353: 1307–1317.

Eggert, T., Ditterich, J. and Straube, A. (2000) Effects of distractors on primary saccade amplitude do not interfere with localization of flashed targets. *Soc. Neurosci. Abstr.*, 1990.

Findlay, J.M. (1982) Global visual processing for saccadic eye movements. *Vision Res.*, 22: 1033–1045.

Findlay, J.M. and Gilchrist, I.D. (1997) Spatial scale and saccade programming. *Perception*, 26: 1159–1167.

Gielen, C., van den Heuvel, P.J. and van Gisbergen, J.A. (1984) Coordination of fast eye and arm movements in a tracking task. *Exp. Brain Res.*, 56: 154–161.

Goldberg, M.E. and Wurtz, R.H. (1972) Activity of superior colliculus in behaving monkey, II. Effect of attention on neuronal responses. *J. Neurophysiol.*, 35: 560–574.

Hayhoe, M., Aivar, P., Shrivastavah, A. and Mruczek, R. (2002) Visual short-term memory and motor planning. In: J. Hyönä, D.P. Munoz, W. Heide and R. Radach (Eds.), *The Brain's Eye: Neurobiological and Clinical Aspects of Oculomotor Research. Progress in Brain Research*, Vol. 140. Elsevier, Amsterdam, pp. 349–363.

Howard, L.A. and Tipper, S.P. (1997) Hand deviations away from visual cues: indirect evidence for inhibition. *Exp. Brain Res.*, 113: 144–152.

Lee, D. (1999) Effects of exogenous and endogenous attention on visually guided hand movements. *Cogn. Brain Res.*, 8: 143–156.

Neggers, S.F. and Bekkering, H. (2000) Ocular gaze is anchored to the target of an ongoing pointing movement. *J. Neurophysiol.*, 83: 639–651.

Ottes, F.P., Van Gisbergen, J.A. and Eggermont, J.J. (1985) Latency dependence of colour-based target vs nontarget discrimination by the saccadic system. *Vision Res.*, 25: 849–862.

Pelz, J., Hayhoe, M. and Loeber, R. (2001) The coordination of eye, head, and hand movements in a natural task. *Exp. Brain Res.*, 139: 266–277.

Sailer, U., Eggert, T., Ditterich, J. and Straube, A. (2002) Global effect of a nearby distracter on targeting eye and hand movements. *J. Exp. Psychol. Hum. Percept. Perform.*, in press.

Schall, J.D. (1995) Neural basis of saccade target selection. *Rev. Neurosci.*, 6: 63–85.

Stuphorn, V., Bauswein, E. and Hoffmann, K.P. (2000) Neurons in the primate superior colliculus coding for arm movements in gaze-related coordinates. *J. Neurophysiol.*, 83: 1283–1299.

Tipper, S.P., Howard, L.A. and Jackson, S.R. (1997) Selective reaching to grasp: evidence for distractor interference effects. *Vis. Cognit.*, 4: 1–38.

Van Sonderen, J.F., Denier van der Gon, J.J. and Gielen, C.C. (1988) Conditions determining early modification of motor programmes in response to changes in target location. *Exp. Brain Res.*, 71: 320–328.

Watt, R.J. (1987) Scanning from coarse to fine spatial scales in the human visual system after the onset of a stimulus. *J. Opt. Soc. Am. A.*, 4: 2006–2021.

Werner, W., Hoffmann, K.P. and Dannenberg, S. (1997) Anatomical distribution of arm-movement-related neurons in the primate superior colliculus and underlying reticular formation in comparison with visual and saccadic cells. *Exp. Brain Res.*, 115: 206–216.

CHAPTER 24

Visual short-term memory and motor planning

Mary Hayhoe [1,*], Pilar Aivar [2], Anurag Shrivastavah [1] and Ryan Mruczek [3]

[1] *Center for Visual Science, University of Rochester, Rochester, NY 14627, USA*
[2] *Department of Neuroscience, Erasmus University, P.O. Box 1738, 3000 DR Rotterdam, The Netherlands*
[3] *Department of Neuroscience, Brown University, Providence, RI 02912, USA*

Abstract: Despite extensive experimental work showing that memory for visual information in prior fixations is limited, the nature and content of the information maintained across fixations, when vision functions in its natural context, is not well determined. To gain insight into what memory representations might be needed to support vision in the natural world, we examined eye and hand movements while subjects made a sandwich and while they copied a toy model in a virtual environment. Patterns of eye–hand coordination and fixation sequences suggest the need for planning and coordinating movements over a period of a few seconds. Since the movement plan is initiated when the eye is in a different position from that when the movement itself is made, the planning must be in a coordinate frame that is independent of eye position. Movement planning thus requires a representation of the spatial structure in a scene that is built up over different fixations.

Introduction

To understand the consequences of saccadic eye movements on vision, we must address the relationship between visual perception and short-term visual memory. Vision operates seamlessly across sequences of fixations and this requires the coordination of information in both space and time. Traditionally, this question has been addressed in terms of the perceived stability of the visual world and the extent to which information is integrated across saccades (Rayner and Pollatsek, 1983; Irwin, 1991). Experiments have focused on whether there is an integrated representation of a visual scene, and on what the contents of that representation might be. The conclusion from a large body of previous work is that the representation of information acquired in prior fixations is very limited. Evidence for limited memory from prior fixations is provided by the finding that observers are extremely insensitive to changes in the visual image during an eye movement (Irwin et al., 1990; Irwin, 1991; Henderson, 1992; O'Regan, 1992; Pollatsek and Rayner, 1992; Henderson and Hollingworth, 1999). An eye movement is not necessary to demonstrate this minimal memory. Any transient such as a blank field, a film cut, or a blink will do as well (Hochberg, 1986; Simons, 1996; Levin and Simons, 1997; Rensink et al., 1997; O'Regan et al., 1999). This insensitivity to changes has been described as 'change blindness', and many of these studies have been reviewed by Simons and Levin (1997) and Simons (2000). Since detection of a change requires a comparison of the information obtained at different points in time from different fixations, change blindness has been interpreted as evidence that only a small part of the information in the scene is retained across fixations. Irwin suggests that it is limited by the capacity of working memory, that is, to a small number of individual items, typically about four or five, whose iden-

* Correspondence to: M. Hayhoe, Center for Visual Science, University of Rochester, Rochester, NY 14627, USA. Tel.: +1-716-275-8673; Fax: +1-716-271-3043; E-mail: mary@cvs.rochester.edu

tity is remembered better than their location (Irwin, 1996).

When vision functions in its natural context, the nature and content of the information maintained across fixations is not well determined, despite extensive investigation in standard experimental paradigms. O'Regan, Irwin, and their coworkers (O'Regan and Levy-Schoen, 1983; Irwin et al., 1990; Irwin, 1991, 1992; O'Regan, 1992) postulated the existence of some kind of sparse, post-categorical scene representation that does not include detailed spatial information, consistent with the strict capacity limits set by working memory. However, recent evidence suggests that information about precise spatial relationships between scene objects may also be preserved. For example, subjects encode spatial relationships of 'bystander' objects that are not the target of a saccade (De Graef et al., 2001; Verfaille et al., 2001), and Melcher and Kowler (2001) have shown that memory for both the identity and location of about eight objects in multiple scenes following inspection periods of a few seconds. This memory was of longer duration and greater capacity than typical short-term memory estimates. Chun and Jiang (1998) demonstrated memory for the spatial structure of images by showing that visual search is facilitated (by 60–80 ms) by prior exposure to complex visual contexts associated with the target. They called this 'contextual cueing'. Coding of spatial relationships between groups of objects, larger than the limit of four or five items, in short-term visual memory has also been demonstrated by Jiang et al. (2000). This memory appears to be implicit (that is, revealed in performance measures rather than conscious report), so it would not be revealed by many of the change blindness experiments, which usually require verbal report of the change. Chun and Jiang (1998, 1999) suggest that subjects are sensitive to the structure in a scene, which remains invariant across multiple gaze points. Chun and Nakayama (2000) have suggested that implicit memory for aspects of the spatial structure and features of scenes is important for guiding attention and eye movements to key locations that provide access to, or index into, more detailed information in the scene. They proposed that both contextual cueing and 'priming of pop-out' might be two such mechanisms. Priming of popout is the reduction of both search time and saccade latencies to locations or features that have been recently presented (Maljkovic and Nakayama, 1994; McPeek et al., 2000). Such mechanisms do not require conscious intervention, and exhibit greater memory capacity, longer durability, and greater discriminability than explicit short-term visual memory.

Few studies have examined change blindness in the real world (Simons and Levin, 1998). A satisfactory answer to the question of what information is retained across fixations requires an investigation of natural behavior. There are several reasons that this is necessary. First, the image content of natural scenes places very different demands on the observer than those typically used in experiments. Typical displays are either simple arrays of letters or geometric figures, or pictorial representations of scenes, and cover only a small portion of the visual field. An important difference between these displays and the normal world is that of spatial scale and spatial extent. Observers must deal with the entire visual field of 180°, as well as the space that is currently out of view, whereas typical displays rarely exceed about 30°. The spatial scale of most displays is not matched to the real world. The visual angle subtended by an image of a room in a typical experimental display, for example, is very different from a real room, and it is not clear how such infidelities in spatial scale might affect observers' representations of the spatial structure of the scene. In addition, real world scenes are three-dimensional, whereas most experimental displays are two-dimensional. This introduces an additional level of spatial complexity in normal vision. Another critical difference is the observer's behavioral goals. We are essentially ignorant of the informational requirements of normal vision. While most experiments embody reasonable assumptions about informational needs, they almost certainly do not match up in detail, because most experiments emphasize one particular computation at the expense of all others. In standard paradigms, a single visual or motor operation is examined over repeated trials, and observers almost certainly fine-tune their behavior to the experimental demands. For example, observers are very sensitive to the probabilistic structure of the trials, and match the distribution of attention to expected events (Mack and Rock, 1996; Gibson and Jiang, 1998). In natural behavior, the observer performs a sequence of different computations, and the initiation and timing of visuomotor operations is controlled by the observer, not by the experimenter. This active initiation of behaviors is likely to be important. For example, viewing a picture of a scene is very different from acting within that scene, simply because the observer needs different information. Some evidence for the importance of the observer's actions is given by Wallis and Bulthoff (2000), who showed that drivers and passengers in a virtual environment have different sensitivity to changes in the scene. Other evidence also suggests the importance of the immediate task in determining what is noticed (Folk et al., 1992; Hayhoe et al., 1998).

Chun and Nakayama (2000) pointed out the potential importance of implicit memory structures for guiding attention and eye movements around a scene. They argue that such guidance requires continuity of visual representations across different fixation positions. Such memory is also likely to be important for guiding hand, head, and body movements as well. Motoric interaction with the environment is an important requirement in any situation, and to understand how this requirement is subserved by vision, it is necessary to look at natural performance. Active participation by the observer, and appropriate spatial dimensions are likely to be critical in understanding such performance.

Natural performance

It is now possible to investigate natural behavior, because of the recent availability of eye trackers that can be mounted on the head, and do not require fixing the head on a bite bar, allowing observers to move relatively freely. On first examination, investigation of vision in the natural world has revealed that much of what the visual system has to do can be handled by the acquisition of information within a fixation. That is, memory across fixations may not be necessary for many of the computations that vision has to perform. In natural tasks, the pattern and duration of the fixations are highly specialized for each situation. In driving, Land has shown that drivers reliably fixate the tangent point of the curve to control steering around the curve (Land and Lee, 1994). The angle of gaze with respect to the observer specifies the steering command. In cricket, players exhibit very precise fixation patterns, fixating the bounce point of the ball just ahead of its impact (Land and McCleod, 2000). The angle and speed of the ball after the bounce allows the batsman to guide the bat. A similar pattern is seen in table tennis (Land and Furneaux, 1997). Experiments on the pattern of fixations made while observers copy block patterns showed that subjects make very frequent fixations on the model patterns in preference to using memory, often making two fixations on a single block in the course of copying that block, one to acquire color, and the other for location in the pattern (Ballard et al., 1995). The specialized nature of fixations is also revealed by the finding of Epelboim et al. (1995) that fixations when tapping a sequence of locations on a table are of a different duration than when simply looking at them. In tea making (Land et al., 1999), observers' fixations are tightly linked, step-by-step, with task performance. Land et al. (1999) described these as "object related actions". Thus the sequence: pick up an object, move it to a new location, put the object down, would constitute an object-oriented action, where fixation would be required for picking up, then for targeting the location for placement and guiding the placement. To pick up an object, observers fixate the point on the object where the hand makes contact. Similar step-by-step control of hand actions by fixation at a specific locus in the scene has been demonstrated under more controlled circumstances by Johansson et al. (2001). Thus observers actively select the specific information required for the momentary cognitive goal. Such moment-by-moment extraction suggests a large degree of independence of the visual computations within individual fixations, to the extent that the particular information extracted does not depend on information from prior fixations. This conclusion is consistent with the prior work indicating limited memory across fixation positions. For at least some proportion of the task, observers appear to access the information explicitly at the point of fixation, at the time when it is needed, as opposed to relying on information from prior fixations. This behavior is consistent with O'Regan's suggestion that the scene serves as a kind of external memory that can be quickly accessed when needed (O'Regan, 1992; Ballard et al., 1995). However, some aspects of natural behavior cannot be accounted for this way. Land and Furneaux (1997) noted the need for some kind of visual buffer both in driving, where the current information controls the steering action about 800 ms later, and in piano playing, where the fixations lead the note played by about a second. In the tea-making task, Land et al. (1999) also noted a number of instances where objects were found more easily when they had been fixated a few seconds previously. In the experiments described below, we find further evidence that memory across fixations is needed as a basis for motor planning and coordination.

Sandwich making

In our laboratory, we have observed the eye and hand movements of 11 subjects while they made sandwiches. One goal was to gain insight into the extent to which visual operations within a fixation are independent, and the extent to which information acquired in previous fixations is required for the current operation. We observed several aspects of performance that point to the need for some representation of the spatial structure of the scene that is built up over different fixations. Patterns of eye–hand coordination and fixation sequences suggest the need for planning and coordinating movements over a period of a few seconds. Since the movement plan is initiated when the eye is in a different position from that when the movement itself is made, the planning must be in a coordinate frame that is independent of eye position. (Since the head and body are free to move, it is most plausible that this coordinate frame is allocentric, or external to the body, rather than head centered.) Movement planning thus requires a representation of the spatial structure in a scene that is built up over different fixations.

Subjects wore an eyetracker mounted on the head, and were seated at a table with the items required for making a sandwich, as shown in Fig. 1. This scene had the items necessary for making the sandwich and pouring the soda, together with several background items. A second, more cluttered, scene, containing 10–15 irrelevant items interspersed with the task-relevant ones, was used for four subjects. The scene was covered with a black cloth prior to the begin-

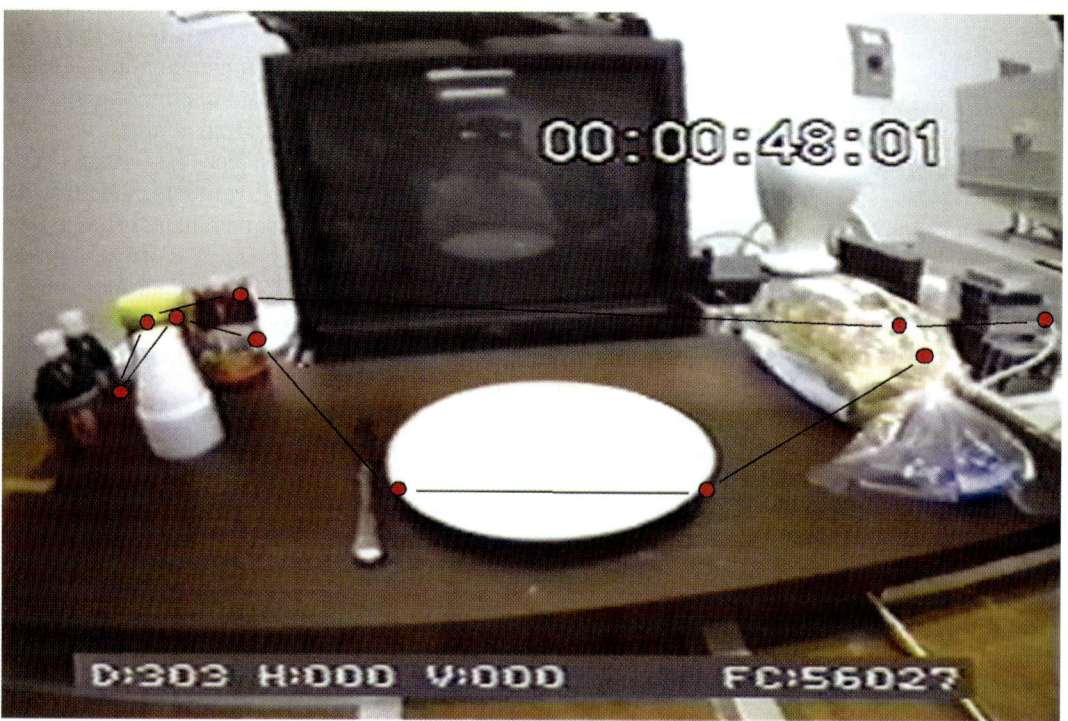

Fig. 1. A frame from the scene camera mounted on the subject's head, showing the layout of the area where the sandwich was made. The dots show the loci of fixations made in the first few seconds after the scene was revealed.

ning of the task. Monocular (left) eye position was monitored with either an Applied Science Laboratories 501 or an ISCAN eyetracker. Both are headband mounted, video-based, IR reflection eyetrackers that track pupil center and corneal reflection. They have an accuracy of about 1° and temporal resolution of 60 Hz. Both systems have a camera aimed at the scene, on or close to the line of sight, providing a 30-Hz video record of the scene from the subject's viewpoint, with a cursor indicating eye position superimposed on the image of the scene. Because the scene-camera moves with the head, the eye-in-head signal indicates the gaze point with respect to the world. Subjects were thus free to make natural movements. No instructions were given except to make a peanut butter and jelly sandwich and to pour a glass of soda. Following calibration, and the instructions, the cloth was removed and the subject began the task.

Initial fixations

In most ordinary environments observers have prolonged exposure to the scene, and multiple opportunities to accumulate information. In 10 min on a park bench, for example, an observer will make on the order of 1000 fixations. This is very different from experimental paradigms, which often compare only two brief exposures. Thus, in ordinary circumstances, observers may be able to build up quite extensive perceptual representations of scenes, despite the capacity limits of visual short-term memory. We were therefore interested to observe what subjects look at when they first view a novel scene. Do they, in fact, make a series of exploratory eye movements as we might expect if they are building a representation of scene layout for later use? We therefore examined the fixations made by subjects after the scene was initially exposed following removal of the calibration display, and before the first reaching movement, which indicated that they had begun the task. We found that on the initial exposure, subjects scan the scene and make a series of fixations on the objects, before the first reaching movement is initiated. For 11 subjects, the mean number of fixations was about 9. An example of one subject's fixations on first view is given in Fig. 1. This subject makes a series of short fixations on the bread, the plate, the jelly, the peanut butter, the coke, and then back to the bread and to a stack of tapes at the edge of the scene. She then returns to fixate the bread bag and reach for the bread. When the scene was made more cluttered by adding a number of irrelevant objects, such as tools and other food items, these initial fixations were distributed fairly equally between relevant and irrelevant objects. During task performance, however, the proportion of fixations on irrelevant objects was sharply reduced. This suggests that subjects are doing something different in the initial fixations.

Since subjects invariably make these 'scanning' fixations, it seems plausible that they perform some useful function, presumably in providing information about the identity and location of objects in the scene. Since there are only on the order of 10 fixations, this finding is consistent with O'Regan and Irwin's suggestion for the existence of a sparse representation of the objects and their locations in a scene, accumulated over different eye positions (O'Regan and Levy-Schoen, 1983; Irwin et al., 1990; Irwin, 1991; O'Regan, 1992). It is also consistent with Pylyshyn's suggestion that observers 'mark' a small number of locations in a scene (Pylyshyn, 1989). It does not tell us much about the level of spatial precision, however, or the extent of the information accrued from each individual fixation, but it does provide prima facie evidence that observers need to establish some kind of integrated scene representation.

Fixation durations

A feature of fixation behavior that has significance for spatial representations is the frequency of very short fixations. The frequency distributions for one of the subjects is shown in Fig. 2, calculated from a frame-by-frame analysis of the 30-Hz video records. (Since a transient track loss might appear like the termination of a fixation, we verified the fixation duration measurements by inspection of an image of the eye superimposed on the record from the scene camera. Movement of the eye during the track loss can be observed directly in the eye image.) The frequency distribution in Fig. 2 shows a number of very short fixations of two to four video frames (66–133 ms). These short fixations do not appear to play a single specialized role. We examined all the fixations

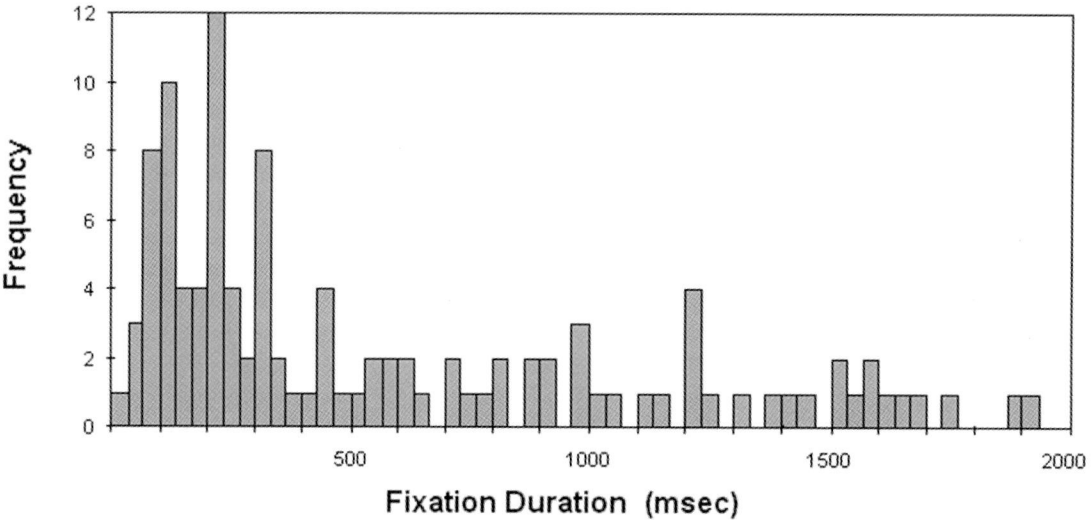

Fig. 2. Frequency distribution of fixation durations for one subject while making the sandwich.

of 100 ms or less and attempted to categorize them according to the context. Very short fixations have previously been observed between the primary and corrective saccade to a target (Becker and Fuchs, 1969). In our experiment, only about 10% of the short fixations could be classified as preceding a corrective saccade. We classified corrective saccades as those where the eye landed on an object (for example the bottle), and then moved to an adjacent location on the object (the neck), followed by an action involving the object (pouring). The occurrence of the action allows us to identify the second fixation locus as the intended target. Of the other short fixations, about one quarter were at the target point of a reaching movement, either for picking up or placement. Some were on an object located more or less on the path of the saccade, between the presaccadic position and the location of the target item that was manipulated next. Notably these objects were ones needed at some other point in the task. For example, a brief fixation might occur on the knife, positioned between plate and bread, as the subject moved from plate to bread to open the bread bag. However, nearly half the fixations could not be obviously classified. Thus short fixations occur on a variety of occasions and are not limited to the interval before a corrective saccade.

Pelz et al. (2000) also noted frequent fixations under 100 ms in several tasks (evaluation of image quality, map reading, model building, and hand washing). In the image evaluation task, 18% of the fixations were less than 166 ms in duration. Such short fixations are of particular interest because the time to program a saccade is reliably found to be in the 200–250-ms range. Consequently, in a fixation of 100 ms or less there, is not enough time to program the saccade based on visual information acquired during that fixation. Therefore the saccade programming must have been initiated prior to the fixation, when the eye is in a different position (Becker and Jurgens, 1979). Consequently the planning cannot be done in a retinal coordinate frame, and the partially programmed second saccade must take account of the first movement. Thus preprogrammed sequences of saccades point to the existence of a representation in spatial coordinates, independent of eye position. Zingale and Kowler (1987) suggested that saccades can be preprogrammed by showing that the latency for the initial saccade increased with the number of saccades in the sequence. Very brief fixations have also been observed in circumstances where two targets are in competition, such as a double-step task (Becker and Jurgens, 1979). Theeuwes and colleagues (Theeuwes et al., 1998, 1999; Irwin et al., 2000) observed short fixations to a distractor stimulus that was suddenly presented when subjects were preparing to target an oddball stimulus. They interpreted these brief fixations as the consequence of a concurrently programmed second saccade to the target, which terminated the fixation on the distractor. McPeek et al. (2000) also demonstrated concurrent programming of saccades in a search task for an oddball stimulus. Saccades to the wrong stimulus were often followed by a second saccade to the correct stimulus with a very brief intersaccadic interval. The initial saccade was usually hypometric, reflecting an influence of the programming of the second saccade on the execution of the first saccade. McPeek and Keller (2001) repeated this finding in monkeys, and subsequently observed that neurons in the superior colliculus show activity related to preparation of the second saccade even while the first saccade is still in progress (McPeek and Keller, 2002). Thus neural activity for more than one saccade can be maintained concurrently, even at levels close to the motor output, and the neural activity for the second saccade must be able to take into account the eye displacement by the first saccade.[1]

The frequency of very short fixations we observed in the sandwich task described here, indicate that preprogramming, or concurrent programming of more than one saccade, is a common occurrence in ordinary movements, and not restricted to particular experimental situations, such as those when two potential targets are presented simultaneously. The significance of preplanning is that programming of the second (and subsequent) saccade in a sequence must initially occur in a reference frame that is independent of the eye, and the second saccade is using information acquired prior to the immediately preceding fixation. This implies the existence of some form of spatial memory representation in natural vision, which is precise enough to support saccadic targeting.

Under special conditions, the latency of saccades evoked by a flashed stimulus can be in the 70–130-ms range, comparable to the fixation durations observed here. These are called express saccades (Fischer and Ramsperger, 1984). These are seen when the fixation point is turned off before the stimulus appears. Usually the stimulus is in one of two positions left or right of fixation. These saccades are commonly thought to be a special kind of saccade that by-passes high level cortical control mechanisms (Fischer and Breitmeyer, 1987). However, if planning is a ubiquitous feature of saccade programming, then it seems likely that the short latencies observed in the express saccade paradigm are simply a result of motor planning, as suggested by Kowler (1991), since motor preparation can occur even in the presence of uncertainty about target location.

Eye–hand coordination in reaching

Reaching movements provide other clues that a representation of the locations of objects is preserved across fixations. Little is known about the targeting of reaches in natural behavior. A straightforward way in which reaches might be targeted is for the subject to visually search the peripheral retina for the desired object, and then to program both the reach and the accompanying saccade on the basis of this information. However, in a typical experiment the target is usually presented at the onset of the trial, and there is little opportunity to locate the target ahead of time, unlike the natural world, where objects are continuously available. When the target is continuously present, observers have the opportunity to plan subsequent arm movements. Such planning is an essential component of motor behavior, and allows speedier movements as well as coordination with other movements, such as the other hand or the body.

We measured the relative timing of eye and hand movements for all the reaches (for picking up or placement, with either hand) that subjects made. (For a small number of the reaches the hand was not visible in the video record at the beginning of the movement and these were omitted.) Most (84%) of the reaching movements were accompanied by a fixation on the target. However, there was substantial

---

[1] The existence of pre-planned sequences of saccades does not distinguish between the various kinds of non-retinotopic frame (head-centered, body-centered, or allocentric). Since the head and trunk are free to move, however, an allocentric frame seems most plausible. We do not attempt to distinguish between a strictly allocentric or exocentric reference frame and one where allocentric behavior is achieved by updating a retinotopic signal following an eye movement (Colby, 1998). Since recent evidence suggests that the cells in the superior colliculus code gaze location in space, not retinal error (Freedman et al., 1996) it seems most straightforward at this point to describe the memory representation as spatial, or allocentric, as opposed to retinal.

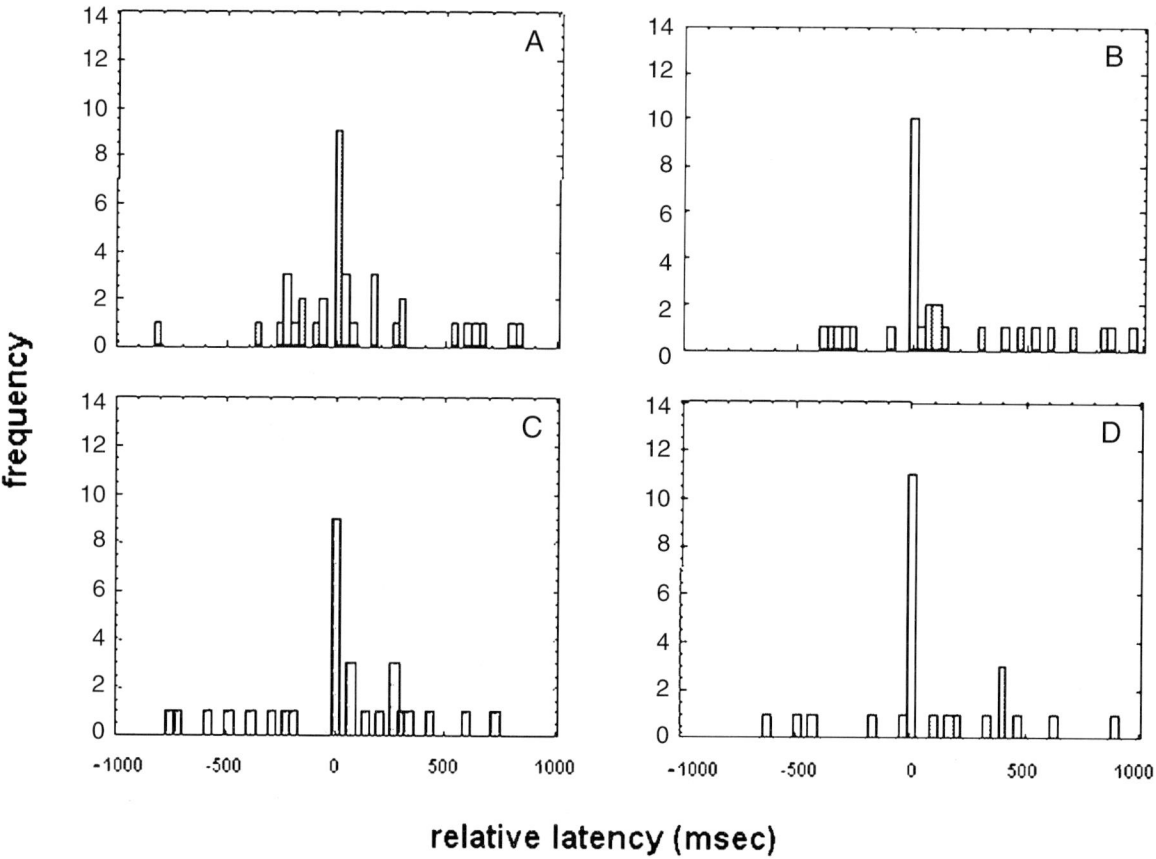

Fig. 3. Relative latencies of the eye and hand movements toward targets to be picked up or locations for object placement on the table. Latency is measured from the initiation of the eye movement to the initiation of the hand movement. Negative values indicate that the hand movement preceded the eye movement.

flexibility in the stage of the reach when the fixation occurred.[2] The frequency distributions of eye–hand relative latencies for four subjects are shown in Fig. 3. Although the predominant strategy is for eye and hand to depart close together in time, there are a significant number of reaches that are initiated as much as a second before the eye movement is made to the target, to guide the end stage of the reach. Similarly, the eye frequently fixates the object for as much as a second before the initiation of the reach. These large lags and leads appear to result from the interweaving of visual control of the two hands, with some reaching movements starting while the eye is supervising the other hand's action. An example of this can be seen in Fig. 4, where the movement of the left hand towards the lid begins at the same time that the eye and right hand move to put down the knife, about 800 ms after the start of the record. The eye does not move to fixate the lid to guide the left hand for another 600 ms (at the 1400-ms mark), after the right hand movement is complete. These long relative latencies suggest that the next eye or hand movement may be planned as much as

---

[2] When the hand movement was not accompanied by a fixation, it was almost always for placing an object on the table. Even when the reach was accompanied by a fixation, gaze was often not on the target for a substantial fraction of the reach. Either the reach was initiated well ahead of the fixation, as shown in Fig. 3, or else gaze departed before contact was made. Presumably, these reaches could be completed without further visual input, or with peripheral guidance.

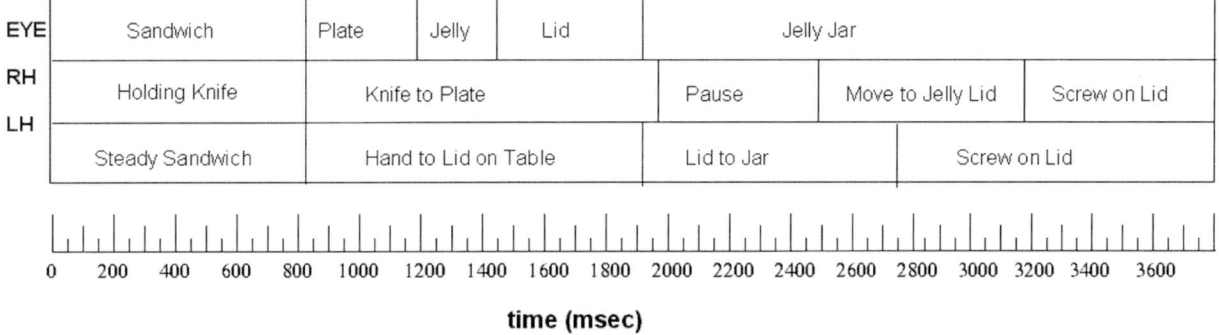

Fig. 4. Example of the interleaving of visual control of the two hands. The top row shows the sequence of fixation loci. The middle row shows the right hand action, and the bottom row the left hand action. While the left hand moves to the lid on the table, gaze first controls the right hand, then moves to the jelly jar, then to the lid just at the point when the left hand makes contact.

a second ahead of time. For example, if fixation of an object is required for final guidance of the reach, it is likely that the fixation is planned to some extent when the reach is initiated, so as to be there at the critical moment. Since several fixations may intervene between the eye and hand movement to the object, this planning must occur in a representation that is independent of eye position. An example can be seen in Fig. 4. While the left hand moves to the jelly lid, the eye guides the knife placement on the plate with the right hand, departing before putdown is complete. The eye then fixates the jelly for 200 ms, then saccades to the jelly lid, arriving just at the point when fixation is required for lid pickup. There must be some way of controlling the timing of the three fixations in order to coordinate so precisely with the two hand movements. This makes it likely that the fixation sequence (plate-jar-lid) is planned as a unit. As discussed in the preceding section, this suggests the existence of a representation independent of eye position as a basis for planning the saccade sequence. There is also the question of what is used for programming and controlling the reaches. The left hand movement in Fig. 4 might have been controlled using the peripheral retina. However, it is also plausible that the hand movement programming and control used the same spatial representation as that used for the eye movement sequence. If this were true, it would be inconsistent with neurophysiological evidence from cells in the intraparietal sulcus that suggests that reaching movements are programmed in an eye-centered coordinate frame (Batista et al., 1999).

Land et al. (1999) also measured eye–hand latencies in their tea-making task. Although they observed some long lead times for the hand, their distribution was strongly biased toward positive values, where the eye leads the hand. On average the eye lead time was about 600 ms. A possibly crucial difference between the tasks is that our subjects were seated, whereas Land et al.'s subjects moved around the room, so that reaching movements were often a component of a whole-body movement that brought the target of interest into the visual field. This raises the possibility that planning reaches requires the target to be in the visual field.

Another feature of the reaching movements is of interest. We examined all the reaches in 11 subjects. For each reach, we looked to see when (or if) that object or location had been fixated on a previous occasion. We found that nearly a third of the reaches were preceded by a fixation on that object in the recent past (less than 8 s). (This fixation is prior to the fixation on the object that guides the actual reach.) An example of this is given in Fig. 5. About 600 ms after the beginning of the record, the subject briefly fixates the peanut butter. About 1700 ms later (at the 2300-ms mark), the peanut butter is fixated again, to guide pickup with the left hand at about 3300 ms. These fixations on objects that were to be picked up shortly afterwards may indicate that the subject is planning a reach, and is looking to the object to acquire its spatial location for guiding the next movement. Similar 'look-ahead' fixations were observed by Pelz and Canosa (2001) in a hand-washing context. As subjects approached the

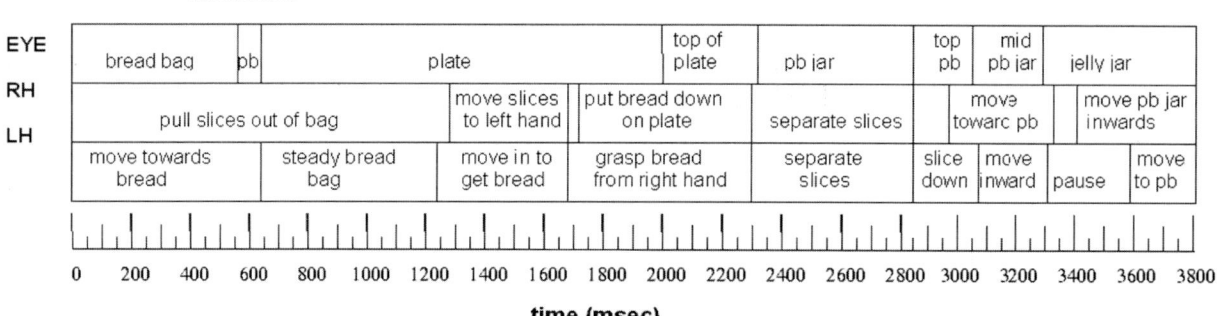

Fig. 5. Example of look ahead fixations. A brief fixation on the peanut butter is made about 1700 ms before the fixation used to guide pickup with the right hand.

wash-basin, they often fixated the tap, soap, and paper towels, before returning to fixate the tap to guide contact with the hand. Pelz et al. interpreted these look-ahead fixations in terms of their perceptual role, suggesting that they provide continuity of perceptual experience. It also seems likely that fixating the location of a future target facilitates the programming of the saccade, and perhaps initiates programming the reach. Evidence for this is given by McPeek et al. (1999), who showed that saccades to colored targets have shorter latency if a target of the same color has been presented on the previous trial. Similar reduced latencies are observed in the responses of frontal eye field neurons in monkeys performing a comparable task (Bichot and Schall, 1999). Similarly, Zelinsky showed that a 1-s preview of a search array prior to the search task led to faster search times and fewer saccades (Zelinsky et al., 1997) to reach the target. Epelboim et al. (1995) found that the time taken to tap a specified sequence of colored lights arrayed on a table rapidly decreased as the task was repeated, suggesting that repeated fixations of the locations facilitated the tapping movements. It is known that accurate saccades can be made on the basis of memory for stimulus location when the original stimulus is no longer present (e.g. Miller, 1980; Gnadt et al., 1991; Hayhoe et al., 1992; Colby, 1998). However, in normal viewing, the target is continuously present in the peripheral retina, and can be located on the basis of stimulus features, so it is not obvious that spatial memory would be useful in target selection. Its usefulness becomes more apparent when the need for motor planning is taken into account. In the case of reaching movements, the slower velocity of the arm relative to eye movements makes early initiation of the arm movements particularly useful.

While not definitive, these observations make a plausible case for visual representations that span fixations and are maintained over a period of a second or more, to coordinate visually guided movements. The frequency of look-ahead fixations in the present task, as well as their observation by Land et al. (1999) in tea-making, and by Pelz and Canosa (2001) in hand-washing, suggest that maintaining such a representation is a ubiquitous aspect of natural behavior. Similarly, the broad range of eye–hand latencies, ranging from a 1-s lag to a 1-s lead, shows that both eye and hand movements are sometimes planned a second ahead of the other. This suggests the need for some kind of visual memory buffer of a second or two. Land has shown that driving and piano playing also need a memory buffer of the order of a second in duration (Land, 1996; Land and Furneaux, 1997). The wide range of eye–hand latencies is very different from the usual single trial experiments where the eye–hand latency is about 100 ms (Jeannerod, 1988). Such experimental contexts do not provide an opportunity for preplanning. Despite the wide range, it is interesting to note the marked predominance of latencies close to zero, suggesting a preference for simultaneously initiated movements. In general, the relationship between eye and hand movements is much more flexible than expected on the basis of previous experimental work on single movements.

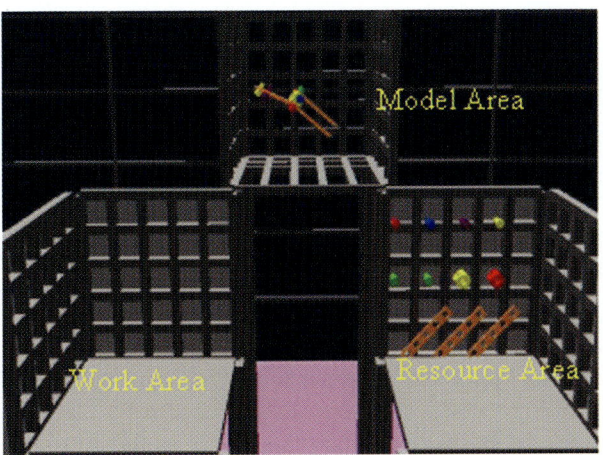 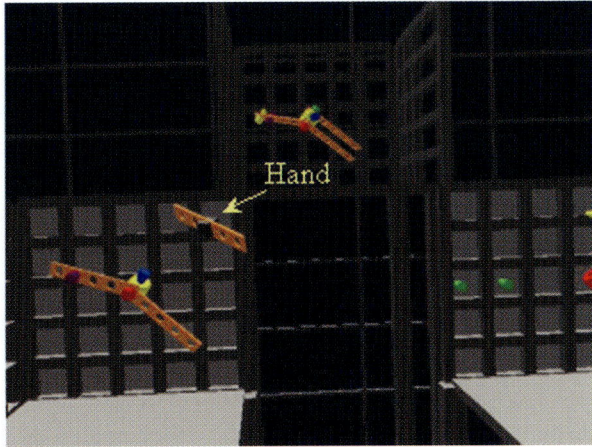

Fig. 6. The Baufix environment. The Model is on the top, the Resource area is on the right, and the Workspace is on the left.

Model building in a virtual environment

Observations of natural behavior, as described here, provide an important and necessary validation of hypotheses formulated in more controlled experiments. They are, however, intrinsically limited, in that they allow only indirect inferences. One way to preserve some of the advantages of natural behavior, while allowing more experimental control, is to use virtual environments that are as close as possible to real ones, where the stimulus can be controlled and manipulated (Loomis et al., 1999; Bulthoff and van Veen, 2001). Therefore we have investigated the hypothesis that observers accumulate a precise enough visual memory representation across saccades to serve as a basis for targeting movements in a virtual environment.

The environment we used simulates wooden parts from a toy construction set, called Baufix, shown in Fig. 6. There are three regions, the Model area in the center, the Resource area on the right, and the Workspace, on the left. The subject's task was to pick up pieces in the Resource region on the right side of the display and move them to the other side of the display to make a copy of the model construction at the top of the display. The virtual wooden parts were picked up and moved using a Fastrack sensor as a 3D mouse. Objects were highlighted when the sensor came in contact with them and the observer picked the objects up using the keyboard. The separation between the workspace and model, and resource and model, was about 30°. The individual regions subtended about 18°. This varied during the experiment with the position of the observer's head in the environment. The horizontal field of view of the head mounted display was 54°. This is not ecological in that it is substantially smaller than the normal field of view. However, the virtual environment is 3-dimensional, and subjects actively interact with objects in the environment as they do in normal environments, so it is plausible that they manage spatial behavior in the normal way.

The visual display was delivered via a Virtual Research V8 head mounted display, updated at 60 Hz, with a resolution of 640 × 480 pixels. The stereo image was generated by a Silicon Graphics Onyx II with four 250-MHz processors and two Infinite Reality 2 graphics boards. Head position was monitored with a Polhemus Fastrack, 6 degrees of freedom, magnetic tracking device. The latency of image updating in this system is about 50 ms. An ASL series 501 infra-red video eye tracker was integrated into the optics of the helmet and used to monitor position of the left eye. The ASL signal was recorded in the data stream and in addition, a 30-Hz video record of the display with eye position superimposed was recorded. An image of the observer's eye provided by the ASL was overlaid on the video scene record containing the location of gaze.

The focus of this experiment was on the saccades to the Resource area for picking up pieces. How were these saccades targeted? If the visual system functions in a memory-less way, the observer would locate the piece on the basis of a visual search for pieces of a particular color, and use this to target the saccade. Alternatively, subjects might use visual memory for the piece's location acquired in prior fixations, or some combination of the two might be used. To test if spatial memory was used, on some trials the locations of the pieces were scrambled when subjects looked away from the Resource area in order to place pieces in the Workspace area. If the remembered location is used in targeting the return saccades, such a manipulation should interfere with the process of locating the next piece. To make the display changes, direction of gaze was computed on line, and a random rearrangement of the pieces was triggered at the point where the Resource area was outside the field of view of the helmet.

Subjects copied the model 10 times. On the first five copies, there were no manipulations of the display. In the next five trials, the Resource pieces were randomly rearranged when the subject's gaze was directed away from the resource following a pickup. The changes occurred on about 80% of the pickups. The three large pieces were not moved so that subjects' attention would not be drawn to the changes.

None of the subjects were aware of the changes on questioning subsequent to the experiment.

Saccades to the Resource area were categorized using a frame-by-frame analysis of the video records. The categories are shown in Fig. 7. The Resource area is frequently out of the field of view of the helmet, at least partially, when the subjects initiate the saccade. On many of the pickups, subjects landed in the Resource area after a large saccade from the Workspace or Model area, and then made several fixations before picking up a piece. In these cases, it is not clear what the basis of the targeting process is, because the search can be made on the basis of color once the eye is in the Resource area, whether or not spatial memory is contributing to the search. On some pickups, however, in trials where the pieces were changing position, the subject landed first on the old location of a particular piece, that is, its location before the subject looked away on the previous pickup. The subject then fixated the new location of the piece, and picked it up. We called these 'Old–New location' searches and they are schematized in Fig. 7. On these trials, it seems likely that the initial fixation was made on the basis of spatial memory information. This happened on

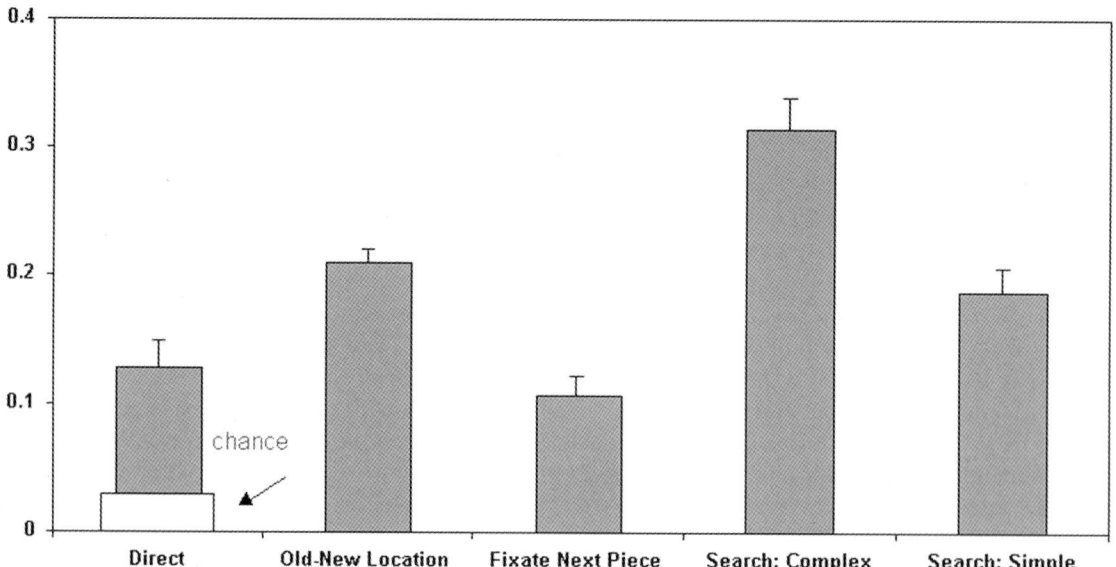

Fig. 7. Frequency of various categories of targeting strategy for pickup in the Resource. Categories are described in the text.

21% of the pickups, so it is a common, but by no means a dominant strategy. On about 13% of pickups, the saccade landed on the piece that was picked up, without any prior fixations. These were called 'Direct fixation' searches and are also illustrated in Fig. 7. On most of these trials, the piece had not moved from its location on the previous visit to the model, so these trials may also indicate spatial memory use. This cannot be claimed with any certainty, however, because the target was visible at the edge of the display on many of these trials, so targeting could also have been on the basis of color or shape. The trials where subjects land on the old location and then correct are therefore most diagnostic. On a small fraction of the Direct fixations (3%), the piece was in fact in a new location, even though the saccade was made directly to the piece. We can use this fraction as an estimate of the likelihood that the Old–New and Direct fixations are chance occurrences. Since the fraction is very small, it seems likely that the Old–New fixations, and perhaps some of the Direct fixations, which together make up over 30% of the targeting sequences, are not chance occurrences. Further support for this is the finding that subjects tended to build the copy in the same order from one trial to the next, so the piece that is picked up is probably actively searched for. Thus Old–New fixations are probably targeted on the basis of spatial information acquired in prior fixations, either in the current trial or on earlier trials. Spatial memory may also be involved in the Direct fixations.

Performance in the virtual environment supports the idea that some representation of the spatial structure of the scene is built up over different fixations and used for targeting saccades to the Resource area. It is not clear how important such memory representations are, however. On the one hand, the majority of pickup movements involved multiple fixations and no evidence for use of spatial memory, even in trials where the pieces remained in the same position from trial to trial. Over five trials without changes, subjects made on the order of 100 fixations in the Resource area, providing much more exposure to spatial context than in the experiments of Chun and Jiang (1998, 1999) so one might have expected a larger proportion of trials would indicate memory use. The facilitatory influence of spatial memory when feature information is also available may be quite subtle, however. Chun and Jiang observed a speeding up of the search by about 60–80 ms. In the Old–New searches, subjects must target the initial fixation exclusively on memory. Other trials may well be facilitated by memory, but such facilitation would not be revealed in the current measures. Experiments by Hayhoe et al. (1998), using a similar paradigm, showed that changing the color of pieces in the model area lead to increases of 100–200 ms in the duration of the subsequent fixation. This increase might have been caused by a disruption of the targeting mechanism. Thus a more careful examination of targeting performance is required to better define the extent of the role of spatial memory.

Conclusions

We have argued in this chapter that it is necessary to observe natural behavior in order to understand the temporal dependencies of vision. Standard experimental paradigms cannot reveal the whole story, because they focus on small time-slices, and single visual operations or movements. The natural world places a very different set of demands on the visual system than those we usually investigate in more controlled paradigms. The primary finding is that motor planning is a ubiquitous aspect of performance. Both eye and hand (or arm) movements appear to use visual information acquired in fixations a second or two prior to the current action. This is in agreement with other observations of natural behavior by Land and colleagues (Land and Furneaux, 1997; Land et al., 1999). Our findings support the suggestion made by Chun and Nakayama (2000), that, despite the compelling evidence of change blindness, and the strict capacity limits of visual short-term memory, there must be some implicit memory mechanisms for guiding attention and gaze around a scene that have higher capacity for spatial information. Several features of natural performance demonstrate that it is necessary to preserve information about spatial structure that can serve as a basis for planning and targeting eye and hand movements. O'Regan (1992) and Irwin (1991) have postulated that there is some integrated representation of the scene, but supposed that the spatial information is imprecise and that the representation is semantic in nature. While many aspects of the trans-saccadic representation of the scene may indeed be ill-defined, the spatial information cannot be imprecise, but must be able to support the targeting of eye and hand movements. Thus measures of trans-saccadic memory that rely on conscious report do not reveal the extent to which memory is required for ordinary behavior.

Acknowledgements

This work was supported by NIH Grants EY 05729 and RR06853. Thanks to Chris Chizk for assistance with the experiments.

References

Ballard, D., Hayhoe, M. and Pelz, J.B. (1995) Memory representations in natural tasks. *Cogn. Neurosci.*, 7: 66–80.

Batista, A., Buneo, C., Snyder, L. and Andersen, R. (1999) Reach plans in eye-centered coordinates. *Science*, 285: 257–260.

Becker, W. and Fuchs, A.F. (1969) Further properties of the human saccadic system: eye movements and correction saccades with and without visual fixation points. *Vision Res.*, 9: 1248–1258.

Becker, W. and Jurgens, R. (1979) An analysis of the saccadic system by means of double-step stimuli. *Vision Res.*, 19: 967–983.

Bichot, N.P. and Schall, J.D. (1999) Effects of similarity and history on neural mechanisms of visual selection. *Nat. Neurosci.*, 2: 549–554.

Bulthoff, H. and van Veen, H. (2001) Vision and action in virtual environments: modern psychophysics in spatial cognition research. In: M. Jenkin and L. Harris (Eds.), *Vision and Attention*. Springer-Verlag, New York, pp. 233–252.

Chun, M. and Jiang, Y. (1998) Contextual cueing: implicit learning and memory of visual context guides spatial attention. *Cogn. Psychol.*, 36: 28–71.

Chun, M. and Jiang, Y. (1999) Top-down attentional guidance based on implicit learning of visual covariation. *Psychol. Sci.*, 10: 360–365.

Chun, M. and Nakayama, K. (2000) On the functional role of implicit visual memory for the adaptive deployment of attention across scenes. *Vis. Cogn.*, 7: 65–82.

Colby, C.L. (1998) Action-oriented spatial reference frames in cortex. *Neuron*, 20: 15–24.

De Graef, P., Verfaille, K. and Lamote, C. (2001) Transsaccadic coding of object position: effects of saccadic status and allocentric reference frame. *Psychol. Belg.*, 41: 29–54.

Epelboim, J., Steinman, R., Kowler, E., Edwards, M., Pizlo, Z., Erkelens, C. and Collewijn, H. (1995) The function of visual search and memory in sequential looking tasks. *Vision Res.*, 35: 3401–3422.

Fischer, B. and Breitmeyer, B. (1987) Mechanisms of visual attention revealed by saccadic eye movements. *Neuropsychologia*, 25: 78–83.

Fischer, B. and Ramsperger, E. (1984) Human express saccades: extremely short reaction times of goal directed eye movements. *Exp. Brain Res.*, 57: 191–195.

Folk, C., Remington, R. and Johnston, J. (1992) Involuntary covert orienting is contingent on attentional control settings. *J. Exp. Psychol.*, 18: 1030–1044.

Freedman, E., Stanford, T. and Sparks, D. (1996) Combined eye–head gaze shifts produced by electrical stimulation of the superior colliculus in rhesus monkeys. *J. Neurophysiol.*, 76: 927–952.

Gibson, B. and Jiang, Y. (1998) Surprise! An unexpected color singleton does not capture attention in visual search. *Psychol. Sci.*, 9: 176–182.

Gnadt, J., Bracewell, R. and Andersen, R. (1991) Sensorimotor transformation during eye movements to remembered visual targets. *Vision Res.*, 31: 693–715.

Hayhoe, M., Lachter, J. and Moeller, P. (1992) Spatial memory and integration across saccadic eye movements. In: K. Rayner (Ed.), *Eye Movements and Visual Cognition: Scene Perception and Reading*. Springer-Verlag, New York, pp. 130–145.

Hayhoe, M., Bensinger, D. and Ballard, D. (1998) Task constraints in visual working memory. *Vision Res.*, 38: 125–137.

Henderson, J.M. (1992) Visual attention and eye movement control during reading and picture viewing. In: K. Rayner (Ed.), *Eye Movements and Visual Cognition*. Springer, Berlin, pp. 261–283.

Henderson, J. and Hollingworth, A. (1999) The role of fixation position in detecting scene changes across saccades. *Psychol. Sci.*, 10: 438–443.

Hochberg, J. (1986) Representation of motion and space in video and cinematic displays. In: K. Boff, L. Kauffman and J. Thomas (Eds.), *Handbook of Perception and Human Performance*, Vol. 1. Wiley, New York, pp. 22.21–22.64.

Irwin, D. (1991) Information integration across saccadic eye movements. *Cogn. Psychol.*, 23: 420–456.

Irwin, D. (1992) Memory for position and identity across eye movements. *J. Exp. Psychol.: Learn. Mem. Cogn.*, 18: 307–317.

Irwin, D. (1996) Integrating information across saccadic eye movements. *Curr. Dir. Psychol. Sci.*, 5: 94–100.

Irwin, D., Zacks, J. and Brown, J. (1990) Visual memory and the perception of a stable visual environment. *Percept. Psychophys.*, 47: 35–46.

Irwin, D., Colcombe, A., Kramer, A. and Hahn, S. (2000) Attentional and oculomotor capture by onset, luminance, and color singletons. *Vision Res.*, 40: 1443–1458.

Jeannerod, M. (1988) *The Neural and Behavioral Organization of Goal-Directed Movements*. Oxford Psychology Series No. 15, Clarendon Press, Oxford.

Jiang, Y., Olsen, I. and Chun, M. (2000) Organization of visual short-term memory. *J. Exp. Psychol.: Learn. Mem. Cogn.*, 26: 683–702.

Johansson, R., Wrestling, G., Backstrom, A. and Flanagan, J.R. (2001) Eye–hand coordination in object manipulation. *J. Neurosci.*, 21: 6917–6932.

Kowler, E. (1991) The role of visual and cognitive processes in the control of eye movement. In: E. Kowler (Ed.), *Eye Movements and Their Role in Visual and Cognitive Processes. Reviews of Oculomotor Research*, Vol. 4. Elsevier, Amsterdam, pp. 1–70.

Land, M. (1996) The time it takes to process visual information while steering a vehicle. *Invest. Ophthalmol. Vis. Sci.*, 37: B248.

Land, M. and Furneaux, S. (1997) The knowledge base of the oculomotor system. *Phil. Trans. R. Lond. Soc. B.*, 352: 1231–1239.

Land, M.F. and Lee, D.N. (1994) Where we look when we steer. *Nature*, 369: 742–744.

Land, M.F. and McLeod, P. (2000) From eye movements to actions: how batsmen hit the ball. *Nature Neurosci.*, 3: 1340–1345.

Land, M.F., Mennie, N. and Rusted, J. (1999) Eye movements and the roles of vision in activities of daily living: making a cup of tea. *Perception*, 28: 1311–1328.

Levin, D. and Simons, D. (1997) Failure to detect changes to attended objects in motion pictures. *Psychon. Bull. Rev.*, 4: 501–506.

Loomis, J., Blascovich, J. and Beall, A. (1999) Immersive virtual environment technology as a basic research tool in psychology. *Behav. Res. Methods Instr. Comput.*, 31: 557–564.

Mack, A. and Rock, I. (1996) *Inattentional Blindness*. MIT Press, Cambridge.

McPeek, R. and Keller, E. (2001) Short-term priming, concurrent processing, and saccade curvature during a target selection task in the monkey. *Vision Res.*, 41: 785–800.

McPeek, R.M. and Keller, E.L. (2002) Superior colliculus activity related to concurrent processing of saccade goals in a visual search task. *J. Neurophysiol.*, 87: 1805–1815.

McPeek, R., Maljkovic, V. and Nakayama, K. (1999) Saccades require focal attention and are facilitated by a short-term memory system. *Vision Res.*, 39: 1555–1565.

McPeek, R., Skavenski, A. and Nakayama, K. (2000) Concurrent processing of saccades in visual search. *Vision Res.*, 40: 2499–2516.

Maljkovic, V. and Nakayama, K. (1994) Priming of pop-out: I. Role of features. *Mem. Cogn.*, 22: 657–672.

Melcher, D. and Kowler, E. (2001) Visual scene memory and the guidance of saccadic eye movements. *Vision Res.*, 41: 3597–3612.

Miller, J. (1980) The information used by the perceptual and oculomotor systems regarding the amplitude of saccadic and pursuit eye movements. *Vision Res.*, 20: 59–68.

O'Regan, J.K. (1992) Solving the 'real' mysteries of visual perception: the world as an outside memory. *Can. J. Psychol.*, 46: 461–488.

O'Regan, J.K. and Levy-Schoen, A. (1983) Integrating visual information from successive fixations: does trans-saccadic fusion exist? *Vision Res.*, 23: 765–769.

O'Regan, J.K., Rensink, R.A. and Clark, J.J. (1999) Change-blindness as a result of 'mudsplashes'. *Nature*, 398: 34.

Pelz, J.B. and Canosa, R. (2001) Oculomotor behavior and perceptual strategies in complex tasks. *Vision Res.*, 41: 3587–3596.

Pelz, J.B., Canosa, R., Babcock, J., Kucharczyk, D., Silver, A. and Konno, D. (2000) Portable eyetracking: a study of natural eye movements. *Proceedings SPIE, Human Vision and Electronic Imaging*, SPIE, San Jose, CA.

Pollatsek, A. and Rayner, K. (1992) In: K. Rayner (Ed.), *Eye Movements and Visual Cognition: Scene Perception and Reading*. Springer-Verlag, New York, pp. 166–191.

Pylyshyn, Z. (1989) The role of location indices in spatial perception: a sketch of the FINST spatial-index model. *Cognition*, 32: 65–97.

Rayner, K. and Pollatsek, A. (1983) Is visual information integrated across saccades? *Percept. Psychophys.*, 34: 39–48.

Rensink, R.A., O'Regan, J.K. and Clark, J.J. (1997) To see or not to see: the need for attention to perceive changes in scenes. *J. Psychol. Sci.*, 8: 368–373.

Simons, D. (1996) In sight, out of mind: When object representations fail. *Psychol. Sci.*, 7: 301–305.

Simons, D.J. (2000) *Change Blindness and Visual Memory. A Special Issue of Visual Cognition*. Psychology Press, Hove.

Simons, D. and Levin, D. (1997) Change blindness. *Trends Cogn. Sci.*, 1: 261–267.

Simons, D. and Levin, D. (1998) Failure to detect changes to people in real-world interactions. *Psychon. Bull. Rev.*, 5: 644–649.

Theeuwes, J., Kramer, A., Hahn, S. and Irwin, D. (1998) Our eyes do not always go where we want them to go: capture of the eyes by new objects. *Psychol. Sci.*, 9: 379–385.

Theeuwes, J., Kramer, A., Hahn, S., Irwin, D. and Zelinsky, G. (1999) Influence of attentional capture on oculomotor control. *J. Exp. Psychol.: Hum. Percept. Peform.*, 25: 1595–1608.

Verfaille, K., De Graef, P., Germeys, F., Gysen, V. and Van Eccelpoel, C. (2001) Selective transsaccadic coding of object and event-diagnostic information. *Psychol. Belg.*, 41: 89–114.

Wallis, G. and Bulthoff, H. (2000) What's scene and not seen: influences of movement and task upon what we see. *Vis. Cogn.*, 7: 175–190.

Zelinsky, G., Rao, R., Hayhoe, M. and Ballard, D. (1997) Eye movements reveal the spatiotemporal dynamics of visual search. *Psychol. Sci.*, 8: 448–453.

Zingale, C. and Kowler, E. (1987) Planning sequences of saccades. *Vision Res.*, 27: 1327–1341.

CHAPTER 25

Commentary: Coordination of eye and hand in time and space

Harold Bekkering [1] and Uta Sailer [2,*]

[1] *Department of Experimental and Work Psychology, University of Groningen, Grote Kruisstraat 2/1, 9712 TS Groningen, The Netherlands*
[2] *Klinikum Grosshadern, Department of Neurology, Center for Sensorimotor Research, Marchioninistr. 23, D-81377 Munich, Germany*

Abstract: Every day of our lives starts with a succession of actions that require eye–hand coordination. From the time we try to turn off the alarm clock and get dressed, to putting toothpaste on the brush and preparing coffee: all these goal-directed hand movements need to be coordinated with the information from the eye. When performing such simultaneous goal-directed eye and hand movements, both the time and location at which eye and hand land on the object need to be harmonized. For better localizing the alarm clock, we need to see it before we hit it. In order to use this visual information for an accurate hand movement, we need the eye to land on the same position, i.e. eye and hand both need to be on the alarm clock instead of the water glass. These two aspects, temporal and spatial coordination, have encouraged a great deal of research. On the following pages, we will summarize a number of findings on how this coordination could be achieved.

Temporal order and organization of eye and hand

Historically, studies on eye–hand coordination first dealt with its temporal aspect. Typically, the eye is on target before the hand (e.g. Abrams et al., 1990). More specifically, the primary saccade is completed around the time the hand achieves peak velocity (e.g. Helsen et al., 2000). In this way, important visual information for movement correction can be picked up and used for an online adjustment of hand movements. Other results indicate that this yoking of hand to eye is not a one-way street. Neggers and Bekkering, 2000 (discussed in greater detail in Carey et al., 2002, this volume) found that saccade onset to a second target was delayed until an arm movement to the first target was completed. This finding shows that not only is the hand dependent on the eye, but also the eye is waiting for the hand.

Recently, the investigation of the temporal organization of eye and hand has been extended to real-life situations. As Hayhoe et al. (2002, this volume) elaborate on, the behavior induced by the restricted laboratory may be different from that in the natural environment because the environments' spatial extent, involved dimensions and behavioral goals differ. The authors found that in natural contexts a large number of hand movements were directed to objects that had been fixated in the recent past. In these cases, the object may be fixated in order to acquire its spatial location for planning the hand movement towards it. The time difference for initiating an eye and hand movement towards the same target could be as much as a second. Thus, eye and hand movements seem to be planned a second ahead of time. Therefore, a visual representation or memory buffer lasting at least a second is required. As there may be several fixations in between the eye and hand move-

---

*Correspondence to: U. Sailer, Klinikum Grosshadern, Department of Neurology, Center for Sensorimotor Research, Marchioninistr. 23, D-81377 Munich, Germany. E-mail: usailer@nefo.med.uni-muenchen.de

ment to the target object, this representation has to be independent from eye position.

Based on the investigation of temporal order in natural tasks, Hayhoe et al. (2002, this volume) show that motor planning is based on spatial representations of the scene, thus tapping into spatial coupling as the second main topic of eye–hand coordination.

Common or separate start signals and target representations?

Early studies investigated the question of whether one common or two separate command signals initiate eye and hand movements. This question was suggested because there was evidence for eye and head being controlled by one common command. Because of the reduced amount of computation necessary, it would be handy if this command were used also to control hand movements (Fischer, 1989). However, already the initial studies on this question showed that it cannot be answered as easily. For example, the high correlation (>0.60) between eye and hand latencies reported by Herman et al. (1981) has later been attributed to methodological artefacts (Bekkering et al., 1995). Other studies replicated these high correlations only in part (Frens and Erkelens, 1991) or not at all (Biguer et al., 1982). Generally, the correlation of eye and hand latencies is higher with non-visual targets than with visual targets. This has been shown both for auditory (Mather and Fisk, 1985) and kinesthetic (Neggers and Bekkering, 1999) as well as for remembered targets (Sailer et al., 2000). It is assumed that in these cases, eye and hand share more transformations or information.

One major question in the domain of spatial eye–hand coordination is whether eye and hand use the same spatial representation of the target or not. Initial studies on this question rather spoke for the use of a common target representation. For instance, Gielen et al. (1984) reported similar responses for eye and hand movements to double-step targets. Eye and hand also always moved towards the same target when there were two simultaneous targets. This led the authors to conclude that there is a common command signal for specifying the end position of eye and hand movements. This conclusion can be reformulated as the use of a shared target representation.

Similar conclusions were reached by changes of spatial parameters in one motor system being caused by changes in the other system. A popular paradigm used for this approach is the saccadic adaptation paradigm (e.g. McLaughlin, 1967; Abrams et al., 1992). When the target is displaced during the saccade, subjects initially acquire the displaced target by means of a second, corrective saccade. After a number of trials, however, subjects land directly on the position of the displaced target. It is believed that this shift in end positions results from a gradual shift of the target representation towards the final position of the target (Gielen et al., 1984). Consequently, if eye and hand shared one target representation, the end positions of hand movements should also be gradually shifted towards the position of the displaced target. Such a result was indeed found by Bekkering et al. (1995). When the target was displaced to a less eccentric position during the saccade, not only the eye adapted and went directly to the final target position, but the hand also showed similarly shortened amplitudes. Comparable results were found by De Graaf et al. (1995) using a similar paradigm. However, they put their results into perspective again in 1999, concluding that a transfer of saccadic adaptation to the hand motor system could not be proven consistently.

A different example of the effect of spatial information manipulated in one motor system on the responses of the other motor system was given by Van Donkelaar, 1997 (Van Donkelaar et al., 2002, this volume). Subjects had to look and point to the same targets while eye movements either started from the same position or from a position that required larger saccades than hand movements. It was found that saccadic amplitude and hand amplitude are not independent from each other, as hand amplitudes increased with saccadic amplitude. Thus, information about saccade amplitude is integrated into the response of hand movements.

But not only the saccadic signal influences hand movements, but hand movements also influence saccades. Eye trajectories towards a target in the presence of distracters were influenced by simultaneous reaches to the target (Tipper et al., 2001).

What all of these studies show is that at least some spatial target information is shared by eye and hand. However, Sailer et al. (2002, this volume) argue that although eye and hand exchange spatial target information, evidence speaks against the use of a shared target representation. If a nearby distracter acted on the same target representations of eye and hand, the distracter would be expected to always influence eye and hand responses in a similar way. Instead, based on the differential effect of a nearby distracter on eye and hand movements in some conditions, they favor the interpretation of eye and hand being based on two separate target representations and selection mechanisms that exchange information.

Sources of spatial information

If eye and hand are assumed to interact by an exchange of information, one should have a closer look at the nature of this information: what sources of spatial target information do eye and hand use and how does it influence the other motor system?

Retinal and extraretinal signals

A considerable number of studies have shown that prohibiting foveal vision of the target reduces the accuracy of hand movements (e.g. Vercher et al., 1996). Abrams et al. (1990) compared the behavior of the hand in a condition where fixation of the target was allowed with a condition where it was not (subjects had to fixate a central fixation spot instead). Fixation of the target enabled larger error corrections of ongoing hand movements (Abrams et al., 1990). Similarly, extinguishing the target at hand movement onset resulted in decreased accuracy (e.g. Prablanc et al., 1986).

On the one hand, fixating the target provides retinal information about the target. There are a number of explanations why that leads to more accurate hand movements. The most obvious reason is that visual resolution is better on the fovea. The more accurate information taken when the target is on the fovea can be used for a better modification of the ongoing hand movement.

On the other hand, fixating the target provides extraretinal information about eye position. It has been suggested that eye position (extraretinal gaze signals) serves as target for the hand. In other words: the hand points to where the eye is looking. According to this account, subjects try to match the end position of their hand movements to the end position of the eye. This so-called 'final gaze hypothesis' (Adam et al., 1993) can be reformulated to whether the hand uses the target representation of the eye. Arguments in favor of this hypothesis come from a study of Soechting et al. (2001) who found that pointing errors and errors at the final gaze position were highly correlated, even when saccades had drifted to this final position. However, these findings are in strong contrast with those of several other authors who did not find a correlation of eye and hand end positions (Biguer et al., 1984; Delreux et al., 1991; Sailer et al., 2000). Thus, as Soechting et al. (2001) themselves remarked, a gaze signal serving as target for the hand is not obligatory. Thus, extraretinal signals can, but need not necessarily be integrated into the hand motor response.

Whether extraretinal signals are used efficiently by the hand motor system or not may depend on the presence of retinal stimulation. In completely dark environments, subjects are not so good at pointing in the direction of their gaze (Enright, 1995; Blouin et al., 2002). Thus, extraretinal information appears to be used better by the hand motor system when retinal stimulation is present as well, particularly, if the amount of visual information is increased (Blouin et al., 2002).

Proprioceptive signals from the hand

Proprioception is an important source for accurate reaching movements. In pointing movements to visual targets, subjects without proprioception were found to have extensive directional errors compared to those with unaffected proprioception (Gordon et al., 1995). Moreover, these errors could not be detected by the subjects themselves when the lights were turned off.

Such proprioceptive information from the hand seems also to be used by the eye, particularly with tracking movements when more proprioceptive information is present. Already in 1969, it was found that tracking a target with the eyes was improved with concurrent hand movements (Steinbach, 1969). This improvement was replicated with regard to the delay of the eye to the target, tracking velocity (Gauthier et al., 1988), and smoothness, i.e. the number of saccades during tracking (Koken and Erkelens,

1992), although the improvement in the latter study was dependent on the predictability of the target.

However, like with simultaneous saccades and pointing movements, the parameters of eye and hand changed differently with changes in conditions. This applied both to latencies to sudden target changes (Bock, 1987) and the gain (Mather and Putchat, 1983). These findings again support the idea that eye and hand are controlled by parallel but interacting mechanisms. Lazzari et al. (1997) proposed a model which assumes that both motor systems are completely independent but exchange information, mediated by sensory (vision, hand muscle proprioception) and hand motor signals. The model assumes that the characteristics of the hand are stored and considered by the eye. However, the findings of two deafferented subjects indicate that proprioception does not seem to be necessary for reducing the time between the onset of eye and hand tracking (Vercher et al., 1996). Instead, the role of proprioception may lie in the information it provides about the arm's inertia (Ghez et al., 1990). Thus, proprioception is necessary for building up a representation about the dynamical properties of the arm (Scarchilli and Vercher, 1999).

Coordinates of spatial target representations

A number of studies have analyzed end point variability of hand movements to determine whether variable error patterns reveal the nature and origin of the coordinate system in which the movements were planned. In pointing to memorized targets, a gaze-centered reference frame was found when vision of the hand was available, whereas a hand-centered reference frame was found without vision of the hand (McIntyre et al., 1997). Similarly, using kinesthetic cues, Flanders et al. (1992) found evidence for a hand-centered reference frame.

Thus, hand movements are coded in a hand-centered frame of reference (Gordon et al., 1994; Vindras and Viviani, 1998), but eye movements in an eye-centered frame of reference. This raises the question on how an exchange of information between the motor systems of eye and hand could take place. Investigating the nature of the visual representations in space (Henriques et al., 1998; Henriques et al., 2002, this volume) showed that open-loop pointing movements in near and far space are coded in an eye-centered coordinate frame. This means that the internal representations of visual targets are remapped for each eye movement. It is suggested that these representations apply to an early stage of hand movement control, i.e. initial perception. Only targets selected for action are thought to be transformed further into head- or hand-centered frames of reference. This suggests that the target representation in terms of a visual map of space consists only of those representations on which we choose to act. In fact, such a strategy seems attractive because of its economic efficiency.

In this sense, the visual representations independent of eye position assumed by Hayhoe et al. (2002, this volume) may be the result of such a more elaborate, later transformation process.

Brain areas involved in eye–hand coordination

The question arises as to where in the brain this transformation of eye-centered into hand-centered coordinates is performed. Neurophysiological studies have revealed the crucial role of the posterior parietal cortex in such a transformation. Reach-related activity in the posterior parietal area was found to be modulated by gaze direction in monkey (Batista et al., 1999) as well as in humans (Baker et al., 1999). However, activity during saccadic delay in the parietal reach region (PRR) in monkey posterior parietal cortex does not reflect the animal's plans to move the eye with the arm or the arm alone. Therefore, although PRR subserves visually guided reaching, there is no evidence for the direct coordination of eye and hand in PRR (Snyder et al., 2000). Saccade-related activity in PRR was seldom presaccadic. One interpretation of the authors holds that this activity reflects the maintenance of target position in an eye-centered frame of reference, if the eyes move after target appearance but before reaching.

Whereas spatial locations for hand movements are coded in an eye-centered frame of reference in the posterior parietal cortex (e.g. Colby et al., 1995), other data suggest that they are coded in a hand-centered frame of reference in the premotor cortex (Graziano, 1999). The TMS data of Van Donkelaar et al. (2002, this volume) support the findings of these physiological studies. TMS over the premotor cortex resulted in an increased influence of the saccadic signal on hand movements. In contrast, TMS over the posterior parietal cortex resulted in a decreased influence of saccades on hand movements. Thus, the two reference frames appear to compensate for each other, with TMS reducing the amount of compensation. However, the results of other studies hint at the distinction being less clear. Gaze signals have also been shown to influence the premotor areas (Mushiake et al., 1997; Boussaoud et al., 1998; Baker et al., 1999). Instead of a stage-wise transformation of coordinates from one frame into another, multiple reference frames may exist in parallel which are integrated in both the parietal and frontal cortex (Battaglia-Mayer et al., 1998; Graziano and Gross, 1998). For example, the common coordinate frame in the posterior parietal lobe would allow the integration of different forms of spatial representations (Andersen et al., 1998).

Another neural structure that has been proposed to play a role in coordinating eye and hand control signals is the superior colliculus (SC). Recently, activity in SC neurons has been reported not only in saccadic eye movements, but also in arm movements (Stuphorn et al., 2000), although the respective neuronal populations do not overlap. Forty percent of the reach cells in the SC were found to modulate their activity with gaze. As these cells provide a signal of the difference between the eye and hand target, they are well suitable for the on-line correction of hand movements. Stuphorn et al. (2000) further discuss that the SC in turn is inhibited by cortical structures, because lesions in the premotor cortex, frontal and supplementary eye field result in an inability to dissociate eye and hand targets, a condition similar to the magnetic misreaching case found in humans (Carey et al., 2002, this volume).

A further candidate area for eye–hand coordination is the cerebellum. Miall and colleagues (Miall, 1998); Miall et al., 2001) report functional imaging data of subjects tracking targets with their eyes alone, their hand alone, or both. Compared to the single-task conditions, cerebellar areas were significantly more activated when the subjects performed a combined eye and hand movement. These findings speak for the involvement of the cerebellum in eye–hand coordination. Reciprocal interactions between the eye and hand motor systems have also been reported by Van Donkelaar and Lee (1994). In this study, cerebellar subjects were slower in initiating eye and hand movements (see also Brown et al., 1993) and had considerably more variable hand movements than control subjects. Also, this variability could be reduced by restricting eye movements.

In monkeys, lesioning the cerebellar dentate nucleus and measuring the outcome on tracking task performance, the correlation between eye and hand movements decreased and the delay between target and eyes increased (Vercher and Gauthier, 1988). Eye movements in the combined task were no longer different from those in the eye-alone task. Thus, after the lesion, the eye movement system could no longer use information from the hand motor system to enhance its performance. These results indicate the role of the cerebellum in coordinating eye and hand signals.

Clinical applicability of transformation accounts

Although such transformational accounts sound theoretically attractive, they also need to pass the empirical test of explaining clinical cases. This is what Buxbaum and Coslett (1997, 1998) have attempted to do with optic ataxia, a deficit in reaching under visual guidance and thus an intriguing clinical example of a breakdown of eye–hand coordination. Buxbaum and Coslett (1997, 1998) have attributed optic ataxia to failures in the transformation of retinal to hand-centered coordinates. More specifically, as parietal neurons could be responsible for this transformation (e.g. Batista et al., 1999; Ferraina et al., 2001), it has been proposed that optic ataxia can be explained by a failure of parietal neurons to combine directional eye and hand information (Battaglia-Mayer and Caminiti, 2002).

However, Carey et al. (2002, this volume) show that the transformational account fails to explain why some cases of optic ataxia are restricted to targets in the periphery. Thus, this crucial condition of this phenomenon is simply not accounted for.

An alternative explanation for the deficits observed in optic ataxia is that it mainly represents a deficit in making fast on-line corrections (Pisella et al., 2000). Such on-line corrections are particularly important in peripheral vision, because then the movement is programmed on the basis of coarse peripheral visual information. In contrast, foveal vision provides enough precise visual information for an accurate programming of the movement and therefore, on-line correction is less important. Thus, this account can well explain why some patients display optic ataxia to peripheral targets only. The role of the posterior parietal cortex in movement correction has also been stressed elsewhere (Debowy et al., 2001; Desmurget et al., 2001). Using a saccadic adaptation paradigm, the brain areas responsible for a modification of eye and hand movements to the displaced targets were investigated using PET (Desmurget et al., 2001). Such updated movements were shown to be mediated by a network involving the PPC, cerebellum, and primary motor cortex.

A further example for a patient with impaired eye–hand coordination is 'magnetic misreaching' (Carey et al., 2002, this volume). This patient failed to reach to extrafoveal targets. However, the authors argue that magnetic misreaching cannot be subsumed under the term of optic ataxia, because in this patient reaching to proprioceptive and auditory targets was also impaired. Instead, they suggest that magnetic misreaching results from the disruption of sensorimotor loops in the posterior parietal cortex with foveation remaining the only functioning route to goal-directed reaching.

Outline

Summary

This short overview could provide only exemplary insights into the research in the field of eye–hand coordination. However, two points may have become evident: first, the main questions in the field of eye–hand coordination are straightforward and can be roughly separated into questions about temporal and spatial coordination, respectively. That is, whether eye and hand use one common or two separate command signals to initiate their movements, and, whether eye and hand use the same spatial representation of the target. Second, the answers to these questions are not as simple as they first seem. For instance the question whether the coordination principle runs from eye to hand or from hand to eye (see also Carey, 2000) depends strongly on the task demands involved. Factors such as target modality (visual versus tactile) and action intentions (do I need information from the eyes for my ongoing hand movement, or do I need it later on), clearly affect both the temporal as well as the spatial coordination between the eye and the hand. Yet, this complexity also enables the enormous flexibility of the system that allows us to effectively interact with our environment.

Trends

What are the fields that can be expected to deliver major new insights in the domain of eye–hand coordination in the near future?

Neurophysiology

Clearly, to gain more insights into the neurophysiological substrates underlying eye–hand coordination, we need additional evidence from human neuroimaging experiments. At the moment, most of our knowledge derives from single-cell experiments in monkeys. Besides some well-known problems with this method such as limited generality of these findings at a more global system level (e.g. activity in the superior colliculus reflects a retinotopic organization of target representation, but is this organization also valid for other cortical areas involved in initiating eye and/or hand movements), and the comparison that has to be made between monkey and human primate brain, a maybe even more severe problem has to be taken into account. If one of the messages of this commentary is true, that the organization of eye–hand coordination is very much task-dependent, findings from more primitive tasks in monkeys might preclude theoretical insights in the underlying mechanisms of eye–hand coordination in more complex human tasks. At the moment, major efforts are undertaken to solve technical problems necessary to perform straightforward experiments with fMRI and EEG that can incorporate hand and eye movements during the neurophysiological measurements. These techniques should deliver new insights into the brain mechanisms of eye–hand coordination next to the ones reported here from recent PET and TMS studies.

Neuropsychology

Some fascinating findings have been reported in this book about patients with optic ataxia and magnetic misreaching that provided new insights into the coordination mechanisms of eye and hand movements in general. We strongly favor a neuropsychological approach to investigate this issue, but emphasize the need to perform well controlled, well-designed and well-measured experiments in these patient groups to add the necessary information about what goes wrong with the coordination of eye and hand after specific brain damages.

Behavioral

Over the years, a clear trend can be seen to include more natural environments in the eye–hand coordination studies (e.g. illuminated rooms, 3D objects). We also strongly advocate this direction. However, including an enriched environment can easily lead to a weakly controlled, less well-designed and hard-to-measure-dependent-variables experiment, from which only tentative conclusions can be drawn. If this is true, this might be too high a price to pay.

Acknowledgements

This chapter reflects equal contributions of both authors and was written when U.S. visited the Department of Experimental and Work Psychology of the University Groningen. U.S. was supported by the Deutsche Forschungsgemeinschaft, SFB 462 'Sensomotorik'. H.B. was supported by the Deutsche Forschungsgemeinschaft, SPP 1001 'Sensomotorische Integration'.

References

Abrams, R.A., Meyer, D.E. and Kornblum, S. (1990) Eye–hand coordination: oculomotor control in rapid aimed limb movements. *J. Exp. Psychol. Hum. Percept. Perform.*, 16: 248–267.

Abrams, R.A., Dobkin, R.S. and Helfrich, M.K. (1992) Adaptive modification of saccadic eye movements. *J. Exp. Psychol. Hum. Percept. Perform.*, 18: 922–933.

Adam, J.J., Ketelaars, M., Kingma, H. and Hoek, T. (1993) On the time course and accuracy of spatial localization: basic data and a two-process model. *Acta Psychol. Amst.*, 84: 135–159.

Andersen, R.A., Snyder, L.H., Batista, A.P., Buneo, C.A. and Cohen, Y.E. (1998) Posterior parietal areas specialized for eye movements (LIP) and reach (PRR) using a common coordinate frame. *Novartis Found. Symp.*, 218: 109–122.

Baker, J.T., Donoghue, J.P. and Sanes, J.N. (1999) Gaze direction modulates finger movement activation patterns in human cerebral cortex. *J. Neurosci.*, 19: 10044–10052.

Batista, A.P., Buneo, C.A., Snyder, L.H. and Andersen, R.A. (1999) Reach plans in eye-centered coordinates. *Science*, 285: 257–260.

Battaglia-Mayer, A. and Caminiti, R. (2002) Optic ataxia as a result of the breakdown of the global tuning fields of parietal neurons. *Brain*, 125: 225–237.

Battaglia-Mayer, A., Ferraina, S., Marconi, B., Bullis, J.B., Lacquaniti, F., Burnod, Y., Baraduc, P. and Caminiti, R. (1998) Early motor influences on visuomotor transformations for reaching: a positive image of optic ataxia. *Exp. Brain Res.*, 123: 172–189.

Bekkering, H., Abrams, R.A. and Pratt, J. (1995) Transfer of saccadic adaptation to the manual motor system. *Hum. Mov. Sci.*, 14: 155–164.

Biguer, B., Jeannerod, M. and Prablanc, C. (1982) The coordination of eye, head, and arm movements during reaching at a single visual target. *Exp. Brain Res.*, 46: 301–304.

Biguer, B., Prablanc, C. and Jeannerod, M. (1984) The contribution of coordinated eye and head movements in hand pointing accuracy. *Exp. Brain Res.*, 55: 462–469.

Blouin, J., Amade, N., Vercher, J.L., Teasdale, N. and Gauthier, G.M. (2002) Visual signals contribute to the coding of gaze direction. *Exp. Brain Res.*, 144: 281–292.

Bock, O. (1987) Coordination of arm and eye movements in tracking of sinusoidally moving targets. *Behav. Brain Res.*, 24: 93–100.

Boussaoud, D., Jouffrais, C. and Bremmer, F. (1998) Eye position effects on the neuronal activity of dorsal premotor cortex in the macaque monkey. *J. Neurophysiol.*, 80: 1132–1150.

Brown, S.H., Kessler, K.R., Hefter, H., Cooke, J.D. and Freund, H.J. (1993) Role of the cerebellum in visuomotor coordination. I. Delayed eye and arm initiation in patients with mild cerebellar ataxia. *Exp. Brain Res.*, 94: 478–488.

Buxbaum, L.J. and Coslett, H.B. (1997) Subtypes of optic ataxia: reframing the disconnection account. *Neurocase*, 3: 159–166.

Buxbaum, L.J. and Coslett, H.B. (1998) Spatio-motor representations in reaching: evidence for subtypes of optic ataxia. *Cogn. Neuropsychol.*, 15: 279–312.

Carey, D.P. (2000) Eye–hand coordination: eye to hand or hand to eye? *Curr. Biol.*, 10: 416–419.

Carey, D.P., Della Sala, S. and Ietswart, M. (2002) Neuropsychological perspectives on eye–hand coordination in visually guided reaching. In: J. Hyönä, D.P. Munoz, W. Heide and R. Radach (Eds.), *The Brain's Eye: Neurobiological and Clinical Aspects of Oculomotor Research. Progress in Brain Research*, Vol. 140. Elsevier, Amsterdam, pp. 311–327.

Colby, C.L., Duhamel, J.R. and Goldberg, M.E. (1995) Oculocentric spatial representation in parietal cortex. *Cereb. Cortex*, 5: 470–481.

De Graaf, J.B., Pelisson, D., Prablanc, C. and Goffart, L. (1995) Modifications in end positions of arm movements following short-term saccadic adaptation. *NeuroReport*, 6: 1733–1736.

Debowy, D.J., Ghosh, S., Ro, J.Y. and Gardner, E.P. (2001) Comparison of neuronal firing rates in somatosensory and

posterior parietal cortex during prehension. *Exp. Brain Res.*, 137: 269–291.
Delreux, V., Vanden-Abeele, S., Crommelinck, M. and Roucoux, A. (1991) Interactions between goal-directed eye and arm movements: arguments for an interdependent motor control. *J. Mot. Behav.*, 23: 147–151.
Desmurget, M., Grea, H., Grethe, J.S., Prablanc, C., Alexander, G.E. and Grafton, S.T. (2001) Functional anatomy of nonvisual feedback loops during reaching: a positron emission tomography study. *J. Neurosci.*, 21: 2919–2928.
Enright, J.T. (1995) The nonvisual impact of eye orientation on eye–hand coordination. *Vision Res.*, 35: 1611–1618.
Ferraina, S., Battaglia, M.A., Genovesio, A., Marconi, B., Onorati, P. and Caminiti, R. (2001) Early coding of visuomanual coordination during reaching in parietal area Pec. *J. Neurophysiol.*, 85: 462–467.
Fischer, B. (1989) Visually guided eye and hand movements in man. *Brain Behav. Evol.*, 33: 109–112.
Flanders, M., Helms Tillery, S.I. and Soechting, J.F. (1992) Early stages in a sensorimotor transformation. *Behav. Brain Sci.*, 15: 309–362.
Frens, M.A. and Erkelens, C.J. (1991) Coordination of hand movements and saccades: evidence for a common and a separate pathway. *Exp. Brain Res.*, 85: 682–690.
Gauthier, G.M., Vercher, J.L., Mussa, I.F. and Marchetti, E. (1988) Oculo-manual tracking of visual targets: control learning, coordination control and coordination model. *Exp. Brain Res.*, 73: 127–137.
Ghez, C., Gordon, J., Ghilardi, M.F., Christakos, C.N. and Cooper, S.E. (1990) Roles of proprioceptive input in the programming of arm trajectories. *Cold Spring Harbor Symp. Quant. Biol.*, 55: 837–847.
Gielen, C., van den Heuvel, P.J. and van Gisbergen, J.A. (1984) Coordination of fast eye and arm movements in a tracking task. *Exp. Brain Res.*, 56: 154–161.
Gordon, J., Ghilardi, M.F. and Ghez, C. (1994) Accuracy of planar reaching movements. I. Independence of direction and extent variability. *Exp. Brain Res.*, 99: 97–111.
Gordon, J., Ghilhardi, M.F. and Ghez, C. (1995) Impairments of reaching movements in patients without proprioception. I. Spatial errors. *J. Neurophysiol.*, 73: 347–360.
Graziano, M.S. (1999) Where is my arm? The relative role of vision and proprioception in the neuronal representation of limb position. *Proc. Natl. Acad. Sci. USA*, 96: 10418–10421.
Graziano, M.S. and Gross, C.G. (1998) Spatial maps for the control of movement. *Curr. Opin. Neurobiol.*, 8: 195–201.
Hayhoe, M., Aivar, P., Shrivastavah, A. and Mruczek, R. (2002) Visual short-term memory and motor planning. In: J. Hyönä, D.P. Munoz, W. Heide and R. Radach (Eds.), *The Brain's Eye: Neurobiological and Clinical Aspects of Oculomotor Research. Progress in Brain Research*, Vol. 140. Elsevier, Amsterdam, pp. 349–363.
Helsen, W.F., Elliott, D., Starkes, J.L. and Ricker, K.L. (2000) Coupling of eye, finger, elbow, and shoulder movements during manual aiming. *J. Mot. Behav.*, 32: 241–248.
Henriques, D.Y., Klier, E.M., Smith, M.A., Lowy, D. and Crawford, J.D. (1998) Gaze-centered remapping of remembered visual space in an open-loop pointing task. *J. Neurosci.*, 18: 1583–1594.
Henriques, D.Y.P., Medendorp, W.P., Khan, A.Z. and Crawford, J.D. (2002) Visuomotor transformations for eye–hand coordination. In: J. Hyönä, D.P. Munoz, W. Heide and R. Radach (Eds.), *The Brain's Eye: Neurobiological and Clinical Aspects of Oculomotor Research. Progress in Brain Research*, Vol. 140. Elsevier, Amsterdam, pp. 329–340.
Herman, R., Herman, R. and Maulucci, R. (1981) Visually triggered eye–arm movements in man. *Exp. Brain Res.*, 42: 392–398.
Koken, P.W. and Erkelens, C.J. (1992) Influences of hand movements on eye movements in tracking tasks in man. *Exp. Brain Res.*, 88: 657–664.
Lazzari, S., Vercher, J.L. and Buizza, A. (1997) Manuo-ocular coordination in target tracking. I. A model simulating human performance. *Biol. Cybern.*, 77: 257–266.
Mather, J.A. and Fisk, J.D. (1985) Orienting to targets by looking and pointing: parallels and interactions in ocular and manual performance. *Q. J. Exp. Psychol. A.*, 37: 315–338.
Mather, J.A. and Putchat, C. (1983) Parallel ocular and manual tracking responses to a continuously moving visual target. *J. Mot. Behav.*, 15: 29–38.
McIntyre, J., Stratta, F. and Lacquanti, F. (1997) Viewer-centered frame of reference for pointing to memorized targets in three-dimensional space [published errata appear in *J. Neurophysiol.* 1998, 79: preceding 1135 and 1998 Jun, 79: 3301], *J. Neurophysiol.*, 78: 1601–1618.
McLaughlin, S.C. (1967) Parametric adjustment in saccadic eye movements. *Percept. Psychophys.*, 2: 359–362.
Miall, R.C. (1998) The cerebellum, predictive control and motor coordination. *Novartis Found. Symp.*, 218: 272–284.
Miall, R.C., Reckess, G.Z. and Imamizu, H. (2001) The cerebellum coordinates eye and hand tracking movements. *Nat. Neurosci.*, 4: 638–644.
Mushiake, H., Tanatsugu, Y. and Tanji, J. (1997) Neuronal activity in the ventral part of premotor cortex during target-reach movement is modulated by direction of gaze. *J. Neurophysiol.*, 78: 567–571.
Neggers, S.F. and Bekkering, H. (1999) Integration of visual and somatosensory target information in goal-directed eye and arm movements. *Exp. Brain Res.*, 125: 97–107.
Neggers, S.F. and Bekkering, H. (2000) Ocular gaze is anchored to the target of an ongoing pointing movement. *J. Neurophysiol.*, 83: 639–651.
Pisella, L., Grea, H., Tilikete, C., Vighetto, A., Desmurget, M., Rode, G., Boisson, D. and Rossetti, Y. (2000) An 'automatic pilot' for the hand in human posterior parietal cortex: toward reinterpreting optic ataxia. *Nat. Neurosci.*, 3: 729–736.
Prablanc, C., Pelisson, D. and Goodale, M.A. (1986) Visual control of reaching movements without vision of the limb. I. Role of retinal feedback of target position in guiding the hand. *Exp. Brain Res.*, 62: 293–302.
Sailer, U., Eggert, T., Ditterich, J. and Straube, A. (2000) Spatial and temporal aspects of eye–hand coordination across different tasks. *Exp. Brain Res.*, 134: 163–173.
Sailer, U., Eggert, T. and Straube, A. (2002) Implications of dis-

tractor effects for the organization of eye movements, hand movements and perception. In: J. Hyönä, D.P. Munoz, W. Heide and R. Radach (Eds.), *The Brain's Eye: Neurobiological and Clinical Aspects of Oculomotor Research. Progress in Brain Research*, Vol. 140. Elsevier, Amsterdam, pp. 341–348.

Scarchilli, K. and Vercher, J.L. (1999) Oculo-manual coordination: taking into account the dynamicals properties of the arm. *Exp. Brain Res.*, 124: 42–52.

Snyder, L.H., Batista, A.P. and Andersen, R.A. (2000) Saccade-related activity in the parietal reach region. *J. Neurophysiol.*, 83: 1099–1102.

Soechting, J.F., Engel, K.C. and Flanders, M. (2001) The Duncker illusion and eye–hand coordination. *J. Neurophysiol.*, 85: 843–854.

Steinbach, M.J. (1969) Eye tracking of self-moved targets: the role of efference. *J. Exp. Psychol.*, 82: 366–376.

Stuphorn, V., Bauswein, E. and Hoffmann, K.P. (2000) Neurons in the primate superior colliculus coding for arm movements in gaze-related coordinates. *J. Neurophysiol.*, 83: 1283–1299.

Tipper, S.P., Howard, L.A. and Paul, M.A. (2001) Reaching affects saccade trajectories. *Exp. Brain Res.*, 2: 241–249.

Van Donkelaar, P. (1997) Eye–hand interactions during goal-directed pointing movements. *NeuroReport*, 8: 2139–2142.

Van Donkelaar, P. and Lee, R.G. (1994) Interactions between the eye and hand motor systems: disruptions due to cerebellar dysfunction. *J. Neurophysiol.*, 72: 1674–1685.

Van Donkelaar, P., Lee, J.-H., and Drew, A.S. (2002) Cortical frames of reference for eye–hand coordination. In: J. Hyönä, D.P. Munoz, W. Heide and R. Radach (Eds.), *The Brain's Eye: Neurobiological and Clinical Aspects of Oculomotor Research. Progress in Brain Research*, Vol. 140. Elsevier, Amsterdam, pp. 301–310.

Vercher, J.L. and Gauthier, G.M. (1988) Cerebellar involvement in the coordination control of the oculo-manual tracking system: effects of cerebellar dentate nucleus lesion. *Exp. Brain Res.*, 73: 155–166.

Vercher, J.L., Gauthier, G.M., Guedon, O., Blouin, J., Cole, J. and Lamarre, Y. (1996) Self-moved target eye tracking in control and deafferented subjects: roles of arm motor command and proprioception in arm–eye coordination. *J. Neurophysiol.*, 76: 1133–1144.

Vercher, J.L., Magenes, G., Prablanc, C. and Gauthier G.M. (1994) Eye-head-hand coordination in pointing at visual targets: spatial and temporal analysis. *Exp. Brain Res.*, 99: 507–523.

Vindras, P. and Viviani, P. (1998) Frames of reference and control parameters in visuomanual pointing. *J. Exp. Psychol. Hum. Percept. Perform.*, 24: 569–591.

SECTION V

Clinical aspects of eye movement research

Section Editor: W. Heide

CHAPTER 26

Visual search in long-term cannabis users with early age of onset

Lynn Huestegge [1,*], Ralph Radach [1], Hans-Juergen Kunert [2] and Dieter Heller [1]

[1] *Technical University of Aachen, Institute of Psychology, Jaegerstrasse 17–19, 52056 Aachen, Germany*
[2] *Technical University of Aachen, Clinic for Psychiatry and Psychotherapy, Pauwelstrasse 30, 52057 Aachen, Germany*

Abstract: The present research tested the hypothesis that there is a specific deficit in visual scanning in chronic users of cannabis with early onset of their drug consumption (age 14 to 16). 17 users and 20 control participants were asked to search for targets on a 5×5 stimulus array while their eye movements were monitored. Cannabis users showed less effective search behavior, including longer response times and more fixations at about the same error level. Search patterns were more conservative and included more frequent reinspections of previously fixated areas. In sum, the results point to two loci of adverse effects: an impairment in visual short-term memory, and less effective visual processing at a more strategic, top down controlled level.

Introduction

Cannabis is the most widely used illicit drug today. Especially young people increasingly consume *Cannabis sativa* with its most important ingredient, Δ-9-tetrahydrocannabinol (THC). Smoked marijuana interacts with an endogenous cannabinoid receptor system in the human brain. The density of this frequent and widely distributed receptor type varies over different brain regions. Detailed distribution maps for mammal brains are provided, for instance, by Herkenham et al. (1991a,b); Herkenham (1992). Some of the regions with high cannabinoid receptor density are directly linked to motor areas, such as basal ganglia, hippocampus, and cerebellum. However, the specific functions of this receptor system still remain unclear.

McLaughlin and Abood (1993) demonstrated a down-regulation of THC-receptor density after chronic THC consumption in rats. Stiglick and Kalant (1985) reported data indicating that chronic exposure of immature rats to cannabinoids may result in irreversible changes of brain morphology as well as of behavior, an effect that did not appear using mature animals. These data suggest that a specific vulnerability for adverse effects of THC may exist during distinct phases of human development. This idea provided one of the major motivations for the present study. Our intention was to compare participants who had begun their chronic use of cannabis early in life, between age 14 and 16, with normal control subjects. Participants were asked to complete a visual search task that in prior research by Ehrenreich et al. (1999) has proven to be sensitive to impaired visual processing performance in early-onset users.

This chapter is divided into four parts. We will first provide more theoretical background and take a look at some of the rich literature on mental and behavioral effects of cannabis. The second part will discuss some relevant previous research on eye movements in visual search, and in the third part methodology and main results of the experiment will be reported.

---

* Correspondence to: L. Huestegge, Technical University of Aachen, Institute of Psychology, Jaegerstrasse 17–19, 52056 Aachen, Germany. Tel.: +49-241-809-3993; E-mail: lynn.huestegge@post.rwth-aachen.de

The concluding discussion will include suggestions for further research on cannabis effects on visual processing and eye movements.

Effects of cannabis on cognition and behavior

Short-term effects of cannabis

Effects of cannabis on human mental functions and behavior that are manifest until a few hours after the drug is ingested will be referred to as short-term effects. They range from emotional and perceptual to cognitive and motor skill changes (see Ashton, 2001, for a recent discussion). There is a rich literature on short-term effects of cannabis, especially with respect to basic neuropsychological processes. Impairments of mental and psychomotor functions due to acute consumption of cannabis have been demonstrated in studies examining body sway, hand steadiness, rotary pursuit, driving and flying simulation, divided attention, sustained attention, the digit–symbol substitution test as well as complex driving and flight simulations (Chait and Pierri, 1992). Although various adverse consequences of cannabis consumption are unquestioned, there is substantial disagreement on the weight of positive versus negative effects. For example, research on effects of cannabis on cognitive functions and motor skills in the context of driving has led to mixed results. Several studies clearly suggested negative effects on driving-relevant abilities, such as deficits in tracking and eye–hand coordination as well as attentional drop-outs (Moskowitz, 1973). On the other hand, there is evidence indicating that these deficits can to some extent be compensated (or even over-compensated) in terms of a reduction in driving velocity. Careful behavior of drivers under the influence of cannabis appears to be due to a subjective impression of impairment. This is in clear contradiction to the pattern of self-perception reported for subjects that were intoxicated with alcohol rather than THC (Robbe, 1994; Berghaus and Krueger, 1998).

Although the measurement of eye movements is a common methodology in drug research, there are only a few studies on short-term effects of cannabis on eye movements. As an example, Fant et al. (1998) looked for performance effects of smoking a single marijuana cigarette on ten volunteers who reported recent use of cannabis. Along with other physiological parameters, smooth-pursuit eye-tracking performance significantly decreased with a peak after 2 hours. However, all effects had completely disappeared after 24 hours, indicating that the residual effects of smoking a single marijuana cigarette are minimal.

Early research on long-term effects

Research efforts on long-term effects of cannabis have so far been of rather moderate extent. These persisting effects were not in the focus of interest, possibly because the pharmacology of THC interactions with brain metabolism and physiology had remained elusive. An excellent review of neuropsychological research up to the mid nineties has been provided by Pope et al. (1995). Following their line of discussion, a distinction can be made between experimental studies in which cannabis is administered to subjects in a controlled fashion, and quasi-experimental, naturalistic studies examining subjects with a specific drug history. An advantage of the experimental approach is that confounding variables like socio-demographic status, social history, or IQ differences can often be reasonably well controlled. However, most of these experiments included participants with a history of modest prior marijuana use, and in some cases the abstinence period before experimental intoxication was not controlled. Therefore, it remains unclear whether changes in behavior were exclusively a consequence of the administered dose of cannabis. Also, for ethical reasons this type of research allows to study drug effects only with respect to limited doses and times of intoxication. Nonetheless, using an experimental design, Leirer et al. (1991) observed significant performance deficits in a flight simulator task over a period of 48 hours.

The vast majority of early research on long-term effects consisted of quasi-experimental studies, in which heavy users without psychiatric disorders were tested on various neuropsychological measures (such as memory, concentration and attention tasks) after acute effects had dissipated. Interestingly, about half of these studies did not find any differences at all between users and non-users. Among those who reported evidence for adverse effects is a study by Varma et al. (1988), who examined subjects with an average period of 7 years of chronic cannabis use. In several perceptuomotor tasks they found increased response times after 12 hours of acute intoxication but no differences in memory and intelligence tests. Research by Block et al. (1990) and Block and Ghoneim (1993) indicated effects on response times and various measures of visuomotor and memory performance over periods longer than 12 hours and Mendhiratta et al. (1988) even claimed to have found deficits 10 years after the last intoxication. Millsaps et al. (1994) reported data pointing to a subtle memory impairment after an abstinence period of about 1 month. Finally, a study of Schwartz et al. (1989) suggested a 6-week effect on a visual retention task and on a Wechsler memory scale for prose passages in eight users vs. nine controls.

Taken together, the results gathered in this early phase of research are quite heterogeneous and methodological problems as well as the lack of an adequate theoretical foundation are apparent. Examples for typical methodological limitations are: missing control groups, confounding socio-economic status and intelligence differences, unknown or brief abstinence periods, an unclear history of other drugs, insufficient group matching and small sample sizes (see Pope et al., 1995, for a detailed discussion). The variables in question are most often not derived from a theoretical framework but rather seem to be randomly chosen. In sum, until the middle of the nineties there was an obvious lack of knowledge about potential persistent effects of cannabinoids on brain functions.

Recent research on long-term effects

In recent years, studies concerning neuropsychological long-term effects became more solid in their methodological foundation. An issue that has moved into the focus of attention is whether potential effects are due to a residue of the drug in the system or, alternatively, due to a long-lasting CNS alteration even after the drug has left the body. Especially in chronic users, the metabolite accumulation in fat stores may be slowly released back into the circulation, a process which can take days after cessation of intoxication (Pope et al., 2001). Therefore, a distinction between residual vs. irreversible effects has become common.

Pope and Yurgelun-Todd (1996) demonstrated an adverse effect on word list memory and mental flexibility after one day of abstinence among 65 heavy-smoking participants in comparison to infrequent smokers. Fletcher et al. (1996) found deficits in word list memory even after three days as well as impairments in selective and divided attention among older, but not younger users. In contrast, Lyketsos et al. (1999) found no differences in the degree of 'cognitive decline' between heavy, light, and non-users during a 12-year longitudinal study. In an impressive recent study Pope et al. (2001) examined 108 subjects (current and former users vs. controls) over an 28-day observation period and found deficits exclusively in current users with respect to visual retention (only at begin of the study), word list memory (only up to 7 days) and card sorting (up to 24 days). Former users did not show any such deficits at all. Pope et al. interpret their results in terms of reversible residual effects rather than long-lasting neurotoxic damage.

Of particular interest for the present research are studies pointing to EEG abnormalities after cannabis intoxication (Struve et al., 1999; Patrick and Struve, 2000). They reported deviating patterns of results in various EEG measures one day after intoxication that were related to the duration of long-term consumption duration. Solowij (1998) conducted an experiment where subjects had to discriminate complex auditory patterns while event-related potentials (ERP) were recorded. She examined P300 delays and processing negativity, a measure reflecting attention processes, in this task after more than 12 hours of drug abstinence. The main result was that users were not only less successful in solving the discrimination task but also showed a larger processing negativity to complex irrelevant stimuli. Surprisingly, in a subsequent experiment where the abstinence period was at a mean of two years, subjects still showed poorer performance as well as higher processing negativity for irrelevant items, with effects that were still about a half of those reported before. This finding suggests a rather long-lasting neurotoxic effect.

Pope et al. (2001) discuss the results obtained by Solowij (1998), and note that "the possibility remains that more sophisticated neurocognitive assessment measures, such as electroencephalographic or functional magnetic resonance imaging measures, might reveal deficits in long-term cannabis users below the threshold detectable with our neuropsychological test battery" (Pope et al., 2001, p. 915). It is exactly at this point where the measurement and analysis of eye movements can come into play. It provides a methodology that can go beyond the scope of classic neuropsychological testing and may reveal subtle abnormalities in basic oculomotor behavior, visual information processing, visual working memory and/or higher cognitive abilities (visual strategies) that are all relevant for success in solving complex visual tasks.

Long-term effects on visual processing and early age of onset

As noted above, the present study is based on the idea that performance in visual tasks may be impaired in long-term cannabis users who have started their consumption of the drug during their adolescence. Evidence in favor of this hypothesis was provided in a prior study conducted while the third author of this chapter was at the University of Göttingen. Ehrenreich et al. (1999) used a computer-assisted battery of neuropsychological tests to examine performance in 99 exclusive cannabis users in comparison to 50 control subjects. The last cannabis use was at a mean of about 30 hours prior to testing. The groups were matched with respect to age, sex, educational and socio-demographic status, and intelligence level. Individuals with psychiatric diseases, head injury or previous or present use of drugs other than cannabis were excluded.

The test battery addressed a broad spectrum of cognitive and attentional functions and consisted of the following tasks (Zimmermann and Fimm, 1993): alertness (response times with or without an acoustic warning signal), divided attention (a dual detection task for visual and acoustic input), flexibility (a task where subjects respond either to a specific letter or digit), working memory (consecutively presented digits to be compared with the one previously presented), and a visual scanning task. In visual scanning, the subject was asked to indicate via key press the presence or absence of a fixed critical item in a 5×5 matrix of squares with one open side (see Fig. 4).

Results indicated that there were virtually no performance differences in all tasks except for visual scanning. Subjects with relatively late onset of cannabis consumption (age 17 or older, $n = 51$) were as successful as normal controls in the visual scanning task. However, subjects with early onset (age 16 or younger, $n = 48$) were significantly slower in response to both target present and target absent trials. Ehrenreich et al. discussed the possibility that these effects were due to residual intoxication rather than a persistent effect related to the early onset of drug abuse. To counter this objection, they showed that in stepwise regression analyses over the whole sample of 99 users, age of onset was a very good predictor of performance, whereas indicators of acute intoxication and cumulative toxicity were not. In supplementary analyses of variance, sex, age (which was lower in the early onset group), blood level of THC and estimated life dose were entered as covariates; nevertheless the group differences persisted. The response time measures reported by Ehrenreich et al. (1999) triggered our interest in asking a number of more detailed questions about characteristics of visual processing and eye movement control in cannabis users solving the visual scanning task. Before reporting the experiment, a brief look at some relevant evidence on eye movements in visual search will be taken.

Eye movements in visual search

The fundamental finding that eye fixations are not equally distributed over a picture represents one of the landmarks of early oculomotor research (Buswell, 1935; Yarbus, 1967). Fixation locations clearly depend on the informativeness of specific regions, an effect that emerges already during the first few seconds of scanning (Mackworth and Morandi, 1967). Even in tasks with a rather homogeneous target area, fixations are neither evenly distributed nor randomly spread. According to Ford et al. (1959), they tend to be underrepresented in the center as well as in the periphery of the search screen. The systematicity of visual search in the scanning of faces under degraded conditions was examined by Noton and Stark (1971), indicating that subjects used stereotypical scan paths in this task. A more theoretical and quantitative approach to this phenomenon was developed by Groner et al. (1984) and Groner and Menz (1985). They introduced a distinction between a local scan path guided by bottom-up processing and a global scan path that appeared to be guided by strategic planning and top down processing. This approach allowed to generate quantitative hypotheses about scanning behavior in naturalistic scenes or pictures, but it appears rather difficult to transfer the idea to scanning tasks that consisted of rather homogenous search arrays or backgrounds.

Gordon (1969) first demonstrated in a letter search task that there is a systematic relation between task difficulty and saccade amplitudes, with more difficult tasks leading to smaller saccades. Jacobs (1986) proposed a model where an increasing amount of visual information to be processed could either lead to a reduction of saccade amplitude, an increase in fixation duration, or both. Hooge and Erkelens (1996) conducted an experiment where expected low discriminability of targets caused strategically prolonged fixation durations. Furthermore, a reinspection analysis for targets in this study revealed that results of foveal target analysis were not used in the preparation of the subsequent saccade. This suggests a pre-programmed control of fixation duration, using estimations of the foveal analysis time of previous fixated stimulus elements (see also Hooge and Erkelens, 1998).

Performance in visual search should depend on visual acuity and discrimination in the periphery (Bloomfield, 1975). The area within which a certain degree of visual detail can be discriminated has been termed conspicuity area, functional visual field, useful field of view or visual lobe (see Findlay and Gilchrist, 1998, for a discussion). On a very general level, the purpose of eye movements is to bring regions or objects of interest outside the functional field of view close to foveal vision. It directly follows that individual effectiveness of extrafoveal processing should co-determine visual search performance. This prediction was tested by Nies et al. (1999), who studied eye movements of novice and expert subjects while searching for very small targets within a homogeneous background. They mapped the spatial extent of the useful field of view (UFV) for trials with target present. This was accomplished by discriminating between fixations around the target that immediately led to detection and those that were not successful. Fitting ellipses corresponding to 70% detection performance led to estimated individual UFVs differing substantially in size as well as horizontal and vertical extent. The validity of this technique was subsequently confirmed in a psychophysical detection experiment. Most importantly, within the sample of 15 subjects examined by Nies et al., the estimated size of the UFV showed a correlation of $r = 0.73$ with search performance. Hence, extrafoveal visual discrimination can be seen as a good predictor of effective search.

On the other hand, the amount of information that can be extracted from the periphery may also be a function of fixation duration. However, in an experiment by Hooge and Erkelens (1999), subjects were not able to strategically vary fixation durations in response to a task variation that required intensive peripheral information processing. This corresponds to a recent analysis of eye movements in reading by Radach and Heller (2000). They found no evidence in support of the hypothesis that a longer fixation duration, possibly allowing for more parafoveal processing, should lead to a longer subsequent saccade amplitude.

There is substantial evidence suggesting that features of the task determine scanning behavior. In addition to basic effects, such as the influence of distractor heterogeneity and target–distractor similarity (Duncan and Humphreys, 1989), recent experiments demonstrated a specific influence of search type ('serial' vs. 'parallel') on eye movement behavior. Gilchrist et al. (1999) found that in serial search subjects showed a greater stereotypical scanning behavior than in a search task where targets 'popped out'. In a series of experiments including both parallel vs. serial search, Zelinsky and Sheinberg (1997) found a substantial correlation between saccade number and response time, but only a weak correlation between average fixation duration and response time. This suggests that fixation durations more likely depend on stimulus factors than on differences in search type (serial vs. parallel) or task difficulty. Today, the distinction between serial and parallel processing as a strict dichotomy is generally seen as a useful, but fictitious heuristic (Wolfe, 1996).

In the current literature on visual search there is a lively debate about the role of memory processes. In response to a provocative study by Horowitz and Wolfe (1998), claiming that 'visual search has no memory', Gilchrist and Harvey (2000) measured eye movements while subjects had to scan an array of letters for a specific item. A reinspection[1] analysis showed that subjects relatively often returned to previously fixated items and that this pattern did not fit in a model of chance. Similarly, Peterson et al. (2001), who were also monitoring eye movements during a visual search task, showed that some items were reinspected during search and that the pattern of reinspections was incompatible with a memory-less search model. A large proportion of reinspections were directed to the target, indicating that subjects memorized which items were not adequately identified. In a dual task paradigm, Woodman et al. (2001) found that independent of the visual working memory load (2 vs. 4 items) visual search remains efficient.

An experimental manifestation of low-level short-term memory for locations already fixated has been termed the 'inhibition of saccade return' effect (Hooge and Frens, 2000), based on the concept of inhibition of return for spatial attention (Posner and Cohen, 1984; see Klein, 2000, for a recent discussion). In the critical experiment, subjects had to fixate a number of dots in accordance to a pre-specified scanning pattern. In this paradigm, reinspection saccades are part of the normal scan path. Interestingly, the duration of the preceding fixations were increased by up to 40%, a result that Hooge and Frens take as evidence for the proposed inhibition. This is in contradiction to eye movement patterns in reading, where the duration of fixations before regressive saccades back to positions to the left of the current fixation is short in comparison to fixations followed by progressions (Radach and Heller, 2000).

Methodology

The present experiment was carried out as part of a series of experimental tasks including a number of oculomotor standard paradigms whose results are not reported in this chapter. It used the visual scanning task developed by Zimmermann and Fimm (1993). As in the prior research discussed above (Ehrenreich et al., 1999), a group of cannabis users and a group of healthy controls were compared. However, there are two major differences between these two studies. First, in the present research, the cannabis group exclusively consisted of users with early onset of chronic drug consumption, in fact many of these users started already at the age of 14. Second, during the present experiment eye movements were recorded while participants were solving the task. Based on the evidence discussed in the previous sections, oculomotor irregularities in cannabis users can be expected in various respects. The neural control of eye movements is organized in terms of a hierarchy of control levels, from elementary, purely automatic control, to 'automated' control in terms of overlearned scanning routines (as found in reading), and to more top-down-based, strategic control (see Findlay and Walker, 1999, for a comprehensive review). The visual scanning task has the advantage that all of these levels are involved in generating appropriate oculomotor behavior such that analyses of eye movement parameters may generate evidence pointing to possible loci of adverse drug effects.

Participants

17 healthy pure cannabis users (14 male, 3 female) were recruited by advertisements in a local newspaper and by word of mouth. Mean age of participants in this group was 24.9 years (SD = 7.8) with a minimum of 19 years and a maximum of 45 years. The minimum requirement for long-term regular use of cannabis was a 4-year consumption period of about one joint per 1 or 2 days. Mean consumption duration amounted to 9.3 years (SD = 7.4; min. = 4, max. = 28). Participants smoked on average 10.5 joints per week (SD = 9.0; min. = 2, max. = 28) and had accumulated a mean life dose of 3526 joints (SD = 2210.8; min. = 728, max. = 7280). Most importantly, their age of onset of chronic cannabis consumption was low and quite homogeneous, ranging between age 14 and 16 (mean = 15.4; SD = 0.7). Users were free from any drug consumption between 16 and 40 hours before testing (mean = 30.9 hours; SD = 7.9 hours).

---

[1] In research on eye movements in visual search such as Gilchrist and Harvey (2000) a return to a previously fixated item is often called a 'refixation'. In basic oculomotor research the same term is used to describe the generation of a single, goal directed saccade (e.g. see Deubel et al., 2002, this volume) and in reading research it commonly refers to successive fixations on the same word (Inhoff and Radach, 1998). To avoid confusion, we decided to use the neutral term 'reinspection' instead.

Samples were taken from each user for (a) blood analysis of routine laboratory parameters, (b) urine screening using immunological routine methods for drugs (benzodiazepines, barbiturates, amphetamines, alcohol, cocaine and opiates), (c) determination of blood concentrations of Δ9THC and its major metabolites, THCOH and THCCOOH, by gas chromatography/mass spectrometry, and (d) measurement of total THC metabolites in urine by fluorescent polarization immunoassay (FPIA) (Moeller et al., 1992). Moreover, subjects underwent a semistructured psychiatric interview and a psychopathometric test (MMPI) to exclude individuals with depression or other psychopathological conditions potentially affecting test results. Cannabis users were also IQ-tested (mean = 118.1, SD = 9.9; min. = 107, max. = 137). The control group consisted of 20 healthy participants, matched in age and sex and without any past or present drug history including cannabis. Both groups consisted mainly of university students, all were socially integrated, successful individuals with comparable educational and socio-demographic status. Alcohol consumption was limited to a modest amount of about four beers per week (or equivalent) in both groups. All subjects took part in standard optometric testing to exclude participants with degraded visual acuity.

Task and procedure

The visual scanning task was developed by Zimmermann and Fimm (1993) as part of a computer-assisted neuropsychological test battery. Participants are asked to respond to the presence vs. absence of a prespecified fixed target appearing in a random position within a 5×5 matrix of squares. The squares all have an opening towards one side, thus there are four different possible stimuli in one matrix. During trials, the target stimulus is permanently presented in the left upper corner of the screen (see Fig. 4). There were 50 trials with and 50 trials without target, presented in fixed random order. Following the original instruction suggested by Zimmermann and Fimm (1993) and also used by Ehrenreich et al. (1999), subjects were explicitly asked to scan each matrix in a reading-like fashion line-by-line until they would either find a target or reach the end of the matrix.

Apparatus

Eye movements were recorded using an SR Research Ltd. EyeLink infrared eye tracking system at a sampling rate of 250 Hz (4 ms temporal resolution). The relative accuracy of the system is in the order of a few minutes of arc. Absolute accuracy in terms of short-term repeatability of fixation position mapping (McConkie, 1981) was estimated in independent test sessions to be better than $0.5°$ for a two-dimensional stimulus field. The on-line saccade detector of the eye tracker was set to detect saccades using an acceleration threshold of $9500°/s^2$ and a velocity threshold of $30°/s$. Stimuli were displayed on a 21 inch EyeQ monitor subtending a visual angle of $34°$ horizontally and $25°$ vertically at a viewing distance of 67 cm. Each stimulus square was 16.5 mm wide and the effective visual angle amounted to $1.4 \times 1.4°$ for each stimulus square and $9.6 \times 9.6°$ for the whole 5×5 search array. The display was generated using a 'Matrox Millennium' video card running at a refresh rate of 100 Hz.

Results

General results

The drug screening applied to urine samples taken before the experiment indicated that none of the participants in the cannabis group had consumed any drugs in addition to cannabis. Their blood level of THC + THCOH was 1.7 ng/ml plasma (SD = 1.7, min. = 0, max. = 7.6). This value is quite low and very similar to the mean value of 1.9 (SD = 3.7) reported in Ehrenreich et al. (1999). In the analyses of response times and mean number of fixations, outliers of three or more standard deviations from the group mean were excluded, leading to the elimination of one control participant.[2] Subjects in the group of cannabis users with early age of onset were significantly slower in their responses in comparison to normal controls (see Fig. 1). This difference amounted to 316 ms ($F(1,34) = 6.24$,

---

[2] This altered the mean values for the control group in these two measures but did not change significance levels in the statistical tests.

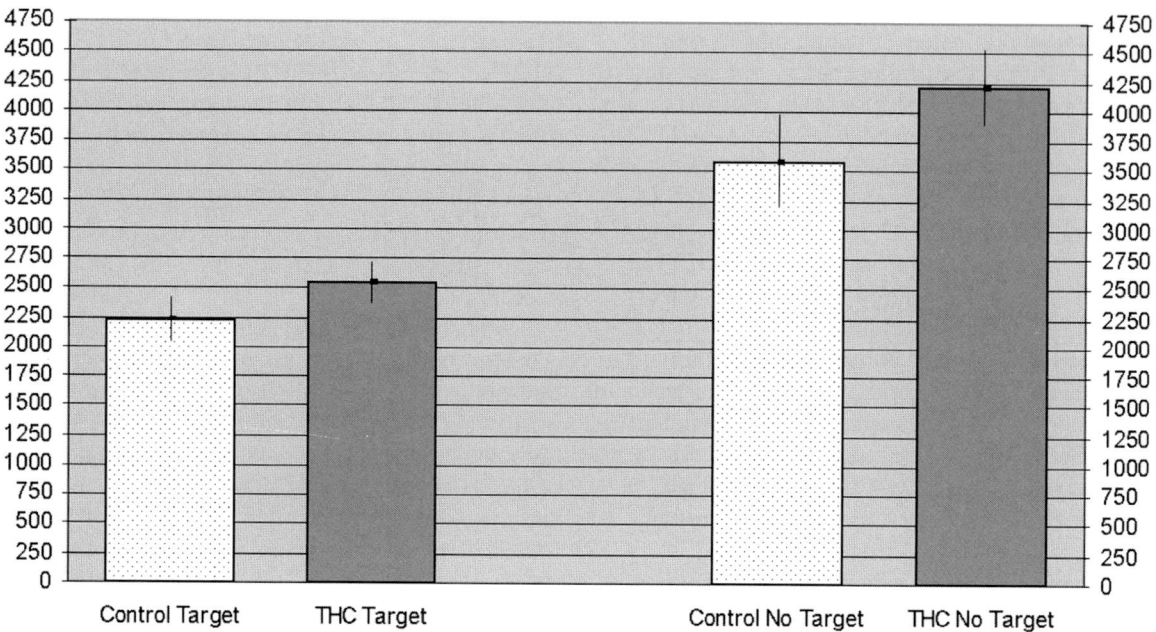

Fig. 1. Mean response times of cannabis users (dark columns) in comparison to normal controls (bright columns) in trials with target present (left columns) and trials with target absent (right columns). Vertical bars represent the standard error of the means.

TABLE 1

General results for participants in the control group vs. THC group

		RT, target (ms)	RT, no target (ms)	Fixation duration (ms)	Saccade amplitude (°)	Fixations per item (N)	Correct answers (N)
Control	mean	2225	3584	224	3.37	12.86	90.25
	SD	394	793	29	0.43	2.58	0.07
THC	mean	2541	4209	221	3.81	14.67	90.51
	SD	361	647	29	0.72	1.91	0.04

Group means are computed on the basis of subject means. SDs indicate the standard deviation of the subject means.

$p < 0.05$) in the target present condition and 625 ms ($F(1, 34) = 6.62$, $p < 0.05$) in the target absent condition. There was no difference in the proportion of correct answers between the two groups (THC 91% vs. controls 90%; $F(1, 35) = 0.02$). Mean fixation durations did not differ (THC 221 ms; controls 224 ms; $F(1, 35) = 0.09$), but saccade amplitudes were significantly larger in the THC group (3.81° vs. 3.37°; $F(1, 35) = 5.17$, $p < 0.05$). A significant difference was also present in the mean number of fixations per item. On average, cannabis users made 14.7 fixations on a 5 × 5 square stimulus page as opposed to 12.9 fixations in controls ($F(1, 34) = 5.66$, $p < 0.05$). Table 1 gives an overview of these general performance and eye movement parameters.

Saccade peak velocities

The velocity of saccadic eye movements in relation to their amplitude is often seen as a key indicator to "access the overall neurologic integrity of the saccadic eye movement system" (Ciuffreda and Tannen,

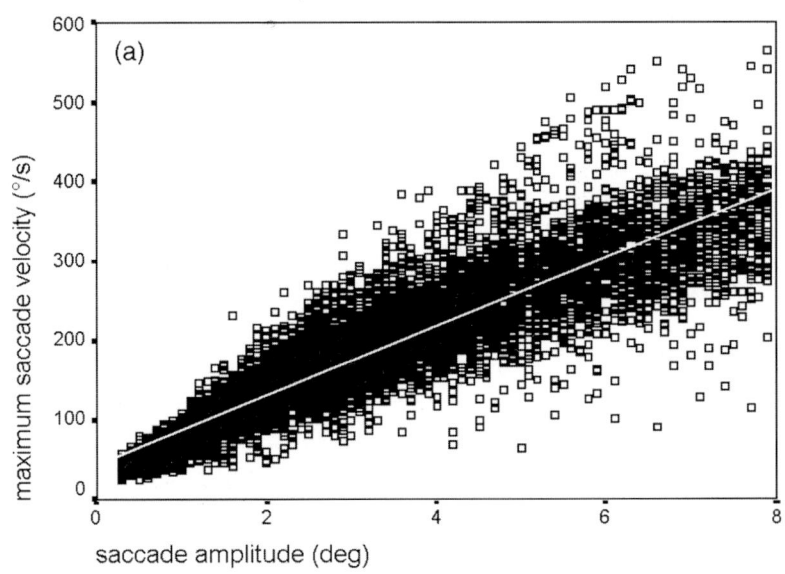

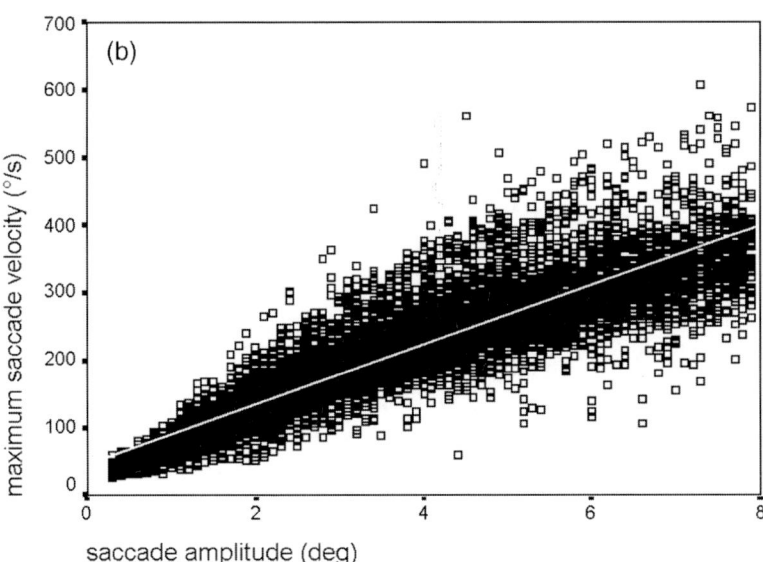

Fig. 2. Scatterplots of main sequence relations between saccade amplitude (°) and maximum velocity for participants in the control group (upper panel) and cannabis users (lower panel).

1994). This relation has been called the "main sequence" (Bahill et al., 1975) and reflects the pulse component of the pulse–step controller signal for saccade generation. Among the possible causes for decreased saccade peak velocities are drugs that reduce alertness (alcohol, barbiturates and diazepam), with most studies examining effects of acute alcohol intoxication (e.g. Heller and Lücke, 1987; see Moser et al., 1998 and Holdstock and de Witt, 1999, for recent discussions).

Fig. 2 presents scatterplots for both groups of the relation between saccade amplitude and peak velocity for saccades made in any direction within the search array (up to 8°). It is apparent from the figure that this relation is linear both for control participants (upper panel) and cannabis users (lower panel). The slopes of the linear regression curves are 43.27 for controls and 43.58 for users ($F(1,35) = 0.004$, $p > 0.05$), and the respective intercepts are 45.02 and 46.42 ($F(1,35) = 0.156$, $p > 0.05$). The mean correlation between saccade amplitude and maximum velocity is $r = 0.91$ in both groups. From these data it is evident that the main sequence relation is virtually identical for cannabis users and control participants. Separate analyses for horizontal, vertical and oblique saccades led to the same results. This can be taken as evidence that the neurophysiological machinery generating the pulse signal for saccades (see Sprenger et al., 2002; Munoz et al., 2002) is intact in chronic cannabis users with early onset.

Relations between saccade amplitudes and fixation durations

In a detailed analysis of a large corpus of reading data, Radach and Heller (2000) examined relations between spatial and temporal eye movement parameters. They found that fixations durations generally do not predict the extent of subsequent saccades. On the other hand, there was a significant relation between the amplitude of incoming saccades and the following fixation duration. This result is in harmony with prior observations in sentence reading tasks (Heller and Müller, 1983; Pollatsek et al., 1986) and was recently replicated in another study on a large corpus of reading data (Vitu et al., 2001). The interpretation suggested by Radach and Heller for this phenomenon is straightforward: the further away from its target an eye movement has been launched, the less opportunity for extrafoveal processing of the target object can be assumed. In the context of the present study this allows for an indirect assessment of extrafoveal processing. If cannabis users have a deficit in peripheral processing (target–nontarget discrimination), this should be manifest in longer fixations as a function of incoming saccade

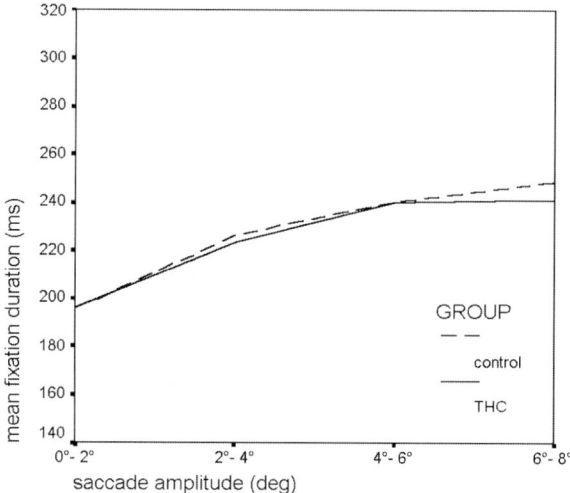

Fig. 3. Relation between saccade amplitude and subsequent fixation duration for control subjects vs. cannabis users. Group means are computed on the basis of subject means. One data point represents at least 5000 observations and each subject contributed at least 50 observations to the group means.

amplitude. Fig. 3 shows this relation for saccade amplitude ranges of up to 2°, 2–4°, 4–6° and 6–8°, including a total of more than 40,000 observations. As the figure indicates, fixation durations are longer following larger incoming saccades, replicating the results found by Radach and Heller (2000) in reading ($F(3,105) = 106.82$, $p < 0.01$). Most importantly, the two groups do not differ significantly ($F(1,35) = 0.148$, $p > 0.05$).

Scan path analyses

In the present visual scanning task, participants were asked to scan a 5 × 5 array of potential targets sequentially in a reading-like fashion. A straightforward indicator for the degree to which viewing behavior corresponded to this instruction is the correlation between the ordinal number of each fixation with the 'line' in the stimulus array that is currently fixated.[3] Interestingly, this correlation is

---

[3] This is similar to a suggestion in the original test documentation by Zimmermann and Fimm (1993). They propose for all items in the target present condition to compute a correlation between response time and the ordinal number of the line in which the target occurred.

Fig. 4. Typical examples of individual scan paths on a search array; item without critical target. The upper panel shows a sequential, reading-like scanning pattern and the lower panel depicts a more holistic and 'parallel' pattern.

substantially larger for the group of cannabis users ($r = 0.52$; $p < 0.01$) than for the controls ($r = 0.44$; $p < 0.01$). This appears to indicate, somewhat surprisingly, that scan paths in cannabis users were more 'systematic' or 'regular', and in better agreement with the instruction. Independent visual inspection of all scan paths produced in this study by two experts (the first two authors of this chapter) suggested that most participants adopted a coherent scanning pattern throughout the experiment. These individual scanning patterns can be grouped into two classes, a sequential line by line pattern and a more holistic (or 'parallel') pattern with only one or two fixations on each line. In the second class of scanning patterns there were several, intraindividually stable types of scan paths, for example moving from the center of the first line to the center of the last line or moving around the search array in one u-shaped scan path. Two typical examples are given in Fig. 4.

In the control group, both patterns were almost evenly represented, with 9 subjects scanning rather sequentially and 8 in a more holistic way, while 3 participants appeared to have no clear strategy. However, in the group of chronic cannabis users 14 of 17 subjects were classified 'sequential scanners', and 3 showed more unsystematic patterns. These observations, together with the finding that control subjects made significantly less fixations per item, suggest that, contrary to the correlation analysis reported above, their scanning behavior was not necessarily more unsystematic or irregular. Instead, many of the control subjects appeared to have developed their own, more effective way to solve the task. A comparison of subjects in the control group classified as 'sequential' vs. 'holistic' scanners indicted that the latter were markedly more efficient. On average, they responded to items with target absent 1297 ms faster (3012 ms vs. 4309 ms for 'sequential' scanners; $F(2, 15) = 11.22$, $p < 0.01$) and to items with target present 653 ms faster (1918 ms vs. 2571 ms for 'sequential' scanners; $F(2, 15) = 14.86$, $p < 0.01$) than subjects scanning in a more sequential way. Remarkably, this better search performance was achieved at almost the same error level (89% as opposed to 92.1% in serial scanners; $F(1, 15) = 1.09$, $p > 0.05$).

In an attempt to assess scan systematicity and to quantify group differences we used a method proposed by Ponsoda et al. (1995). In a first step of analysis, a probability vector was computed that represents the relative number of saccades targeted towards each of eight direction categories (north, northeast, east and so forth). In a second step, for each fixation incoming and outgoing saccades are set into relation to create a transition matrix representing conditional direction vectors. Every entry in this matrix displays the proportion of outgoing saccades to a specific direction relative to a certain incoming saccade direction. This technique is relatively simple but provides an effective tool to determine quantitatively how systematic the scanning behavior is in a given subject. For example, if scanning is systematic in terms of a reading-like sequential pattern, most of the saccades coming from the west should be succeeded by saccades directed to the east, or, in the case of 'returns sweeps' to the beginning of the text line, saccades to the west or southwest. If a subject scans the search array in a u-like fashion starting in the left upper corner, saccades coming from the north should regularly be followed by saccade going to the south or the east, etc. As opposed to the regular patterns described above, unsystematic scanning would produce a random distribution of saccades over the different direction vectors and conditional vectors.

The frequency distribution of saccade directions, as expressed in angular saccade vectors, is presented in Fig. 5. Both show a relatively systematic scanning behavior, with most of the saccades being directed to the east (controls 35.4%; THC 36.9%). In the figure, this large peak somewhat obscures significant group differences in westward and northwestward saccades. Subjects in the cannabis group made significantly more saccades directed to the west (25% vs. 22.4% for controls; $F(1, 35) = 5.62$, $p < 0.05$), and significantly less saccades directed to the northwest (6.4% vs. 7.6% for controls; $F(1, 35) = 6.45$, $p < 0.05$), corresponding to a more reading-like type of scanning.

In a second step of analysis, conditional transition vectors of saccade direction were computed, expressing the relative frequency of a specific direction pairing relative to all pairs beginning with a specific direction. Of the 64 pairs that could be analyzed in the respective transition matrix, we focused on the horizontal directions, as they were most frequent and also promised to provide some additional information regarding the differences in westward saccade frequencies mentioned above. Looking at saccade pairs starting with an eastward saccade (reading direction), it turned out that many of them were followed by a saccade in the opposite direction (Table 2). This effect was substantially stronger in the cannabis group (THC 45%; controls 38%; $F(1, 35) = 4.58$, $p < 0.05$). This means that after an eastward saccade, THC subjects were more likely to continue with a saccade in the opposite direction. A subsequent eastward saccade was slightly less likely (38% for both groups; $F(1, 35) = 0.01$, $p > 0.05$). A second significant group difference was present

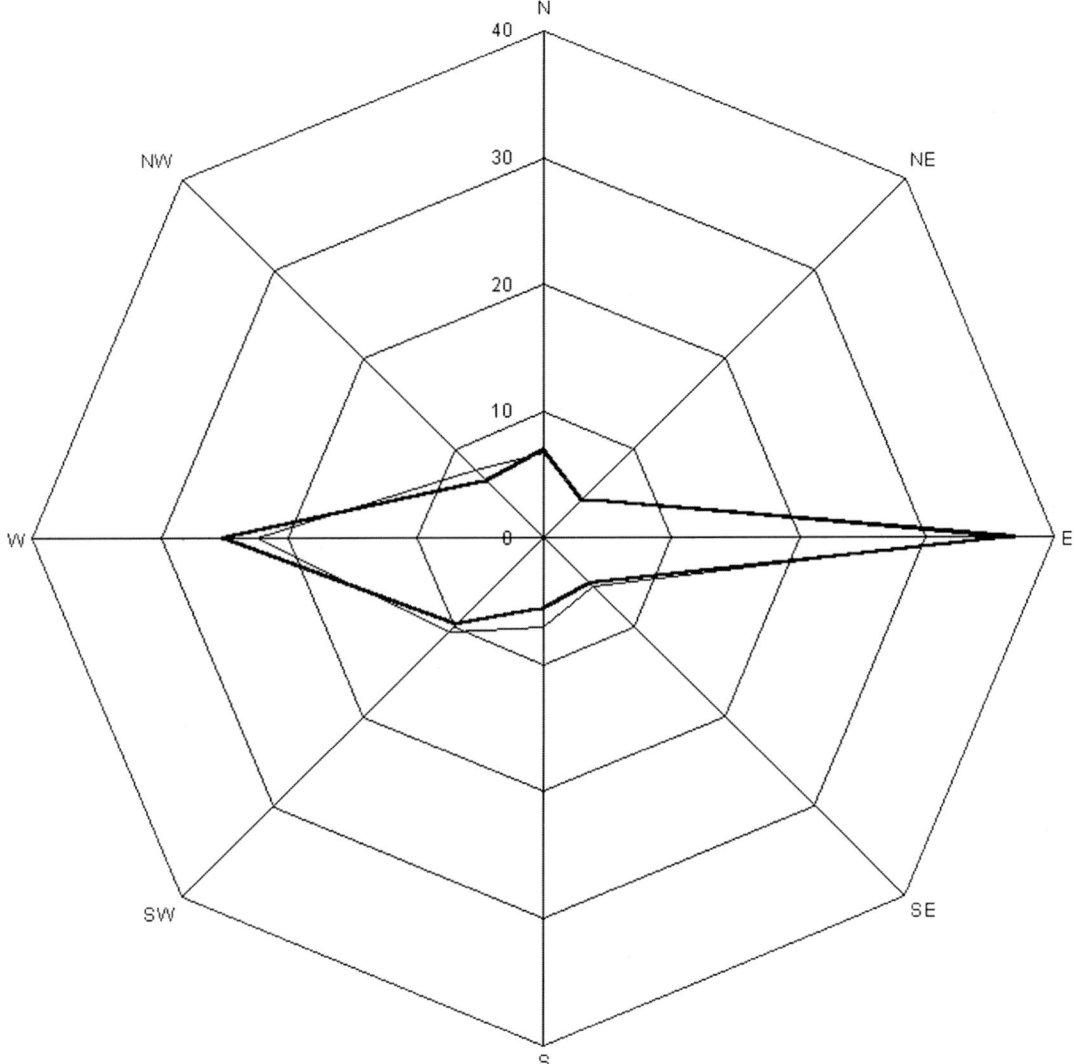

Fig. 5. Spatial distribution of relative vector probability of saccade direction. The thick line represents the THC group, and the thin line represents the control group.

in south-going subsequent saccades (THC 8%; controls 14%; $F(1,35) = 4.71$, $p < 0.05$). Saccades to the north did not differ between the groups. In pairs starting with a westward saccade about half were followed by a saccade to the east, which was significantly more frequent in the THC group (63% vs. 54% for controls; $F(1,35) = 4.67$, $p < 0.05$). On the other hand, control subjects significantly more often continued with a saccade to the north (16% vs. 11% for THC; $F(1,35) = 4.80$, $p < 0.05$). Subsequent saccades to the west did not differ between the groups, and saccades to the south were slightly more frequent in the control group (13% vs. 10% for THC; $F(1,35) = 1.99$, $p > 0.05$), without producing a significant difference.

In general, this analysis provides a quantitative base for the group differences reported above. First, it shows that control subjects are significantly more

TABLE 2

Relative frequencies of conditional saccade direction pairs (see text for further explanations)

		First saccade eastward				First saccade westward			
Second saccade (percent):		north	east	south	west	north	east	south	west
Control	mean	10	38	14	38	16	54	13	17
	SD	8.5	14.4	11.1	7.3	8.5	15.2	9.1	7.0
THC	mean	9	38	8	45	11	63	10	16
	SD	5.9	12.9	5.9	12.2	4.7	11.0	6.2	5.9

likely to continue an incoming horizontal saccade with a vertical saccade. Second, it indicates that cannabis users, following an incoming horizontal saccade more frequently continue to make a saccade into the opposite direction. It needs to be noted that this last figure includes both reinspection saccades going back to locations on the current and 'return sweeps' going to the beginning of the scan path on the next line in the search array. In an attempt to address the question of reinspections in a more direct way, we computed the probability with which the same stimulus element was returned to after the eyes had scanned another element. Due to the nature of the task (fairly easy discrimination of only four possible stimuli), usually more than one element was processed during one fixation and the total number of reinspections is relatively small. In the control group this frequency was 4.5% (SD = 2.3) and in the cannabis group it amounted to 6.4% (SD = 2.3). Despite these small probabilities of reinspection, the group difference was significant ($F(1,35) = 6.35$, $p < 0.05$).

Discussion

The present chapter started with reviewing some of the literature on long-term effects of cannabis on human cognition and behavior. This discussion indicated that much of the earlier literature suffered from various methodological and theoretical problems, but that recent research is more solid in its methodology and theoretical base. However, the results of this literature review are also not conclusive in that many of the studies show no differences between cannabis users and controls, while others appear to demonstrate massive performance deficits in various tasks. In some cases such deficits may be caused by residual intoxication, but there are also a few observations that point to the possibility of permanent damage to the nervous system.

One of the studies supporting the idea of long-term impairments due to cannabis was the research by Ehrenreich et al. (1999). They developed the novel hypothesis that there may be a specific vulnerability for cannabis in terms of interactions between THC and other cannabis metabolites and the human brain's cannabinoid receptor system at a peripubertal age. The empirical part of this chapter again tested their suggestion that visual search performance is degraded in cannabis users with early onset of their drug consumption. This hypothesis was confirmed in showing that cannabis users needed substantially more time than controls to complete a visual scanning task at about the same error level.

In our analyses of eye movements while participants were solving the task, several aspects were considered. First, we examined the 'main sequence relation' of saccade velocity as a function of saccade amplitude and found in both groups a linear relation with virtually identical slopes and intercepts. This indicates that the step component of the pulse–step signal in the saccade generation is not affected by chronic use of cannabis. This finding may be generalized to the claim that the basic brainstem machinery of saccade generation (see Sprenger et al., 2002; Munoz et al., 2002) is intact. This corresponds to results of recent experiments in our laboratory involving the same groups of subjects but using the standard gap and overlap paradigms. Here saccade velocity was also identical for the two groups, but latencies were significantly slower in cannabis users.

In a second stage of analysis we considered the relation between saccade amplitude and the duration of the subsequent fixation. Consistent with earlier findings on eye movements in reading (Radach and Heller, 2000), fixation duration increased substantially following saccades that came from more distant locations. This effect has recently been replicated by Vitu et al. (2001) who termed it the 'saccade distance effect'. These observations are in harmony also with supplementary unpublished analyses of a data set by Nies et al. (1999) on visual search of small targets over an unstructured (in half of the cases empty) stimulus field, where we found the same relation. In the current experiment, there were no group differences between control subjects and cannabis users with respect to the saccade distance effect. Following the logic suggested in the section on visual search and eye movements, this can be taken to suggest that chronic cannabis consumption does not result in an impairment of extrafoveal discrimination. A more modest interpretation would be that the use of extrafoveal information is not degraded to the degree that this information is used to determine the subsequent fixation duration. This includes the possibility that it is not the immediate use of processing results from extrafoveally acquired information that determines the duration of the following fixation. Instead, it is possible that information about the saccade amplitude or launch distance is utilized to pre-determine a fixation duration that is likely to allow for successful search (Hooge and Erkelens, 1998).

Our analysis of scan paths started with the observation that the correlation between ordinal number of fixation and the number of the line in the stimulus array that is being fixated is larger in cannabis users. This suggested that these participants scanned the search array in a more regular way and in better correspondence with the instruction. However, visual inspection of scan paths appeared to indicate that many of the control subjects used a more holistic strategy including more parallel processing of adjacent elements. Several aspects of these observations were subsequently confirmed in a quantitative analysis of conditional transition vectors of saccade direction. Most importantly, this analysis suggests that cannabis users may have made more reinspection saccades to regions in the stimulus array that had been previously processed. This hypothesis was tested in a more direct way by computing the frequency of returns to single elements, with the result that indeed cannabis users made more such reinspections.

In many search tasks, participants have to deal with two concurrent sources of memory load. One is to memorize the relevant target and one is to keep track of the regions or objects that have already been processed. The first kind of memory load can be considered minimal in the present experiment since the critical element that participants are asked to find never changed. In fact, subjects in both groups almost never fixated the comparison target. However, the second source of visual short-term memory load is present in this task, and the data indicate that participants in the cannabis group have greater difficulties to deal with it. The suggestion that cannabis users may have a deficit in visual short-term memory nicely corresponds to results of a recent experiment examining the same subjects in a memory guided saccade paradigm. We asked participants to delay a response to a target that disappeared after a short presentation duration. In the group of cannabis users, saccades towards the former target locations were substantially hypermetric relative to controls. Similarly, saccades were also hypermetric in the standard antisaccade task that requires a spatial re-mapping of stimulus coordinates.

Taken together, the results of the present study indicate that long-term cannabis users with early age of onset are substantially less efficient in visual scanning. In line with Ehrenreich et al. (1999), we assume that early and massive use of cannabis starting at peripubertal age (up to age 16) is causing specific impairments in visual processing and that these deficits are due to permanent neurotoxic damage as opposed to residual effects of recent drug use. This interpretation is also backed by the fact that there was no suggestion of any alteration in the saccade amplitude–velocity relation for the cannabis group which could have been diagnostic for behaviorally relevant residual effects. Two possible loci of adverse effects have been identified in this study. One is at the level of visual short-term memory, and one at a more strategic, top down controlled level of individual search patterns.

It is not easy to conclude on the basis of our data whether the observed differences in search patterns are of clinical importance. One may claim that although cannabis users were significantly less efficient, their visual search behavior was not nearly as dramatically disrupted as seen in patients with damage to specific brain areas in the visual and oculomotor systems (e.g. see the research on consequences of visual neglect after parietal lesions by Husain et al., 2001, or Sprenger et al., 2002). However, the observed conservatism of cannabis users in visual scanning strategies takes on a different aspect when seen in the context of the classic "a-motivational syndrome hypothesis" (McGlothlin and West, 1968). This hypothesis states that regular use of marijuana in young people may contribute to the development of passive, inward-turning, a-motivational personality characteristics.[4] An alternative or complementary idea is that conservative scanning may have developed *in response* to a self-perceived, neurotoxically caused reduction in visual processing efficiency. This argument could be based on the observations made in the present experiment pointing to problems with visual short-term memory and on results recently obtained in our laboratory using the memory-guided saccade paradigm (s.a.). These hypotheses will need to be addressed in future research.

References

Ashton, C.H. (2001) Pharmacology and effects of cannabis: a brief review. *Br. J. Psychiatry*, 178: 101–106.

Bahill, A.T., Clark, M.R. and Stark, L. (1975) The main sequence, a tool for studying human eye movements. *Math. Biosci.*, 24: 194.

Berghaus, G. and Krueger, H.P. (1998) *Cannabis im Strassenverkehr*. Fischer, Stuttgart.

Block, R.I. and Ghoneim, M.M. (1993) Effects of chronic marijuana use on human cognition. *Psychopharmacology*, 110: 219–228.

Block, R.I., Farnham, S., Braverman, K., Noyes Jr., R. and Ghoneim, M.M. (1990) Long-term marijuana use and subsequent effects on learning and cognitive functions related to school achievement: preliminary study. *NIDA Res. Monogr. Ser.*, 101: 96–111.

Bloomfield, J.R. (1975) Theoretical approaches to visual search. In: C.G. Drury and J.G. Fox (Eds.), *Human Reliability in Quality Control*. Taylor and Francis, London, pp. 19–29.

Buswell, G.T. (1935) *How People Look at Pictures: A Study of Psychology of Perception in Art*. University of Chicago Press, Chicago, IL.

Chait, L.D. and Pierri, J. (1992) Effects of smoked marijuana on human performance: a critical review. In: L. Murphy and A. Bartke (Eds.), *Marijuana/Cannabinoids: Neurobiology and Neurophysiology*. CRC Press, Boca Raton, FL, pp. 387–424.

Ciuffreda, K.J. and Tannen, B. (1994) *Eye Movement Basics for the Clinician*. Mosby, St. Louis.

Deubel, H., Schneider, W.X. and Bridgeman, B. (2002) Transsaccadic memory of position and form. In: J. Hyönä, D.P. Munoz, W. Heide and R. Radach (Eds.), *The Brain's Eye: Neurobiological and Clinical Aspects of Oculomotor Research*. Progress in Brain Research, Vol. 140, Elsevier, Amsterdam, pp. 165–180.

Duncan, J. and Humphreys, G.W. (1989) Visual search and stimulus similarity. *Psychol. Rev.*, 96: 433–458.

Ehrenreich, H., Rinn, T., Kunert, H.J., Moeller, M.R., Poser, W., Schilling, L., Gigerenzer, G. and Hoehe, M.R. (1999) Specific attentional dysfunction in adults following early start of cannabis use. *Psychopharmacology*, 142(3): 295–301.

Fant, R.V., Heishman, S.J., Bunker, E.B. and Pickworth, W.B. (1998) Acute and residual effects of marijuana in humans. *Pharmacol. Biochem. Behav.*, 60(4): 777–784.

Findlay, J.M. and Gilchrist, I.D. (1998) Eye guidance during visual search. In: G. Underwood (Ed.), *Eye Guidance While Reading and While Watching Dynamic Scenes*. Elsevier, Amsterdam, pp. 295–312.

Findlay, J.M. and Walker, R. (1999) A model of saccade generation based on parallel processing and competitive inhibition. *Behav. Brain Sci.*, 22(4): 661–674.

Fletcher, J.M., Page, J.B., Francis, D.J., Copeland, K., Naus, M.J., Davis, C.M., Morris, R., Krauskopf, D. and Satz, P. (1996) Cognitive correlates of long-term cannabis use in Costa Rican men. *Arch. Gen. Psychiatry*, 53: 1051–1057.

Ford, A., White, C.T. and Lichtenstein, M. (1959) Analysis of eye movements during free search. *J. Opt. Soc. Am.*, 49: 287–292.

Gilchrist, I.D. and Harvey, M. (2000) Refixation frequency and memory mechanisms in visual search. *Curr. Biol.*, 10: 1209–1212.

Gilchrist, I.D., Csete, A.A.E. and Harvey, M. (1999) Evidence for strategic scanning in serial visual search. *Abstract at the 10th European Conference on Eye Movements*.

Gordon, I.E. (1969) Eye movements during search through printed lists. *Percept. Mot. Skills*, 29: 683–686.

Groner, R. and Menz, C. (1985) The effect of stimulus characteristic, task requirements and individual differences on scanning patterns. In: R. Groner, G.W. McConkie and C. Menz (Eds.), *Eye Movements and Human Information Processing*. Elsevier, Amsterdam, pp. 239–250.

Groner, R., Walder, F. and Groner, M. (1984) Looking at faces: Local and global aspects of scanpaths. In: A.G. Gale and

---

[4] In the laboratory, participants in the group of cannabis users portrayed themselves not as suffering from an addiction but rather as people pursuing a certain way of life. They appeared extremely motivated, asserting that they were eager to show that people who take cannabis are 'not stupid'. It is possible that in our study this extra motivation has acted to counterbalance deficits that may well make a larger difference in real life.

F. Johnson (Eds.), *Theoretical and Applied Aspects of Eye Movement Research*. Elsevier, Amsterdam, pp. 523–533.

Heller, D. and Lücke, S. (1987) Time related effects of alcohol on saccade velocity. In: G. Lueer and U. Lass (Eds.), *Proceedings of the 4th ECEM*. Hogrefe, Göttingen, pp. 160–163.

Heller, D. and Müller, H. (1983) On the relationship between saccade size and fixation duration in reading. In: R. Groner, C. Menz, D. Fischer and R.A. Monty (Eds.), *Views*. Erlbaum, Hillsdale, NJ, pp. 287–302.

Herkenham, M. (1992) Cannabinoid receptor localization in brain: relationship to motor and reward systems. *Ann. N.Y. Acad. Sci.*, 654: 19–32.

Herkenham, M., Lynn, A.B., de Costa, B.R. and Richfield, E.K. (1991a) Neuronal localization of cannabinoid receptors in the basal ganglia of the rat. *Brain Res.*, 547: 267–274.

Herkenham, M., Lynn, A.B., Johnson, M.R., Melvin, L.S., de Costa, B.R. and Rice, K.C. (1991b) Characterization and localization of cannabinoid receptors in rat brain: a quantitative in vitro autoradiographic study. *J. Neurosci.*, 11: 563–583.

Holdstock, L. and de Witt, H. (1999) Ethanol impairs saccadic and smooth pursuit eye movements without producing self-reports of sedation. *Alcohol Clin. Exp. Res.*, 23(4): 664–672.

Hooge, I.T.C. and Erkelens, C.J. (1996) Control of fixation duration in a simple search task. *Percept. Psychophys.*, 58(7): 969–976.

Hooge, I.T.C. and Erkelens, C.J. (1998) Adjustment of fixation duration in visual search. *Vision Res.*, 38(9): 1295–1302.

Hooge, I.T.C. and Erkelens, C.J. (1999) Peripheral vision and oculomotor control during visual search. *Vision Res.*, 39: 1567–1575.

Hooge, I.T.C. and Frens, M.A. (2000) Inhibition of saccade return (ISR): spatio-temporal properties of saccade programming. *Vision Res.*, 40: 3415–3426.

Horowitz, T.S. and Wolfe, J.M. (1998) Visual search has no memory. *Nature*, 394: 575–577.

Husain, M., Mannan, S., Hodgson, T., Wojciulik, E., Driver, J. and Kennard, C. (2001) Impaired spatial working memory across saccades contributes to abnormal search in parietal neglect. *Brain*, 124(5): 941–952.

Inhoff, A. and Radach, R. (1998) Definition and computation of oculomotor measures in the study of cognitive processes. In: G. Underwood (Ed.), *Eye Guidance in Reading and Scene Perception*. Elsevier, Oxford, pp. 29–45.

Jacobs, A.M. (1986) Eye movement control in visual search: how direct is visual span control? *Percept. Psychophys.*, 39: 47–58.

Klein, R.M. (2000) Inhibition of return. *Trends Cogn. Sci.*, 4: 138–147.

Leirer, V.O., Yesavage, J.A. and Morrow, D.G. (1991) Marijuana carry-over effects on aircraft pilot performance. *Aviat. Space Environ. Med.*, 62: 221–227.

Lyketsos, C.G., Garrett, E., Liang, K.Y. and Anthony, J.C. (1999) Cannabis use and cognitive decline in persons under 65 years of age. *Am. J. Epidemiol.*, 149: 794–800.

Mackworth, M.H. and Morandi, A.J. (1967) The gaze selects informative details within pictures. *Percept. Psychophys.*, 2: 547–552.

McConkie, G.W. (1981) Evaluating and reporting data quality in eye movement research. *Behav. Res. Methods Instrum.*, 13: 97–106.

McGlothlin, W.H. and West, L.J. (1968) The marihuana problem: an overview. *Am. J. Psychiatry*, 125: 126–134.

McLaughlin, C.R. and Abood, M.E. (1993) Developmental expression of cannabinoid receptor mRNA. *Dev. Brain Res.*, 76: 75–78.

Mendhiratta, S.S., Varma, V.K., Dang, R., Malhorta, A.K., Das, K. and Nehra, R. (1988) Cannabis and cognitive functions: a re-evaluation study. *Br. J. Addict.*, 83: 749–753.

Millsaps, C.L., Azrin, R.L. and Mittenberg, W. (1994) Neuropsychological effects of chronic cannabis use on the memory and intelligence of adolescents. *J. Child Adolesc. Subst. Abuse*, 3(1): 47–55.

Moeller, M.R., Doerr, G. and Warth, St. (1992) Simultaneous quantitation of D9-tetrahydrocannabinol (THC) and 11-Nor-9-carboxy-delta-9-tetrahydrocannabinol (THC-COOH) in serum by GC/MS using deuterated internal standards and its application to a smoking study and forensic cases. *J. Forensic Sci.*, 37: 969–983.

Moser, A., Heide, W. and Kömpf, D. (1998) The effect of oral ethanol consumption on eye movements in healthy volunteers. *J. Neurol.*, 245(8): 542–550.

Moskowitz, H. (1973) Psychological tests and drugs. *Pharmacopsychiatry*, 6: 114–126.

Nies, U., Heller, D., Radach, R. and Bedenk, B. (1999) Eye movements during free search on a homogenous background. In: W. Becker, H. Deubel and T. Mergner (Eds.), *Current Oculomotor Research: Physiological and Psychological Aspects*. Plenum Publishers, New York, pp. 269–278.

Noton, D. and Stark, L. (1971) Scanpaths in saccadic eye movements while viewing and recognizing patterns. *Vision Res.*, 11: 929–942.

Patrick, G. and Struve, F.A. (2000) Reduction of auditory P50 gating response in marihuana users: further supporting data. *Clin. Electroencephalogr.*, 31: 88–93.

Peterson, M.S., Kramer, A.F., Wang, R.F., Irwin, D.E. and McCarley, J.S. (2001) Visual search has memory. *Psychol. Sci.*, 12(4): 287–292.

Pollatsek, A., Rayner, K. and Balota, D.A. (1986) Inferences about eye movement control from the perceptual span in reading. *Percept. Psychophys.*, 40: 123–130.

Ponsoda, V., Scott, D. and Findlay, J.M. (1995) A probability vector and transition matrix analysis of eye movements during visual search. *Acta Psychol.*, 88: 167–185.

Pope Jr., H.G. and Yurgelun-Todd, D. (1996) The residual cognitive effects of heavy marijuana use in college students. *JAMA*, 275: 521–527.

Pope Jr., H.G., Gruber, A.J. and Yurgelun-Todd, D. (1995) The residual neuropsychological effects of cannabis. *Drug Alcohol Depend.*, 38: 25–34.

Pope Jr., H.G., Gruber, A.J., Hudson, J.I., Huestis, M.A. and Yurgelun-Todd, D. (2001) Neuropsychological performance in long-term cannabis users. *Arch. Gen. Psychiatry*, 58: 909–915.

Posner, M.I. and Cohen, Y. (1984) Components of visual orienting. In: H. Bouma and D. Bouwhuis (Eds.), *Attention and Performance X*. Erlbaum, London, pp. 531–556.

Radach, R. and Heller, D. (2000) Relations between spatial and temporal aspects of eye movement control. In: A. Kennedy, R. Radach, D. Heller and J. Pynte (Eds.), *Reading as a Perceptual Process*. Elsevier, Oxford, pp. 165–192.

Robbe, H.W.J. (1994) *Influence of Marijuana on Driving*. Institute for Human Psychopharmacology, University of Limburg, Maastricht.

Schwartz, R.H., Gruenewald, P.J., Klitzner, M. and Fedio, P. (1989) Short-term memory impairment in cannabis-dependent adolescents. *Am. J. Dis. Child*, 143: 1214–1219.

Solowij, N. (1998) *Cannabis and Cognitive Functioning*. Cambridge University Press, Cambridge.

Sprenger, A., Kömpf, D. and Heide, W. (2002) Visual search in patients with left visual hemineglect. In: J. Hyönä, D.P. Munoz, W. Heide and R. Radach (Eds.), *The Brain's Eye: Neurobiological and Clinical Aspects of Oculomotor Research*. Progress in Brain Research, Vol. 140, Elsevier, Amsterdam, pp. 395–416 (this volume).

Stiglick, A. and Kalant, H. (1985) Residual effects of chronic cannabis treatment on behaviour in mature rats. *Psychopharmacology*, 85: 346–349.

Struve, F.A., Straumanis, J.J., Patrick, G., Leavitt, J., Manno, J.E. and Manno, B.R. (1999) Topographic quantitative EEG sequelae of chronic marihuana use. *Drug Alcohol Depend.*, 56: 167–179.

Varma, V.K., Malhorta, A.K., Dang, R., Das, K. and Nehra, R. (1988) Cannabis and cognitive functions: a prospective study. *Drug Alcohol Depend.*, 21: 147–152.

Vitu, F., McConkie, G.W., Kerr, P. and O'Regan, J.K. (2001) Fixation location effects on fixation durations during reading: an inverted optimal viewing position effect. *Vision Res.*, 41: 3513–3533.

Wolfe, J.M. (1996) Visual search. In: H. Pashler (Ed.), *Attention*. University College London Press, London.

Woodman, G.F., Vogel, E.K. and Luck, S.J. (2001) Visual search remains efficient when visual working memory is full. *Psychol. Sci.*, 12(3): 219–224.

Yarbus, A.L. (1967) *Eye Movements and Vision*. Plenum, New York.

Zelinsky, G.J. and Sheinberg, D.L. (1997) Eye movements during parallel–serial visual search. *J. Exp. Psychol. Hum. Percept. Perform.*, 23(1): 244–262.

Zimmermann, P. and Fimm, B. (1993) Diagnosis of attentional deficits: theoretical considerations and presentation of a test battery. In: F.J. Stachowiak (Ed.), *Developments in the Assessment and Rehabilitation of Brain Damaged Patients*. Narr Verlag, Tübingen, pp. 3–30.

CHAPTER 27

Visual search in patients with left visual hemineglect

A. Sprenger, D. Kömpf and W. Heide *

Department of Neurology, Medical University, D-23538 Lübeck, Germany

Abstract: In patients with hemi-spatial neglect eye movement patterns during visual search reflect not only inattention for the contralesional hemi-field, but interacting deficits of multiple visuo-spatial and cognitive functions, even in the ipsilesional hemi-field. Evidence for these deficits is presented from the literature and from saccadic scan-path analysis during feature and conjunction search in 10 healthy subjects and in 10 patients with manifest or recovered left visual neglect due to right-hemispheric stroke. Deficits include (1) a rightward shift of spatial representation, (2) deficient spatial working memory and failure of systematic search strategies, leading to multiple re-fixations, more after frontal lesions, and (3) a reduced spotlight of attention and a deficient pop-out effect of color, more after temporo-parietal lesions.

Introduction: visual neglect

The main feature of hemi-spatial neglect (Vallar, 1998; Bisiach and Vallar, 2000; Kerkhoff, 2001) is the disability to react or respond to stimuli presented in the hemi-space contralateral to a cerebral hemispheric lesion and to actively explore that side of space. Instead, patients are not aware of these stimuli and have a strong tendency to orientate their focus of attention, their eye fixations, and their manual exploration into the ipsilesional hemi-space, in spite of preserved visual fields and intact motor systems. Causative cerebral lesions involve the temporo-parietal junction (often the superior temporal gyrus) and, less frequently, the fronto-premotor cortex, most often in the right hemisphere (Karnath et al., 2001; Vallar, 2001). Although neglect predominately concerns the visual domain, it has been demonstrated for stimuli of various sensory modalities, such as acoustic or tactile, for mental imagery, and for spatial exploration in total darkness. Thus neglect is not a disorder of primary sensory processing, such as hemianopia, nor of spatially directed motor responses, but of spatial cognition. It can refer to multiple frames of spatial reference, i.e. to the allocentric representation of visual objects (object-based neglect), to the patient's own body (hemiasomatognosia and motor neglect), and to the egocentric representation of extrapersonal or near peripersonal space (space-based neglect), oriented according to the retinal midline (retinocentric), to the current direction of gaze (oculocentric), or to the midline of the head (head-centered) or trunk (body-centered). According to a recent study on saccadic latencies (Behrmann et al., 2002b), the oculocentric reference and a modulatory influence of eye-in-head position appeared to be most important for spatial coding in visual neglect.

Mechanisms involved in hemi-spatial neglect

Although a large amount of literature on neglect has piled up during the last decades, its basic mechanisms are still a matter of lively discussion. Most of the proposed models explain only certain aspects of the syndrome and cannot account for the whole variety of clinical and neuropsychological findings in neglect patients (Vallar, 1998; Bisiach and Val-

---

* Correspondence to: W. Heide, Department of Neurology, Medical University, Ratzeburger Allee 160, D-23538 Lübeck, Germany. Tel.: +49-451-500-3472; Fax: +49-451-500-2489; E-mail: heide_w@neuro.mu-luebeck.de

lar, 2000; Kerkhoff, 2001). There has been a long debate, if neglect is a disorder of spatial attention or of spatial representation. There is evidence for both: it has been shown that in left visual neglect the patient's internal egocentric spatial reference is rotated by about 15° into the ipsilesional right hemi-space (Ventre et al., 1984), and there is a loss of awareness and mental representation for parts of left visual hemi-space (Bisiach et al., 1981). This deficit can be modulated (enhanced or released) by sensory stimuli that shift the egocentric spatial midline into a specific horizontal direction, such as vestibular, proprioceptive, or optokinetic stimulation (Ventre et al., 1984; Karnath, 1994a; Vallar, 1998). In addition, there is evidence for disorders of spatial attention in neglect. Not only inattention for the left visual hemi-field, but also a deficit in disengaging attention from an ipsilesional focus towards a new stimulus on the contralesional side (Posner et al., 1984; Posner and Driver, 1992), a deficit in orienting spatial attention and motor intention towards the contralesional side, with a sharp boundary between neglected and attended regions and 'directional hypokinesia' into the neglected hemi-field (Heilman et al., 1993), alternatively a pathological bias of the orienting of attention, with a continuous gradient of neglect along the horizontal axis running from the contralesional to the ipsilesional side and leading to ipsilesional 'hyperattention' (Kinsbourne, 1993). Further, neglect is associated with non-spatial impairment of sustained attention (Robertson et al., 1997, 1998). In the framework of a 'premotor theory of attention', hemineglect has been interpreted as an imbalance of spatial representations that control motor programs, producing an attentional deficit (Rizzolatti and Berti, 1993). Visual extinction of the left-hemi-field stimulus in case of bilateral simultaneous visual stimulation is another attentional disorder, often associated with neglect, particularly in patients with parieto-temporal and subcortical lesions (Vallar et al., 1994). In addition to these mechanisms, deficits of spatial working memory and of motor planning (deficient search strategies, motor perseveration) also contribute to symptoms of hemi-spatial neglect and might modulate neglect behavior (Na et al., 1999; Wojciulik et al., 2001). Nowadays there is general agreement that not a single fundamental deficit, but different pathological mechanisms, or damage to discrete spatial representations or maps, and attentional systems, may account for the multifaceted manifestations of neglect.

Diagnostic assessment and eye movement analysis in hemi-spatial neglect

The presence of visual neglect can be inferred from behavior, if the patient is always orienting towards right ipsilesional hemi-space and only exploring this part of space, even in response to contralesional sensory stimuli. Thus a neglect patient may eat only the right half of his plate or shave only the right half of his face. If neglect behavior is less severe, the diagnosis of neglect has to be confirmed by simple paper–pencil tests, such as the standardized behavioral inattention test (BIT; Wilson et al., 1987). Such a battery has to include visuo-constructive tasks such as drawing or copying, further tasks of perceptual judgments such as line bisection (the midpoint of a long horizontal line has to be marked), and tasks of visuo-spatial scanning and exploration, such as reading and cancellation tasks. The latter include the widely used letter and star cancellation task, that require the identification and manual cancellation of a target letter or a target shape among a variety of distracters. These have been shown to be the most sensitive neglect tests (Weintraub and Mesulam, 1988; Ferber and Karnath, 2001).

The process of visuo-spatial exploration can be monitored more accurately by recording saccadic eye movements during visual search for targets among distracters. The distribution of visual fixations across the visual scene or visual field is regarded to reflect not only the patient's internal representation of visual space, but also the distribution of attention across this scene. Accordingly in previous studies, neglect patients' saccadic scan paths during visual search have been demonstrated to be very sensitive in reflecting hemi-spatial neglect of the contralesional half of the display (Chédru et al., 1973; Rizzo and Hurtig, 1992; Behrmann et al., 1997). In addition, however, these studies have shown that the pathological saccadic search behavior of neglect patients depends on a variety of stimulus-related (bottom-up) and cognitive (top-down) variables as well as on the location of lesions in either the parieto-temporal lobe or in the fronto-premotor cortex (Heide and

Kömpf, 1998). Stimulus-related variables were the use of natural versus abstract visual scenes, and in the latter a variable degree of similarity between target and distracters (Harvey et al., 2002). As confounding factors, previous authors (Zihl and Hebel, 1997; Husain et al., 2001) discussed deficits of spatial working memory for locations of targets that have already been visited, compulsive motor perseveration, particularly in patients with frontal lesions, further a loss of search strategies, an impaired inhibition of return towards already fixated locations (Bartolomeo et al., 2001), and cortical oculomotor deficits, concerning the initiation and planning of saccades in contralesional directions (Behrmann et al., 2002a). Thus eye movement analysis during visual search might disclose the differential contribution of the various visuo-spatial and cognitive mechanisms contributing to hemi-spatial neglect. In the following paragraphs of this chapter we will summarize the main results of these studies and then present our own recent results of saccadic scan-path analysis during feature and conjunction search in patients with manifest or recovered hemi-spatial neglect, due to frontal or parieto-temporal lesions. It will be demonstrated, how the saccade data reflect the different stimulus-related, lesion-related and cognitive factors, influencing neglect patients' behavior during visual search.

Visual search in hemi-spatial neglect: previous research

Eye movements in visual search

In everyday life it is often necessary to search for a specific target among distracters in a visual environment. Based on task instructions and previous knowledge (top-down influences) we have expectations about the shape and possible location of the target object thus restricting search efforts to certain areas of interest. If the target 'pops out' due to a single salient visual feature, e.g. color (bottom-up influences), it is identified pre-attentively and attention is captured in a fast, reflex-like manner. According to the Feature Integration Theory proposed by Treisman and Gelade (1980), search duration tends to be independent of the total number of items, indicating parallel processing of target locations, because the salient feature of all targets (e.g. the color) is perceptually integrated across the whole display. If, however, the target only differs by non-salient features, e.g. form, or by a conjunction of features, which cannot be integrated across the display, attention has to be shifted intentionally from one object to the next, following an efficient systematic search strategy. This serial mode of search is more time-consuming, and search duration increases with the total number of items.

Thus, as outlined in Fig. 1, active visual search can be performed in two modes: a pre-attentive fast parallel mode dominated bottom-up by 'pop-out' features of the visual stimulus, and an attentive slow serial mode, mainly driven by a number of top-down influences, such as task instruction, previous knowledge, individual search strategies, spatial working memory, and an internal spatial representation of the stimulus. Other investigators have shown that this dichotomy is not strict, but shows a continuous transition between the parallel and the serial mode. Even in serial tasks like conjunction search, the search process is guided by the most salient feature, such as color ('Guided Search' model; Wolfe, 1994). Visual search has two output systems that are intimately related to each other: shifts of visuo-spatial attention and saccadic eye movements. During the last years, analysis of saccadic scan paths during visual search has shown that the eye movement patterns reflect the distribution of attention and the underlying parallel and serial search processes quite accurately (Findlay and Walker, 1999). Saccade targets are selected from a visual 'salience map', that also guides shifts of attention. Search duration is proportional to the number of saccades, and no evidence has been found for (covert) attentive scanning during fixation intervals (Findlay, 1997; Williams et al., 1997; Zelinsky and Sheinberg, 1997; Motter and Belky, 1998a; Scialfa and Joffe, 1998; Maioli et al., 2001). In normal subjects, refixations of targets that had already been visited occurred in a very low percentage. This can be attributed to the following three mechanisms: (1) a systematic geometrical search strategy reflected in the saccadic scan path (Noton and Stark, 1971; Zangemeister et al., 1995); (2) spatial working memory for locations of targets that had already been found; and (3) inhibition of return to previously fixated items (Horowitz and Wolfe, 1998; Gilchrist and Harvey, 2000; Hooge and

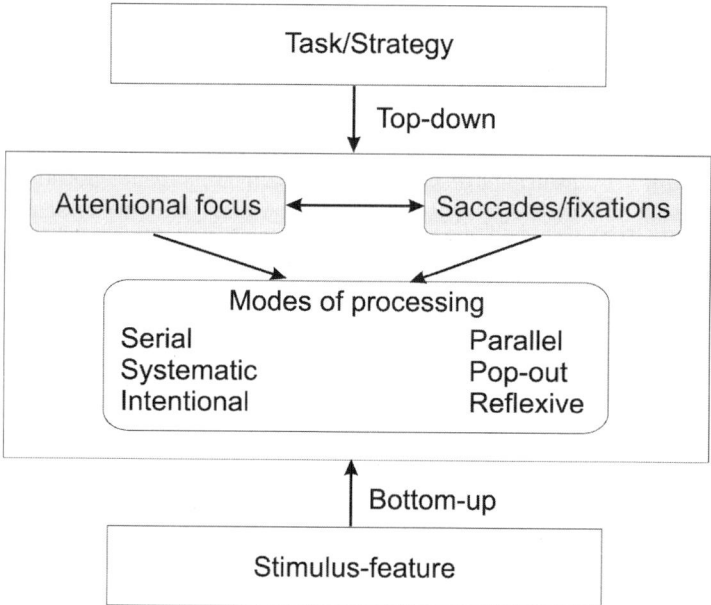

Fig. 1. Mechanism influencing saccadic scan paths during visual search.

Frens, 2000; Peterson et al., 2001). Which of these mechanisms contributes most, remains controversial. The significance of eye movements in visual search is outlined in some more details in the preceding chapter (Huestegge et al., 2002, this volume).

In a recent study in our lab (Sprenger et al., 2001) we could show that saccadic scan paths during color, form and conjunction search of abstract displays reflect low-level (bottom-up) features of the visual display as well as high-level (top-down) cognitive influences in terms of strategies and attention. More serial search tasks — like form or conjunction search — induced systematic geometrical scanning patterns of a circular, '8'-like or line-wise shape that were characteristic for each individual subject, with a predominance of horizontal and vertical saccades. The pop-out effect of color appeared to overrule these internally generated search strategies in color search, where the attention focus (useful field of view) was wider than in form or conjunction search, more items could be processed during each single fixation, and large targeting saccades were performed across the stimulus. Although high numbers of items (40, 60, 80) were presented, inhibition of return obviously worked: only a small number of items was visited twice, indicating an intact working memory of the scan path. We wondered which of these different mechanisms might be impaired in neglect patients with deficits of visual exploration due to cerebral hemispheric lesions.

Visual search in neglect: influences of lesion location and search modes

Neglect patients' visual search behavior in bedside cancellation tests has shown that left hemi-spatial neglect is much more severe when targets are presented in both halves of the visual display, when distracters are introduced, when the stimuli are presented in an unstructured array, and when there is a high similarity between targets and distracters, requiring serial search behavior (Weintraub and Mesulam, 1988; Eglin et al., 1991). Thus, in a number of studies (Grabowecky et al., 1993; Aglioti et al., 1997; Hildebrandt et al., 1999) neglect patients were mainly impaired in attentive serial search, whereas pre-attentive search was more or less preserved in most of these cases, apart from a few exceptions (Esterman et al., 2000). However, these studies did not measure search behavior by means of eye movement recordings, nor did they find an influence of lesion location (Eglin et al., 1991). Also, neglect in most of these patients was rather mild, and these authors did not exactly correlate visual search performance with the severity of neglect. In another study (Husain and Kennard, 1997), increasing the discriminability of targets and distracters and reducing the number of distracters facilitated more efficient and faster (more parallel) search mechanisms and improved performance in a neglect patient with a frontal lesion, but not in another with a fronto-parietal lesion. This study indicated for the first time that besides task difficulty lesion location does contribute to the impairment of visual search in neglect: whereas serial search was impaired in both frontal and parietal lesions, parallel (pre-attentive) search appeared to be more deficient after parieto-temporal lesions. This hypothesis needs to be confirmed in systematic studies in the future. At least, such a view is supported by recent results of functional magnetic resonance imaging: in addition to overlapping fronto-parietal activation in all search tasks, parallel spatial integration (perceptual grouping) of similar distracters across the display specifically activated the right temporo-parietal cortex (Wilkinson et al., 2002), whereas a serial conjunction search caused higher activity in the frontal eye fields (FEF) and in the parieto-occipital junction (Donner et al., 2002). Consequently, future research should address the question whether neglect patients' deficits of parallel and serial search critically depend on the location of cerebral hemispheric lesions or just on the severity of neglect. In such studies, quantitative assessment of attentive search strategies and of pre-attentive pop-out mechanisms might be achieved by an exact analysis of eye movements and scan paths. This issue will be dealt with in our own study presented later in this chapter.

Eye movement recordings during visual exploration of natural scenes or during line bisection (Ishiai et al., 1987, 1996; Rizzo and Hurtig, 1992; Karnath, 1994b; Kim et al., 1997; Barton et al., 1998) have shown that neglect patients in contrast to normal subjects and brain-damaged patients without neglect immediately orient their eye fixations into the right ipsilesional half of the display and rarely return back to the midline or into the left hemi-field. Such a leftward orienting of eye fixations as well as perceptual awareness for the left half of the scene may be facilitated either bottom-up by stimulus features (e.g. connecting elements between both hemi-fields), or by top-down influences (e.g. specific instructions, non-specific phasic alerting; Robertson et al., 1998), or by the semantic contents of the scene, if adequate visual perception can only be achieved when the whole stimulus is scanned. The latter is true for face stimuli. There may, however, be a dissociation between the oculomotor and the perceptual level: patients can perform leftward searching saccades, without awareness for that portion of space and without improvement in line bisection performance.

The influence of lesion location has been investigated in one of our earlier studies (Heide and Kömpf, 1998): neglect patients with lesions around the right frontal eye field (FEF) were most severely impaired in exploring an abstract visual display of colored squares, in terms of complete left-sided neglect and increased duration of single fixations. However, their performance was much better, when they had to explore a natural visual scene, such as a cookie theft in the kitchen. In contrast, parietal neglect patients were more impaired in the natural scanning task and in the initiation of reflexive visually triggered saccades into the contralesional hemi-field, but performed better in the systematic serial scanning of the abstract display of colored squares. We concluded that the FEF predominantly controls systematic voluntary exploration of space (serial search), whereas the parieto-temporal lobe is more important for reflexive orienting of attention and eye movement as well as for spatial exploration in the presence of visual elements that attract attention.

Horizontal distributions of eye fixations: spatial bias or attentional gradient?

A number of visual search studies (De Renzi et al., 1989; Hildebrandt et al., 1999) demonstrated a gradual increase of detected targets along the horizontal meridian of the display, from its left to its right uttermost end, with even a tendency to repeated cancellations of the same targets on the right end. These findings were interpreted as evidence for the gradient model (Kinsbourne, 1993) of attentional distribution in hemi-spatial neglect. Further evidence for this assumption was presented by Behrmann et al. (1997), who performed detailed eye movement analysis during visual search of a letter among distracters. They obtained a gradual increase in the proportion of ocular fixations along the horizontal meridian, extending between 22.5° of left and right horizontal eccentricities. However, the authors admitted that the peak of maximum fixations was not on the extreme right as predicted by a strict gradient model, but slightly more medial, at about 18° of right horizontal eccentricity. In contrast to these results, saccadic exploration of space in total darkness (Hornak, 1992; Karnath and Fetter, 1995; Karnath, 1997) yielded almost symmetrical, bell-shaped distributions of ocular fixations around the subjective egocentric midline, which was rotated around an earth-vertical axis into the right hemi-space by about 15°, with respect to the body's mid-sagittal plane. The authors argued that this distribution of fixations reflects the pathological representation of space in neglect or an abnormal transformation of sensory signals into a spatial coordinate system. Pure attentional models can hardly explain these findings, as spatial exploration in total darkness cannot be modulated by the attraction or disengagement of visual attention. In a subsequent study, Karnath et al. (1998) were able to replicate these findings for visual search in the light, where a random configuration of letters was presented on the inner surface of a sphere surrounding the subjects and permitting free exploratory eye and head movements. It should be noted that the center of spatial exploration by eye and head movements was located far more rightwards than the whole stimulus used by Behrmann et al. (1997), where the restricted horizontal dimension of the search display misled to the assumption of a gradient-like distribution. Actually, the average orientation of gaze was centered around 14.6° rightwards, head orientation around 26.3° rightwards and eye-in-head orientation around 13.2° rightwards, thus demonstrating the rightward bias of spatial representation for eye-, head- and body-centered coordinate frames. Unfortunately, the authors do not comment on how these results were related to the severity of neglect or to the location of lesions.

Do saccadic scan paths in neglect reflect oculomotor deficits or directional hypokinesia?

Quantitative analysis of saccades during visuo-spatial exploration in neglect has consistently demonstrated not only the rightward bias of spatial exploration with fewer fixations and shorter total fixation times in the left hemi-field, but also hypometric amplitudes of exploratory saccades and prolonged mean durations of single fixations (Chédru et al., 1973; Ishiai et al., 1987; Walker et al., 1996; Zihl and Hebel, 1997), more pronounced after FEF lesions than after temporo-parietal lesions (Heide and Kömpf, 1998). However, the latter deficits were non-directional and not lateralized, i.e. hypometria of saccadic amplitudes concerned leftward and rightward saccades to an equal amount and the longer duration of single fixations was distributed uniformly across the horizontal meridian. Also the frequency of rightward and leftward saccades was about the same (Behrmann et al., 1997; Barton et al., 1998; Niemeier and Karnath, 2000; Husain et al., 2001). Thus the non-spatial deficits of exploratory saccades cannot account for the rightward spatial bias, and there is no evidence for directional hypokinesia or impaired programming of internally triggered exploratory saccades into the left hemi-space, nor for a direction-specific deficit to disengage attention from current fixation (Posner and Driver, 1992). In contrast, reflexive visually triggered saccades in parietal neglect patients have been shown to be delayed and sometimes hypometric into the contralesional hemi-field, in correlation with the severity of neglect (Girotti et al., 1983; Braun et al., 1992; Heide and Kömpf, 1998). Walker et al. (1996) had provided good evidence that this abnormal eye movement pattern is a consequence of neglect rather than its cause. It affects primarily the initiation and planning of leftward saccades, not their execution (Behrmann et al., 2002a). It is coded relative to the current position of gaze (oculocentrically), but modulated by eye-in-head position (Behrmann et al., 2002b).

What causes multiple re-fixations in the ipsilesional field?

Already in simple cancellation tests (Weintraub and Mesulam, 1988), neglect patients perform their search inefficiently, without any obvious search strategy and with repeated re-cancellations of targets in the right half of the display. Recently, Wojciulik et al. (2001) tested a patient with right inferior frontal and basal ganglia damage with cancellation tasks. The marks were either visible — just as in bedside tests — or invisible. The stimulus consisted of meaningful objects and of meaningless circles. In the visible condition, some targets on the left side were missed, but there were nearly no re-cancellations. In the invisible condition, cancellation of meaningful objects was comparable to the visible condition, but the meaningless circles were re-cancelled quite often, more on the right than on the left side. Wojciulik et al. concluded that non-spatial working memory (for meaningful objects) was intact, but spatial working memory could not retain the location of items already cancelled, if they were of the same shape (circles). Deficient spatial working memory could be an independent causative factor which, in addition to the rightward spatial bias, contributes to asymmetric visual search in neglect.

As an oculomotor correlate of these re-cancellations, multiple re-fixations of locations already searched in the ipsilesional half of the display have been found in quantitative eye movement studies of visual search in neglect by Behrmann et al. (1997) and by Zihl and Hebel (1997). The latter authors attributed them to a possible impairment of spatial working memory for target locations across saccadic eye movements. They found them predominantly in patients with frontal lesions, in association with a deficit in planning efficient search strategies. In contrast, parietal neglect patients were more impaired in taking advantage of perceptual grouping in dot displays to improve the visuo-spatial guidance of their scan path.

The finding of multiple re-fixations and impaired spatial working memory was addressed in detail by Husain et al. (2001) in a parietal neglect patient, performing serial search tasks (for the letters T among Ls) of various display sizes and various numbers of targets and distracters, thus of variable spatial working memory load. They found the re-fixation rate of targets correlated with the severity of neglect. Furthermore, subjects had to indicate each target by a mouse click, and the re-click rate of targets that had already been visited correlated not only with the severity of neglect, but also with the working memory load of the task. Thus a non-lateralized deficit of spatial working memory for target locations across the whole display appears to contribute to the neglect behavior of this patient, exacerbating the rightward bias by keeping him busy re-fixating and re-clicking on target locations in the right ipsilesional hemi-field that had already been searched before. The deficit of spatial working memory was confirmed by neuropsychological testing, whereas object-related working memory was found intact. The deficit might specifically affect transsaccadic spatial memory, i.e. the ability to update the spatial representation of targets for saccade-induced shifts of their retinal position and to retain these target locations in working memory across saccadic eye movements. This function is specifically controlled by an area in the right posterior parietal cortex, located lateral to the intraparietal sulcus, as was demonstrated by lesion and fMRI studies in humans (Heide et al., 1995, 2001).

In conclusion, abnormal exploration of space in left visual neglect is not restricted to the left contralesional hemi-field, but also involves the right ipsilesional hemi-field, which obviously is not 'healthy' like in homonymous hemianopia. Apart from 'hyperattention' for the ipsilesional field (Kinsbourne, 1993) and from deficient spatial working memory, the multiple re-fixations and re-clicks of ipsilateral targets might reflect compulsive motor perseveration, which has been documented in neglect patients with frontal or subcortical brain lesions (Na et al., 1999; Rusconi et al., 2002). However, Husain et al. (2001) present good evidence against this assumption, as multiple saccades and an average time interval of 15 s intervened between a click and a re-click on the same target. However, the question remained open if re-fixations could alternatively reflect two other deficits that have been found in neglect patients: first, a high-level deficit of motor planning, in terms of deficient search strategies (Weintraub and Mesulam, 1988; Zangemeister et al., 1995); second, a low-level deficit of exogenous attentional orienting, in terms of an impaired inhibition of return (Klein and MacInnes, 1999; Gilchrist and Harvey, 2000; Bartolomeo et al., 2001).

Conclusions and outstanding questions

It has become obvious during the last years that hemi-spatial neglect is a heterogeneous, multi-component and multi-modal disorder of spatial cognition, spatial orientation, and spatial exploration, resulting from damage to a number of cerebral structures, predominantly in the right parieto-temporal and frontal lobes. Neglect includes various visuo-perceptual, visuo-motor and cognitive deficits. As saccadic eye movements reflect the perceptual and cognitive processes underlying visual search for targets among distracters (Liversedge and Findlay, 2000), their recording permits the investigation of such processes involved in neglect and the determination of factors that guide visuo-spatial exploration. Previous research provides evidence that the following neglect-associated deficits might contribute to the abnormal pattern of exploratory saccades (scan path) during visual search: (1) an abnormal allocation of attention along the horizontal dimension, possibly following a left-to-right gradient; (2) a constant or variable rightward bias of spatial representation; (3) deficits of low-level mechanisms for reflexive orienting of attention: (a) an impaired pop-out effect in simple feature search, e.g. for color; (b) an impaired inhibition of return to locations already searched; (4) impaired spatial working memory for target locations across saccades; (5) loss of high-level strategies for systematic serial search, following a geometric scan path; (6) compulsive motor perseveration in the right hemi-field; (7) additional oculomotor deficits, e.g. hypometric exploratory saccades.

Now it remains to assess the differential contribution of these various mechanisms, their possible interactions, their relation to the severity of neglect, and the influence of lesion location in the fronto-premotor or temporo-parietal cortex. That was the objective for our study on 10 patients with manifest or recovered left visual hemineglect, due to right hemispheric stroke-induced cortical lesions. For color, form, and conjunction search we used abstract visual displays with different numbers of target and distracter items, thus keeping the difficulty and spatial working memory load of the task variable. This stimulus is appropriate for investigating the influence of different low-level (bottom-up) and high-level (top-down) factors on search performance and saccadic scan paths, activating both the fast (parallel) and the slow (serial) search mode, as outlined in Fig. 1. In contrast to previous studies we used color for feature search, because its strong pop-out effect induces nearly parallel processing mechanisms in healthy subjects (Treisman and Gelade, 1980; Wolfe et al., 1990; Wolfe, 1998). It is still unknown how this pop-out effect is affected in patients with hemi-spatial neglect. That might have a practical consequence: if the pop-out effect of color is still present in neglect, patients could improve their orientation in the home environment by coloring strategic points.

Methods

Subjects

In this study 10 patients and 10 healthy adult control subjects participated. All patients (mean age 63, range 31 to 77 years) had left visual neglect due to strokes in the territory of the right middle cerebral artery that had happened between 10 days and 2 years prior to investigation. Postischemic lesions were located either in the posterior temporo-parietal cortex (5 cases) or in the frontal lobe (5 cases), damaging either the FEF in the middle portion of the precentral gyrus or its efferences in the internal capsule. The severity of neglect was assessed using the German version of the Behavioral Inattention Test (BIT; Wilson et al., 1987). Accordingly, 5 patients (3 frontal, 2 parietal lesions) had moderate visual hemineglect, with a BIT score ranging between 80 and 160 (normal limit > 166; maximum score 170). The remaining 5 patients had already recovered from clinically manifest neglect and visual extinction, but most of them exhibited discrete symptoms during testing (BIT scores ranging between 161 and 170). All patients had a visual acuity above 0.7 and normal color perception (tested by means of Ishihara tables), 4 of them had moderate left hemiparesis. The control group consisted of 10 healthy adults with a visual acuity of at least 1.0 and normal color vision, and without any neurological or ophthalmic disease. All participants were naive with respect to the object of the study and gave their informed written consent, according to the Declaration of Helsinki. The experiment was performed in one session.

Stimuli and tasks

Visual stimuli were presented on a Sony Multiscan 17se II monitor at a 100 Hz refresh rate, generated by the Visual Stimulus Generator (VSG 2/4, Cambridge Research Systems Ltd.). The eye-to-screen distance was 60 cm. Visual features of presented stimulus items presented were color and form. Color was defined by CIE coordinates (red 0.601, 0.322; green 0.218, 0.579; blue 0.147, 0.07) as used by Zelinsky (1996). The objects' form feature was either a triangle, a square or a circle, each subtending 0.5° of visual angle. The objects were presented at a luminance of 5 cd/m^2 on a dark background (0.1 cd/m^2) in a dark room. The stimuli for visual search consisted of 40, 60, or 80 items, among which 0, 1, 4, or 8 targets had to be detected. The items were distributed randomly across the whole screen, subtending an area of 32 × 22°, with a distance of at least 1° between neighboring items. For the testing, a set of 84 different screens was created, each of them was presented once so that the whole session consisted of 84 single trials.

The task was to search for all targets with a specified feature such as color or form, or with a conjunction of color and form. Each test trial started with the presentation of the target, while subjects are fixating a central fixation point, followed by the presentation of the stimulus. Thus the ocular scan path of saccadic search started always from the center of the display. The subjects were instructed to search for all targets as accurately and fast as possible. In case of detecting a target, they had to press the left mouse button. After finishing the search in each trial, subjects had to press the right mouse button, and the stimulus disappeared. Subjects could now take a short break, and then start the next trial with a mouse click. Thus the test was self-paced. As subjects were wearing a scleral search coil during the testing, total recording time was limited to 30 min. All subjects performed the search tasks within this time. However, as the patients were impaired in these tasks and had deficits of sustained attention in addition to their neglect, they needed much more time than the controls. So many of them could perform only a limited number of trials, between 20 and 84 (mean 50), depending on their state.

Recording procedure

Eye and head movements were recorded in a 6-ft-diameter scleral search coil system (CNC Engineering, Seattle) using standard eye coils (Skalar, Delft, NL). The subject's head was not fixed tightly, but rested comfortably on a neck support during the experiment. Therefore head movements were recorded with a second search coil — which was attached to subject's head — and used to correct the data that were affected by head movements.

At the beginning of the session, the cornea of the subject's dominant eye (usually the right eye) was anaesthetized by a local anesthetic (Novesine®). The subject was now informed about the task and performed 12 test trials. Then the search coil was inserted and calibrated. At the end of the session a second calibration was performed. Then search coil was removed, not later than 30 min after its insertion, and the subjects were interviewed concerning their impressions and strategies.

Data storage and calibration

Eye movement data were digitized with a sampling rate of 500 Hz and stored in a binary format on the recording PC. Visual stimuli and the subjects' responses (per mouse click) were stored on the stimulus PC. The communication between the PCs guaranteed exact timing and joining both data files in the off-line analysis. In order to achieve highly accurate eye position data, a 9-point calibration was performed at the beginning and the end of the test run. Small non-linear distortions were corrected by means of a neural network algorithm using a parametric self-organizing map (PSOM) (Pomplun et al., 1994). The spatial accuracy of recorded eye position with respect to the stimulus display was always better than 0.4°, usually 0.15°.

Results

Fig. 2 shows typical saccadic scan paths during conjunction (Fig. 2a,b) and color search (Fig. 2c,d) of a normal subject (Fig. 2a,c) and two patients with manifest neglect, one with a right frontal and the other with a right parietal lesion (Fig. 2b,d, respectively). Saccadic scanning starts always from the center. Each single fixation is surrounded by an open circle, the size of which is proportional to the duration of fixation. In conjunction search for the green circle, the normal subject uses a line-wise back-and-forth strategy of systematic serial scanning. Nevertheless his search is guided by the pop-out effect of the color, as on his way he fixates also green squares or

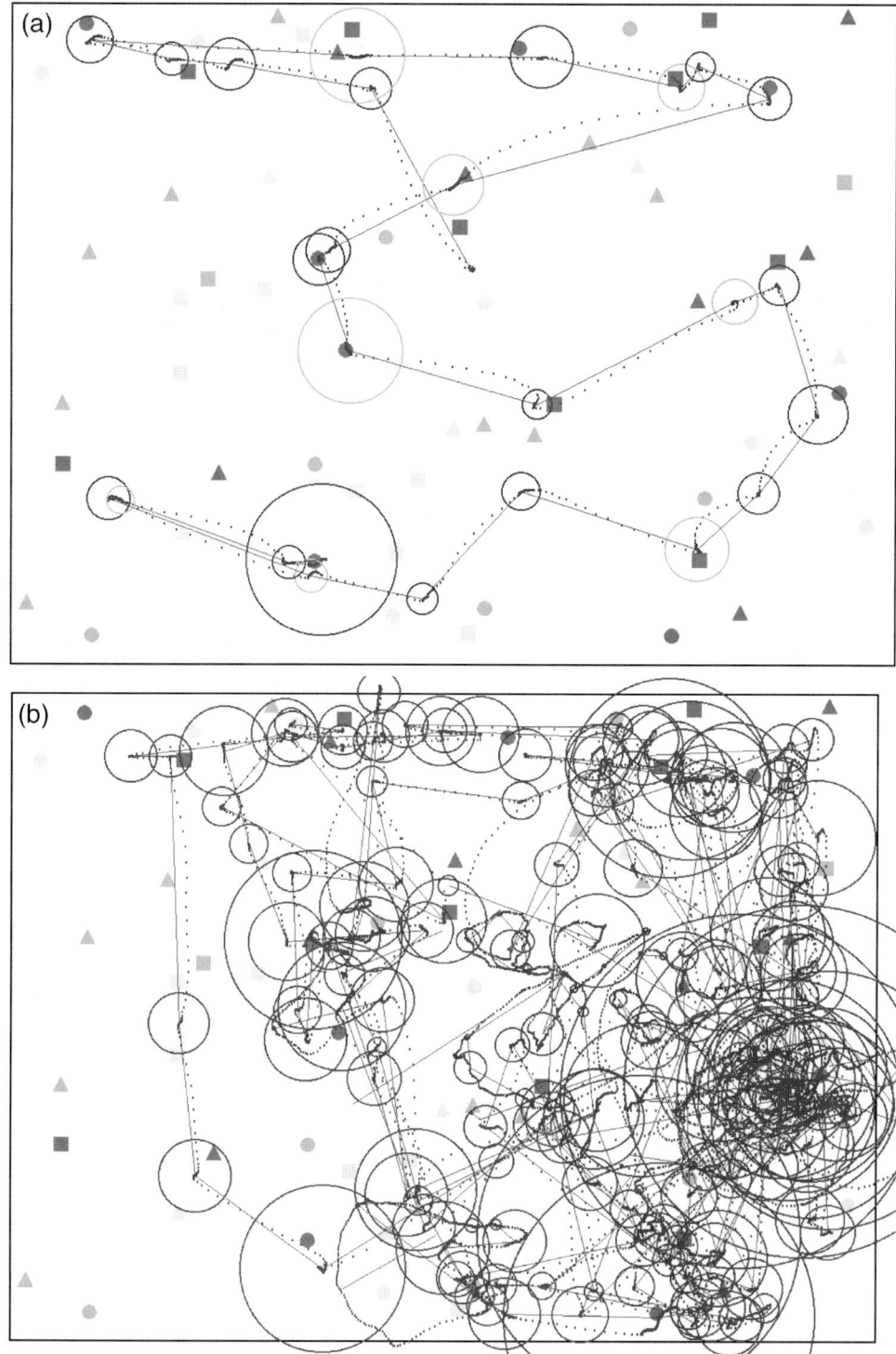

Fig. 2. (a–d) Examples of saccadic scan paths recorded during visual search in a control subject (a,c), in a patient with a right frontal lesion around the FEF (b), and in a patient with a right parieto-temporal lesion (d). Tasks were conjunction search (green circle) in a,b and color search (all green items) in c,d. The display size was $32 \times 24°$ of visual angle. In the gray-scale plot, the darkest objects were

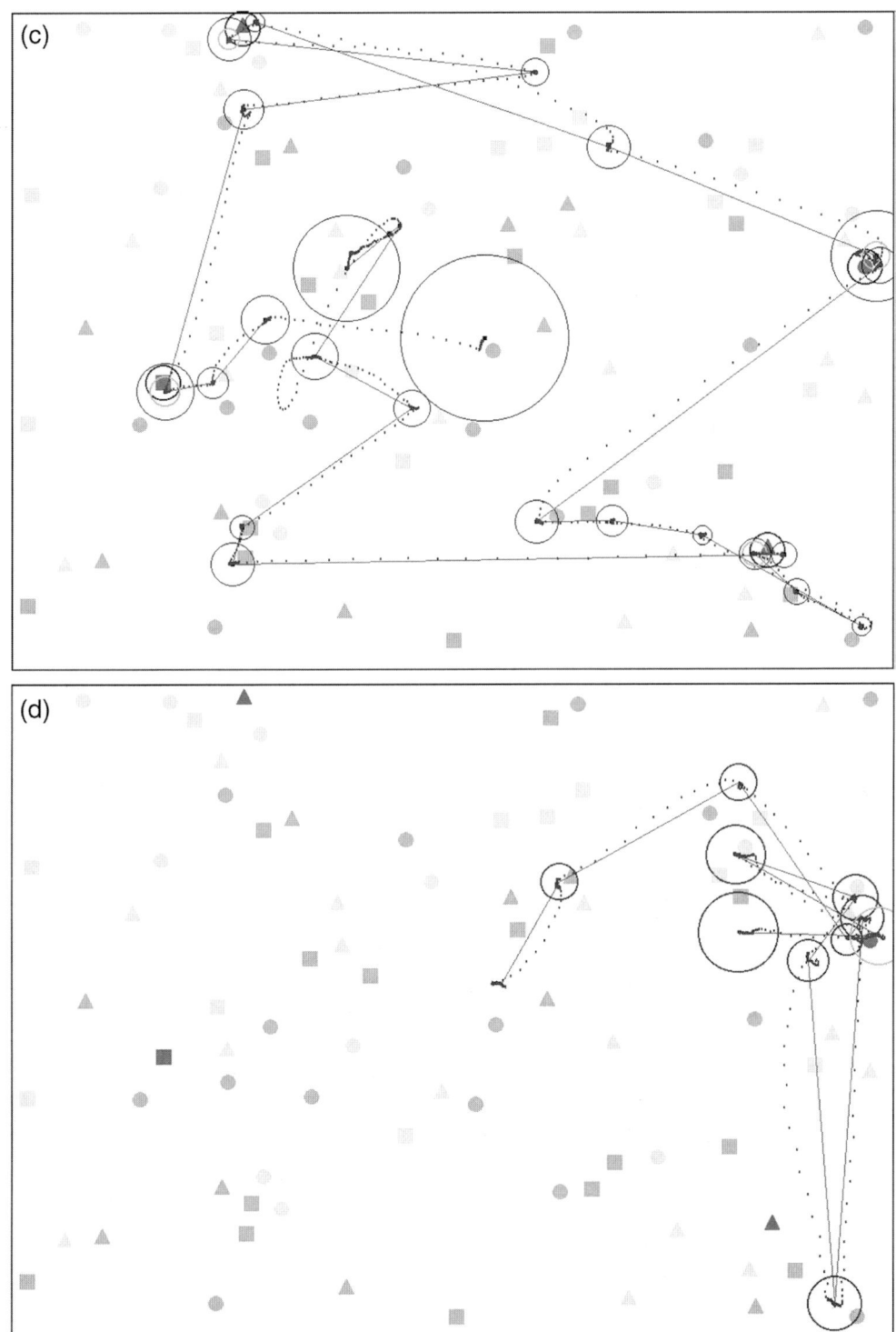

originally green, other objects were red and blue. The dotted lines plot the two-dimensional eye movement traces, superimposed on the stimulus. Solid lines were added to connect single fixations, for the sake of clarity. Circles around dots indicate the duration of single fixations.

triangles. His color search (for green items, Fig. 2c) uses about the same number of fixations, but for double the number of items, thus being more efficient than conjunction search. The scan path (circular) is less regular than in conjunction search, because it is interrupted by large saccades towards the green targets, induced by their pop-out effect. In both tasks, all targets were fixated and clicked upon once, without any re-fixations.

In contrast, the parietal patient (Fig. 2d) fixates only one out of four targets during color search and completely neglects the left half of the display, in spite of two pop-out targets. Obviously the pop-out effect was lost for left hemi-space and reduced for the right, as there were hardly any large targeting saccades. Her scan path reflects a strong rightward bias: starting from the center she immediately orients rightwards and performs a few re-fixations near the right edge. The patient with the right FEF lesion exhibited a totally different behavior in conjunction search (Fig. 2b): he scanned almost the whole display, except its uttermost left portion, and fixated seven out of eight targets, but nevertheless his scan path reflects a strong rightward bias, because he performed a tremendous number of re-fixations predominantly in the right hemi-field, in a chaotic manner, without any obvious search strategy. Re-fixations culminate around a target located near the right edge of the display so frequently that perseverative behavior cannot be excluded. The patient appears unable to retain the location of this target in working memory, as well as the fact that he had already searched there, thus indicating deficient spatial working memory across saccades. This assumption is supported by the elevated re-click rate of 0.57 (number of re-clicks per number of clicked targets). Due to the high number of saccades and to the much longer duration of single fixations, his total search time was massively prolonged. Nevertheless his scan path was obviously guided by the pop-out effect of any green target, and in color search he performed much better. Thus in contrast to the parietal patient, pop-out search appears to be largely preserved after frontal lesions. To confirm these single-case observations we will now present quantitative results of behavioral performance and eye movement analysis for the whole group.

Search duration

Search duration was measured from the appearance of the stimulus to the moment when subjects pressed the right mouse button to indicate that the search was finished. For statistics, the design of the study required a $3 \times 4 \times 3 \times 2$ ANOVA (three different quantities of items, four different quantities of targets, three different tasks, two groups [controls and patients]). These data revealed significant differences for the factors 'group' ($F(1, 1245) = 515.04$, $p < 0.001$), 'task' ($F(2, 1245) = 90.36$, $p < 0.001$), 'number of targets' ($F(3, 1245) = 27.89$, $p < 0.001$), and 'number of items' ($F(2, 1245) = 9.37$, $p < 0.001$). There were significant interactions between the factors 'group' and 'number of targets' ($F(3, 1245) = 7.65$, $p < 0.001$) and 'group' by 'task' ($F(2, 1245) = 12.98$, $p < 0.001$), but not between other factors. This means that search duration was generally prolonged in the patients, by about a factor of 3, but the strength of this effect depended on the task (more pronounced in color search). For patients and controls, search duration increased with increasing numbers of items or targets, thus with the spatial working memory load of the task. This was true for all tasks including color search, indicating that even pop-out search is not completely parallel, neither in control subjects nor in neglect patients. Analyzing the effect of the task on patients' search duration yielded only a few significant differences: search duration was shorter for color search compared to form or conjunction search in the 60-item condition with targets absent ($F(2, 40) = 5.08$, $p < 0.01$; see Table 1) and in the 80-item condition with targets absent ($F(2, 33) = 10.79$, $p < 0.001$). In all other conditions the patients' search duration did not differ significantly between the tasks, indicating that the patients were impaired in taking advantage of the pop-out effect of color. In contrast, in the control group search duration was always shorter for color search compared to form or conjunction search (always $p < 0.001$).

Rightward bias of eye fixations

To quantify the rightward bias of spatial representation and to reflect the allocation of visuo-spatial attention across the stimulus display, we plotted the relative distribution of eye fixations along the hor-

TABLE 1

Mean total search duration (in s) — standard deviations are given in brackets

	Controls			Patients		
Set size:	40	60	80	40	60	80
Color	1.9 (0.8)	2.4 (1.1)	3.0 (2.9)	6.8 (3.6)	7.2 (5.6)	5.7 (4.9)
Conjunction	4.3 (1.6)	5.1 (1.7)	6.0 (1.5)	12.6 (7.2)	13.8 (6.8)	16.9 (5.8)
Form	5.4 (1.1)	6.4 (1.8)	7.3 (2.1)	15.6 (12.2)	16.9 (10.2)	13.4 (6.5)

izontal meridian in Fig. 3, in terms of the relative frequency (percentage) of postsaccadic eye positions within each 1°-interval of horizontal eccentricity, weighted by the duration of fixations. When assessed accordingly, the median horizontal eye position is significantly shifted rightwards by about 5° in patients with manifest neglect, compared to control subjects and patients in remission whose distribution of fixations was symmetrical, centered around primary position [ANOVA 3 × 3 × 3 (neglect × task × set size), $F(2, 171) = 147.3$, $p < 0.001$]. The slope of the asymmetrical distribution of eye positions in manifest neglect (Fig. 3C) shows a continuous gradient from left to right, but — in contrast to Kinsbourne's model — reaches its maximum not at the right edge of the stimulus, but already at about 13° rightward eye position. It should be noted that the rightward bias was not invariant across the search tasks, but increased (by about 2°) with the spatial working memory load of the task, in terms of set size (number of items). However, though being significant for single trials within subjects, this set size effect did not reach the level of significance ($p = 0.162$) for the whole group, due the low number of subjects. The same was true for the number of targets. The three different tasks, however, did not at all modulate the rightward bias: neither did the pop-out effect of right targets induce more right fixations in color search, compared to the other tasks, nor did the high similarity of targets and distracters in the more difficult form search increase the rightward bias. Further, there was no significant influence of lesion location.

In accordance with the rightward bias, the difference of mean total fixation duration between the two hemi-fields was only significant for the group of patients with manifest neglect in color search ($T = -4.7$, df = 6, $p = 0.003$) and in conjunction search ($T = -2.5$, df = 6, $p = 0.048$).

Duration of single fixations

Following Kinsbourne's gradient model of attentional allocation in neglect, with the assumption of hyperattention in the ipsilesonal hemi-field, it would be plausible to expect longer durations of single fixations in the right hemi-field, compared to the left. This might have been true for the patient's performance in Fig. 2b and possibly for some of the cases reported by Behrmann et al. (1997), but there was no significant ($p > 0.25$) hemi-field effect in our groups of subjects and patients, neither in the different subgroups. However, mean fixation duration was significantly ($p < 0.0005$) prolonged in patients with manifest neglect, more in the frontal (328 ± 52 ms) than in the parietal group (303 ± 25 ms), compared to the control group (229 ± 26 ms) and to patients with recovered neglect (227 ± 21 ms). In accordance with earlier studies (Heide and Kömpf, 1998), we interpret this as a non-spatial deficit of initiating exploratory saccades. Though being maximal in frontal neglect, the deficit is more associated with the presence of manifest neglect than with lesion location. Also the type of search task did not modulate fixation duration in our patients, only the control subjects tended to fixate a bit longer in color search, in association with larger saccadic amplitudes, compared to the other tasks.

Direction of saccades while searching

As shown by Gilchrist and Harvey (2000) or in our previous study (Sprenger et al., 2001) as well as in the preceding chapter of this book by Huestegge and co-workers, a systematic serial search induces more saccades in orthogonal directions, predominantly horizontal, whereas in pop-out (color) search a more uniform distribution of saccades across or-

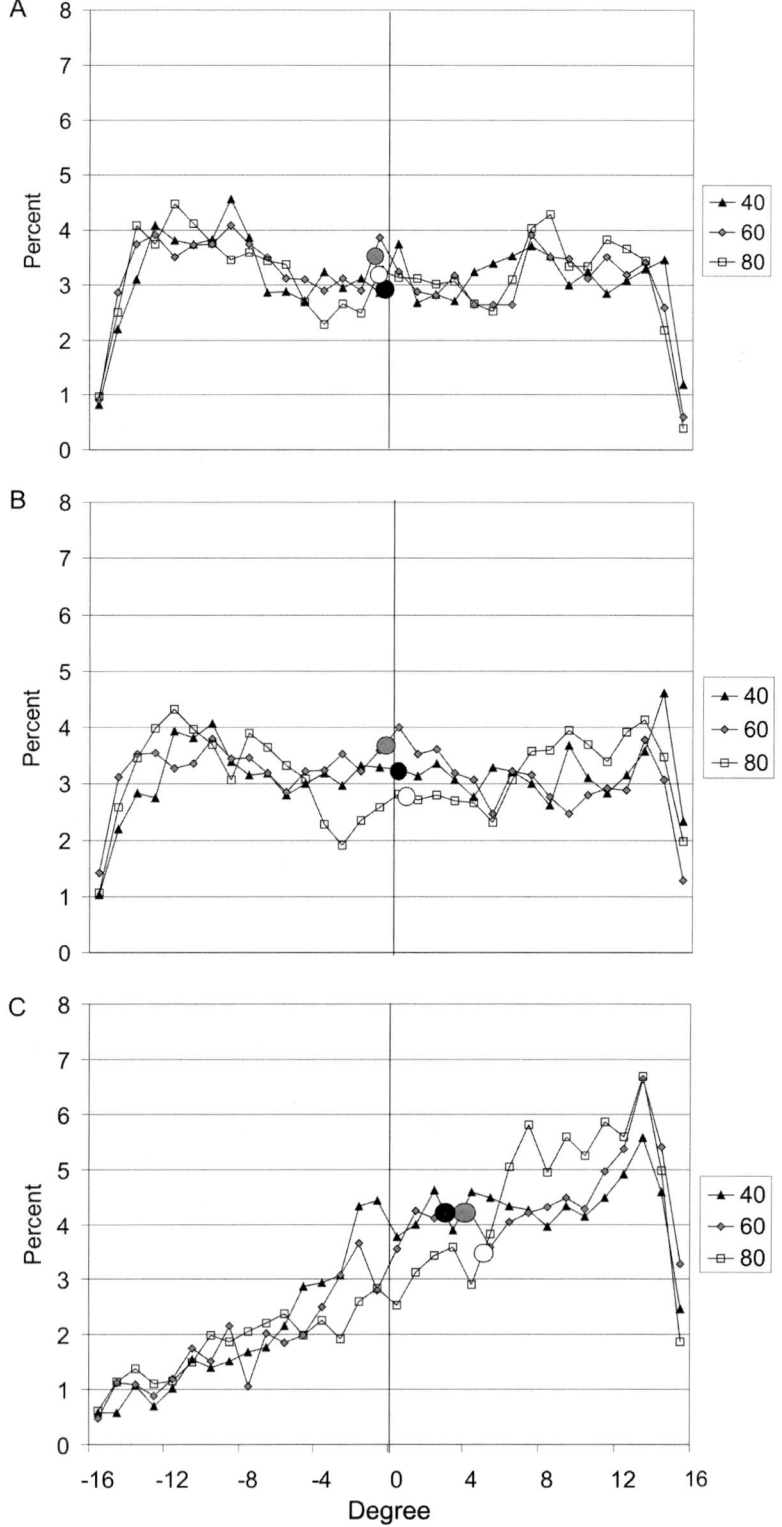

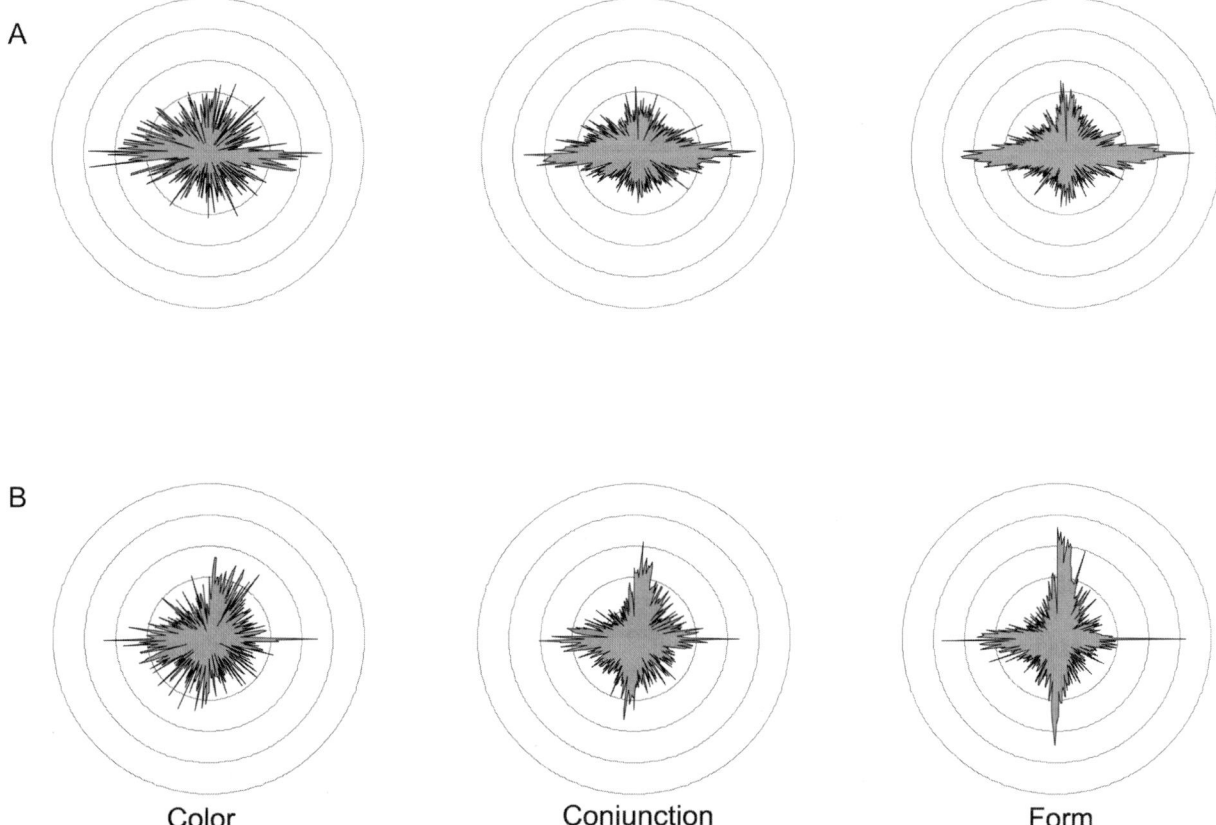

Color Conjunction Form

Fig. 4. Relative frequency of saccades (in percent of the total number of saccades) by direction: (A) control subjects, (B) patients. Each circle indicates 0.2%, so the outer circle represents 1%.

thogonal and oblique directions can be observed (Fig. 4A). Our neglect patients show similar results with a distinct overrepresentation of saccades into the right-upwards direction (Fig. 4B).

This presentation of data in polar plots is one possible attempt to quantify search strategies, but it requires cautious interpretation. Gilchrist and Harvey (2000) concluded that a nearly equal distribution of saccades by direction indicates an unsystematic irregular search, but a systematic circular scanning strategy would produce the same distribution. Even though our neglect patients show a clear orthogonal structure of their saccade distribution in conjunction and form search (Fig. 4B), with only a tendency of fewer horizontal saccades than the control group, hardly any structured search strategies could be found during visual inspection of their scan paths. The loss of geometric strategies was most pronounced in patients with frontal neglect and multiple re-fixations.

It has been a matter of debate whether patients with unilateral visual neglect perform less saccades

---

Fig. 3. Left–right distribution of the mean frequency of postsaccadic horizontal eye positions (plotted on the y-axis in percent relative to the total number of saccades), for each fixation weighted by its duration, sampled in 1°-intervals of horizontal eccentricity (plotted on the x-axis): (A) control group, (B) patients with recovered or subclinical neglect, (C) patients with manifest neglect. Large dots indicate the median horizontal eye positions for each set size (40, 60, and 80 items).

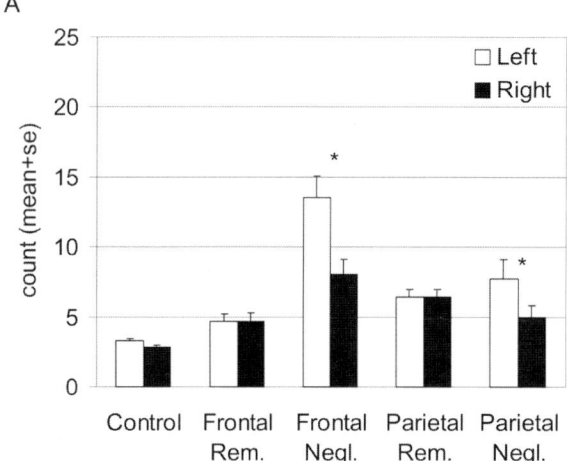
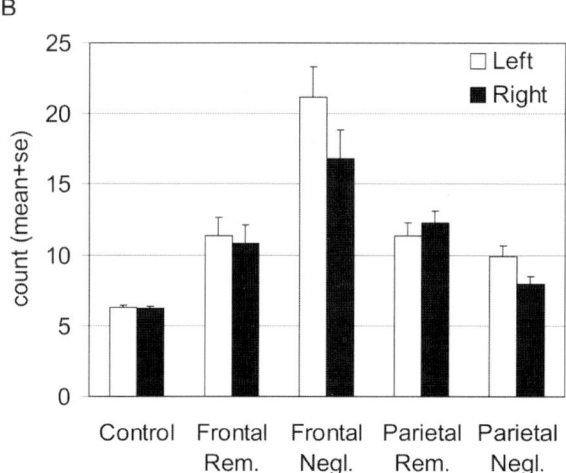
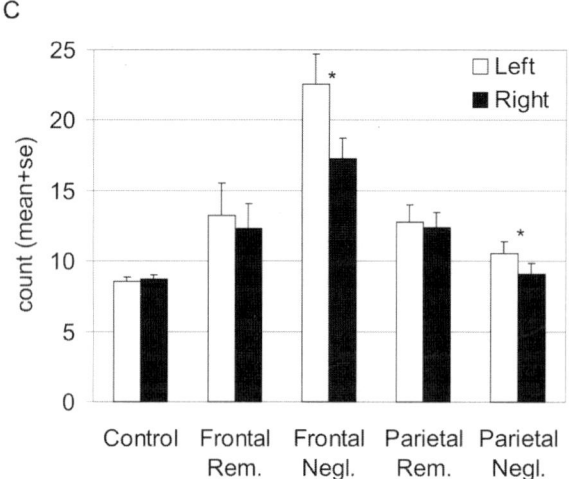

into the neglected hemi-field during visual exploration in a search task or rather multiple small-amplitude saccades (Chédru et al., 1973; Ishiai et al., 1987; Behrmann et al., 1997; Niemeier and Karnath, 2000). We categorized all saccades depending on which of the four orthogonal directions was predominant. The four classes were separated by the four oblique (45°) axes. A comparison of left- and rightward saccades (Fig. 5) shows a significantly ($p < 0.05$) larger number of leftward saccades in the subgroups of patients with manifest neglect in color and form search, most pronounced in the frontal group. This implies a higher frequency of small-step leftward saccades, depending primarily on the presence of manifest neglect and, less critically, on the frontal lesion site, thus not constituting a primary oculomotor deficit. Apart from this, compared to the control group, all groups of patients performed significantly more saccades in both directions, most obviously in frontal neglect. Statistical analysis of saccadic amplitudes yielded no significant directional differences between leftward and rightward saccades, in accordance with the study by Niemeier and Karnath (2000). There was only a mild tendency for hypometric leftward saccades during color search in patients with manifest neglect.

Amplitudes of target saccades reflect the pop-out effect of color

Besides quantifying search strategies, it is important to find an eye movement parameter for quantifying the pop-out effect in color search. As mentioned in Fig. 2c, the pop-out effect of the target color attracts the focus of attention even over large distances towards the current fixation point. Therefore large-amplitude saccades towards the targets ('target saccades') can be expected. However, it is not trivial to categorize a saccade as a target-saccade. Husain et al. (2001) as well as Gilchrist and Harvey (2000) defined a distance of less than 1° between the

Fig. 5. Mean number of saccades (on the *y*-axis) for both horizontal directions, including all saccades directed between 45° upwards and 45° downwards. Top (A): color search; middle (B): conjunction search; bottom (C): form search; * indicates a significant difference between left- and rightward saccades ($p < 0.05$).

endpoint of a saccade and the target to classify the saccade as target-related. Maioli et al. (2001) considered saccades as foveation saccades when they landed in a circular area of 3.66° around the item or the target (twice the diameter of the stimulus item). These methods assume that the focus of attention ('spotlight') has a circular shape, which is still an unproven hypothesis. The size of this circle has been shown to depend not only on target size, but also on the duration of fixation, on the density of items and on possible pop-out effects. At minimum, its size may be derived from the size of the fovea centralis, which is usually about 2° in diameter. Nevertheless, humans are able to shift their attention covertly, i.e. without eye movements (Hoffman, 1998), to objects that are further away than 1° while keeping the eyes fixating. As a compromise, we defined the size of the circle by 2° radius modulated by the duration of fixation: at a duration of 200 ms the size was unchanged, lower durations reduced the size down to 1°, longer fixations increased it up to 4° radius. This is in line with monkey data by Motter and Belky (1998a,b) whose measurements of detection performance during active visual search identified a zone of focal attention with a radius of about twice the average nearest neighbor distance (which ranged between 1° and 2° in our study), thus being controlled by the density of items. In addition, items with a pop-out color were available to guide search even from outside the region of focal attention.

Hence, we computed the items and targets within the calculated focus of attention for each saccade and thus managed to identify saccades towards targets. When doing this, it must be taken into account that target saccades with large amplitudes may be succeeded by one or two corrective saccades. Therefore the critical target saccade, induced by the pop-out feature of the target, may be one of the three last saccades towards target location. So we took the maximum amplitude out of these three saccades as the amplitude of the target saccade. The mean amplitudes of target saccades for each subgroup are plotted in Fig. 6 for the color, conjunction, and form search, respectively. In the control group the pop-out effect of color search is obviously reflected in significantly ($p < 0.0005$) larger amplitudes, compared to the other two tasks (11.5° versus 8.6°). This effect is preserved in both frontal groups ($p < 0.01$), dimin-

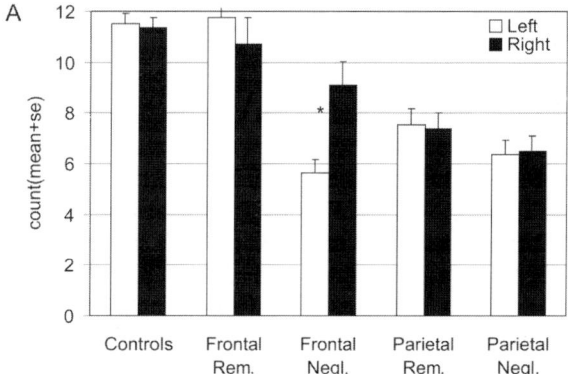
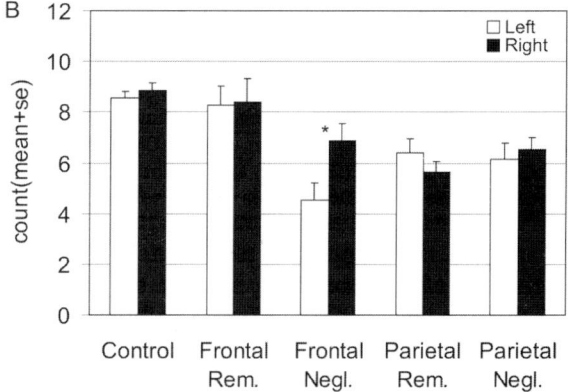
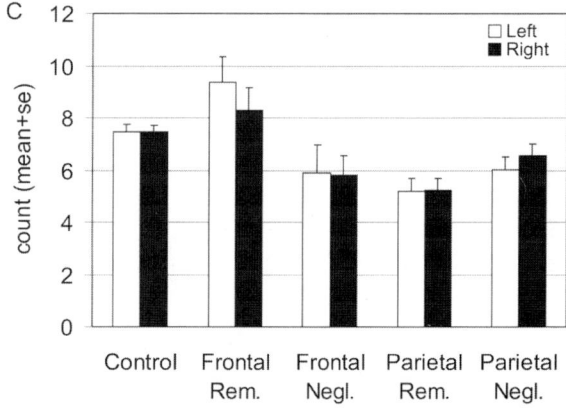

Fig. 6. Mean amplitudes of targeting saccades, calculated from the largest amplitude out of the three last saccades towards each target: (A) color search task, (B) conjunction search task, (C) form search task.

ished in the recovered parietal group, but completely absent in the parietal neglect group for both leftward and rightward saccades. This important finding indicates a non-directional loss of the pop-out effect in patients with right parieto-temporal lesions, which is evident even after recovery from manifest neglect, reflected in a significantly reduced amplitude of target saccades in color search, compared to normal subjects and to patients with frontal lesions. This deficit of reflexive attentional orienting might be critical for these patients' search performance, inducing a more serial search strategy and acting together with the rightward spatial bias to exacerbate neglect. Another finding was a directional deficit in terms of reduced amplitudes of leftward target saccades in patients with manifest frontal neglect ($p < 0.05$). This specific effect has not been reported in earlier search studies and might be explained as a consequence of the right FEF lesion resulting in hypometric voluntary saccades into the contralesional direction.

Re-fixations of items and targets

Control subjects scanned the serial search stimuli in a systematic manner, using a geometric strategy (scan path) and keeping the scanned locations in their working memory. Hence only a few number of re-fixations of items can be observed. Patients with hemineglect re-fixate items and target often, more in frontal than in parietal neglect (Fig. 2; Husain et al., 2001; Zihl and Hebel, 1997). Quantitative data analysis revealed that all our patient groups had elevated re-fixation rates, compared to controls, but patients with manifest frontal neglect performed significantly more re-fixations than all the other groups (Fig. 7). Their re-fixation rate increased with increasing working memory load of the task, reflected in an increasing number of targets.

This finding argues against the view that motor perseveration might cause these re-fixations, for two reasons: first, the number of targets is not immediately visible or obvious for the patient, so there is no reason why it should increase motor perseveration; second, the correlation with the working memory demands indicates rather a deficit of spatial working memory across saccades, most prominent in patients with frontal neglect, but present also in the other groups. In line with this, functional imaging studies have shown that spatial working memory is represented in a widely distributed network of fronto-parietal cortical areas (LaBar et al., 1999). As the deficit was still present when manifest neglect had recovered, we consider it as an independent factor that, in combination with the rightward bias, exacerbates neglect behavior in visual search. Such a deficit has been documented also with classical neuropsychological testing (Husain et al., 2001). In how far also an impaired inhibition of return (as

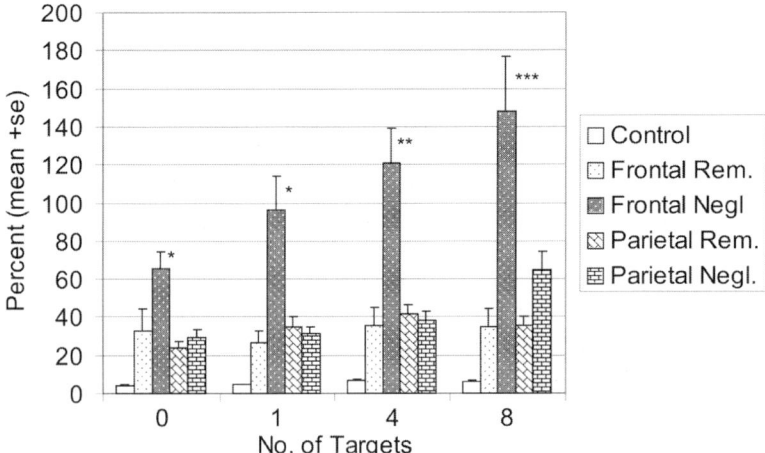

Fig. 7. Refixation rate of items, relative to the number of fixated items, plotted separately for the different numbers of targets, thus for different spatial working memory load. Control subjects re-fixated items significantly less than all groups of patients ($p < 0.01$). The group with frontal neglect has significantly (see stars) higher re-fixation rates than all other groups, and they increase significantly with the number of targets ($p = 0.032$).

demonstrated in neglect by Bartolomeo et al., 2001) contributes to the high re-fixation rate, cannot be decided from our data and requires further research. In frontal neglect, the deficit of working memory appears to coincide with a profound impairment in using systematic strategies for visual search. These two deficits exacerbate each other: the less a patient can rely on high-level strategies, the more he has to rely on spatial working memory to avoid repeated scanning of visited locations (Gilchrist and Harvey, 2000). This might be the reason why patients with frontal neglect performed so badly in this respect. Their abnormal search behavior cannot be attributed to impaired spatial updating of target locations across saccades based on deficient efference copy information, as this deficit has been found specifically in patients with posterior parietal lesions (Heide et al., 1995).

Final conclusions

Several recent studies on visual search in neglect have demonstrated that the eye movement analysis of the saccadic scan path provides insight into various perceptual, cognitive and visuo-motor processes underlying the multifaceted syndrome of hemi-spatial neglect. There is multiple evidence that the disorder of visual hemineglect is not restricted to the contralesional left hemi-field, but implies profound deficits of visual exploration and spatial cognition also in the right ipsilesional field. Using standardized visual displays of non-semantic items and distracters, we could modify a number of bottom-up and top-down influences on visual search in a controlled manner and measure how these factors are reflected in the saccadic scan paths. According to our data, the following mechanisms contribute to left hemineglect in visual search. Though probably arising from independent sources, influenced by the location of lesions, they are intimately related to each other and interact in contributing to the manifestation of neglect.

(1) The rightward bias of spatial orientation is not invariant, but increases with the working memory load of the task. The distribution of attention and eye fixations along the horizontal meridian appears to mimic a continuous left-to-right gradient, if only the central 20° of horizontal eccentricity are investigated, like in our study. Other studies (Karnath et al., 1998) measured the complete field of gaze and found a bell-shaped distribution around the shifted egocentric midline.

(2) Multiple refixations, most pronounced in frontal neglect, reflect dysfunction of systematic search strategies and of transsaccadic spatial working memory, even after recovery from manifest neglect. In how far these effects are confounded by impaired inhibition of return, requires further research. However, there was no clear evidence that compulsive motor perseveration causes the re-fixations. Anyway, these results confirm the critical role of the FEF for intentional serial search.

(3) In contrast, neglect after parieto-temporal lesions is specifically associated with impaired reflexive orienting of attention, reflected in a deficient popout effect and hypometric targeting saccades, thus a shrunken zone of focal visual attention, that can be found even after recovery from manifest neglect.

(4) Neglect-like saccadic exploration during visual search cannot generally be attributed to primary oculomotor deficits. However, there was evidence for an increased number of hypometric leftward exploratory saccades specifically in patients with manifest frontal neglect, following lesions around the FEF. Previous investigators did not find this deficit (Niemeier and Karnath, 2000; Husain et al., 2001), as they examined primarily parietal neglect patients.

Some of our questions remain open so far. Last but not least, this might be because groups of neglect patients are always heterogeneous, and some of the patients are not able to cooperate throughout the whole testing session, due to their limited resources of sustained attention. By applying specific paradigms of visual search to larger numbers of patients, future research should continue to disentangle the contribution of multiple mechanisms to the syndrome of visual neglect, and to identify underlying critical deficits that can be a basis for rehabilitative training, according to the specific manifestation of the syndrome in each individual patient.

References

Aglioti, S., Smania, N., Barbieri, C. and Corbetta, M. (1997) Influence of stimulus salience and attentional demands on visual search patterns in hemispatial neglect. *Brain Cogn.*, 34: 388–403.

Bartolomeo, P., Siéroff, E., Decaix, C. and Chokron, S. (2001) Modulating the attentional bias in unilateral neglect: the effects of the strategic set. *Exp. Brain Res.*, 137: 432–444.

Barton, J.S.J., Behrmann, M. and Black, S. (1998) Ocular search during line bisection. The effects of hemi-neglect and hemianopia. *Brain*, 121: 1117–1131.

Behrmann, M., Watt, S., Black, S.E. and Barton, J.J. (1997) Impaired visual search in patients with unilateral neglect: an oculographic analysis. *Neuropsychologia*, 35: 1445–1458.

Behrmann, M., Ghiselli-Crippa, T. and Di Matteo, I. (2002a) Impaired initiation, but not execution of contralesional saccades in hemispatial neglect. *Behav. Neurol.*, 13: 1–16.

Behrmann, M., Ghiselli-Crippa, T., Sweeney, J.A., Di Matteo, I. and Kass, R. (2002b) Mechanisms underlying spatial representation revealed through studies of hemispatial neglect. *J. Cogn. Neurosci.*, 14: 272–290.

Bisiach, E. and Vallar, G. (2000) Unilateral neglect in humans. In: F. Boller, J. Grafman and G. Rizzolatti (Eds.), *Handbook of Neuropsychology*. 2 ed., Vol. 1, Elsevier, Amsterdam, pp. 459–502.

Bisiach, E., Capitani, E., Luzzatti, C. and Perani, D. (1981) Brain and conscious representation of outside reality. *Neuropsychologia*, 19: 543–551.

Braun, D., Weber, H., Mergner, T. and Schulte-Monting, J. (1992) Saccadic reaction times in patients with frontal and parietal lesions. *Brain*, 115: 1359–1386.

Chédru, F., Léblanc, M. and Lhermitte, F. (1973) Visual searching in normal and brain damaged subjects: contributions to the study of unilateral inattention. *Cortex*, 9: 94–111.

De Renzi, E., Gentilini, M., Faglioni, P. and Barbieri, C. (1989) Attentional shift towards the rightmost stimuli in patients with left visual neglect. *Cortex*, 25: 231–237.

Donner, T.H., Kettermann, A., Diesch, E., Ostendorf, F., Villringer, A. and Brandt, S.A. (2002) Visual feature and conjunction searches of equal difficulty engage only partially overlapping frontoparietal networks. *Neuroimage*, 15: 16–25.

Eglin, M., Robertson, L.C. and Knight, R.T. (1991) Cortical substrates supporting visual search in humans. *Cereb. Cortex*, 1: 262–272.

Esterman, M., McGlinchey-Berroth, R. and Milberg, W. (2000) Preattentive and attentive visual search in individuals with hemispatial neglect. *Neuropsychology*, 14: 599–611.

Ferber, S. and Karnath, H.O. (2001) How to assess spatial neglect — line bisection or cancellation tasks? *J. Clin. Exp. Neuropsychol.*, 23: 599–607.

Findlay, J.M. (1997) Saccade target selection during visual search. *Vision Res.*, 37: 617–631.

Findlay, J.M. and Walker, R. (1999) A model of saccade generation based on parallel processing and competitive inhibition. *Behav. Brain Sci.*, 22: 661–721.

Grabowecky, M., Robertson, L.C. and Treisman, A. (1993) Preattentive processes guide visual search: evidence from patients with unilateral visual neglect. *J. Cogn. Neurosci.*, 5: 288-302.

Gilchrist, I.D. and Harvey, M. (2000) Refixation frequency and memory mechanisms in visual search. *Curr. Biol.*, 10: 1209–1212.

Girotti, F., Casazza, M., Musicco, M. and Avanzini, G. (1983) Oculomotor disorders in cortical lesions in man: the role of unilateral neglect. *Neuropsychologia*, 21: 543–553.

Harvey, M., Olk, B., Muir, K. and Gilchrist, I.D. (2002) Manual responses and saccades in chronic and recovered hemispatial neglect: a study using visual search. *Neuropsychologia*, 40: 705–717.

Heide, W. and Kömpf, D. (1998) Combined deficits of saccades and visuo-spatial orientation after cortical lesions. *Exp. Brain Res.*, 123: 164–171.

Heide, W., Blankenburg, M., Zimmermann, E. and Kömpf, D. (1995) Cortical control of double-step saccades — implications for spatial orientation. *Ann. Neurol.*, 38: 739–748.

Heide, W., Binkofski, F., Seitz, R.J., Posse, S., Nitschke, M.F., Freund, H.-J. and Kömpf, D. (2001) Activation of frontoparietal cortices during memorized triple-step sequences of saccadic eye movements: an fMRI study. *Eur. J. Neurosci.*, 13: 1177–1189.

Heilman, K.M., Watson, R.T. and Valenstein, E. (1993) Neglect and related disorders. In: K.M. Heilman and E. Valenstein (Eds.), *Clinical Neuropsychology*. 3rd ed., Oxford University Press, New York, pp. 279–336.

Hildebrandt, H., Giesselmann, H. and Sachsenheimer, W. (1999) Visual search and visual target detection in patients with infarctions of the left or right posterior or the right middle brain artery. *J. Clin. Exp. Neuropsychol.*, 21: 94–107.

Hoffman, J.E. (1998) Visual attention and eye movements. In: H. Pashler (Ed.), *Attention*. Psychology Press, Hove, pp. 119–153.

Hooge, I.T. and Frens, M.A. (2000) Inhibition of saccade return (ISR): spatio-temporal properties of saccade programming. *Vision Res.*, 40: 3415–3426.

Hornak, J. (1992) Ocular exploration in the dark by patients with visual neglect. *Neuropsychologia*, 30: 547–552.

Horowitz, T.S. and Wolfe, J.M. (1998) Visual search has no memory. *Nature*, 394: 575–577.

Huestegge, L., Radach, R., Kunert, H.-J. and Heller, D. (2002) Visual search in long-term canabis users with early age of onset. In: J. Hyönä, D.P. Munoz, W. Heide and R. Radach (Eds.), The Brain's Eye: Neurobiological and Clinical Aspects of Oculomotor Research. Progress in Brain Research, Vol. 140, Elsevier, Amsterdam, pp. 377–394.

Husain, M. and Kennard, C. (1997) Distractor-dependent frontal neglect. *Neuropsychologia*, 35: 829–841.

Husain, M., Mannan, S., Hodgson, T., Wojciulik, E., Driver, J. and Kennard, C. (2001) Impaired spatial working memory across saccades contributes to abnormal search in parietal neglect. *Brain*, 124: 941–952.

Ishiai, S., Furukawa, T. and Tsukagoshi, H. (1987) Eye-fixation patterns in homonymous hemianopia and unilateral spatial neglect. *Neuropsychologia*, 25: 675–679.

Ishiai, S., Seki, K., Koyama, Y. and Gono, S. (1996) Ineffective leftward search in line bisection and mechanisms of left unilateral spatial neglect. *J. Neurol.*, 243: 381–387.

Karnath, H.O. (1994a) Subjective body orientation in neglect and the interactive contribution of neck muscle proprioception and vestibular stimulation. *Brain*, 117: 1001–1012.

Karnath, H.O. (1994b) Spatial limitation of eye movements during ocular exploration of simple line drawings in neglect syndrome. *Cortex*, 30(2): 319–330.

Karnath, H.O. (1997) Spatial orientation and the representation of space with parietal lobe lesions. *Philos. Trans. R. Soc. Lond. B Biol. Sci.*, 352: 1411–1419.

Karnath, H.O. and Fetter, M. (1995) Ocular space exploration in the dark and its relation to subjective and objective body orientation in neglect patients with parietal lesions. *Neuropsychologia*, 33: 371–377.

Karnath, H.O., Niemeier, M. and Dichgans, J. (1998) Space exploration in neglect. *Brain*, 121: 2357–2367.

Karnath, H.O., Ferber, S. and Himmelbach, M. (2001) Spatial awareness is a function of the temporal not the posterior parietal lobe. *Nature*, 411: 950–953.

Kerkhoff, G. (2001) Spatial hemineglect in humans. *Prog. Neurobiol.*, 63: 1–27.

Kim, M., Anderson, J.M. and Heilman, K.M. (1997) Search patterns using the line bisection test for neglect. *Neurology*, 49: 936–940.

Kinsbourne, M. (1993) Orientational bias model of unilateral neglect: evidence from attentional gradients within hemispace. In: I.H. Robertson and J. Marshall (Eds.), *Unilateral Neglect: Clinical and Experimental Studies*. Erlbaum LEA Publishers, Hove, pp. 63–86.

Klein, R.M. and MacInnes, W.J. (1999) Inhibition of return is a foraging facilitator in visual search. *Psychol. Sci.*, 10: 346–352.

LaBar, K.S., Gitelman, D.R., Parrish, T.B. and Mesulam, M. (1999) Neuroanatomic overlap of working memory and spatial attention networks: a functional MRI comparison within subjects. *Neuroimage*, 10: 695–704.

Liversedge, S.P. and Findlay, J.M. (2000) Saccadic eye movements and cognition. *Trends Cogn. Sci.*, 4: 6–14.

Maioli, C., Benaglio, I., Siri, S., Sosta, K. and Cappa, S. (2001) The integration of parallel and serial processing mechanisms in visual search: evidence from eye movement recording. *Eur. J. Neurosci.*, 13: 364–372.

Motter, B.C. and Belky, E.J. (1998a) The zone of focal attention during active visual search. *Vision Res.*, 38: 1007–1022.

Motter, B.C. and Belky, E.J. (1998b) The guidance of eye movements during active visual search. *Vision Res.*, 38: 1805–1815.

Na, D.L., Adair, J.C., Kang, Y., Chung, C.S., Lee, K.H. and Heilman, K.M. (1999) Motor perseverative behavior on a line cancellation task. *Neurology*, 52: 1569–1576.

Niemeier, M. and Karnath, H.O. (2000) Exploratory saccades show no direction-specific deficit in neglect. *Neurology*, 54: 515–518.

Noton, D. and Stark, L. (1971) Scanpaths in saccadic eye movements while viewing and recognizing patterns. *Vision Res.*, 11: 929–942.

Peterson, M.S., Kramer, A.F., Wang, R.F., Irwin, D.E. and McCarley, J.S. (2001) Visual search has memory. *Psychol. Sci.*, 12: 287–292.

Pomplun, M., Velichkovsky, B. and Ritter, H. (1994) An artificial neural network for high precision eye movement tracking. In: B. Nebel and L. Dreschler-Fischer (Eds.), *Lecture Notes in Artificial Intelligence: AI-94 Proceedings*. Springer, Berlin, pp. 63–69.

Posner, M.I. and Driver, J. (1992) The neurobiology of selective attention. *Curr. Opin. Neurobiol.*, 2: 165–169.

Posner, M.I., Walker, J.A., Friedrich, F.J. and Rafal, R.D. (1984) Effects of parietal injury on covert orienting of attention. *J. Neurosci.*, 4: 1863–1874.

Rizzo, M. and Hurtig, R. (1992) Visual search in hemineglect: What stirs idle eyes? *Clin. Vis. Sci.*, 7: 39–52.

Rizzolatti, G. and Berti, A. (1993) Neural mechanisms of spatial neglect. In: I.H. Robertson and J.C. Marshall (Eds.), *Unilateral Neglect: Clinical and Experimental Studies*. Erlbaum LEA Publishers, Hove, pp. 87–105.

Robertson, I.H., Manly, T., Beschin, N., Daini, R., Haeske-Dewick, H., Homberg, V., Jehkonen, M., Pizzamiglio, G., Shiel, A. and Weber, E. (1997) Auditory sustained attention is a marker of unilateral spatial neglect. *Neuropsychologia*, 35: 1527–1532.

Robertson, I.H., Mattingley, J.B., Rorden, C. and Driver, J. (1998) Phasic alerting of neglect patients overcomes their spatial deficit in visual awareness. *Nature*, 395(6698): 169–172.

Rusconi, M.L., Maravita, A., Bottini, G. and Vallar, G. (2002) Is the intact side really intact? Perseverative responses in patients with unilateral neglect: a productive manifestation. *Neuropsychologia*, 40: 594–604.

Scialfa, C.T. and Joffe, K.M. (1998) Response times and eye movements in feature and conjunction search as a function of target eccentricity. *Percept. Psychophys.*, 60: 1067–1082.

Sprenger, A., Kompf, D., Moschner, C. and Heide, W. (2001) Saccadic scan paths during visual search. In: J.A. Sharpe (Ed.), *Neuro-ophthalmology at the Beginning of the New Millennium*. Medimond, Englewood, NJ, pp. 191–206.

Treisman, A.M. and Gelade, G. (1980) A feature-integration theory of attention. *Cognit. Psychol.*, 12: 97–136.

Vallar, G. (1998) Spatial hemineglect in humans. *Trends Cogn. Sci.*, 2: 87–97.

Vallar, G. (2001) Extrapersonal visual unilateral spatial neglect and its neuroanatomy. *Neuroimage*, 14: S52–S58.

Vallar, G., Rusconi, M.L., Bignamini, L., Geminiani, G. and Perani, D. (1994) Anatomical correlates of visual and tactile extinction in humans: a clinical CT scan study. *J. Neurol. Neurosurg. Psychiatry*, 57: 464–470.

Ventre, J., Flandrin, J.M. and Jeannerod, M. (1984) In search for the egocentric reference. A neurophysiological hypothesis. *Neuropsychologia*, 22: 797–806.

Walker, R., Findlay, J.M., Young, A.W. and Lincoln, N.B. (1996) Saccadic eye movements in object-based neglect. *Cogn. Neuropsychol.*, 13: 569–615.

Weintraub, S. and Mesulam, M.M. (1988) Visual hemispatial inattention: stimulus parameters and exploratory strategies. *J. Neurol. Neurosurg. Psychiatry*, 51: 1481–1488.

Wilkinson, D.T., Halligan, P.W., Henson, R.N., Dolan, R.J. (2002) The effects of interdistracter similarity on search processes in superior parietal cortex. *Neuroimage*, 15: 611–619.

Williams, D.E., Reingold, E.M., Moscovitch, M. and Behrmann, M. (1997) Patterns of eye movements during parallel and serial visual search tasks. *Can. J. Exp. Psychol.*, 51: 151–164.

Wilson, B., Cockburn, J. and Halligan, P. (1987) Development of a behavioral test of visuospatial neglect. *Arch. Phys. Med. Rehabil.*, 68: 98–102.

Wojciulik, E., Husain, M., Clarke, K. and Driver, J. (2001) Spatial working memory deficit in unilateral neglect. *Neuropsychologia*, 39: 390–396.

Wolfe, J.M. (1994) Guided search 2.0 — a revised model of visual-search. *Psychonom. Bull. Rev.*, 1: 202–238.

Wolfe, J.M., Yu, K.P., Stewart, M.I., Shorter, A.D., Friedman-Hill, S.R. and Cave, K.R. (1990) Limitations on the parallel guidance of visual search: color × color and orientation × orientation conjunctions. *J. Exp. Psychol. Hum. Percept. Perform.*, 16: 879–892.

Zangemeister, W.H., Oechsner, U. and Freksa, C. (1995) Short-term adaptation of eye movements in patients with visual hemifield defects indicates high level control of human scanpath. *Optom. Vis. Sci.*, 72: 467–477.

Zelinsky, G.J. (1996) Using eye saccades to assess the selectivity of search movements. *Vision Res.*, 36: 2177–2187.

Zelinsky, G.J. and Sheinberg, D.L. (1997) Eye movements during parallel–serial visual search. *J. Exp. Psychol. Hum. Percept. Perform.*, 23: 244–262.

Zihl, J. and Hebel, N. (1997) Patterns of oculomotor scanning in patients with unilateral posterior parietal or frontal lobe damage. *Neuropsychologia*, 35: 893–906.

CHAPTER 28

Saccadic adaptation in neurological disorders

Michael R. MacAskill [1,2,*], Tim J. Anderson [1,2,3] and Richard D. Jones [1,2,4]

[1] *Christchurch Movement Disorders and Brain Research Group, Christchurch, New Zealand*
[2] *Department of Medicine, Christchurch School of Medicine and Health Sciences, P.O. Box 4345, Christchurch, New Zealand*
[3] *Department of Neurology, Christchurch Hospital, Private Bag 4710, Christchurch, New Zealand*
[4] *Department of Medical Physics and Bioengineering, Christchurch Hospital, Private Bag 4710, Christchurch, New Zealand*

Abstract: The role of saccadic adaptive processes in recovery from the effects of various neurological disorders, such as myasthenia gravis, extraocular muscle palsies, and age-related macular degeneration, is reviewed. Studies of clinical populations (e.g. cerebellar disease, mild closed head injury, and opsoclonus) in which intrasaccadic displacement of visual targets has been used to stimulate adaptation are also reviewed. Our own data from such a study of 12 subjects with Parkinson's disease are presented, showing that visually guided adaptation is preserved in PD while memory-guided adaptation is impaired. This supports a model in which different brain regions subserve adaptation in different tasks.

The need for adaptive tuning of motor output

The ability to make accurate movements is vital for successful functioning. For movements of a duration greater than one reaction time, sensory feedback can be used to monitor the trajectory in-flight and to make any necessary corrections while the movement is ongoing. Movements which are rapid enough to be completed in less than one reaction time cannot be corrected in-flight, and are known as ballistic or open-loop movements because they cannot be controlled during their execution using closed-loop perceptual feedback. To accurately perform ballistic movements, the brain must maintain a precise model of the efferent commands required to achieve a movement of a given amplitude. As this 'gain' of efference to amplitude will change over time, due to factors such as illness or aging, there must be a compensatory adaptive mechanism by which the brain can amend its gain model over time.

Adaptive control of ocular velocity

Adaptive processes are necessary throughout the nervous system to ensure that appropriate actions are taken in response to perceptual information. Even relatively simple systems such as the vestibular system must be capable of adaptive changes in order to maintain their accuracy:

"A fairly common example of the brain repairing itself is the recovery from a sudden peripheral vestibular lesion. Spontaneous nystagmus and dizziness result. These symptoms diminish over the next two to three weeks and, in a few months, not a trace of the disorder remains... Some part of the brain must sense it if our responses are no longer appropriate to the stimuli... It not only detects dysmetria but sets about at once to correct it... Such a process is adaptive because it restores proper function; it is plastic because the changes in behavior are semipermanent and it is a primitive form of learning by the brain." (Robinson, 1975, p. 413)

---

* Correspondence to: Department of Medicine, Christchurch School of Medicine, P.O. Box 4345, Christchurch, New Zealand. Tel.: +64-3-3640-640 extension 88138; Fax: +64-3-3640-935;
E-mail: michael.macaskill@ chmeds.ac.nz

Such adaptation does not occur solely in response to lesions of the nervous system. The simple act of putting on strong glasses can necessitate a similar correction (Robinson, 1975). The human VOR is so adaptable that in response to prolonged wearing of lateral reversing prisms, even its sign can be changed, resulting in compensatory eye movements in the *same* direction as head movements (Gonshor and Melvill Jones, 1976).

Adaptive control of the ocular position signal

A saccade to a given position requires a 'pulse' of innervation to drive the eyes to the target and an ongoing 'step' of innervation to maintain them there. If the size of the pulse and step are not matched, then the eyes will drift at the end of the saccade until they reach the position dictated by the step signal. A pulse–step mismatch can be simulated by making the visual field drift slowly at the end of a saccade, mimicking the effects of post-saccadic drift (Optican and Miles, 1985). Kapoula et al. (1989) found that their human subjects adapted to this stimulation (after 10,000–20,000 saccades) by developing a zero-latency post-saccadic drift in the same direction as the pattern motion. This presumably indicated that the step signal, indicating intended eye position following a saccade, can be adapted separately from the pulse signal, indicating the amplitude of the saccade.

Generally, however, the pulse and step signals are in agreement (Kommerell et al., 1976), and most studies of adaptation in the saccadic system assume that the phasic and tonic components of the neural saccade signal will change in concert with each other. It is this adaptation of overall saccade amplitude that is the concern of the remainder of this paper. Adaptive control of other eye movements (pursuit, vergence, and torsion) has been discussed recently by Takagi et al. (2001).

Adaptive control of saccade amplitude in central and peripheral disorders

In many motor tasks, we can choose to perform either fast or slow movements. The velocities of saccades, however, are not under conscious control (Bahill et al., 1975), and because they are too brief to be modified in-flight, saccades are always open-loop (unless slowed grossly by disease; Zee et al., 1976; MacAskill et al., 2000). There is, therefore, a unique requirement for the saccadic system to rely completely on open-loop learning processes to maintain its accuracy.

There are a number of neurological illnesses which reveal the action of adaptive processes attempting to maintain saccadic metricity. Myasthenia gravis, for example, is an autoimmune disease which attacks the acetylcholine receptor, leading to failed neuromuscular transmission and subsequent muscle weakness. Ocular manifestations of myasthenia gravis include ptosis, diplopia, and hypometria of large saccades (Leigh and Zee, 1999). That adaptive processes can at least partially counteract extraocular muscle weakness is shown by administration of edrophonium, which temporarily improves neuromuscular transmission. Following edrophonium, saccades often become hypermetric, as "the central nervous system has adaptively increased the size of the saccadic pulse in an attempt to overcome the myasthenic weakness... If the brain had been standing idly by, edrophonium would merely have caused refixations to become orthometric" (Leigh and Zee, p. 378).

A similar adaptation process was observed in a person subject to the sudden onset of a medial rectus paresis secondary to a partial third nerve palsy (Abel et al., 1978). Saccades made by the affected eye were initially hypometric but recovered to normal size over several days during which the patient was forced to use the affected eye while the good eye was patched. Similar results were found by Optican et al. (1985) in four patients with ocular muscle weakness. As the weak eye returned to normal accuracy, the patched, normal, eye became correspondingly overactive, indicating the presence of a central signal to both eyes (an effect also demonstrated by Kommerell et al., 1976). Optican et al. showed that this overactivity also occurred in pursuit movements: when the weak eye became able to follow a target moving at $15°/s$, the patched eye reached speeds of up to $50°/s$. Adaptive changes observed in the normal eye varied as a function of eye position and movement direction, consistent with the way in which the effects of ocular muscle weakness also vary with orbital position and with whether the muscle acts as an agonist or antagonist. The adaptation process cannot, therefore, arise from a simple global parametric change in innervation.

The purpose of a saccade is to direct the fovea to the intended point of fixation, and thus adaptation of saccade size may be required in response to sensory as well as motor pathology. An example is age-related macular degeneration, which is the leading cause of blindness among the elderly in Europe and North America (Cheraskin, 1992). The scotoma formed in central vision usually causes people to adopt a consistent extrafoveal preferred retinal location (PRL) to fixate objects (Whittaker and Cummings, 1988; White and Bedell, 1990). Although each person consistently uses a single PRL, its location depends upon the shape and size of their scotoma (Timberlake et al., 1986). There is a tendency to form a PRL in the lower visual field (i.e. retinally superior to the fovea), perhaps because most important information for primates is gained from the lower visual field (Bertera and Timberlake, 1988; Heinen and Skavenski, 1992). Following changes in preferred fixation locus, saccades should also adapt so as to direct the PRL rather than the fovea to the target. In order to control for the inherent variability among human subjects with naturally occurring maculopathy, Heinen and Skavenski (1992) examined saccades and fixation in monkeys following precisely administered bilateral foveal lesions induced by laser photocoagulation. They found that adaptation in the fixation system occurred almost overnight, while adaptation of saccades was slower and incomplete. The different time constants suggested that their mechanisms were also different, and different from mechanisms underlying saccadic adaptation in other situations.

Fortunately, another technique exists so that scotomata can be induced experimentally in a non-invasive fashion. Bertera and Timberlake (1988) used an eyetracker to project an artificial, retinally stabilised 'scotoma' upon the fovea of healthy human subjects. They found that a PRL developed, visually below the scotoma, within a few minutes in all subjects. Unfortunately this work has not been reported in full, but the technique is of particular value as adaptation findings in monkeys do not always generalise to humans, an observation to which we shall return shortly. Hence Heinen and Skavenski's claim that the saccadic adaptation seen in response to macular degeneration is different to other forms of saccadic adaptation remains to be confirmed by further human studies.

A number of neurological conditions, sensory and motor, stimulate the adaptive repair mechanism of the saccadic system. In the case of myasthenia gravis, this adaptive capacity may not always be sufficient to compensate for the degree of impairment. Other disorders, such as Parkinson's disease and cerebellar disease, also result in enduring saccadic dysmetria (see Fig. 1). It is not clear whether this is again due to impairments that are too large to be completely compensated for by adaptation, or if the adaptive process itself is impaired, or even if stable dysmetria may be independent of standard adaptive processes (Harris, 1995; Mezey, 2000). To resolve these issues in such chronic disorders, it is necessary to measure the responses of these patients using an experimental technique designed to stimulate observable short-term adaptation.

The laboratory-induced model of saccadic adaptation

McLaughlin (1967) pioneered a visual manipulation which stimulates the adaptive modification of saccade size. As subjects made a saccade to a target, the target was shifted back slightly in the opposite direction. Such intrasaccadic movements are not perceived consciously (Dodge, 1900), provided that they are not too large (Bridgeman et al., 1975; McConkie and Currie, 1996; MacAskill et al., 1999). Despite the imperceptibility of the second movement, the motor system responds appropriately, executing a corrective saccade to bring the fovea to the new target location. Over a number of trials, saccadic amplitude alters, reducing or even eliminating the need for a corrective saccade. If the intrasaccadic step is of a consistent size and direction, then the eyes are eventually directed toward the final target position rather than to where the target was when the saccade was initiated. Adaptation is stimulated by visual error at the end of a saccade rather than by the occurrence of corrective saccades, and results in changed motor output rather than a perceptual remapping (Wallman and Fuchs, 1998).

Adaptation in response to intrasaccadic target steps occurs rapidly (within several hundred saccades for humans and within fifteen hundred for monkeys; Fuchs et al., 1996). Their differing rates of adaptation might suggest that adaptation in response

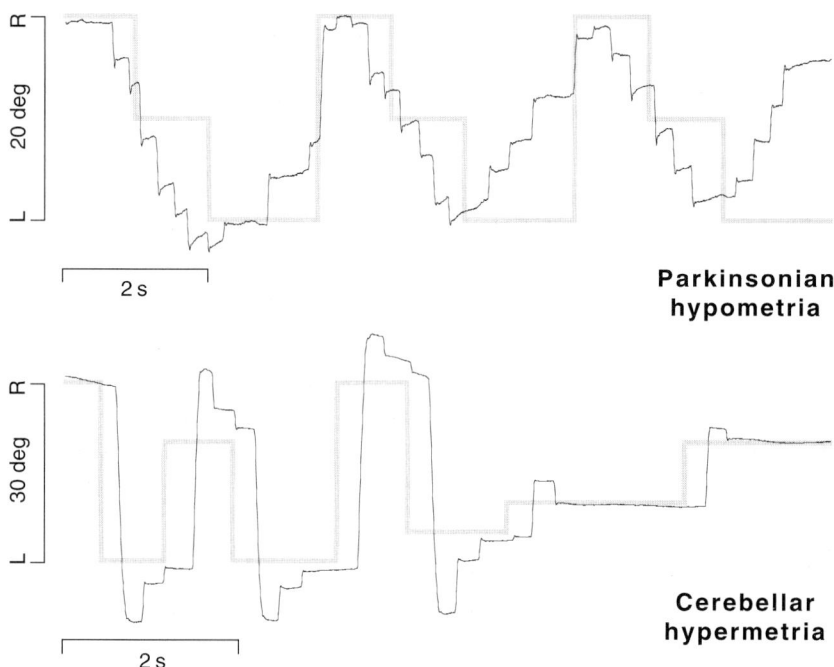

Fig. 1. Example saccades made by people with enduring saccadic dysmetria in response to moving targets (grey lines). (Top) Grossly hypometric saccades made by a middle-aged man with PD while following a repetitive three-step target sequence (due to the target predictability, all initial saccades precede their corresponding target steps). (Bottom) Hypermetric saccades made by a teenage girl while following a randomly stepping target, some years after resection of a cerebellar tumour.

to visual manipulation is not a good model of adaptation in response to muscular weakening (Optican and Robinson, 1980). Scudder et al. (1998), however, showed that the two phenomena do access the same adaptive process. As adaptation occurs independently for different saccade amplitudes (Deubel, 1987; Frens and van Opstal, 1994; Albano, 1996), Scudder et al. reasoned that adaptation to eye muscle weakening should take longer as all saccade amplitudes are affected and need to be adjusted, in a variety of behavioural circumstances. The laboratory-induced technique merely appears to produce adaptation faster, as subjects are exposed only to the limited subset of saccade amplitudes and tasks decided upon by the investigator (see also Miller et al., 1981). Scudder et al. validated their hypothesis in monkeys which either underwent surgical weakening of the extraocular muscles or experienced McLaughlin's illusory dysmetria. The number of visual targets was equated in each paradigm and the rates of adaptation were indeed found to be equal. The nonparametric nature of saccadic adaptation was further confirmed by varying the size of the intrasaccadic displacement as a function of orbital position, mimicking the way in which the effects of a weakened muscle are not constant in different gaze positions. Once more the groups performed similarly, again indicating that adaptation in response to visual manipulation relies upon the same neural processes as that in response to weakness of the extraocular muscles.

Although the high speed of laboratory-induced saccadic adaptation should not generate suspicion that subjects are employing a conscious strategy rather than a natural adaptive capacity, when exceptionally fast adaptive changes occur (for example, within several trials in Erkelens and Hulleman, 1993), it seems likely that subjects are aware of the intrasaccadic displacements. Generally, however, saccadic adaptation does not seem to be a conscious process. In an experiment where the target was displaced intrasaccadically when it appeared as a green cross but not when it appeared as a red circle, Deubel (1995a) showed that even for subjects made aware of this distinction, all saccades were adapted, regardless of the target to which they were directed. Fuchs et al. (1996) studied the adaptation of saccadic gain in seven macaques. They argued that the adaptation seen was evidence of a "real neuronal reorganisation" (p. 2523) and not a cognitive strategy, as (1) the adaptation had a gradual time course (800–1200 saccades), (2) readaptation to normal gain had a similar time course to the initial adaptation (see also Straube et al., 1997), and (3) adaptation persisted after 20 h in a darkened room.

The primate model of human saccadic adaptation

It should be noted, however, that observations in monkeys can differ from human findings. The time course for human adaptation is considerably shorter (Deubel, 1995a; Fuchs et al., 1996), perhaps due to stronger cortical involvement in saccade generation in humans than in macaques (Frens and van Opstal, 1997). It has also been argued that the difference is due to monkeys being exposed to a greater number of targets (Desmurget et al., 2000), which, as we have seen, can slow the adaptation process.

Other differences between adaptation in humans and monkeys are that recalibration in humans can take longer than the initial adaptation (Deubel, 1995a), and that adaptation of saccades in monkeys transfers to head movements (Phillips et al., 1997) whereas in humans it does not (Kröller et al., 1996). Most significant, however, are the differences in gain transfer between saccade types. Following adaptation of saccades in one behavioural task, the alteration in saccade size in another task can be measured. Fuchs et al. (1996) demonstrated substantial adaptation transfer between reflexive and memory-guided saccades in monkeys (never less than 69%). In humans little or no transfer occurs: only 2.4% of the change in size of reflexive saccades transferred to memory-guided saccades, with only 17% transfer in the opposite direction (Deubel, 1999). Fuchs et al. were "forced to conclude that humans and monkeys simply employ different mechanisms of adaptation to solve apparently identical problems of saccadic gain control" (p. 2534).

On the basis of saccade dynamics, Frens and van Opstal (1994) speculated that different neural pathways underlie adaptation in humans and monkeys. Adapted saccades in the rhesus monkey can have decreased peak velocities relative to same-sized normal saccades (Fitzgibbon et al., 1985; Frens and van Opstal, 1997; Straube et al., 1997), while Frens and van Opstal's (1994) data showed that saccade dynamics are not altered in humans. There is conflicting evidence on this point, however, as two other studies (Abrams et al., 1992; Straube and Deubel, 1995) have shown that human saccade dynamics are altered by the adaptation process.

In summary, although there is debate on some findings, the non-human primate model of saccadic adaptation currently has significant limitations in approximating human processes. There is, therefore, a value in examining adaptation in human populations with neurological disorders, as lesion studies in non-human primates may not generalise to humans. We will discuss human clinical studies after first discussing some of the brain regions thought to be important in the adaptive control of saccades.

The cerebellum and adaptation

There is a great deal of evidence from the experimental literature which implicates the cerebellum in the adaptive control of saccades. Optican and Robinson (1980) studied adaptation following surgical weakening of the lateral recti of rhesus monkeys, some of which also underwent partial or total cerebellectomies. Total ablation abolished adaptation. Partial ablation revealed that the midline cerebellum (vermis, paravermis, and fastigial nuclei) was important in adaptive control of saccadic dysmetria (i.e. the pulse of saccadic innervation). The flocculus, meanwhile, was said to be responsible for adapting the step of innervation (i.e. compensating for post-saccadic drift). Takagi et al. (1998) also showed that lesions of the dorsal cerebellar vermis in monkeys resulted in an inability to adapt the size of the saccadic pulse, resulting in pulse-size dysmetria. Optican et al. (1986) confirmed that floccular lesions abolished adaptive control of post-saccadic ocular drift in primates, resulting in enduring pulse–step mismatch dysmetria.

Desmurget et al. (1998, 2000) conducted PET studies of healthy human subjects performing reflexive saccades with intrasaccadic steps. These steps were either of a consistent size and direction, leading to adaptation, or of random size and direction, forming a non-adaptation control condition. In the adaptation condition they found a focal region of rCBF increase in the medioposterior cerebellar cortex, more marked on the side ipsilateral to the direction of the adapted saccades. No significant activation occurred in the deep cerebellar nuclei, the frontal eye field or the superior colliculus. Impressively, there was a correlation between increased activation and the amount of adaptation.

Straube and Deubel (1995) claimed that the dynamics of human saccades are altered when they undergo adaptation, which implicates the cerebellum in the adaptive process as its caudal fastigial nucleus (cFN) has a role in the acceleration and deceleration of visually guided saccades (as described by Robinson, 1995). Although Desmurget et al.'s (1998) data did not show the direct involvement of the cFN in adaptation, it is possible that cerebellar disease could impair adaptation by disrupting the input to the cFN from vermal oculomotor cells.

It seems indisputable that the cerebellum is involved in the adaptation of saccades in some way. It should be noted, however, that almost all experimental work on adaptation has examined only reflexive visually guided saccades. It may be that the cerebellum is less involved in adapting the size of saccades made in other situations.

Saccadic adaptation in neurologically impaired humans

Saccadic adaptation probably exists to counteract gradual changes in muscle efficiency as a result of aging, and possibly also to aid in the initial acquisition of accurate saccades in infancy (the saccades of young babies are grossly hypometric, Aslin and Salapatek, 1975). As we have seen, this latent adaptive capacity can also aid in counteracting the effects of neurological illness, although this is unlikely to be the teleological reason for its existence. Studying saccadic adaptation in clinical populations is of value because of the insight it yields both into the underlying disorder and into the adaptation process itself. A number of such studies are reviewed below.

Cerebellar disease

Given the importance of the cerebellum as revealed by experimental studies, investigations of saccadic adaptation in people with cerebellar disorders have been surprisingly limited until very recently.

Waespe and Baumgartner (1992) examined adaptation of visually guided reflexive saccades in two patients with cerebellar cortical atrophy and an enduring saccadic hypermetria. They did not exhibit any adaptive changes in saccade gain following 160–200 centripetal double-step reflexive trials.

Straube et al. (1995) examined a human subject with a midline cerebellar tumour and showed that this bilateral deep cerebellar nuclei lesion had differential effects upon externally and internally triggered saccades: hypermetria was greater for reflexive saccades to suddenly appearing targets than it was for 'scanning' saccades to continuously visible targets. It appears that damage to the cerebellum impaired the maintenance of the metricity of the reflexive saccades only.

The most comprehensive study of saccadic adaptation in people with cerebellar disease was conducted recently by Straube et al. (2001). They examined nine patients with cerebellar degeneration, five with cerebellar infarcts, and two with congenital malformations. The degeneration group showed no significant adaptation of reflexive saccades, although individual performance within this group was highly variable. Both the infarct and congenital groups exhibited a significant adaptive gain change although the magnitude of this change was still significantly less than that of the control group. Primary saccade accuracy in cerebellar conditions is extremely variable from trial to trial, and it is possible that it is this variability, rather than the cerebellar damage itself, which impairs the adaptive process. Straube et al. found, however, that there was no correlation between the variability of saccade gain at baseline and the subsequent degree of adaptive gain change. It was concluded that cerebellar lesions impair the adaptation of saccades, although there is large variation between subjects due to differing lesion extent and location.

Extracerebellar lesions disrupting cerebellar pathways

Waespe and Baumgartner (1992) also examined 13 patients with ischaemia in the lateral medulla or the cerebellar territory of the posterior inferior cerebellar artery (although the former had a lesion outside the cerebellum, it interrupted olivo-cerebellar pathways). Unlike their two patients with cerebellar atrophy, some adaptation occurred but was less than that achieved by controls. The lesions were unilateral and a lateralised effect was seen in some subjects: adaptation was decreased only for ipsilaterally directed saccades. Many of the patients showed an enduring dysmetria of saccades at baseline, which was also lateralised (ipsilaterally directed saccades hypermetric, contralateral saccades hypometric).

Although the cerebellum is clearly important for maintaining adaptive control of visually guided saccades, it is likely that cortical areas may also be involved in adaptation, particularly in other, more volitional, saccade types (Deubel, 1995b, 1999). Gaymard et al. (2001) reasoned that this would require cerebellar communication with cortical oculomotor areas via the thalamus and in particular the ventrolateral thalamic nuclei. They examined four patients with focal lesions of the thalamus, two with cerebellar signs and two without (the latter presumably involving non-cerebellar areas of the thalamus). All subjects underwent a gain-shortening paradigm of reflexive visually guided saccades. The non-cerebellar subjects reduced gain normally. The cerebellar subjects reduced the gain of their saccades but in an atypical fashion: saccades made in a direction ipsilateral to the lesion decreased in gain significantly less than did control saccades, while those in the contralateral direction showed a significantly *larger* decrease in gain than did control saccades. Once again implicating the ipsilateral cerebellum in adaptive saccade control, this study was also notable for demonstrating the importance of cerebello-thalamo-cortical communication.

Mild closed head injury

Heitger et al. (2001), in the largest study to date involving saccadic adaptation, examined 30 people with mild closed head injury (CHI) and 30 matched controls. Neuropsychological tests revealed impairments of explicit cognitive learning in the CHI group. The CHI subjects also showed deficits on a range of anti-saccade and memory-guided saccade measures, and produced a smaller number of self--paced saccades in a given time period. All of those impairments are consistent with the primarily frontal lobe damage caused by mild CHI. The extent and rate of reflexive saccade adaptation, however, did not differ between the groups. That saccadic adaptation following CHI is normal is consistent with studies that have shown deficits on other, frontal-reliant, cognitive learning tasks whereas implicit learning was preserved (McDowall and Martin, 1996; Shum et al., 1996).

Interestingly, approximately a third of both the control and CHI subjects did not show an exponential decrease in saccade gain during the adaptation phase but instead exhibited a linear decrease. Straube et al. (2001) reported a similar phenomenon in an unspecified number of their subjects. It appears that the classic exponential learning 'curve' of saccadic adaptation (Straube et al., 1997) is not a universal feature, in humans at least. We speculate that this may be due to the large inter-trial variability in gain frequently seen in subjects, which acts to mask the shape of any underlying function. Additionally, breaking the long adaptation phase into several discrete blocks of trials can introduce discontinuities into the data due to the small amount of 'unlearning' which can occur in these brief periods (unpublished observations).

Post-opsoclonus syndrome

Mezey (2000) studied adaptation of reflexive saccades in seven children with a history of opsoclonus. Opsoclonus consists of high frequency saccadic oscillations with vertical, horizontal and torsional components, and is consequently also known as saccadomania or dancing eye syndrome (Leigh and Zee, 1999). The opsoclonus had resolved in Mezey's seven subjects although five had ongoing neurological deficits, including two with abnormal saccadic hypermetria and two with hypometria. Six of the seven children showed a saccadic gain decrease within the normal range, including the two with pre-existing hypermetria. The only one to not adapt saccade size was a child with a gross pre-existing hypometria (mean baseline gain = 0.63). Mezey concluded that, as three of the four subjects with pre-existing baseline dysmetria had a preserved ability to alter saccadic gain, the absolute baseline gain level may be at least partially independent of the mechanism to change that level. It has been proposed that the saccadic system operates to minimise the flight time taken to reach a target (Harris, 1995). Consequently, the saccadic system will tend to undershoot targets rather than overshoot. For subjects with a large variability in saccade amplitude, the theory predicts that their mean gain will tend to be more hypometric than normal. Such a strategy ensures that the majority of their corrective saccades are in the same direction as the primary saccade, hence minimising total flight time. Therefore the presence of abnormally hypometric saccades does not necessarily imply the impairment of adaptive control mechanisms: abnormally sized primary saccades may in fact indicate a preserved capacity to optimise saccadic gain in response to high variability of gain. This has important implications for the study reported below, in which we examined subjects with Parkinson's disease who had a pre-existing saccadic hypometria.

Saccadic adaptation in Parkinson's disease

As was mentioned in the discussion of Gaymard et al.'s (2001) thalamic lesion study, cortical regions may play a significant role in adjusting the accuracy of saccadic movements. The preponderance of evidence indicating the importance of the cerebellum may be due to most experiments measuring adaptation only in response to reflexive, visually guided saccades, in which the cerebellum is particularly involved. Exceptions have been Deubel (1995b, 1999) and Erkelens and Hulleman (1993), who found that reflexive saccades and other, more volitional, saccade tasks appear to be adapted somewhat independently. That is, adapting the size of saccades in one behavioural task does not necessarily transfer to the size of saccades performed immediately afterward in another context. Deubel (1999) factorially assessed the degree of transfer of adaptation between reflexive, scanning, overlap, and memory-guided saccades, leading to a multiple-locus model in which at least three brain regions are involved in controlling the accuracy of saccades. As might be expected, reflexive visual saccades were said to be adapted by the cerebellum, but the adaptation of more volitional saccades was said to involve the frontal cortex (in the region of the dorsolateral prefrontal cortex for memory-guided saccades and the region of the frontal eye fields for scanning and overlap saccades).

In this context, we decided it would be pertinent to measure the adaptation of reflexive and memory-guided saccades in Parkinson's disease (PD). PD is a disorder of basal ganglia function (see Lang and Lozano, 1998a,b for a broad introduction), particularly characterised by motor slowing, rigidity, tremor, and hypometria. Oculomotor deficits have been thoroughly investigated and although results are often in conflict due to the variability of symptom severity in different samples, memory-guided saccades are usually impaired (Hodgson et al., 1999). Simple reflexive saccades tend to be impaired only in more severely affected subjects (MacAskill et al., 2002).

PD is particularly relevant to the study of saccadic adaptation as:

(1) The basal ganglia are involved in extensive feedback loops with cortical, and especially frontal cortical, areas (Alexander et al., 1990). Hence it might be expected that disordered basal ganglia operation might impair the proposed adaptation pathways (Deubel, 1999) between frontal cortical adaptation zones and brainstem and superior colliculus oculomotor centres. Such an impairment should be more evident in memory-guided rather than reflexive saccades as the latter should rely more upon the cerebellum for adaptation.

(2) People with PD show an enduring saccadic hypometria, particularly of memory-guided saccades (Crawford et al., 1989; Lueck et al., 1990). We therefore wished to assess any asymmetry in the degree of gain-increasing and gain-decreasing adaptation.

(3) There is evidence that the basal ganglia themselves may be important in feedback and error correction in a variety of domains (Brainard and Doupe, 2000; Lawrence, 2000).

Method

Subjects

Nine men and three women with idiopathic PD were tested off-medication. Symptom severity was mild to moderate as assessed by Hoehn and Yahr staging and the Unified Parkinson's Disease Rating Scale. Mean age was 61 (range 44–72). A control group of seven male and five female subjects was recruited, with a mean age of 63 (range 44–73).

Apparatus

Eye movements were recorded using a Skalar IRIS infrared limbus tracker (Reulen et al., 1988) at 200 Hz. A computer-generated stimulus (a red square target subtending 0.75° on a homogeneous background) was video front-projected (refresh rate 70 Hz) on to a large screen 1.70 m in front of the seated subject, whose head was restrained by use of a bite bar or chin rest.

Procedures

Sessions

Each subject performed both the reflexive (visually guided) and memory-guided saccade tests in different sessions, separated by a week. Session order was balanced across subjects.

Reflexive test

Representative recordings illustrating the three phases (baseline, adaptation, and test) in the reflexive condition are shown in Fig. 2.

Baseline phase. Subjects followed a target which made steps of 12, 14, 16, 18, 20, 22, or 24 degrees left or right from its previous position. This phase consisted of 1 test of 49 trials, lasting approximately 80 s.

Adaptation phase. As for the baseline phase but as soon as the saccade to the new target position was detected (by a real-time eye velocity threshold of 30°/s), the target was displaced by a fixed proportion (12.5%) of the distance between the current and previous target positions. This displacement was either in the same direction as the initial displacement (centrifugal) or in the opposite direction (centripetal), this direction being constant for a given subject. After a random delay (1000–2000 ms), sufficient to allow the subject to re-fixate on the new target position, the cycle repeated. This phase consisted of 245 trials, split into 5 consecutive tests of 49 trials each.

Test phase. As for the baseline phase except that when a subject's saccade towards a new target position was detected, the target was extinguished for 500 ms and then reappeared at the same place. This lack of visual information immediately following the primary saccade slows the recalibration to normal saccadic gain considerably (Deubel, 1999).

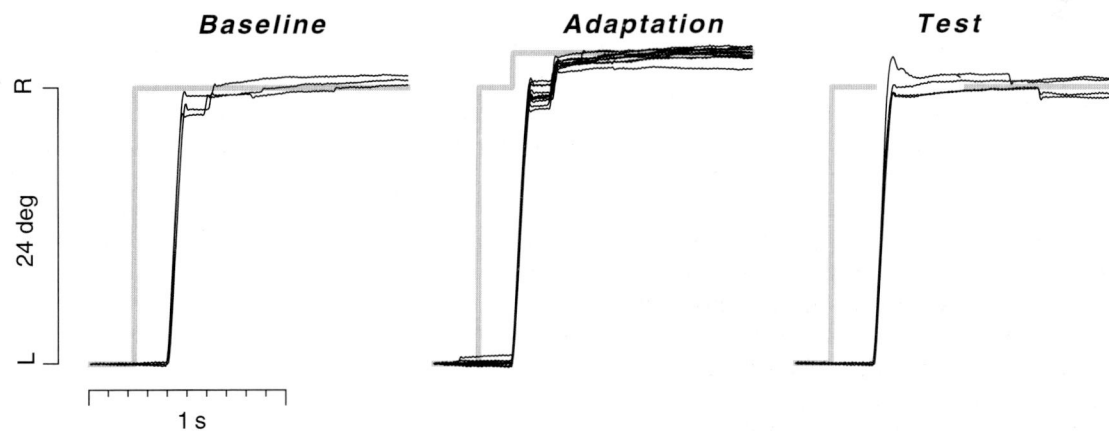

Fig. 2. Recordings of all 24° rightward saccades made by one control subject during each phase (baseline, centrifugal adaptation, and test) in the reflexive condition. Grey lines indicate representative target displacements. In the baseline phase, the primary saccades undershot the target location, requiring corrective saccades to achieve foveation. The adaptation phase increased the apparent hypometria of primary saccades because of the intrasaccadic centrifugal target displacement. The resulting adaptation yielded test-phase primary saccades that were normometric or even hypermetric (the increased corrective saccade latency in this phase was due to the presence of the 500 ms period in which the target was blanked).

Memory-guided test

Baseline phase. After a fixation stimulus had been displayed for 1250 ms, a peripheral target flashed briefly (400 ms duration at 12, 14, 16, 18, 20, 22, or 24 degrees to the left or right of the fixation target). The subject remained fixated on the original target. After a variable period (500–1500 ms) the fixation target disappeared, with a simultaneous tone. The subject then executed a saccade to the remembered location of the peripheral target. Immediately the saccade was detected, the peripheral target reappeared, and the subject made a corrective saccade to it if required. This target then served as the fixation target for the next cycle. This phase consisted of 1 test of 35 trials lasting approximately 100 s.

Adaptation phase. As in the baseline phase, detection of a saccade caused the peripheral target to be re-displayed. However, the new target position was at a location displaced by 12.5% from its original flashed eccentricity, either in a centrifugal or centripetal direction (constant for a given subject). This phase consisted of 245 trials, split into 7 consecutive tests of 35 trials each.

Test phase. As for the baseline condition but with a delay of 500 ms following saccade initiation before the peripheral target reappeared, again to slow the recalibration to normal saccadic gain.

Results

Comparison of baseline saccade gain

Saccade gain was defined as the amplitude of the primary saccade divided by the stimulus amplitude, generally known as primary saccade gain. The gains of primary saccades in the baseline phase were compared by a mixed-design ANOVA. Controls made larger primary saccades than did PD subjects ($F(1, 21) = 5.09$, $p < 0.04$), and, overall, reflexive saccades were larger than memory-guided ones ($F(1, 21) = 12.84$, $p < 0.002$). There was no significant interaction effect; that is, both groups exhibited a similar magnitude difference in gain between the saccade types.

Adaptation of saccades

A mixed-design ANOVA was conducted separately for each saccade type to analyse differences in saccade gain between the baseline and test phases. The between-group variables were Group (PD vs control) and Direction (centripetal vs centrifugal) while the within-group variable was Phase (baseline vs test). The mean gain values are shown in Fig. 3.

Reflexive saccades

There was a main effect of Group ($F(1, 20) = 9.10$, $p < 0.01$), with control saccades larger overall than PD saccades. There was also a main effect for Direction ($F(1, 20) = 9.48$, $p < 0.01$): averaged across the baseline and test, saccades in the centrifugal condition were larger than those in the centripetal condition. Lastly, there was an interaction between Direction and Phase ($F(1, 20) = 24.61$, $p < 0.0001$): saccades increased in size between baseline and test in the centrifugal condition, and decreased in size in the centripetal condition. That is, subjects adapted the size of their saccades in the same direction as that of the intrasaccadic step. There was no interaction between Group and any of the other variables, indicating that there was no difference in the extent of adaptation between the PD and control groups.

Memory-guided saccades

There was again a main effect of Group, with control saccades having a larger gain overall than PD saccades ($F(1, 19) = 5.93$, $p < 0.03$). A main effect for Direction was not present: as Fig. 3 indicates, due to the PD performance, there was not a consistent relationship between the direction of adaptation and the resulting change in saccade gain. There was a main effect of Phase ($F(1, 19) = 7.33$, $p < 0.02$): saccades were smaller overall in the test phase than in the baseline phase, again due to the PD subjects performance. Finally, there was an interaction between Phase and Direction ($F(1, 19) = 6.98$, $p < 0.02$). That is, collapsed across Group, there was negligible change in gain following centrifugal adaptation, but a substantial gain reduction following centripetal adaptation.

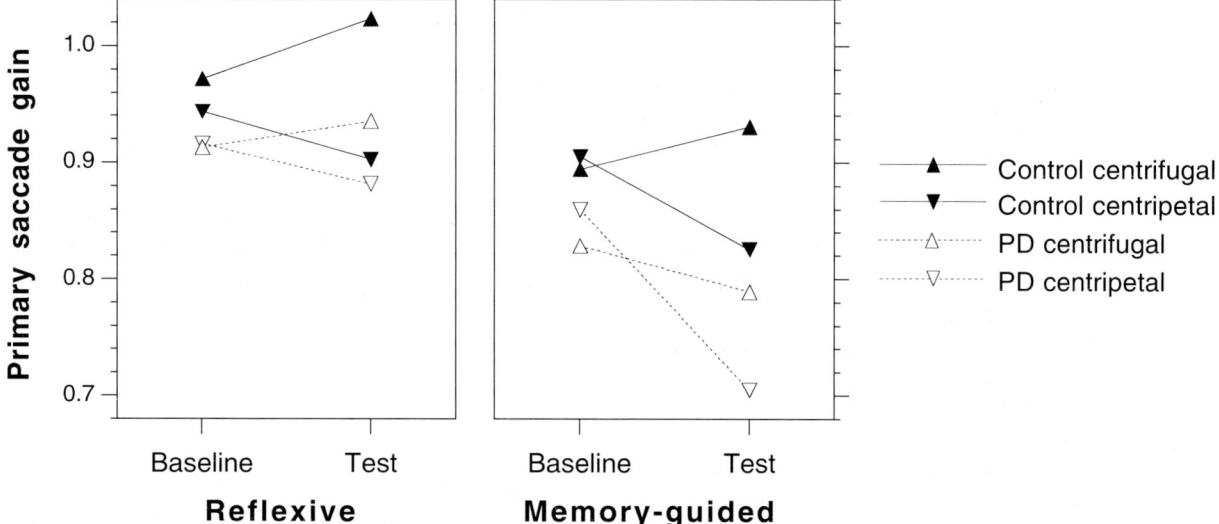

Fig. 3. Primary saccade gain for PD subjects (unfilled symbols) and controls (filled symbols) in the baseline and test phases for each adaptation direction (upward-pointing triangles, centrifugal; downward, centripetal). PD subjects produced smaller reflexive saccades overall, yet adaptation led to appropriate changes in saccade gain for both PD and control subjects (left panel). Adaptation of memory-guided saccades, however (right panel), resulted in appropriate gain changes only for control subjects, while PD subjects showed decreased gain following both centripetal and centrifugal adaptation.

Awareness of intrasaccadic manipulation

Following the baseline test, subjects were instructed to continue performing the saccadic task in the same way, but were told that the procedure would be changed in some way and were asked to report any awareness they had of any such change.

A number of subjects reported erroneous or irrelevant changes (e.g. that the beeps changed in tone or that the inter-trial intervals altered). Nine (three PD and six controls) claimed that the target reappeared in a different position during the test phase in at least one session. As there was no target displacement during the test phase this was also an erroneous report. Nine other subjects (seven PD and two controls) did not report any awareness of intrasaccadic displacements in either session. Three subjects (one PD and two controls) noticed, occasionally to frequently, that their eyes did not land at the target position during the adaptation phase of at least one session. They attributed this to the inaccuracy of their own eye movements, however, rather than to target manipulation. Another PD subject (undergoing centripetal adaptation of memory-guided saccades) reported the impression that his eyes were undershooting the target. This subject exhibited a substantial hypometria in this condition and continually undershot the final target position even though the centripetal target movement should have resulted in saccadic overshooting. That is, in this case the subject was accurately reporting the dysmetria of his own eye movements and not the oppositely directed target displacement, which remained unperceived.

Six subjects (two PD and four controls) did notice intrasaccadic target displacements during at least one of the adaptation phases (one of these was also one of the subjects who reported displacements during the test phase). Their reports of the frequency of the intrasaccadic shifts are given in Table 1.

Discussion

Adaptation of visually and memory-guided saccades in PD

Despite a pre-existing saccadic hypometria, PD subjects showed a normal capacity to adaptively increase or decrease the size of their saccades in response to intrasaccadic target displacements when following a simple stepping visual target (see Fig. 3). As in

TABLE 1

Reports of the frequency of the intrasaccadic shifts

Group	ISS	Reflexive session	Memory-guided session
PD	+	occasional but attributed to self	2/3 of trials
PD	−	2 trials in first block	NIL
Control	+	NIL	1/3 to 1/2 of trials
Control	−	1 trial in fourth block	up to 2/3 but attributed to self
Control	+	3–4 trials per block	2/3 of trials
Control	+	'quite often' but attributed to self	'frequent'

Six subjects reported that they saw the target make a double step or reappear at a different location during one of the adaptation phases. Their descriptions of how often this occurred are given. Three subjects noticed their eyes landing in the wrong location but attributed this to their own inaccuracy rather than to target displacement. 'ISS' indicates the direction of the intrasaccadic step (+ for centrifugal, − for centripetal).

Mezey's (2000) study of opsoclonus, a pre-existing and enduring saccadic dysmetria does not necessarily indicate an impairment of the ability to adaptively modify saccade accuracy. That is, our PD subjects were not impaired at adaptation per se but showed an adaptive deficit that was specific to memory-guided saccades: increased hypometria regardless of the intended direction of adaptation. This adaptive impairment is different to that observed in cerebellar disorders, in which adaptation tends to be either absent or reduced (Waespe and Baumgartner, 1992; Straube et al., 2001). It is similar to the findings of an excessive gain decrease in saccades ipsilateral to lesions of cerebellar thalamic nuclei (Gaymard et al., 2001). In three patients with hemi-Parkinson's disease, Carl and Wurtz (1985) found ipsilaterally directed reflexive saccades to be normal or slowed symmetrically, while ipsilateral memory-guided saccades were slowed or had abnormal trajectories. Our patients, however, were generally affected bilaterally. When categorised as to whether their motor symptoms were predominantly left-sided, right-sided, or equal, no differences were seen.

Our data indicate that the basal ganglia do not have a generalised role in saccadic adaptation. This supports Deubel's (1999) multiple locus model, with basal ganglia impairment possibly impairing the communication from frontal cortical adaptation regions to subcortical oculomotor centres in memory-guided saccades.

Awareness of intrasaccadic displacements

The rate of detection of target double-steps during the reflexive adaptation phase was acceptably low for a study of adaptation. Undoubtedly, if the subjects had been told what the target manipulation was, and were asked to detect it trial by trial in a psychophysical study, they would have been more sensitive.

Few subjects detected that the target reappeared at a new location during the memory-guided adaptation phase. Of concern, however, was their impression that this happened on a large proportion of trials (1/2 to 2/3). For this subset of the subjects, it could be said that the observed adaptation of memory-guided saccades may have been affected at least partially by conscious strategies. Frens and van Opstal (1994) found that the three of their ten subjects who did not exhibit reflexive adaptation were also the only subjects to notice the target shift throughout the adaptation phase. No consistent effects on adaptation were noted in our results and, hence, all subjects were retained in the analysis. Perhaps of note, however, is that the only PD subject who increased rather than decreased the size of his memory-guided saccades following centrifugal adaptation was also the only one to have noticed the target shift.

Saccadic suppression of displacement (SSD, Bridgeman et al., 1975) decreases the probability of detecting a target displacement during a saccade. Preliminary experimentation to establish appropriate thresholds for intrasaccadic displacements in our laboratory (MacAskill et al., 1999) examined detection solely in the reflexive saccade task, and we are not aware of any other study that has investigated SSD thresholds in other saccade types. It might be expected that target shifts would be more detectable in memory-guided saccades than in reflexive saccades, as the memory-guided task effectively includes a period of target blanking. That is, the target appears peripherally, is extinguished for a period, and is then re-illuminated during the saccade toward it. Such a period of blanking can make target displacements more detectable (Deubel and Schneider, 1994; Deubel et al., 1996, 1998). Although only a small number of subjects appeared to perceive the target manipulation during memory-guided saccades, those subjects were quite sensitive to it. This indicates that further studies should be conducted on the detectability of intrasaccadic manipulations during various non-reflexive saccade types. When examining the transfer of adaptation between saccades of different types (Deubel, 1987; Erkelens and Hulleman, 1993; Deubel, 1995b, 1999), it is important to know that similar (that is, unconscious) adaptation processes are being examined.

A sizeable proportion of our subjects (9 of 24) reported that the target was displaced during the test phase of either saccade type, when in fact the target was not displaced at all. This verifies that subjects are capable of spontaneously reporting an impression of unusual target displacement, although in these cases it was erroneous. This illusion of target displacement may have been due to the 500 ms period of target blanking following each saccade. This was introduced to slow re-calibration to baseline gain levels (Deubel, 1999). Deubel et al. (1998) also showed, however, that blanking a target can lead to an impression of displacement even when no displacement occurs. This effect, perhaps in concert with the adaptation-induced inaccuracy of saccade landing position with respect to the target when it reappeared, may have caused the subjects' erroneous perception of displacement.

Conclusion

The oculomotor system, for all its complexity, has been described as a 'cartoon' of motor control (Robinson, 1986), as it is relatively simple and well-understood compared to other motor systems. Studying the adaptation of saccades is relatively easy due to the way in which the oculomotor system can be visually deceived in order to produce compensatory motor learning and the way in which this learning can be assessed in a quantitative and accurate manner. This adaptive system provides at least a caricature of more general motor adaptation processes. In some neurological conditions and in some behavioural tasks, saccades can be made more accurate despite a pre-existing dysmetria. This provides hope that analogous training techniques could also be developed to correct the disturbances of limb and posture control experienced in such disorders.

Abbreviations

cFN	caudal fastigial nucleus
CHI	closed head injury
ISS	intrasaccadic step
PD	Parkinson's disease
PET	positron emission tomography
PRL	preferred retinal location
rCBF	regional cerebral blood flow
SSD	saccadic suppression of displacement
VOR	vestibuloocular reflex

Acknowledgements

The authors gratefully acknowledge the assistance of the New Zealand Neurological Foundation, which funded preliminary work required for the study reported in this chapter. Helpful comments on a possible effect to examine were made by Professor John Sweeney. Parts of the data reported here were originally published in MacAskill et al. (2002) and are reprinted with permission of Oxford University Press.

References

Abel, L.A., Schmidt, D., Dell'Osso, L.F. and Daroff, R.B. (1978) Saccadic system plasticity in humans. *Ann. Neurol.*, 3: 313–318.

Abrams, R.A., Dobkin, R.S. and Helfrich, M.K. (1992) Adaptive modification of saccadic eye movements. *J. Exp. Psychol. Hum. Percept. Perform.*, 18: 922–933.

Albano, J.E. (1996) Adaptive changes in saccade amplitude: oculocentric or orbitocentric mapping? *Vision Res.*, 36: 2087–2098.

Alexander, G.E., Crutcher, M.D. and DeLong, M.R. (1990) Basal ganglia–thalamocortical circuits: parallel substrates for motor, oculomotor, 'prefrontal' and 'limbic' functions. *Prog. Brain Res.*, 85: 119–146.

Aslin, R.N. and Salapatek, P. (1975) Saccadic localization of visual targets by the very young human infant. *Percept. Psychophys.*, 17: 293–302.

Bahill, A.T., Clark, M.R. and Stark, L. (1975) The main sequence, a tool for studying human eye movements. *Math. Biosci.*, 24: 191–204.

Bertera, J.H. and Timberlake, G.T. (1988) Preferred eccentric viewing positions with a simulated scotoma [Abstract]. *Invest. Ophthalmol. Vis. Sci.*, 29(Suppl.): 135.

Brainard, M.S. and Doupe, A.J. (2000) Interruption of a basal ganglia–forebrain circuit prevents plasticity of learned vocalizations. *Nature*, 404: 762–766.

Bridgeman, B., Hendry, D. and Stark, L. (1975) Failure to detect displacement of the visual world during saccadic eye movements. *Vision Res.*, 15: 719–722.

Carl, J.R. and Wurtz, R.H. (1985) Asymmetry of saccadic control in patients with hemi-Parkinson's disease [Abstract]. *Invest. Ophthalmol. Vis. Sci.*, 26(Suppl.): 258.

Cheraskin, E. (1992) Macular degeneration: how big is the problem? *J. Natl. Med. Assoc.*, 84: 873–876.

Crawford, T.J., Henderson, L. and Kennard, C. (1989) Abnormalities of nonvisually guided eye movements in Parkinson's disease. *Brain*, 112: 1573–1586.

Desmurget, M., Pélisson, D., Urquizar, C., Prablanc, C., Alexander, G.E. and Grafton, S.T. (1998) Functional anatomy of saccadic adaptation in humans. *Nat. Neurosci.*, 1: 524–528.

Desmurget, M., Pélisson, D., Grethe, J.S., Alexander, G.E., Urquizar, C., Prablanc, C. and Grafton, S.T. (2000) Functional adaptation of reactive saccades in humans: a PET study. *Exp. Brain Res.*, 132: 243–259.

Deubel, H. (1987) Adaptivity of gain and direction in oblique saccades. In: J.K. O'Regan and A. Lévy-Schoen (Eds.), *Eye Movements: from Physiology to Cognition*. Elsevier North Holland, Amsterdam, pp. 181–190.

Deubel, H. (1995a) Is saccadic adaptation context-specific? In: J.M. Findlay (Ed.), *Eye Movement Research*. Elsevier Science, Amsterdam, pp. 177–187.

Deubel, H. (1995b) Separate adaptive mechanisms for the control of reactive and volitional saccadic eye movements. *Vision Res.*, 35: 3529–3540.

Deubel, H. (1999) Separate mechanisms for the adaptive control of reactive, volitional, and memory guided saccadic eye movements. In: D. Gopher and A. Koriat (Eds.), *Attention and Performance XVII: Cognitive Regulation of Performance*. MIT Press, Cambridge, MA, pp. 697–721.

Deubel, H. and Schneider, W.X. (1994) Perceptual stability and postsaccadic visual information: can man bridge a gap? *Behav. Brain Sci.*, 17: 259–260.

Deubel, H., Schneider, W.X. and Bridgeman, B. (1996) Postsaccadic target blanking prevents saccadic suppression of image displacement. *Vision Res.*, 36: 985–996.

Deubel, H., Bridgeman, B. and Schneider, W.X. (1998) Immediate post-saccadic information mediates space constancy. *Vision Res.*, 38: 3147–3159.

Dodge, R. (1900) Visual perception during eye movement. *Psychol. Rev.*, 7: 454–465.

Erkelens, C.J. and Hulleman, J. (1993) Selective adaptation of internally triggered saccades made to visual targets. *Exp. Brain Res.*, 93: 157–164.

Fitzgibbon, E.J., Goldberg, M.E. and Segraves, M.A. (1985) Short term adaptation in the monkey. In: E.L. Keller and D.S. Zee (Eds.), *Adaptive Processes in the Visual and Oculomotor Systems*. Advances in the Biosciences Vol. 57, Pergamon, Oxford, pp. 329–333.

Frens, M.A. and van Opstal, A.J. (1994) Transfer of short-term adaptation in human saccadic eye movements. *Exp. Brain Res.*, 100: 293–306.

Frens, M.A. and van Opstal, A.J. (1997) Monkey superior colliculus activity during short-term saccadic adaptation. *Brain Res. Bull.*, 43: 473–483.

Fuchs, A.F., Reiner, D. and Pong, M. (1996) Transfer of gain changes from targeting to other types of saccade in the monkey: constraints on possible sites of saccadic gain adaptation. *J. Neurophysiol.*, 76: 2522–2535.

Gaymard, B., Rivaud-Pechoux, S., Yelnik, J., Pidoux, B. and Ploner, C.J. (2001) Involvement of the cerebellar thalamus in human saccade adaptation. *Eur. J. Neurosci.*, 14: 554–560.

Gonshor, A. and Melvill Jones, G. (1976) Extreme vestibuloocular adaptation induced by prolonged optical reversal of vision. *J. Physiol. (Lond).*, 256: 381–414.

Harris, C.M. (1995) Does saccadic undershoot minimize saccadic flight-time? A Monte-Carlo study. *Vision Res.*, 35: 691–701.

Heinen, S.J. and Skavenski, A.A. (1992) Adaptation of saccades and fixation to bilateral foveal lesions in adult monkey. *Vision Res.*, 32: 365–373.

Heitger, M.H., MacAskill, M.R., Anderson, T.J., Jones, R.D., Ardagh, M.W. and Donaldson, I.M. (2001) Subconscious saccadic adaptation is not affected by mild closed head injury [Abstract]. *N. Z. Med. J.*, 114: 480.

Hodgson, T.L., Dittrich, W.H., Henderson, L. and Kennard, C. (1999) Eye movements and spatial working memory in Parkinson's disease. *Neuropsychologia*, 37: 927–938.

Kapoula, Z., Optican, L.M. and Robinson, D.A. (1989) Visually induced plasticity of postsaccadic ocular drift in normal humans. *J. Neurophysiol.*, 61: 879–891.

Kommerell, G., Olivier, D. and Theopold, H. (1976) Adaptive programming of phasic and tonic components in saccadic eye movements: investigations of patients with abducens palsy. *Invest. Ophthalmol.*, 15: 657–660.

Kröller, J., Pélisson, D. and Prablanc, C. (1996) On the short-term adaptation of eye saccades and its transfer to head movements. *Exp. Brain Res.*, 111: 477–482.

Lang, A.E. and Lozano, A.M. (1998a) Parkinson's disease (first of two parts). *N. Engl. J. Med.*, 339: 1044–1052.

Lang, A.E. and Lozano, A.M. (1998b) Parkinson's disease (second of two parts). *N. Engl. J. Med.*, 339: 1130–1143.

Lawrence, A.D. (2000) Error correction and the basal ganglia: similar computations for action, cognition and emotion. *Trends Cogn. Sci.*, 4: 365–367.

Leigh, R.J. and Zee, D.S. (1999) *The Neurology of Eye Movements*. Oxford University Press, Philadelphia, PA.

Lueck, C.J., Tanyeri, S., Crawford, T.J. and Henderson, L. (1990) Antisaccades and remembered saccades in Parkinson's disease. *J. Neurol. Neurosurg. Psychiatry*, 53: 284–288.

MacAskill, M.R., Muir, S.R. and Anderson, T.J. (1999) Saccadic suppression and adaptation: revisiting the methodology. In: W. Becker, H. Deubel and T. Mergner (Eds.), *Current Oculomotor Research: Physiological and Psychological Aspects*. Plenum, New York, pp. 93–96.

MacAskill, M.R., Anderson, T.J. and Jones, R.D. (2000) Saccadic suppression of displacement in severely slowed saccades. *Vision Res.*, 40: 3405–3413.

MacAskill, M.R., Anderson, T.J. and Jones, R.D. (2002) Adaptive modification of saccade amplitude in Parkinson's disease. *Brain*, 125: 1570–1582.

McConkie, G.W. and Currie, C.B. (1996) Visual stability across saccades while viewing complex pictures. *J. Exp. Psychol. Hum. Percept. Perform.*, 22: 563–581.

McDowall, J. and Martin, S. (1996) Implicit learning in closed head injured subjects: evidence from an event sequence learning task. *N. Z. J. Psychol.*, 25: 1–6.

McLaughlin, S.C. (1967) Parametric adjustment in saccadic eye movements. *Percept. Psychophys.*, 2: 359–362.

Mezey, L.E. (2000) *The Adaptive Control of Saccades in Normal and Abnormal Children and Adults*. Unpublished doctoral dissertation, Institute of Child Health, University College London Medical School, London.

Miller, J.M., Anstis, T. and Templeton, W.B. (1981) Saccadic plasticity: parametric adaptive control by retinal feedback. *J. Exp. Psychol. Hum. Percept. Perform.*, 7: 356–366.

Optican, L.M. and Miles, F.A. (1985) Visually induced adaptive changes in primate saccadic oculomotor control signals. *J. Neurophysiol.*, 54: 940–958.

Optican, L.M. and Robinson, D.A. (1980) Cerebellar-dependent adaptive control of primate saccadic system. *J. Neurophysiol.*, 44: 1058–1076.

Optican, L.M., Zee, D.S. and Chu, F.C. (1985) Adaptive response to ocular muscle weakness in human pursuit and saccadic eye movements. *J. Neurophysiol.*, 54: 110–122.

Optican, L.M., Zee, D.S. and Miles, F.A. (1986) Floccular lesions abolish adaptive control of post-saccadic ocular drift in primates. *Exp. Brain Res.*, 64: 596–598.

Phillips, J.O., Fuchs, A.F., Ling, L., Iwamoto, Y. and Votaw, S. (1997) Gain adaptation of eye and head movement components of simian gaze shifts. *J. Neurophysiol.*, 78: 2817–2821.

Reulen, J.P.H., Marcus, J.T., Koops, D., De Vries, F.R., Tiesinga, G., Boshuizen, K. and Bos, J.E. (1988) Precise recording of eye movement: the IRIS technique Part 1. *Med. Biol. Eng. Comput.*, 26: 20–26.

Robinson, D.A. (1975) Editorial: How the oculomotor system repairs itself. *Invest. Ophthalmol.*, 14: 413–415.

Robinson, D.A. (1986) Is the oculomotor system a cartoon of motor control? *Prog. Brain Res.*, 64: 411–417.

Robinson, F.R. (1995) Role of the cerebellum in movement control and adaptation. *Curr. Opin. Neurobiol.*, 5: 755–762.

Scudder, C.A., Batourina, E.Y. and Tunder, G.S. (1998) Comparison of two methods of producing adaptation of saccade size and implications for the site of plasticity. *J. Neurophysiol.*, 79: 704–715.

Shum, D., Sweeper, S. and Murray, R. (1996) Performance on verbal implicit and explicit memory tasks following traumatic brain injury. *J. Head Trauma Rehabil.*, 11: 43–53.

Straube, A. and Deubel, H. (1995) Rapid gain adaptation affects the dynamics of saccadic eye movements in humans. *Vision Res.*, 35: 3451–3458.

Straube, A., Deubel, H., Spuler, A. and Büttner, U. (1995) Differential effect of a bilateral deep cerebellar nuclei lesion on externally and internally triggered saccades in humans. *Neuroophthalmology*, 15: 67–74.

Straube, A., Fuchs, A.F., Usher, S. and Robinson, F.R. (1997) Characteristics of saccadic gain adaptation in rhesus macaques. *J. Neurophysiol.*, 77: 874–895.

Straube, A., Deubel, H., Ditterich, J. and Eggert, T. (2001) Cerebellar lesions impair rapid saccade amplitude adaptation. *Neurology*, 57: 2105–2108.

Takagi, M., Zee, D.S. and Tamargo, R.J. (1998) Effects of lesions of the oculomotor vermis on eye movements in primate: saccades. *J. Neurophysiol.*, 80: 1911–1931.

Takagi, M., Trillenberg, P. and Zee, D.S. (2001) Adaptive control of pursuit, vergence and eye torsion in humans: basic and clinical implications. *Vision Res.*, 41: 3331–3344.

Timberlake, G.T., Mainster, M.A., Peli, E., Augliere, R.A., Essock, E.A. and Arend, L.E. (1986) Reading with a macular scotoma. I. Retinal location of scotoma and fixation area. *Invest. Ophthalmol. Vis. Sci.*, 27: 1137–1147.

Waespe, W. and Baumgartner, R. (1992) Enduring dysmetria and impaired gain adaptivity of saccadic eye movements in Wallenberg's lateral medullary syndrome. *Brain*, 115: 1123–1146.

Wallman, J. and Fuchs, A.F. (1998) Saccadic gain modification: visual error drives motor adaptation. *J. Neurophysiol.*, 80: 2405–2416.

White, J.M. and Bedell, H.E. (1990) The oculomotor reference in humans with bilateral macular disease. *Invest. Ophthalmol. Vis. Sci.*, 31: 1149–1161.

Whittaker, S.G. and Cummings, R.W. (1988) Saccade control without foveal function. *Invest. Ophthalmol. Vis. Sci.*, 29(Suppl.): 135.

Zee, D.S., Optican, L.M., Cooke, J.D., Robinson, D.A. and Engel, W.K. (1976) Slow saccades in spinocerebellar degeneration. *Arch. Neurol.*, 33: 243–251.

CHAPTER 29

Saccade sequences as markers for cerebral dysfunction following mild closed head injury

M.H. Heitger [1,2,*], T.J. Anderson [1,2,3] and R.D. Jones [1,2,4]

[1] *Christchurch Movement Disorders and Brain Research Group, Christchurch, New Zealand*
[2] *Department of Medicine, Christchurch School of Medicine and Health Sciences, P.O. Box 4345, Christchurch, New Zealand*
[3] *Department of Neurology, Christchurch Hospital, Private Bag 4710, Christchurch, New Zealand*
[4] *Department of Medical Physics and Bioengineering, Christchurch Hospital, Private Bag 4710, Christchurch, New Zealand*

Abstract: Diffuse axonal injury caused by mild closed head injury (CHI) is likely to affect the neural networks concerned with the planning and execution of sequences of memory-guided saccades. Thirty subjects with mild CHI and thirty controls were tested on 2- and 3-step sequences of memory-guided saccades. CHI subjects showed more directional errors, larger position errors, and hypermetria of primary saccades and final eye position. No deficits were seen in temporal accuracy (timing and rhythm). These results suggest that computerized tests of saccade sequences can provide sensitive markers of cerebral dysfunction after mild CHI.

Introduction

Closed head injury

Closed head injuries (CHI) are responsible for a vast number of hospital admissions and days of work lost. The annual incidence of mild traumatic brain injury in the United States has been estimated at around 131 cases per 100,000 persons (Kraus and Nourjah, 1988). In addition, Sosin et al. (1996) estimated the yearly rate of mild to moderate brain injury that does not result in institutionalization at 618 per 100,000 persons (1.5 million cases/year in the USA), with most of these being related to head trauma. They stated that 75% of these cases would seek medical attention but only 25% are admitted to hospital. Jennett (1996) reported the annual admission rates for head trauma in Britain at between 210 and 404 per 100,000 and compares this admission rate to numbers of 93–403 per 100,000 in other countries (Australia, France, South Africa, Spain, Sweden, USA). He indicated that around 80% of these admissions were categorized as mild.

The traditional interpretation of the terms 'mild' and 'moderate' CHI includes a brief loss of consciousness in combination with a post-traumatic amnesia (PTA) duration of less than 24 h followed by disturbances of neurological function (Wrightson and Gronwall, 1998). On the Glasgow coma scale (GCS), the most frequently used clinical tool to grade head injury severity, scores between 13 and the maximum of 15 are classified as mild cases, followed by moderate cases with scores between 9 and 12 and severe cases with scores of 8 or less (Richardson, 2000, p. 10).

Alternatively, Jennett and Teasdale, 1981 (p. 90) suggested severity grading based on the duration of post-traumatic amnesia (PTA). On their scale, a PTA duration of less than 1 h represents mild head trauma

---

* Correspondence to: M.H. Heitger, Department of Medicine, Christchurch School of Medicine and Health Sciences, P.O. Box 4345, Christchurch, New Zealand. Tel.: +64-3-364-0640 extension 88138; Fax: +64-3-364-0935; E-mail: marcus.heitger@chmeds.ac.nz

with moderate cases showing PTA durations of up to 24 h. However, PTA can be difficult to assess especially in mild head trauma due to ambiguous information from the patients, who combine own recall and second-hand accounts from witnesses or relatives. In contrast to the GCS, a lack of a standardized procedure in obtaining exact information often makes the PTA scale difficult to use in minor head trauma (Richardson, 2000, pp. 84–86) and there has been debate on where to draw the PTA line for mild cases between 1 h and 24 h post-injury (Alexander, 1995; Wrightson and Gronwall, 1998). Accordingly, Crevits et al. (2000), who studied saccades in mild CHI patients, defined mild CHI as having GCS scores of 13–15 with PTA durations of less than 24 h. We have conformed with this definition in the current study.

Most patients with mild to moderate CHI initially show a disturbance of cognitive functions (slowed information processing, lack of concentration, deficits in attention, learning, short-term memory, etc.) combined with symptoms such as headache, fatigue, dizziness, anxiety, irritability, and increased light or sound sensitivity (Slater, 1989; Wright, 1998). Although these complaints tend to resolve within the first few weeks following CHI, a proportion of CHI patients are at risk of developing post-concussion syndrome (PCS), with persistence of quite disabling symptoms for periods of months or even years beyond the first weeks following the injury (Rutherford et al., 1978; Rimel et al., 1981; Mallinson and Longridge, 1998b).

A combination of psychological and structural factors has been discussed as the underlying cause for PCS (Jane and Rimel, 1982; Jane et al., 1985; Bohnen and Jolles, 1992; Watson et al., 1995) and diffuse axonal damage has been suggested as the cause or at least a contributing factor to PCS (Mittl et al., 1994). Wrightson and Gronwall (1998) suggested that the likelihood of developing persisting problems is unrelated to age, gender or cause of accident.

Neural injury arising from CHI

Even mild CHI can cause extensive neural damage throughout the brain. The contemporary view is that a blow to the head sufficient to cause even brief disturbance of consciousness may produce detectable structural brain damage. Levin et al. (1987) reported on CT and MRI scans undertaken on 20 cases of mild or moderate head injury, 6 of which represented mild cases of head trauma. Lesions were detected in 17 out of 20 patients, with the vast majority of these situated in the frontal and temporal lobes.

Fronto-temporal focal lesions frequently occur in combination with non-focal, 'diffuse brain damage' (Bernad, 1991). The initial forces to the head at the time of the injury produce linear and rotational forces, which cause movement of the brain relative to the skull. This rotation of the brain within the skull does not simply produce contusions at the point of contact between the cerebral hemispheres and the cranium but also produces damaging shearing forces within the brain, which decrease in magnitude from the surface of the brain to its centre (Richardson, 2000, pp. 39–57). Even minor CHIs can induce lesions and diffuse axonal damage or axonal stretching as a result of shearing forces at the time of impact. These diffuse lesions are independent of the original site of impact. Diffuse axonal damage has been well documented in humans (e.g. Blumbergs et al., 1989; Sahuquillo et al., 1989; Crooks et al., 1992; Gieron et al., 1998; Lee et al., 1998; Parizel et al., 1998). CT head scans commonly fail to detect these minute neural lesions but MRI frequently demonstrates diffuse axonal injury following CHI, though predominantly in severely head-injured patients (Levin et al., 1989; Zarkovic et al., 1991; Mendelsohn et al., 1992a,b; Paterakis et al., 2000).

Animal studies have confirmed that even minor blows to the head can result in diffuse axonal damage (Povlishock et al., 1983; Jane et al., 1985). Levin et al. (1992) reported intracranial lesions in patients with mild to moderate CHI. Mittl et al. (1994) showed MRI-based evidence of diffuse axonal injury in patients with mild head injury and normal CT head scans. Most of these lesions were located at the grey–white matter junction with some located in deep white matter. The authors considered that these lesions may represent the pathological substrate underlying the post-concussion syndrome associated with deficits in cognitive functioning. Servadei et al. (1994) described a case of a mild head-injured patient with diffuse axonal injury extending into the brainstem.

At a cellular level, most of the neural damage following CHI is triggered by uncoordinated harming responses resulting from the compromised functional integrity of the CNS as well as the disruption of the intra-cellular balances (Armstead, 1999; Knoblach et al., 1999; Trembovler et al., 1999; Vagnozzi et al., 1999; Morrison et al., 2000). The death of damaged neurons also adversely affects undamaged neurons that have synaptic connections with injured nerve cells. The retraction of synaptic terminals causes anterograde and retrograde transneural degeneration of otherwise undamaged neurons (Kandel et al., 1991, pp. 258–263).

Neural damage and eye movements

Anatomical substrates for the planning and execution of saccades include a vast number of cortical and subcortical areas and pathways such as the frontal eye field (FEF), the dorsolateral prefrontal cortex (DLPFC), the supplementary motor area (SMA), the posterior parietal cortex (PPC), the middle temporal area (MT), and the occipital lobe with the striate cortex. Subcortical structures include the thalamus, superior colliculus (SC) and structures in the brainstem. The complexity and the distribution of this network make it vulnerable to functional deficits caused by neural damage resulting from CHI. Frontal areas, such as the FEF play a crucial role in voluntary eye movements, including memory-guided saccades (e.g. Pierrot-Deseilligny et al., 1991b, 1995; Rivaud et al., 1994; Gaymard et al., 1999). The DLPFC contributes to spatial short-term memory (Gaymard et al., 1998a; Ploner et al., 1999) and suppression of saccades (Pierrot-Deseilligny et al., 1991b). The PPC provides an interface between sensory and motor structures (Andersen, 1995; Connolly et al., 2000; DeSouza et al., 2000) and plays an important role in visuospatial orientation (Heide et al., 1995), important for oculomotor and also limb movement coordination. The interdependency of neural activity in the DLPFC and the PPC shown by Chafee and Goldman-Rakic (2000) in memory-guided saccades illustrates the importance of the functional integrity of the entire neural network necessary for proper eye movement function. The SMA is directly involved in planning and execution of intentional eye movements, including the task of memory-guided sequences of saccades (Gaymard et al., 1990, 1993). Sites involved in oculomotor and limb sensory–motor processing are often co-located within these areas, such as SMA or PPC (Picard and Strick, 1996, 1997; Andersen et al., 1998) and can also show functional involvement in higher cognitive processes such as direction of attention, short-term memory, response inhibition and higher information processing, (Roberts et al., 1994; Corbetta et al., 1998; McPeek et al., 1999; Klein et al., 2000; Nieman et al., 2000; Snyder et al., 2000).

It would be reasonable to expect that the neural damage caused by CHI is likely to disrupt the complex neural networks concerned with the planning and execution of eye movements. In particular, the task of memory-guided sequences, which involves most of the anatomical substrates involved in oculomotor control, is well suited to demonstrate the adverse effects of neural injury. Studies on neurodegenerative disorders such as Parkinson's disease (Crawford et al., 1989; Lueck et al., 1992; Vermersch et al., 1994; Hodgson et al., 1999; Blekher et al., 2000; Rivaud-Pechoux et al., 2000) or neurological disorders such as Tourette's Syndrome (Straube et al., 1997; LeVasseur et al., 2001) have demonstrated the adverse effects of neural dysfunction on oculomotor processing using single memory-guided saccades and memory-guided sequences. Brain lesions caused by infarction have also been shown to affect the planning and execution of memory-guided saccades, including memory-guided sequences (Gaymard et al., 1990, 1993, 1998b, 1999; Pierrot-Deseilligny et al., 1991b; Vermersch et al., 1999).

Closed head injury and eye movements

Only limited attention has been paid to eye movements following CHI. Williams et al. (1997) found saccade deficits in 16 patients with severe traumatic head injury (mean PTA of 43.7 days). Their findings included prolonged latencies of reflexive saccades, antisaccades and simple memory-guided saccades, smaller numbers of self-paced saccades, hypometria of reflexive saccades and increased response errors on antisaccades and simple memory-guided saccades. Glass et al. (1995) reported 'impersistent' execution of saccades in nine moderate–severely head-injured patients (coma duration 1 to 20 days) in terms of number of saccades initiated within 500 ms of stimulus presentation and falling within 50% of the expected target amplitude. Mulhall et al. (1999) studied bedside examinations of antisaccades, single memory-guided saccades and self-paced saccades in a group of 19 cases of head trauma and detected a significant difference only in a lower number of self-paced saccades in the head-injured group. They compared their findings to results from infrared oculographic tests of saccades and concluded that bedside tests of saccades have only limited value in patients with head trauma. Crevits et al. (2000) found no abnormalities of single remembered saccades and antisaccades in 32 patients with mild CHI. Conversely, Mosimann et al. (2000) reported increased latencies and larger position errors in addition to increased response errors on single memory-guided saccades and antisaccades in whiplash patients with persisting symptoms.

Based on evidence of widespread axonal damage in mild CHI (see above) we considered that oculomotor function should be impaired in many cases of mild CHI, despite such deficits not being evident on clinical examination. Although studies on eye movement deficits in neuro-degenerative diseases have shown the utility of sequences of memory-guided saccades to detect adverse effects of neural damage (see above), this study is the first to use this paradigm in the context of head trauma. This study was part of a larger project incorporating tests for eye and upper-limb movements in combination with neuropsychological testing following mild head trauma. We wished to establish whether the expected deficits in oculomotor function would be sufficiently substantial to warrant a prospective study relating motor deficits with the recovery following mild CHI.

Methods

Participants

The study aimed at including mild and moderate cases of CHI, although the final CHI group comprised only mild cases of CHI. Inclusion criteria were: aged 15 to 40 years, documented CHI within the previous 2 days, Glasgow coma scale (GCS) score between 9 and 15, disturbance of consciousness (e.g., stunned or loss of consciousness) of less than 20 min, post-traumatic amnesia (PTA) of less than 24 h, and adequate command of the English language.

Exclusion criteria were: influence of alcohol or psychoactive drugs at time of injury, regular intake of psychoactive drugs or medication, history of current central neurological disorders or presence of a psychiatric condition, evidence of structural brain damage or hematoma on CT head scan (if available as part of the clinical assessment, seven participants had received a CT head scan), oculomotor deficits upon clinical examination, presence of strabismus, skull fractures (including jaw and facial fractures), or past history of severe head injury.

The final CHI group comprised 30 subjects. Causes: rugby (13), motor vehicle accidents (7), horse riding (2), bicycle accidents (2), hit by cricket ball (1), hit by soccer ball (1), assault (1), work accidents (1) and other causes (2). The mean age for the patient group ($N = 30$) was 22.2 years (SD 7.1, range 15–37). The patient mean for years of education was 12.8 (SD 1.86). All patients had a GCS score between 13 and 15 (13: 2 cases; 14: 5 cases; 15: 23 cases). Twenty-five patients had a confirmed loss of consciousness (mean = 2.56 min, SD = 3.27). The duration of the post-traumatic amnesia ranged from 3 min to 4 h (mean = 34.4 min, SD = 60.6). All patients completed the tests within 9 days of their injury (mean 4.2, SD 1.8, range 2–9 days).

The control group consisted of subjects with no prior history of moderate or severe CHI, no current central neurological disorder or psychiatric condition, and no regular intake of psychoactive drugs or medication. The controls were matched to the CHI group with respect to age ($\leq \pm 3$ years for subjects >18 years, $\leq \pm 1$ year for participants <18 years), gender and educational background (years of education, ± 2 years for participants >18, $\leq \pm 1$ year for subjects <18). Over 50% of the control group was recruited from friends or siblings of CHI patients. The mean age for the control group was 22.4 years (SD 7.0, range 15–37). The control mean for years of education was 13.2 (SD 2.1).

Apparatus

Eye movements were recorded using the infra-red scleral reflection oculography technique (Reulen et al., 1988, IROG, Skalar Medical, The Netherlands). Eye position signals were low-pass filtered at 100 Hz, sampled and digitized at 200 Hz, displayed on the operator's computer screen, and recorded on disk for off-line analysis.

Subjects were seated in a darkened room with head movements restrained by a bite bar. Eye movements were generated using a horizontal LED bar 1.5 m in front of the subject. Calibration for each eye was obtained before each test. The tests were generated and recorded by a PC running the *EMMA* (eye movement measurement and analysis) program (Muir et al., 2001).

Saccadic sequences paradigm

A central fixation LED appeared for 2000 ms and then jumped to a pre-defined number of successive horizontal eccentric positions 5° or 15° on either side of the central fixation point, 1000 ms for each position and with the final sequence position always being the centre fixation LED. Subtest A comprised six different sequences with two eccentric target positions (i.e., 2-step sequences) and three practice repetitions per sequence. Subtest B comprised six different sequences with three eccentric target positions (i.e., 3-step sequences) and five practice repetitions per sequence (Fig. 1). During practice, a buzzer sounded coincident with each target relocation. After the last target was extinguished, the subject had to repeat the sequence in darkness and without the buzzer, as accurately as possible in terms of the position and timing of the sequence. Before the start of subtest A, subjects were exposed to a rehearsal sequence to familiarize themselves with the test.

Key measures were the number of directional errors, the number of saccades per step, gain of the primary saccade (G_p), gain of the final eye position (G_f) and the mean position error (PE) for all steps throughout each sequence. Gains and position error for each step were calculated as

$$G_p = EP_p/SP$$
$$G_f = EP_f/SP$$
$$PE = |(EP_f - SP)/SP| \times 100$$

where EP_p is the eye position after the primary saccade, EP_f is the final eye position and SP is the

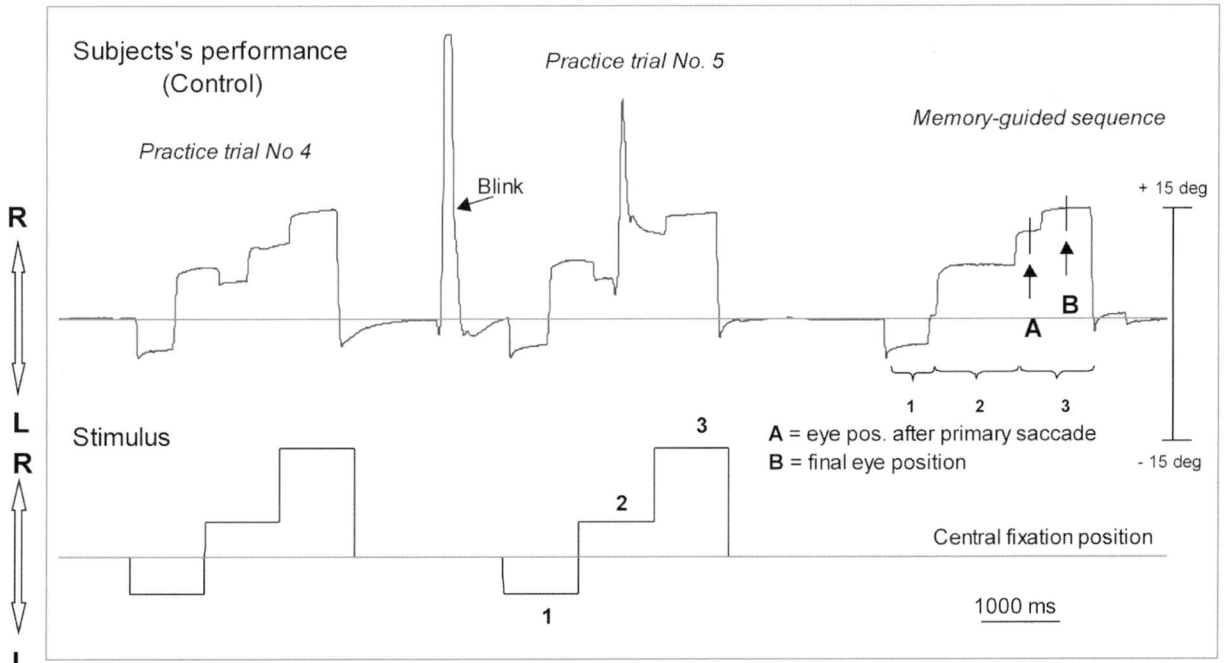

Fig. 1. Paradigm for memory-guided sequences of saccades (subtest B, 3-step sequence)

stimulus position. The mean position error for a sequence j was calculated as

Mean $PE_{\text{sequence } j}$
$$= (PE_{\text{step1} j} + PE_{\text{step2} j} + \ldots + PE_{\text{step} nj})/n$$

An amplitude error was also derived. This approach was based on the view that a sequence of saccades could be perceived as a motor pattern rather than a sequence of locations in 3-dimensional space (Ditterich et al., 1998). That is, the subject is considered to store a sequence of motor commands rather than the independent target positions themselves. This motor pattern of amplitudes and rhythm would then be performed as a series of motor commands independent from spatial validation. The amplitude error represents the deviation (%) from the expected amplitude per step, based on the final amplitudes. The amplitude error (AE) for a step k was calculated as

$$AE\ \text{step}_k = \frac{|(EP_f\text{step}_k - EP_f\text{step}_{k-1})| - |(SP\ \text{step}_k - SP\ \text{step}_{k-1})|}{|(SP\ \text{step}_k - SP\ \text{step}_{k-1})|} \times 100$$

The mean amplitude error for a sequence j was calculated as

Mean $AE_{\text{sequence } j}$
$$= (AE_{\text{step1} j} + AE_{\text{step2} j} + \ldots + AE_{\text{step} nj})/n$$

The absolute time index (ATI) served as a measure of the subject's overall timing.

$$ATI = T_r/T_s$$

where T_r is the subject's total response time, T_s is the duration of the sequence.

The inter-response interval (IRI) served as a measure for the subject's ability to maintain a constant rhythm during a sequence. The IRI for a particular step k was calculated as

$$IRI_k = T_{rk}/T_r - T_{sk}/T_s$$

where T_{rk} is the subject's response time for step k and T_{sk} is the stimulus presentation time for step k. The proportion of one particular step within the whole performance is compared to its expected proportion (subtest A: $T_{sk}/T_s = 0.5$; subtest B: $T_{sk}/T_s = 0.333$), as all stimulus steps are exactly 1.0 s long. Therefore, subjects with a total performance time of, for example, 1.8 s and individual steps of 0.6 s duration would still have a perfect rhythm within their performance. The mean IRI for a sequence j was calculated as

Mean $IRI_{\text{sequence } j}$
$$= (IRI_{\text{step1} j} + IRI_{\text{step2} j} + \ldots + IRI_{\text{step} nj})/n$$

Data analysis

Analysis of the eye movement data used analysis options provided in the *EMMA* program (Muir et al., 2001). Results were then analyzed statistically using *Statistica* (© Statsoft). The data were shown to have differences in variances between the groups, and skewed distributions on most measures. Hence, a non-parametric Wilcoxon Matched-Pairs statistic was used for between-group comparisons. Differences between groups were considered significant for p-values of ≤ 0.05. The analysis comprised 30 matched pairs. ANOVA was used to compare saccade subsets of different amplitudes (5, 10, 15, 20 and 30°), based on the pooled saccades per group for each amplitude tier, independent of the place of particular amplitude steps within sequences.

In the following results, the values presented of PE, AE, G_p, G_f, ATI, IRI, response errors and numbers of saccades are the means of the above values over all sequences in the particular subtest.

Results

Response errors (directional errors)

The CHI group showed a significantly higher number of response errors (directional errors) in the longer sequences of memory-guided saccades (subtest B, three steps, 10.4% vs 2.6%, $p = 0.003$, Table 1), but no difference for short sequences (subtest A, two steps, 4.2% vs 1.7%, $p = 0.183$, Table 1). This likely reflects a relationship between cognitive load and tendency for error.

Number of saccades per sequence

Both groups took, on average, the same number of saccades to reach the final performance (Table 1).

TABLE 1

Saccadic performance — errors, accuracy, timing, number of saccades

Measure		CHI ($n = 30$)		Controls ($n = 30$)		Difference		p-level
		Mean	SD	Mean	SD	Absolute	(%)	
Directional errors (%)								
Subtest A (2 steps)		**4.2**	9.0	**1.7**	5.5	2.5	151	0.183
Subtest B (3 steps)		**10.4**	11.5	**2.6**	5.2	7.8	300	0.003
Accuracy								
Primary saccade gain (G_p):								
Subtest A (2 steps)		**1.06**	0.24	**0.97**	0.14	0.09	9	0.115
Subtest B (3 steps)		**1.11**	0.30	**0.96**	0.18	0.15	16	0.019
Gain final eye position (G_f):								
Subtest A (2 steps)		**1.25**	0.24	**1.12**	0.14	0.13	12	0.020
Subtest B (3 steps)		**1.35**	0.42	**1.13**	0.20	0.22	19	0.016
Position error (PE, %):								
Subtest A (2 steps)		**40**	21	**26**	17	14	53	0.001
Subtest B (3 steps)		**57**	45	**33**	17	24	73	0.006
Amplitude error (AE, %):								
Subtest A (2 steps)		**30**	18	**19**	10	11	59	0.016
Subtest B (3 steps)		**43**	27	**26**	16	17	65	0.005
Absolute time index (ATI)								
Subtest A (2 steps)		**1.11**	0.21	**1.13**	0.15	0.02	2.1	0.585
Subtest B (3 steps)		**1.01**	0.13	**1.02**	0.12	0.01	0.6	0.765
Inter-response interval (IRI)								
Subtest A (2 steps)		**0.1**	0.05	**0.09**	0.04	0.01	12.5	0.130
Subtest B (3 steps)		**0.09**	0.04	**0.08**	0.03	0.01	14.6	0.158
Number of saccades								
Subtest A	step 1	**1.61**	0.53	**1.63**	0.49	0.02	1.2	0.674
	step 2	**2.93**	0.55	**2.8**	0.54	0.13	4.6	0.344
Subtest B	step 1	**1.56**	0.45	**1.43**	0.38	0.13	9.1	0.200
	step 2	**1.58**	0.39	**1.61**	0.38	0.03	2.1	0.981
	step 3	**3.03**	0.65	**2.91**	0.53	0.11	3.8	0.537

Spatial accuracy

The CHI group showed significantly poorer spatial accuracy on final eye position as measured by the position error (subtest A, two steps, 40% vs 26%, $p = 0.001$, Table 1; subtest B, three steps, 57% vs 33%, $p = 0.006$, Table 1). The comparison of individual steps of subtest A and B showed larger position and amplitude errors of the CHI group on all steps (Table 2). Following the split into different saccade amplitudes (5, 10, 15, 20 and 30°) these differences in position error were significant for 10, 15 and 20° amplitudes (Table 3). Increased position errors were mostly matched by abnormally large saccadic gains. The CHI group had hypermetric responses in both subtest A (final gain 1.25 vs 1.12, $p = 0.02$) and subtest B (final gain 1.35 vs 1.13, $p = 0.016$; primary saccade gain 1.11 vs 0.96, $p = 0.019$). These results remained in most cases following the split into either individual sequence steps as well as separate amplitude tiers (Tables 2 and 3). The hypermetria was more pronounced for smaller target amplitudes with group differences in primary saccade gain of 27% (5° amplitudes) and 20% (10° amplitudes), whereas for 30° amplitudes this difference had narrowed to about 3.4% (Table 3), indicating an inverse relationship between amplitude size and magnitude of position errors. A similar trend existed for the gain of the final eye position, with differences of around 27% for 5 and 10° amplitudes and of about 3.9% for 30° steps.

TABLE 2

Saccadic performance — position error and mean gains per individual steps

Measure	CHI ($n = 30$)		Controls ($n = 30$)		Difference		p-level
	Mean	SD	Mean	SD	Absolute	(%)	
Remembered sequences (subtest A)							
Position error (PE, %):							
Step 1	**31.96**	21.5	**19.98**	10.8	11.98	59.96	0.020
Step 2	**46.47**	23.6	**30.83**	17.5	15.64	50.73	0.003
Amplitude error (AE, %):							
Step 1	**31.96**	21.5	**19.98**	10.8	11.98	59.96	0.020
Step 2	**28.76**	15.8	**18.33**	11.1	10.43	56.90	0.013
Primary saccade gain (G_p):							
Step 1	**1.01**	0.29	**0.92**	0.17	0.09	9.78	0.089
Step 2	**1.10**	0.27	**1.01**	0.22	0.09	8.91	0.184
Gain final eye position (G_f):							
Step 1	**1.21**	0.26	**1.08**	0.15	0.13	12.04	0.030
Step 2	**1.29**	0.3	**1.16**	0.21	0.13	11.21	0.028
Remembered sequences (subtest B)							
Position error (PE, %):							
Step 1	**38.33**	22.3	**26.61**	17.1	11.72	44.04	0.011
Step 2	**67.27**	48.3	**42.61**	20	24.66	57.87	0.000
Step 3	**48.98**	38.5	**28.18**	21	20.80	73.81	0.010
Amplitude error (AE, %):							
Step 1	**38.33**	22.3	**26.61**	17.1	11.72	44.04	0.011
Step 2	**39.36**	24.9	**24.45**	13.6	14.91	60.98	0.014
Step 3	**48.73**	34.5	**26.13**	16.3	22.60	86.49	0.003
Primary saccade gain (G_p):							
Step 1	**1.06**	0.23	**0.92**	0.23	0.14	14.85	0.009
Step 2	**1.24**	0.48	**1.06**	0.30	0.18	16.71	0.125
Step 3	**1.07**	0.33	**0.91**	0.24	0.16	17.16	0.044
Gain final eye position (G_f):							
Step 1	**1.25**	0.26	**1.04**	0.24	0.21	19.74	0.002
Step 2	**1.44**	0.60	**1.23**	0.30	0.22	17.51	0.171
Step 3	**1.33**	0.41	**1.12**	0.24	0.21	18.41	0.020

Temporal accuracy (timing and rhythm)

No difference was found on the absolute time index (subtest A: 1.11 vs 1.13, $p = 0.585$, Table 1; subtest B: 1.01 vs 1.02, $p = 0.77$, Table 1). In addition, the ability to keep a steady rhythm within the sequence was not impaired in the CHI group, as evidenced by similar mean inter-response intervals (subtest A: 0.1 vs 0.09, $p = 0.13$, Table 1; subtest B: 0.09 vs 0.08, $p = 0.16$, Table 1).

Discussion

The results indicate that mild CHI can adversely affect the performance of memory-guided sequences of saccades, despite there being no oculomotor deficits on clinical examination. The CHI group showed increased directional errors and impaired spatial accuracy with abnormal hypermetria but no impairments on timing, rhythm or number of saccades per sequence.

Our study is the first to examine memory-guided sequences following head trauma, in contrast to earlier studies which included only tests of single memory-guided saccades (Williams et al., 1997; Crevits et al., 2000; Mosimann et al., 2000). The study of Crevits et al. (2000) is of particular interest, as they incorporated patients with mild CHI only and found no deficits in latencies or response errors in single memory-guided saccades. Their selection cri-

TABLE 3

Accuracy of memory-guided sequences (subtest B) keyed by amplitude (pooled saccade populations)

Amplitude	CHI ($n = 30$)		Controls ($n = 30$)		Difference		p-level
	Mean	SD	Mean	SD	Absolute	(%)	
Position error (PE, %):							
5°	**52.20**	51.08	**37.03**	52.42	15.16	40.95	0.062
10°	**70.84**	85.17	**39.82**	43.95	31.02	77.90	0.000
15°	**25.59**	28.22	**17.13**	14.70	8.46	49.39	0.013
20°	**51.17**	75.57	**34.48**	38.48	16.69	48.40	0.019
30°	**35.18**	32.09	**25.90**	28.37	9.28	35.84	0.103
Primary saccade gain (G_p):							
5°	**1.26**	0.57	**0.99**	0.64	0.27	27.12	0.005
10°	**1.19**	0.79	**0.99**	0.55	0.20	20.14	0.015
15°	**0.87**	0.35	**0.85**	0.26	0.02	2.73	0.618
20°	**1.17**	0.82	**1.00**	0.49	0.17	16.75	0.037
30°	**0.99**	0.46	**0.96**	0.35	0.03	3.35	0.672
Gain final eye position (G_f):							
5°	**1.42**	0.60	**1.12**	0.63	0.30	26.89	0.002
10°	**1.50**	0.99	**1.19**	0.56	0.32	26.65	0.001
15°	**1.09**	0.37	**0.97**	0.22	0.12	12.35	0.010
20°	**1.34**	0.85	**1.20**	0.48	0.13	10.89	0.108
30°	**1.13**	0.46	**1.09**	0.37	0.04	3.86	0.591

teria were similar to our own (GCS 13–15, PTA < 24 h, impaired consciousness) and eventually comprised 25 non-intoxicated mild CHI patients. However, all cases had the maximal GCS score of 15, only 15 had lost consciousness, none exceeded a PTA of 1 h (the mean PTA was not indicated), and 7 patients had no PTA at all. Consequently, it is unclear whether their finding of no oculomotor deficits was due to their having a substantially milder group than our own or was because single memory-guided saccades are less susceptible to the effects of mild CHI than memory-guided sequences. Similar to our findings, Mosimann et al. (2000) found an increased number of unwanted reflexive saccades (response errors) as well as increased position errors on single memory-guided saccades in whiplash patients with persisting symptoms. Whiplash injuries frequently have similar causes to CHI and can occur concomitantly in some cases, especially after motor vehicle accidents. Although the locations of damage can differ from CHI, symptoms are similar to those occurring after mild CHI and can persist for up to several years (Mallinson and Longridge, 1998a,b).

In our study, increased position errors occurred mainly in the form of a pronounced hypermetria (see Tables 1 and 2). Higher position errors on the CHI side were matched by increased amplitude errors on all steps in subtest A and subtest B (Table 2), indicating that deficits in accuracy were not only based on independent errors in spatial accuracy but on the decreased ability of the CHI patients to accurately program and execute a learned motor sequence or motor program. This also implies that the CHI group was less able to benefit from corrective movements to subjectively perceived errors in amplitude.

Ohtsuka et al. (1989) stated that position errors of more than 5° in single memory-guided saccades tend to be followed by a corrective saccade. Ditterich et al. (1998) also discussed the subject's tendency to correct perceived errors with corrective saccades in sequences of memory-guided saccades. We compared the degree to which our groups made a corrective saccade towards the expected target position during the sequences (i.e., the tendency to go further if they had undershot the expected amplitude or to go back if their primary saccade had gone too far). We found that both groups made secondary corrective saccades in the 'correct' direction in about 64% of all saccades (CHI 63.3% vs controls 65.8%), indicating that both groups tended to perceive errors equally well but with the controls being far more able to maintain an accurate performance throughout the sequence. We did not, however, assess the mean magnitude of these corrective movements. Bock et al. (1995) calculated that about 60% of a position error would be corrected and considered this correction mechanism as evidence for the existence of extraretinal inputs to the saccadic generator, which are used to maintain an accurate motor performance. Thus, the deficits found in our CHI group in the memory-guided sequences could be due to difficulty in accurately storing a sequence of saccades, memorizing a faulty motor program, or erroneous input of extraretinal information leading to ineffective correction of perceived errors. Interestingly, there was no difference in the number of saccades in any of the steps of the memory-guided sequences. Similarly, Williams et al. (1997) found no difference in the average number of saccades in single memory-guided saccades in severely head-injured patients.

Hypermetria of memory-guided saccades executed in darkness has been reported (Zingale and Kowler, 1987; Israel, 1992; in Petit et al., 1996). Ohtsuka et al. (1989) also noted that initial memory-guided saccades tend to overshoot the expected amplitude and are frequently followed by a corrective saccade, especially when the position errors exceed 5°. They further suggested a negative correlation between target amplitude and size of position error (amplitude of 20°: position error = $7.7 \pm 5.4°$; 40°: $5.8 \pm 4.5°$; 60°: $6.7 \pm 4.3°$; 80°: $3.2 \pm 3.3°$) which is consistent with the results from our control group showing similar position errors, as well as the CHI group, although with increased position errors. In contrast to the reports of hypermetria in memory-guided saccades in normal subjects, Ploner et al. (1999) observed hypometria in memory-guided saccades in patients with unilateral ischaemic lesions to the frontal eye field (FEF) and the dorsolateral prefrontal cortex (DLPFC). Crawford et al. (1989) reported hypometria in single memory-guided saccades in patients with idiopathic Parkinson's Disease. Similarly, Vermersch et al. (1994, 1999) reported hypometria in single memory-guided saccades in Parkinsonian patients and a patient with a caudate nucleus lesion. Hodgson et al. (1999) found hypometria in sequences of memory-guided saccades in patients with mild to moderate Parkinson's Disease and suggested the disruption of short-term spatial memory representations as underlying cause for the observed saccade deficits.

Cerebral lesions as cause for impaired saccade sequences after mild CHI

It is likely that the deficits in performance of memory-guided sequences are the result of neural damage, which can follow even mild cases of head trauma (e.g. Mittl et al., 1994). The deficits on memory-guided sequences indicate that the proper functioning of the corresponding networks of cortical and subcortical structures was disrupted by mild CHI. The consequent functional impairments likely affected the ability to accurately store or retrieve spatial information as well as the capacity to efficiently program a motor sequence and to relay the motor commands to the eyes.

However, as MRI scanning was not available for this study, we are unable to quantify or localize the extent of neural damage in the patients. Consequently, there is uncertainty about the factor composition triggering the impaired motor output, that is, the question of whether cortical dysfunction or damage to subcortical pathways was primarily responsible for the observed deficits.

The non-focal character of diffuse axonal injury (DAI), in combination with the heterogeneous functional structure of the oculomotor system, makes it difficult to assign eye movement deficits in response accuracy or spatial accuracy in our CHI group to distinct or specific cerebral regions. However, the impaired CHI performance on sequences of memory-guided saccades suggests impaired function of the SEF/SMA in combination with deficits originating in the PEF/PPC, FEF and DLPFC (Pierrot-Deseilligny et al., 1991b; Anderson et al., 1994; Gaymard et al., 1999), as demonstrated by decreased spatial accuracy and increased response errors.

Considerable evidence is available to demonstrate that lesions affecting the proper function of certain cortical areas impair eye movements (e.g. Guitton et al., 1985; Gaymard et al., 1990, 1993; Pierrot-Deseilligny et al., 1991a,b, 1991c; Thier et al., 1991; Keating, 1993). Lesions of PPC, FEF and DLPFC impair single remembered saccades (Guitton et al., 1985; Pierrot-Deseilligny et al., 1991b), whereas sequences of remembered saccades are impaired following lesions of the SMA (Gaymard et al., 1990, 1993), and also the hippocampal formation (Muri et al., 1994a). Muri et al. showed that transcranial magnetic stimulation over the SMA (Muri et al., 1994b, 1995) and the PPC (Muri et al., 1996) adversely affected sequences of memory-guided saccades and single memory-guided saccades with increased errors in amplitude and prolonged latencies. PET studies (Anderson et al., 1994; O'Sullivan et al., 1995; Sweeney et al., 1996) confirm the contribution of the SMA to memory-guided saccades but also support the participation of other areas such as FEF, DLPFC, thalamus or PPC. Research in monkeys confirms the importance of the PPC, in particular the left lateral bank of the intraparietal sulcus for saccade-related sensory–motor transformation in memory-guided saccades (Gnadt and Andersen, 1988; Gnadt et al., 1991). Neural damage to the PPC or its connections with the SC might have contributed to inaccurate memory-guided saccades in the CHI group, although there are indications that inaccuracies of memory-guided saccades can have their origin downstream from the SC (Stanford and Sparks, 1994). The DLPFC contributes to spatial short-term memory (O'Sullivan et al., 1995; Gaymard et al., 1998a) and accuracy of memory-guided saccades is impaired by transcranial magnetic stimulation over the DLPFC (Brandt et al., 1998). Walker et al. (1998) reported impairments of spatial working memory and executive functioning in a patient with lesions to the prefrontal cortex. In general, the FEF and the DLPFC play an important role in the generation and suppression of voluntary saccades (Guitton et al., 1985; Pierrot-Deseilligny et al., 1995; Ploner et al., 1999), including memory-guided saccades. Sakai et al. (1998) pointed out the importance of frontal areas such as the DLPFC and the preSMA for visuomotor sequence learning, which also involves a shift from activation of frontal areas in early learning stages to mainly parietal areas in later stages. These findings support the argument that neural dysfunction originating in frontal and pre-frontal cortical areas may have contributed to the saccade deficits of the CHI group.

It has been shown that most of the diffuse neural damage is located at the grey and white matter junction (Mittl et al., 1994), in some cases extending into the deeper white matter and the brainstem. Important relay pathways within the oculomotor and sensory–motor networks pass through these areas. Diffuse axonal injury (DAI) may cause the disruption of motor network pathways important for intra-cerebral communication and information relay to motor neurons. Several studies on primates and other animals have demonstrated such connections (Tusa and Ungerleider, 1988; Leichnetz, 1989; Andersen et al., 1990; Tian and Lynch, 1996). PET and MRI studies have also helped illuminate the functional anatomy of motor processing in humans, showing that their motor networks involved in oculomotor coordination are in general comparable to the findings from non-human primates (Anderson et al., 1994; Kawashima et al., 1995, 1998). The oculomotor network involves, amongst others, projections from the PPC to the frontal cortex (PEF to FEF/SEF), connections between FEF/SEF and the intramedullary lamina of the thalamus, the SC and the cerebellar vermis in addition to separate projections form the PPC (PEF) to the SC, and direct pathways from the frontal cortex to the saccade generators in the brainstem. Chafee and Goldman-Rakic (2000) found an interdependency of neural activity in the DLPFC and the PPC in memory-guided saccades which underlines the suggestion of considerable intra-cerebral communication and the importance of the corresponding neural pathways for the relay of information and motor commands. Electrophysiologal studies in monkeys (Everling et al., 1999; Everling and Munoz, 2000) have shown that neural activity in cortical areas such as the FEF is closely correlated to neural activity in the SC and the saccadic burst neurons in the brainstem, showing that cortical areas directly regulate neural activation patterns in lower regions (Dorris et al., 1997; Dorris and Munoz, 1998; Everling et al., 1999). Eye movement deficits are to be expected should the functional integrity of the corresponding neural pathways be compromised, as is often the case in CHI.

The subjects were also assessed on several neuropsychological tests with high cognitive loads. The complete neuropsychological data are the subject of a separate publication (in preparation). In essence, the CHI group showed deficits on several of these tests including the Paced Auditory Serial Addition Task, Trail Making Test B, Single Digit Modalities Test, the California Verbal Learning Test, and two subtests of the Wechsler Abbreviated Scale of Intelligence, the Vocabulary Test and Matrix Reasoning. However, we found very few correlations between neuropsychological test results and measures of memory-guided sequences of saccades. This lack of association suggests that the deficits on memory-guided sequences of saccades may incorporate additional aspects of cerebral dysfunction following mild CHI, which appear to be independent from cognitive functions assessed by neuropsychological testing.

The present observation of abnormalities of sequences of memory-guided saccades in combination with reports of deficits on antisaccades and self-paced saccades (Heitger et al., 2001a) as well as impairment of upper-limb sensory–motor function following mild CHI (Heitger et al., 2001b) presents a picture of widespread impairment of motor functions originating in the frontal and the parietal cortex. This picture is consistent with the results of research on the biomechanics of CHI (Wilson, 1990; Ommaya, 1995) and previous studies incorporating neuropsychological testing (Levin et al., 1987, 1992; Mattson and Levin, 1990; Duncan et al., 1997), showing that damage seems to occur mostly in frontal and fronto-temporal parts of the brain, leaving occipital areas and the cerebellum largely unharmed. Further support for this view is the finding that oculomotor smooth pursuit is largely preserved following mild CHI (Heitger et al., 2001a), suggesting that occipital areas and the cerebellum seem to be less affected in mild CHI. Further, the cerebellar vermis mediates the subconscious saccadic adaptation of reflexive saccades (Desmurget et al., 2000), which is unaffected by mild CHI (Heitger et al., 2001c). The absence of deficits on timing and rhythm (i.e., temporal accuracy) on memory-guided sequence performance in our experiment would also appear consistent with this suggestion, as these functions are at least in part mediated by the cerebellum (Ivry et al., 1988).

Concluding remarks

Results from our study indicate that, although oculomotor function may appear normal on clinical examination, mild CHI can cause deficits in the performance of memory-guided sequences of saccades. It is likely that these deficits are caused by neural damage resulting from diffuse cerebral lesions. The observed abnormalities indicate dysfunction originating in frontal and dorso-parietal cortical areas either through direct cortical lesions or through damage to neural pathways originating in or connecting these areas.

Our results suggest that abnormalities of memory-guided saccades may provide sensitive markers of impaired neurophysiological functioning after mild CHI. The deficits on memory-guided sequences add to other evidence of altered motor function following mild CHI, such as impairments of antisaccades, self-paced saccades, and aspects of upper-limb sensory–motor performance. The findings indicate a potential use for computerized eye movement tests to supplement clinical and neuropsychological patient assessment following mild head trauma.

It will be important to determine how soon the deficits in saccades resolve following injury, and whether there is a correlation with the persistence of symptoms and the development of post-concussion syndrome (PCS), as there is currently no accurate mean to determine the likelihood of developing PCS in a patient with mild or moderate CHI.

Abbreviations

ATI	absolute time index
CHI	closed head injury
CT	computer tomography
DAI	diffuse axonal injury
DLPFC	dorsolateral prefrontal cortex
EMMA	eye movement measurement and analysis
FEF	frontal eye field
GCS	Glasgow coma scale
IRI	inter-response interval
LED	light emitting diode
MRI	magnetic resonance imaging
MT	middle temporal area
PCS	post-concussion syndrome
PEF	parietal eye field
PET	positron emission tomography
PPC	posterior parietal cortex
PTA	post-traumatic amnesia
SC	superior colliculus
SD	standard deviation
SEF	supplementary eye field
SMA	supplementary motor area

References

Alexander, M.P. (1995) Mild traumatic brain injury: pathophysiology, natural history, and clinical management. *Neurology*, 45: 1253–1260.

Andersen, R.A. (1995) Encoding of intention and spatial location in the posterior parietal cortex. *Cereb. Cortex*, 5: 457–469.

Andersen, R.A., Asanuma, C., Essick, G. and Siegel, R.M. (1990) Corticocortical connections of anatomically and physiologically defined subdivisions within the inferior parietal lobule. *J. Comp. Neurol.*, 296: 65–113.

Andersen, R.A., Snyder, L.H., Batista, A.P., Buneo, C.A. and Cohen, Y.E. (1998) Posterior parietal areas specialized for eye movements (LIP) and reach (PRR) using a common coordinate frame [discussion 122–128, 171–175]. *Novartis Found. Symp.*, 218: 109–122.

Anderson, T.J., Jenkins, I.H., Brooks, D.J., Hawken, M.B., Frackowiak, R.S. and Kennard, C. (1994) Cortical control of saccades and fixation in man: a PET study. *Brain*, 117: 1073–1084.

Armstead, W.M. (1999) Superoxide generation links protein kinase C activation to impaired ATP-sensitive K^+ channel function after brain injury. *Stroke*, 30: 153–159.

Bernad, P.G. (1991) Neurodiagnostic testing in patients with closed head injury. *Clin. Electroencephalogr.*, 22: 203–210.

Blekher, T., Siemers, E., Abel, L.A. and Yee, R.D. (2000) Eye movements in Parkinson's disease: before and after pallidotomy. *Invest. Ophthalmol. Vis. Sci.*, 41: 2177–2183.

Blumbergs, P.C., Jones, N.R. and North, J.B. (1989) Diffuse axonal injury in head trauma. *J. Neurol. Neurosurg. Psychiatry*, 52: 838–841.

Bock, O., Goltz, H., Belanger, S. and Steinbach, M. (1995) On the role of extraretinal signals for saccade generation. *Exp. Brain Res.*, 104: 349–350.

Bohnen, N. and Jolles, J. (1992) Neurobehavioral aspects of post-concussive symptoms after mild head injury. *J. Nerv. Ment. Dis.*, 180: 683–692.

Brandt, S.A., Ploner, C.J., Meyer, B.U., Leistner, S. and Villringer, A. (1998) Effects of repetitive transcranial magnetic stimulation over dorsolateral prefrontal and posterior parietal cortex on memory-guided saccades. *Exp. Brain Res.*, 118: 197–204.

Chafee, M.V. and Goldman-Rakic, P.S. (2000) Inactivation of parietal and prefrontal cortex reveals interdependence of neural activity during memory-guided saccades. *J. Neurophysiol.*, 83: 1550–1566.

Connolly, J.D., Goodale, M.A., Desouza, J.F., Menon, R.S. and Vilis, T. (2000) A comparison of frontoparietal fMRI activation during anti-saccades and anti-pointing. *J. Neurophysiol.*, 84: 1645–1655.

Corbetta, M., Akbudak, E., Conturo, T.E., Snyder, A.Z., Ollinger, J.M., Drury, H.A., Linenweber, M.R., Petersen, S.E., Raichle, M.E., Van Essen, D.C. and Shulman, G.L. (1998) A common network of functional areas for attention and eye movements. *Neuron*, 21: 761–773.

Crawford, T.J., Henderson, L. and Kennard, C. (1989) Abnormalities of nonvisually-guided eye movements in Parkinson's disease. *Brain*, 112: 1573–1586.

Crevits, L., Hanse, M.C., Tummers, P. and Van Maele, G. (2000) Antisaccades and remembered saccades in mild traumatic brain injury. *J. Neurol.*, 247: 179–182.

Crooks, D.A., Scholtz, C.L., Vowles, G., Greenwald, S. and Evans, S. (1992) Axonal injury in closed head injury by assault: a quantitative study. *Med. Sci. Law*, 32: 109–117.

Desmurget, M., Pelisson, D., Grethe, J.S., Alexander, G.E., Urquizar, C., Prablanc, C. and Grafton, S.T. (2000) Functional adaptation of reactive saccades in humans: a PET study. *Exp. Brain Res.*, 132: 243–259.

DeSouza, J.F., Dukelow, S.P., Gati, J.S., Menon, R.S., Andersen, R.A. and Vilis, T. (2000) Eye position signal modulates a human parietal pointing region during memory-guided movements. *J. Neurosci.*, 20: 5835–5840.

Ditterich, J., Eggert, T. and Straube, A. (1998) Fixation errors and timing in sequences of memory-guided saccades. *Behav. Brain Res.*, 95: 205–217.

Dorris, M.C. and Munoz, D.P. (1998) Saccadic probability influences motor preparation signals and time to saccadic initiation. *J. Neurosci.*, 18: 7015–7026.

Dorris, M.C., Pare, M. and Munoz, D.P. (1997) Neuronal activity in monkey superior colliculus related to the initiation of saccadic eye movements. *J. Neurosci.*, 17: 8566–8579.

Duncan, J., Johnson, R., Swales, M. and Freer, C. (1997) Frontal lobe deficits after head injury: unity and diversity of function. *Cogn. Neuropsychol.*, 14: 713–741.

Everling, S. and Munoz, D.P. (2000) Neuronal correlates for preparatory set associated with pro-saccades and anti-saccades in the primate frontal eye field. *J. Neurosci.*, 20: 387–400.

Everling, S., Dorris, M.C., Klein, R.M. and Munoz, D.P. (1999) Role of primate superior colliculus in preparation and execution of anti-saccades and pro-saccades. *J. Neurosci.*, 19: 2740–2754.

Gaymard, B., Pierrot-Deseilligny, C. and Rivaud, S. (1990) Impairment of sequences of memory-guided saccades after supplementary motor area lesions. *Ann. Neurol.*, 28: 622–626.

Gaymard, B., Rivaud, S. and Pierrot-Deseilligny, C. (1993) Role of the left and right supplementary motor areas in memory-guided saccade sequences. *Ann. Neurol.*, 34: 404–406.

Gaymard, B., Ploner, C.J., Rivaud, S., Vermersch, A.I. and Pierrot-Deseilligny, C. (1998a) Cortical control of saccades. *Exp. Brain Res.*, 123: 159–163.

Gaymard, B., Rivaud, S., Cassarini, J.F., Dubard, T., Rancurel, G., Agid, Y. and Pierrot-Deseilligny, C. (1998b) Effects of anterior cingulate cortex lesions on ocular saccades in humans. *Exp. Brain Res.*, 120: 173–183.

Gaymard, B., Ploner, C.J., Rivaud-Pechoux, S. and Pierrot-Deseilligny, C. (1999) The frontal eye field is involved in spatial short-term memory but not in reflexive saccade inhibition. *Exp. Brain Res.*, 129: 288–301.

Gieron, M.A., Korthals, J.K. and Riggs, C.D. (1998) Diffuse axonal injury without direct head trauma and with delayed onset of coma. *Pediatr. Neurol.*, 19: 382–384.

Glass, I., Groswasser, Z. and Groswasser-Reider, I. (1995) Impersistent execution of saccadic eye movements after traumatic brain injury. *Brain Inj.*, 9: 769–775.

Gnadt, J.W. and Andersen, R.A. (1988) Memory related motor

planning activity in posterior parietal cortex of macaque. *Exp. Brain Res.*, 70: 216–220.

Gnadt, J.W., Bracewell, R.M. and Andersen, R.A. (1991) Sensorimotor transformation during eye movements to remembered visual targets. *Vision Res.*, 31: 693–715.

Guitton, D., Buchtel, H.A. and Douglas, R.M. (1985) Frontal lobe lesions in man cause difficulties in suppressing reflexive glances and in generating goal-directed saccades. *Exp. Brain Res.*, 58: 455–472.

Heide, W., Blankenburg, M., Zimmermann, E. and Kompf, D. (1995) Cortical control of double-step saccades: implications for spatial orientation. *Ann. Neurol.*, 38: 739–748.

Heitger, M.H., Anderson, T.J., Jones, R.D., Ardagh, M.W. and Donaldson, I.M. (2001a) Mild closed head injury and eye movements [abstract]. *N. Z. Med. J.*, 114: 385.

Heitger, M.H., Anderson, T.J., Jones, R.D., Ardagh, M.W. and Donaldson, I.M. (2001b) Deficits in upper-limb visual-motor function following mild closed head injury [abstract]. *N. Z. Med. J.*, 114: 385.

Heitger, M.H., MacAskill, M.R., Anderson, T.J., Jones, R.D., Ardagh, M.W. and Donaldson, I.M. (2001c) Subconscious saccadic adaptation is not affected by mild closed head injury [abstract]. *N. Z. Med. J.*, 114: 480.

Hodgson, T.L., Dittrich, W.H., Henderson, L. and Kennard, C. (1999) Eye movements and spatial working memory in Parkinson's disease. *Neuropsychologia*, 37: 927–938.

Israel, I. (1992) Memory-guided saccades: what is memorized? *Exp. Brain Res.*, 90: 221–224.

Ivry, R.B., Keele, S.W. and Diener, H.C. (1988) Dissociation of the lateral and medial cerebellum in movement timing and movement execution. *Exp. Brain Res.*, 73: 167–180.

Jane, J.A. and Rimel, R.W. (1982) Prognosis in head injury. *Clin. Neurosurg.*, 29: 346–352.

Jane, J.A., Steward, O. and Gennarelli, T. (1985) Axonal degeneration induced by experimental noninvasive minor head injury. *J. Neurosurg.*, 62: 96–100.

Jennett, B. (1996) Epidemiology of head injury. *J. Neurol. Neurosurg. Psychiatry*, 60: 362–369.

Jennett, B. and Teasdale, G. (1981) *Management of Head Injuries*. Davis, Philadelphia, PA.

Kandel, E.R., Schwartz, J.H. and Jessell, T.M. (1991) *Principles of Neural Science*. Appleton and Lange, Norwalk, CT.

Kawashima, R., Roland, P.E. and O'Sullivan, B.T. (1995) Functional anatomy of reaching and visuomotor learning: a positron emission tomography study. *Cereb. Cortex*, 5: 111–122.

Kawashima, R., Tanji, J., Okada, K., Sugiura, M., Sato, K., Kinomura, S., Inoue, K., Ogawa, A. and Fukuda, H. (1998) Oculomotor sequence learning: a positron emission tomography study. *Exp. Brain Res.*, 122: 1–8.

Keating, E.G. (1993) Lesions of the frontal eye field impair pursuit eye movements, but preserve the predictions driving them. *Behav. Brain Res.*, 53: 91–104.

Klein, C., Fischer, B., Hartnegg, K., Heiss, W.H. and Roth, M. (2000) Optomotor and neuropsychological performance in old age. *Exp. Brain Res.*, 135: 141–154.

Knoblach, S.M., Fan, L. and Faden, A.I. (1999) Early neuronal expression of tumor necrosis factor-alpha after experimental brain injury contributes to neurological impairment. *J. Neuroimmunol.*, 95: 115–125.

Kraus, J.F. and Nourjah, P. (1988) The epidemiology of mild uncomplicated brain injury. *J. Trauma*, 28: 1637–1643.

Lee, T.T., Galarza, M. and Villanueva, P.A. (1998) Diffuse axonal injury (DAI) is not associated with elevated intracranial pressure (ICP). *Acta Neurochir. (Wien)*, 140: 41–46.

Leichnetz, G.R. (1989) Inferior frontal eye field projections to the pursuit-related dorsolateral pontine nucleus and middle temporal area (MT) in the monkey. *Vis. Neurosci.*, 3: 171–180.

LeVasseur, A.L., Flanagan, J.R., Riopelle, R.J. and Munoz, D.P. (2001) Control of volitional and reflexive saccades in Tourette's syndrome. *Brain*, 124: 2045–2058.

Levin, H.S., Amparo, E., Eisenberg, H.M., Williams, D.H., High Jr., W.M., McArdle, C.B. and Weiner, R.L. (1987) Magnetic resonance imaging and computerized tomography in relation to the neurobehavioral sequelae of mild and moderate head injuries. *J. Neurosurg.*, 66: 706–713.

Levin, H.S., Amparo, E.G., Eisenberg, H.M., Miner, M.E., High Jr., W.M., Ewing-Cobbs, L., Fletcher, J.M. and Guinto Jr., F.C. (1989) Magnetic resonance imaging after closed head injury in children. *Neurosurgery*, 24: 223–227.

Levin, H.S., Williams, D.H., Eisenberg, H.M., High Jr., W.M. and Guinto Jr., F.C. (1992) Serial MRI and neurobehavioural findings after mild to moderate closed head injury. *J. Neurol. Neurosurg. Psychiatry*, 55: 255–262.

Lueck, C.J., Crawford, T.J., Henderson, L., Van Gisbergen, J.A., Duysens, J. and Kennard, C. (1992) Saccadic eye movements in Parkinson's disease: II. Remembered saccades — towards a unified hypothesis? *Q. J. Exp. Psychol. A.*, 45: 211–233.

Mallinson, A.I. and Longridge, N.S. (1998a) Dizziness from whiplash and head injury: differences between whiplash and head injury [see comments]. *Am. J. Otol.*, 19: 814–818.

Mallinson, A.I. and Longridge, N.S. (1998b) Specific vocalized complaints in whiplash and minor head injury patients [see comments]. *Am. J. Otol.*, 19: 809–813.

Mattson, A.J. and Levin, H.S. (1990) Frontal lobe dysfunction following closed head injury: a review of the literature. *J. Nerv. Ment. Dis.*, 178: 282–291.

McPeek, R.M., Maljkovic, V. and Nakayama, K. (1999) Saccades require focal attention and are facilitated by a short-term memory system. *Vision Res.*, 39: 1555–1566.

Mendelsohn, D., Levin, H.S., Bruce, D., Lilly, M., Harward, H., Culhane, K.A. and Eisenberg, H.M. (1992a) Late MRI after head injury in children: relationship to clinical features and outcome. *Childs Nerv. Syst.*, 8: 445–452.

Mendelsohn, D.B., Levin, H.S., Harward, H. and Bruce, D. (1992b) Corpus callosum lesions after closed head injury in children: MRI, clinical features and outcome. *Neuroradiology*, 34: 384–388.

Mittl, R.L., Grossman, R.I., Hiehle, J.F., Hurst, R.W., Kauder, D.R., Gennarelli, T.A. and Alburger, G.W. (1994) Prevalence of MR evidence of diffuse axonal injury in patients with mild head injury and normal head CT findings. *Am. J. Neuroradiol.*, 15: 1583–1589.

Morrison, B., Eberwine, J.H., Meaney, D.F. and McIntosh, T.K.

(2000) Traumatic injury induces differential expression of cell death genes in organotypic brain slice cultures determined by complementary DNA array hybridization. *Neuroscience*, 96: 131–139.

Mosimann, U.P., Muri, R.M., Felblinger, J. and Radanov, B.P. (2000) Saccadic eye movement disturbances in whiplash patients with persistent complaints. *Brain*, 123: 828–835.

Muir, S.R., MacAskill, M.R., Herron, D., Goelz, H., Jones, R.D. and Anderson, T.J. (2001) EMMA — an Eye-Movement Measurement and Analysis System. *Proc. 23rd Int. Conf. IEEE Eng. Med. Biol. Soc.*, 23: 4 pages (CD-ROM).

Mulhall, L.E., Williams, I.M. and Abel, L.A. (1999) Bedside tests of saccades after head injury [see erratum in J. Neurophthalmol., 20(2): 146]. *J. Neuroophthalmol.*, 19: 160–165.

Muri, R.M., Rivaud, S., Timsit, S., Cornu, P. and Pierrot-Deseilligny, C. (1994a) The role of the right medial temporal lobe in the control of memory-guided saccades. *Exp. Brain Res.*, 101: 165–168.

Muri, R.M., Rosler, K.M. and Hess, C.W. (1994b) Influence of transcranial magnetic stimulation on the execution of memorised sequences of saccades in man. *Exp. Brain Res.*, 101: 521–524.

Muri, R.M., Rivaud, S., Vermersch, A.I., Leger, J.M. and Pierrot-Deseilligny, C. (1995) Effects of transcranial magnetic stimulation over the region of the supplementary motor area during sequences of memory-guided saccades. *Exp. Brain Res.*, 104: 163–166.

Muri, R.M., Vermersch, A.I., Rivaud, S., Gaymard, B. and Pierrot-Deseilligny, C. (1996) Effects of single-pulse transcranial magnetic stimulation over the prefrontal and posterior parietal cortices during memory-guided saccades in humans. *J. Neurophysiol.*, 76: 2102–2106.

Nieman, D.H., Bour, L.J., Linszen, D.H., Goede, J., Koelman, J., Gersons, B.P.R. and de Visser, B.W.O. (2000) Neuropsychological and clinical correlates of antisaccade task performance in schizophrenia. *Neurology*, 54: 866–871.

Ohtsuka, K., Sawa, M. and Takeda, M. (1989) Accuracy of memory-guided saccades. *Ophthalmologica*, 198: 53–56.

Ommaya, A.K. (1995) Head injury mechanisms and the concept of preventive management: a review and critical synthesis. *J. Neurotrauma*, 12: 527–546.

O'Sullivan, E.P., Jenkins, I.H., Henderson, L., Kennard, C. and Brooks, D.J. (1995) The functional anatomy of remembered saccades: a PET study. *Neuroreport*, 6: 2141–2144.

Parizel, P.M., Ozsarlak, A., Van Goethem, J.W., van den Hauwe, L., Dillen, C., Verlooy, J., Cosyns, P. and De Schepper, A.M. (1998) Imaging findings in diffuse axonal injury after closed head trauma. *Eur. Radiol.*, 8: 960–965.

Paterakis, K., Karantanas, A.H., Komnos, A. and Volikas, Z. (2000) Outcome of patients with diffuse axonal injury: the significance and prognostic value of MRI in the acute phase. *J. Trauma*, 49: 1071–1075.

Petit, L., Orssaud, C., Tzourio, N., Crivello, F., Berthoz, A. and Mazoyer, B. (1996) Functional anatomy of a prelearned sequence of horizontal saccades in humans. *J. Neurosci.*, 16: 3714–3726.

Picard, N. and Strick, P.L. (1996) Motor areas of the medial wall: a review of their location and functional activation. *Cereb. Cortex*, 6: 342–353.

Picard, N. and Strick, P.L. (1997) Activation on the medial wall during remembered sequences of reaching movements in monkeys. *J. Neurophysiol.*, 77: 2197–2201.

Pierrot-Deseilligny, C., Rivaud, S., Gaymard, B. and Agid, Y. (1991a) Cortical control of reflexive visually guided saccades. *Brain*, 114: 1473–1485.

Pierrot-Deseilligny, C., Rivaud, S., Gaymard, B. and Agid, Y. (1991b) Cortical control of memory-guided saccades in man. *Exp. Brain Res.*, 83: 607–617.

Pierrot-Deseilligny, C., Rosa, A., Masmoudi, K., Rivaud, S. and Gaymard, B. (1991c) Saccade deficits after a unilateral lesion affecting the superior colliculus. *J. Neurol. Neurosurg. Psychiatry*, 54: 1106–1109.

Pierrot-Deseilligny, C., Rivaud, S., Gaymard, B., Muri, R. and Vermersch, A.I. (1995) Cortical control of saccades. *Ann. Neurol.*, 37: 557–567.

Ploner, C.J., Rivaud-Pechoux, S., Gaymard, B.M., Agid, Y. and Pierrot-Deseilligny, C. (1999) Errors of memory-guided saccades in humans with lesions of the frontal eye field and the dorsolateral prefrontal cortex. *J. Neurophysiol.*, 82: 1086–1090.

Povlishock, J.T., Becker, D.P., Cheng, C.L.Y. and Voughn, G.W. (1983) Axonal change in minor head injury. *J. Neuropathol. Exp. Neurol.*, 42: 225–242.

Reulen, J.P.H., Marcus, J.T., Koops, D., De Vries, F.R., Tiesinga, G., Boshuizen, K. and Bos, J.E. (1988) Precise recording of eye movement: the IRIS technique Part 1. *Med. Biol. Eng. Comput.*, 26: 20–26.

Richardson, J.T.E. (2000) *Clinical and Neuropsychological Aspects of Closed Head Injury*. Psychology Press, Hove.

Rimel, R.W., Giordani, B., Barth, J.T., Boll, T.J. and Jane, J.A. (1981) Disability caused by minor head injury. *Neurosurgery*, 9: 221–228.

Rivaud, S., Muri, R.M., Gaymard, B., Vermersch, A.I. and Pierrot-Deseilligny, C. (1994) Eye movement disorders after frontal eye field lesions in humans. *Exp. Brain Res.*, 102: 110–120.

Rivaud-Pechoux, S., Vermersch, A.I., Gaymard, B., Ploner, C.J., Bejjani, B.P., Damier, P., Demeret, S., Agid, Y. and Pierrot-Deseilligny, C. (2000) Improvement of memory guided saccades in parkinsonian patients by high frequency subthalamic nucleus stimulation. *J. Neurol. Neurosurg. Psychiatry*, 68: 381–384.

Roberts, R.J.J., Hager, L.D. and Heron, C. (1994) Prefrontal cognitive processes: working memory and inhibition in the antisaccade task. *J. Exp. Neuropsychol.*, 123: 374–393.

Rutherford, W.H., Merret, J.D. and McDonald, J.R. (1978) Symptoms at one year following concussion from minor head injuries. *Injury*, 10: 225–230.

Sahuquillo, J., Vilalta, J., Lamarca, J., Rubio, E., Rodriguez-Pazos, M. and Salva, J.A. (1989) Diffuse axonal injury after severe head trauma: a clinico-pathological study. *Acta Neurochir. (Wien)*, 101: 149–158.

Sakai, K., Hikosaka, O., Miyauchi, S., Takino, R., Sasaki, Y. and Putz, B. (1998) Transition of brain activation from frontal to parietal areas in visuomotor sequence learning. *J. Neurosci.*, 18: 1827–1840.

Servadei, P., Vergoni, G., Pasini, A., Fagioli, L., Arista, A. and Zappi, D. (1994) Diffuse axonal injury with brainstem localisation: report of a case in a mild head injured patient. *J. Neurosurg. Sci.*, 38: 129–130.

Slater, E.J. (1989) Does mild mean minor? Recovery after closed head injury. *J. Adolesc. Health Care*, 10: 237–240.

Snyder, L.H., Batista, A.P. and Andersen, R.A. (2000) Intention-related activity in the posterior parietal cortex: a review. *Vision Res.*, 40: 1433–1441.

Sosin, D.M., Sniezek, J.E. and Thurman, D.J. (1996) Incidence of mild and moderate brain injury in the United States, 1991. *Brain Inj.*, 10: 47–54.

Stanford, T.R. and Sparks, D.L. (1994) Systematic errors for saccades to remembered targets: evidence for a dissociation between saccade metrics and activity in the superior colliculus. *Vision Res.*, 34: 193–206.

Straube, A., Mennicken, J.B., Riedel, M., Eggert, T. and Muller, N. (1997) Saccades in Gilles de la Tourette's syndrome. *Mov. Disord.*, 12: 536–546.

Sweeney, J.A., Mintun, M.A., Kwee, S., Wiseman, M.B., Brown, D.L., Rosenberg, D.R. and Carl, J.R. (1996) Positron emission tomography study of voluntary saccadic eye movements and spatial working memory. *J. Neurophysiol.*, 75: 454–468.

Thier, P., Bachor, A., Faiss, J., Dichgans, J. and Koenig, E. (1991) Selective impairment of smooth-pursuit eye movements due to an ischemic lesion of the basal pons. *Ann. Neurol.*, 29: 443–448.

Tian, J.R. and Lynch, J.C. (1996) Corticocortical input to the smooth and saccadic eye movement subregions of the frontal eye field in Cebus monkeys. *J. Neurophysiol.*, 76: 2754–2771.

Trembovler, V., Beit-Yannai, E., Younis, F., Gallily, R., Horowitz, M. and Shohami, E. (1999) Antioxidants attenuate acute toxicity of tumor necrosis factor-alpha induced by brain injury in rat. *J. Interferon Cytokine Res.*, 19: 791–795.

Tusa, R.J. and Ungerleider, L.G. (1988) Fiber pathways of cortical areas mediating smooth pursuit eye movements in monkeys. *Ann. Neurol.*, 23: 174–183.

Vagnozzi, R., Marmarou, A., Tavazzi, B., Signoretti, S., Di Pierro, D., Del Bolgia, F., Amorini, A.M., Fazzina, G., Sherkat, S. and Lazzarino, G. (1999) Changes of cerebral energy metabolism and lipid peroxidation in rats leading to mitochondrial dysfunction after diffuse brain injury. *J. Neurotrauma*, 16: 903–913.

Vermersch, A.I., Rivaud, S., Vidailhet, M., Bonnet, A.M., Gaymard, B., Agid, Y. and Pierrot-Deseilligny, C. (1994) Sequences of memory-guided saccades in Parkinson's disease. *Ann. Neurol.*, 35: 487–490.

Vermersch, A.I., Gaymard, B.M., Rivaud-Pechoux, S., Ploner, C.J., Agid, Y. and Pierrot-Deseilligny, C. (1999) Memory guided saccade deficit after caudate nucleus lesion. *J. Neurol. Neurosurg. Psychiatry*, 66: 524–527.

Walker, R., Husain, M., Hodgson, T.L., Harrison, J. and Kennard, C. (1998) Saccadic eye movement and working memory deficits following damage to human prefrontal cortex. *Neuropsychologia*, 36: 1141–1159.

Watson, M.R., Fenton, G.W., McClelland, R.J., Lumsden, J., Headley, M. and Rutherford, W.H. (1995) The post-concussional state: neurophysiological aspects. *Br. J. Psychiatry*, 167: 514–521.

Williams, I.M., Ponsford, J.L., Gibson, K.L., Mulhall, L.E., Curran, C.A. and Abel, L.A. (1997) Cerebral control of saccades and neuropsychological test results after head injury. *J. Clin. Neurosci.*, 4: 186–196.

Wilson, J.T. (1990) The relationship between neuropsychological function and brain damage detected by neuroimaging after closed head injury. *Brain Inj.*, 4: 349–363.

Wright, S.C. (1998) Case report: postconcussion syndrome after minor head injury. *Aviat. Space Environ. Med.*, 69: 999–1000.

Wrightson, P. and Gronwall, D. (1998) Mild head injury in New Zealand: incidence of injury and persisting symptoms. *N. Z. Med. J.*, 111: 99–101.

Zarkovic, K., Jadro-Santel, D. and Grcevic, N. (1991) Distribution of traumatic lesions of corpus callosum in 'inner cerebral trauma'. *Neurol. Croat.*, 40: 129–155.

Zingale, C.M. and Kowler, E. (1987) Planning sequences of saccades. *Vision Res.*, 27: 1327–1341.

CHAPTER 30

Cognition and the inhibitory control of saccades in schizophrenia and Parkinson's disease

T.J. Crawford [*,1], D. Bennett [1], G. Lekwuwa [2], S. Shaunak [2] and J.F.W. Deakin [3]

[1] *Mental Health and Neural Systems Research Unit, Department of Psychology, Lancaster University, Lancaster, LA1 4YF, UK*
[2] *Lancashire Teaching Hospitals NHS Trust, Neuroscience Directorate, Departments of Neurology and Neurophysiology, Sharoe Green Lane, Preston, PR2 9HT, UK*
[3] *Neurosciences and Psychiatry Unit, University of Manchester, G907, Stopford Building, Oxford Road, Manchester, M13 9PT, UK*

Abstract: Historically, various lines of evidence have converged on the view that the brain expends much of its neural resources on inhibiting its own activity in a critical step towards the cognitive control of behaviour. The loss of inhibitory control is widely reported in neurological and psychiatric disorders; however, the consequences of reduced inhibition in terms of wider cognitive effects on cognitive control operations such as planning, abstract thought, working memory and the ability to appreciate the perspective of others ('theory of mind') has been widely overlooked. The antisaccade paradigm examines the conflict between a prepotent stimulus that produces a powerful urge to fixate the target, and the overriding goal to 'look' in the opposite direction. In this chapter we illustrate how this paradigm is increasingly used to explore the relationship of inhibitory control and cognition in Parkinson's disease, schizophrenia and healthy participants. Evidence is presented that is consistent with the theory of cognitive inhibition as a distinct process that can be dissociated from working memory. We conclude that the inhibitory control of saccadic eye movement should be studied in the wider context of cognitive operations.

Introduction

"If the centres of inhibition, and thereby the faculty of attention, are weak, or present impulses unusually strong, volition is impulsive rather than deliberate. The centres of inhibition being thus the essential factor of attention, constitute the organic basis of all the higher intellectual faculties." (Ferrier, 1876).

In the 19th century a number of physiologists and philosophers became increasingly convinced that mental constructs such as intelligence and the will, were dependent on the capacity to inhibit undesired or inappropriate reflexive activity. The concept of central inhibition has a long, and at times controversial, history in neuroscience. Volkmann (1838) used the concept to account for reflexes that only emerged after decapitation. It was believed that through inhibition, the cerebral control of the lower reflexes was possible and mentally controlled behaviour was formed. Alexander Bain (1859) argued that the inhibition of action was intimately related to cognition and perception. Echoing more recent theories, such as premotor theory (cf. Rizzolatti et al., 1987), he argued that the internal mental representations involved the preparation of a movement that was arrested or suppressed. A visual image was a "train of the rapid movements of the eyes, hither and thither, over voluminous points, lines, and surfaces", . . . the "inward operations for holding a remembered or ideal picture in view were again the very same as the actual examination of the original", except that the movements were prevented from taking place

---

[*] Correspondence to: T.J. Crawford, Mental Health and Neural Systems Research Unit, Department of Psychology, Lancaster University, Lancaster, LA1 4YF, UK. E-mail: t.crawford@lancaster.ac.uk

(Bain, 1859). For Bain, the 'will' controlled attention by preventing activity in the voluntary muscles. This inhibitory component was the principle distinction between thought and action. David Ferrier broadly shared this view. "... We think of form by initiating and then inhibiting the movement of the eyes or hands through which and by which ideas of form had been gained and persist... We recall an object in idea by pronouncing the name in the suppressed manner" (Ferrier, 1876). As a student of Bain's, Ferrier became a powerful advocate of the central physiological and cognitive role of inhibition, arguing that the development of the 'will' depended on the control of motor and inhibitory centres. He provided an anatomical landmark for this inhibition by suggesting that it was housed in the prefrontal cortex.[1]

The problem of self-control

When we chose to fixate on one object rather than another or to avoid fixating on a compelling stimulus, we are engaged in cognitive control. Cognitive control enables us to modulate those aspects of the environment that will be rejected or selected for detailed scrutiny, and to respond or withhold a response to a given stimulus. This ability to influence our own perceptions, thoughts, actions and attentional mechanisms is an important feature of voluntary control. Studies have provided a wealth of information on the component operations in specific tasks, but few have advanced our understanding of the control mechanisms that promote the selection of one task as against another (see Monsell and Driver, 2000).

The antisaccade task: exploring response inhibition

The saccadic eye movement system has provided an important behavioral arena for exploring inhibition in the context of the voluntary and involuntary control of action. Two components can be distinguished: a 'reflexive' component that responds automatically to visual events, and a volitional component that is not dictated by the current stimulus and enables a 'semi-independent' action to be formed. 'Reflexive' saccades, also referred to as prosaccades (PS), are automatic, reflex-like responses generated towards a visible stimulus. In contrast voluntary saccades are generated in response to specific instructions or symbolic cues (Walker et al., 2000). The antisaccade paradigm (Fig. 1B) (Hallet, 1978) has been used widely to explore the programming of volitional eye movements and the inhibition of inappropriate action. Antisaccades are directed towards a spatial position in the opposite visual field to that of the stimulus. The paradigm requires the suppression of a reflexive saccade that would normally be generated in response to a novel visual target, and the generation of a volitional saccade to the mirror position. Compared to visually guided saccades, the mean latency of antisaccades is increased (Forbes and Klein, 1996; Kristjánsson et al., 2001; Walker et al., 2000) and the peak velocity is reduced (Everling and Fischer, 1998). Saccadic inhibition errors, resulting from a failure in the suppression of a reflexive eye movement, have latencies that are comparable to those of visually guided saccades (Fischer and Weber, 1992).

Prefrontal cortex and the inhibitory control of reflexive saccades

In early research on patients with brain lesions (Guitton et al., 1985) a failure of inhibitory control was attributed to a dysfunction of the frontal eye fields (FEF). Subsequently, dorsolateral prefrontal cortex (DLPFC) (Pierrot-Deseilligny et al., 1991a; see also Gaymard et al., 1999) emerged as the critical area. DLPFC and the FEF may have distinct functions in the control of antisaccades. A lesion of DLPFC produced inhibition errors, while a FEF lesion was associated with an increase in the latency of correct antisaccades (Pierrot-Deseilligny et al., 1991a; Rivaud et al., 1994). Single unit recordings in primates have demonstrated an increase in neuronal activity in the FEF during visually guided saccades when compared to antisaccades (Everling and Munoz, 2000). Besides the involvement of the prefrontal cortex, the inhibition of reflexive saccades requires the modulation of the fixation units in the rostral pole of the superior colliculus (SC) (Everling

---

[1] Ferrier's general theory of inhibition was short-lived and did not survive into his 1886 2nd edition of *Functions of the Brain*.

1A. Reflexive Pro saccade

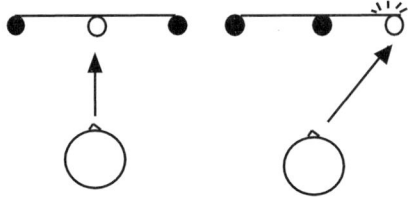

1B. Antisaccade

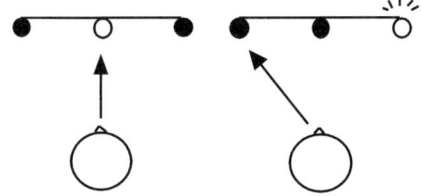

1C. Memory-guided saccade

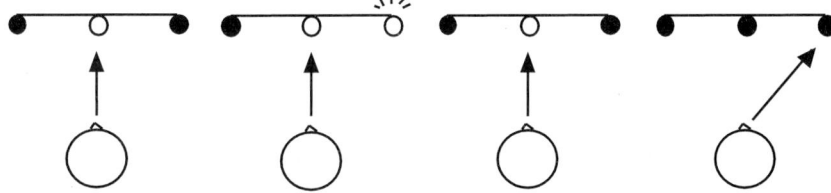

Fig. 1. (A) A visual stimulus is presented in a random sequence to the left or right of a central fixation point and subjects are instructed to respond with a rapid and accurate eye movement. (B) Antisaccades are directed towards a spatial position in the opposite visual field to that of the stimulus. (C) Subjects are instructed to suppress the normal reflexive eye movement in response to a novel stimulus, and to delay the saccade until the offset of the central light. There is no visual information on the location of the previously presented target at the moment of saccadic initiation (modified from Broerse et al., 2001a).

et al., 1999); these units reduce their firing rates prior to and during antisaccades. The important role of the SC for inhibition of reflexive saccades was confirmed by a study in a patient with a SC lesion who showed an increased number of inhibition errors (Pierrot-Deseilligny et al., 1991b). The generation of a correct antisaccade requires the transformation of visuospatial information to the mirror image projection, a process that involves both the PPC and DLPFC (Pierrot-Deseilligny et al., 1995).

Functional imaging studies have identified a number of brain areas in the inhibitory control of reflexive saccades. The study of Sweeney et al. (1996) demonstrated the involvement of the DLPFC. Muri et al. (1998) also reported activation of the DLPFC, and not the FEF. Both results are, however, in conflict with previous studies of Paus et al. (1993) and O'Driscoll et al. (1995), who failed to observe DLPFC activation. The inconsistent observations may be partly explained by the fact that these studies employed different manipulations of stimulus parameters. For example, the O'Driscoll et al. (1995) study employed a brief target flash of 100 ms, which was below the normal reaction time of a saccade. This implied that also in the baseline condition (visually guided saccades) a spatial working memory component was involved which presumably activated the DLPFC.

The evidence on the role of SEF in the inhibitory control of reflexive saccades is conflicting. Patients with SEF lesions showed no abnormality of reflexive or antisaccades (Pierrot-Deseilligny et al., 1991a, 1993). However, neurophysiological studies show that SEF houses different populations of cells that contribute to the complex processes that are required to program an antisaccade (Schlag-Rey et al., 1997). Activity has been recorded in the SEF in relation to a competition between different eye movement responses; these cells appeared to register the behavioral conflicts in choice tasks (Basso and Wurtz, 1997). Neurons in the SEF also displayed significant changes in their activity as subjects learned new and arbitrary stimulus–saccade associations (Chen and Wise, 1995). One population displayed evolving activity as monkeys learned the associations of a novel stimulus with little activity related to familiar stimuli; the response to novel stimuli was reduced as the monkey learned the associations. Another population showed activity that was related to familiar stimuli, which increased as the performance improved. Both types of cell showed marked lability in their directional preferences during these tasks, suggesting a plasticity for integrating sensory input and motor response (Chen and Wise, 1996). Zhang and Barash (2000) recently described a remarkable population of 'paradoxical' visual cells in LIP that apparently switched their directional preference during the antisaccade trials.

Saccadic inhibition and executive function: evidence from schizophrenia research

Patients with severe brain damage are difficult to study with the traditional methods of neuropsychology, since the psychological complications can make it difficult to distinguish the generic cognitive impairments from the secondary effects of the disorder. The "lack of comprehension of the experimental test, lack of ability to execute it, lack of interest, cooperation, and of endurance, all conspire to increase the task of the experimenter and to modify the value of his results." (cf. Diefendorf and Dodge, 1908.) In contrast to most of the traditional neuropsychological tests, where performance is dependent on the development of verbal and manual abilities, saccadic eye movement paradigms allow experimental manipulations that can examine behaviour in infant, adult and animal studies using an identical behavioural response.

A number of recent studies showed that schizophrenics generate prosaccades with normal accuracy and latency (Fukushima et al., 1988, 1990; Clementz et al., 1994; Crawford et al., 1995a,b; Hutton et al., 1998; Karoumi et al., 1998; Maruff et al., 1998; Muller et al., 1999; Straube et al., 1999). In contrast, schizophrenic patients are unable to modulate express saccades, though there is disagreement on the direction of the abnormality (Currie et al., 1993; Sereno and Holzman, 1993; Matsue et al., 1994; Clementz, 1996).

However, studies have agreed on an increase in the frequency of inhibition errors in schizophrenic patients. Compared to healthy controls, schizophrenics generated memory-guided saccades with more inhibition errors (e.g. Crawford et al., 1995a). There is increasing evidence of selective impairments that were positively correlated with cognitive measures using traditional neuropsychological tests. The Wisconsin Card Sort Test (WCST) (Heaton, 1981) examines executive functions such as attention switching, inhibition of mental set, and response monitoring, and is widely regarded as a sensitive measure of prefrontal cognitive impairment. Fig. 2 is based on a reanalysis of the data from Crawford et al. (1995a). Across all patient and control groups the frequency of perseverative errors on the WSCT task was correlated with inhibition errors on the antisaccade task ($r = 0.6$, $p < 0.001$) (see also Rosse et al., 1993). Together with the strong association of antisaccade errors with measures of verbal and nonverbal IQ (Crawford et al., 1995a) this relationship is in line with the 19th century speculations on the involvement of behavioural inhibition in high-level cognitive operations. Hypofunction of the prefrontal cortex may underlie several clinical aspects of schizophrenia (Weinberger et al., 1992). In that study, reduced cerebral blood flow in DLPFC during performance on the WCST correlated with the patients' performance on the task. A similar relationship was observed in patients with Parkinson's disease, and a correlation was found between prefrontal activation and motor behaviour linked to central dopaminergic activity. We discuss the implications for the inhibitory control of saccades in Parkinson's disease below.

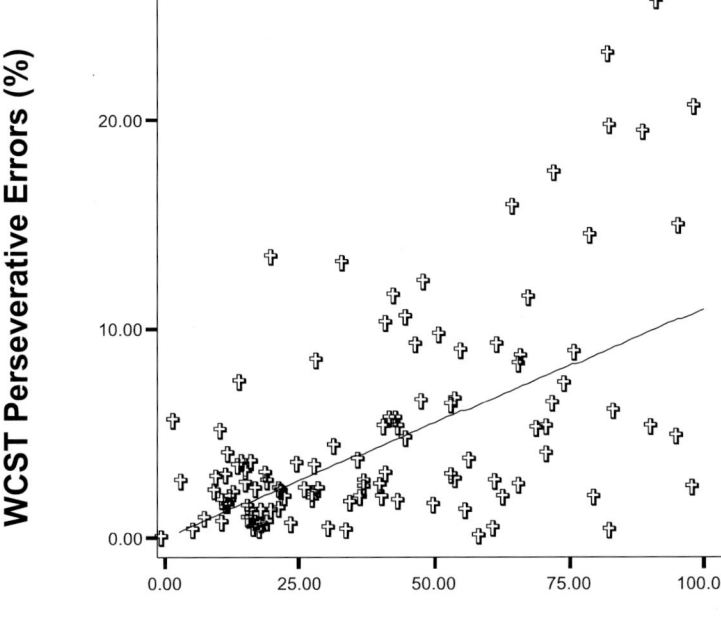

Fig. 2. Antisaccade inhibition errors are correlated with perseverative errors on the Wisconsin Card Sort Test (WCST). The data include schizophrenics, bipolar disorder, neurotics and healthy controls (based on data from Crawford et al., 1995a).

Is there a selective impairment of saccadic inhibition in schizophrenia?

If schizophrenic patients have a selective deficit of inhibitory control, a similar impairment in the inhibitory control of saccades in the memory-guided and antisaccade tasks would be expected, given that inhibition is also required during the delay period in the memory task. Indeed, inhibitory errors are increased in schizophrenia in this task, and these are highly correlated with the antisaccade inhibitory errors (Crawford et al., 1995a). However, given that schizophrenia is associated with abnormal scores in a broad range of tasks, it is important to note the evidence that schizophrenics do not have a global impairment of the generation of saccadic eye movements (cf. Diefendorf and Dodge, 1908). The relative specificity of the saccadic impairments has been demonstrated by the preservation of reflexive and predictive saccades (e.g. Crawford et al., 1995a; Hutton et al., 1998).

Are inhibition errors caused by a failure of working memory?

In the antisaccade paradigm there is a conflict between a compelling urge to fixate the stimulus and the resistance that is required to generate a voluntary eye movement to the opposite side. We will argue that the outcome of this conflict will be determined by the powers of two distinct, but functionally related, subsystems, cognitive inhibition and working memory.

Studies of the effects of prefrontal damage have found evidence that supports a number of distinct functions that include working memory and the inhibition of prepotent responses (e.g. Guitton et al., 1985; Diamond, 1996). We, and others, have inferred that the failure to inhibit reflexive saccades in the antisaccade task reflects, to some degree, a failure of the inhibitory mechanisms of the prefrontal cortex (see Crawford et al., 1995a,b; Pierrot-Deseilligny et al., 1995). However, according to a recent theory these data should not be interpreted in terms a fundamental function of the prefrontal cortex. The most potent evidence for this view comes from a computational model that can account for performance across a range of frontal lobe tasks, without recourse a distinct process of inhibition. According to this unified scheme, a single working system, with no specific inhibitory component, is sufficient to account for the 'prefrontal' errors on inhibition tasks (Kimberg and Farah, 1993, 2000). With admirable clarity Kimberg and Farah (2000, p. 739) leave no room for uncertainty with respect to their position: ". . . We will argue that the contribution of prefrontal cortex to the performance of tasks requiring inhibition is working memory, and that the weakening of working memory leads to disinhibited behaviour." In their view, inhibition errors are a consequence of a failure in working memory (for a related theory see Thelen et al., 2001).

Effects of lorazepam and haloperidol on saccadic inhibition

In assuming that inhibitory control is a by-product of working memory, Kimberg and Farah's (2000) theory yields the prediction that the two constructs should be interdependent. We examined this prediction in a drug study with healthy participants, designed to induce high rates of inhibition errors. Green and King (1998) showed that saccadic inhibition errors were increased in the antisaccade task after single doses of lorazepam. The current study asked whether this effect was dissociated from the measures of spatial accuracy in a saccadic test of working memory. The effects on saccades of the lorazepam, haloperidol (a conventional dopamine-blocking neuroleptic) and placebo were compared to determine whether working memory and inhibition control could be dissociated neuropharmacologically.

Sixteen normal healthy volunteers recruited from a volunteer panel participated in the study. Seven males and nine females, mean age 28 years (SD = 6.4), mean weight 65.9 kg (SD = 6.2). Each volunteer underwent a general medical and psychiatric assessment to exclude neurological or psychological disorder. In a within-subject design all participants received single doses of haloperidol (2 mg), haloperidol (4 mg), lorazepam (2 mg) and matched placebo, at weekly intervals in a crossover design with a balanced Latin-square randomisation. A weekly interval separated the saccadic eye movement sessions. Drugs were administered according to a double-blinded, double-dummy design, which concealed the identity of the drugs from the subject and experimenter. It was assumed that changes in working memory would be reflected by three saccadic parameters in the memory-guided task: (1) amplitude of the primary saccade in relation to the target; (2) the final eye position after all corrective saccade were completed; (3) the frequency of spontaneous corrections following inhibition errors.

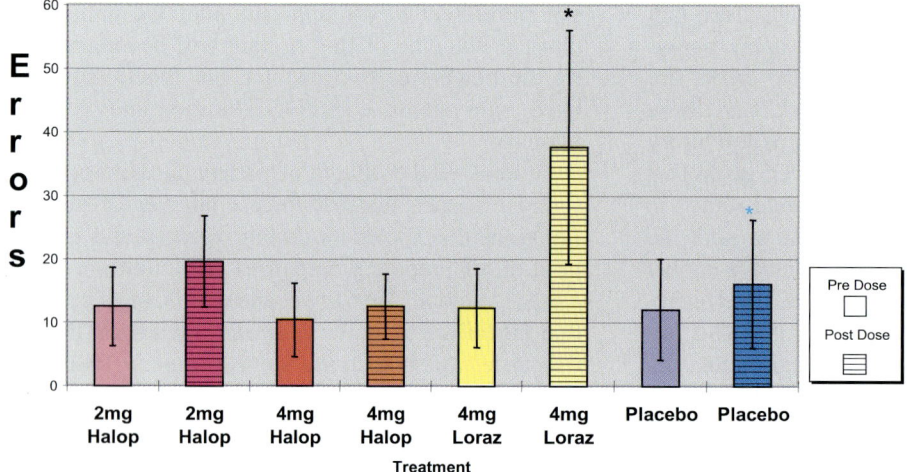

Fig. 3. Mean frequency of inhibition errors (%) in the antisaccade paradigm in pre- and post-treatment trials. Halop, haloperidol; loraz, lorazepam.

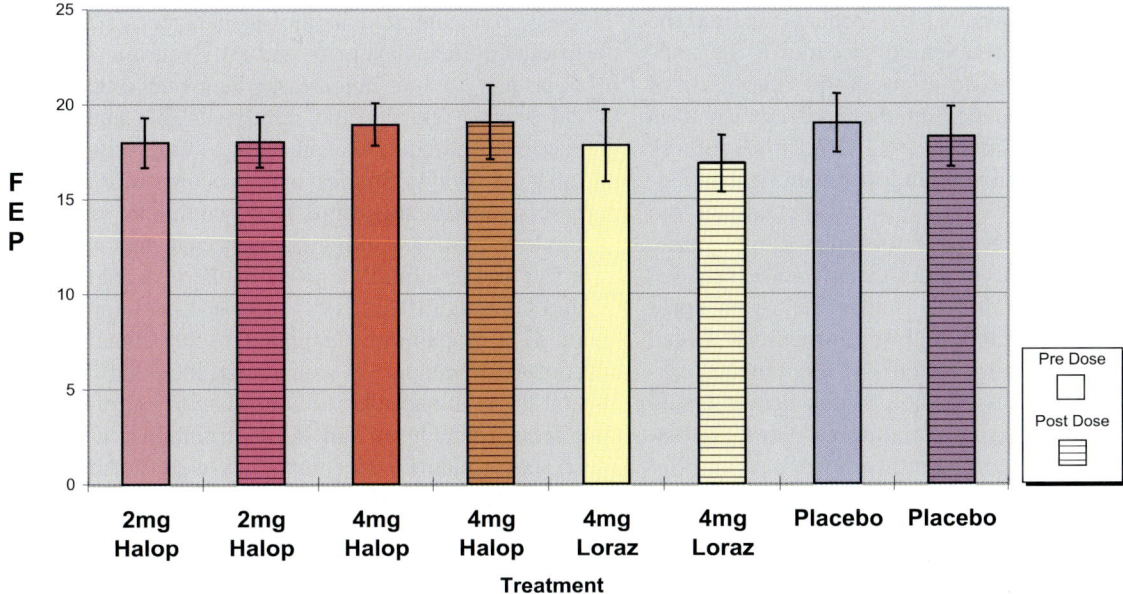

Fig. 4. Mean final eye positions (FEP) of primary saccades at 20 degree target in the memory-guided saccade paradigm.

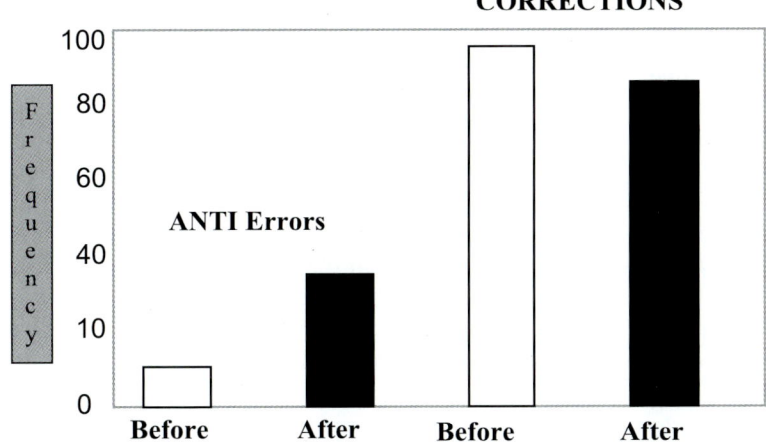

Fig. 5. Mean frequency of reflexive inhibition errors and spontaneous corrections with lorazepam in the antisaccade paradigm.

Saccadic eye movements were examined using the standard pro, antisaccade, and memory-guided tasks (see Crawford et al., 1995a). Fig. 3 shows that there was significant increase ($F = 9.97$, $p < 0.005$) in saccadic inhibition errors during the antisaccade paradigm in the lorazepam treatment condition from pre- to post-drug. Neither of the other treatments significantly altered the frequency of inhibition errors from the pre-drug baseline. With haloperidol (4 mg) inhibition errors were also increased during the memory-guided task from the pre- to post-drug test ($F = 7.51$, $p < 0.01$). Fig. 5 shows that there was a high rate (80%) of spontaneous error correction, despite the increase in inhibition errors with lorazepam. In the working memory task there was no effect of any drug in the memory-guided saccade task on primary saccade amplitude nor final eye position (see Figs. 4 and 5). Lorazepam and haloperidol each produced a dissociation between inhibitory control and spatial working memory. These results can be summarised as follows. (1) Lorazepam impaired the inhibitory control of reflexive saccade in the antisaccade task, but had no effect on the amplitude of the primary saccade nor on the final eye position of memory-guided saccades. (2) The high rate of spontaneous corrections with lorazepam is also consistent with preserved memory and mental set, and suggests that non-specific factors such as motivation or sedation were not a confounding factor (see also Crawford et al., 1995b). (3) Haloperidol (4 mg) produced increased inhibition errors in memory-guided task, yet the final eye position and spontaneous corrections were unaffected. The results demonstrated that working memory and inhibitory control are dissociable[2], thus undermining the view that inhibitory errors are dependent on the efficiency of working memory.

We briefly consider the possible major neuropharmacological influences on the inhibitory control of saccades.

Dopamine and inhibitory control

Several lines of evidence suggest that dopamine plays an important role in regulating the functions of the prefrontal cortex. The concentration of dopamine is higher in the prefrontal cortex than in other cortical areas (Brown et al., 1979) and afferent dopamine fibres are known to terminate in prefrontal cortex (Berger et al., 1988). Direct oculomotor evidence comes from the findings that local infusion of dopamine to prefrontal cortex enhanced the activity of neurons in the delayed response task (Sawaguchi et al., 1990). Conversely depletion of dopamine by 6-hydroxydopamine or 1-methyl-4-phynyl-1,2,3,6-tetrahydropyridine (MPTP) impaired performance in similar tasks (Brozoski et al., 1979; Schneider and Kovelowski, 1990); these deficits were reversed by administration of apomorphine or L-Dopa. There is a higher concentration of D_1-dopamine receptors than D_2-dopamine receptors in prefrontal cortex (Williams and Goldman-Rakic, 1993), concentrated in the deep layers of the prefrontal cortex (layers 5 and 6). Neurons in layer 5 project to the caudate nucleus and other cortical areas (Yeterian and Pandya, 1994, and to the superior colliculus via inhibitory striato-nigro-collicular pathways. Studies of the oculomotor delayed response task suggest that D_1-dopamine receptors mediate spatial working memory and may also play a role in the inhibition phase of the task (Sawaguchi and Goldman-Rakic, 1991, 1994). Local application of a D_1-dopamine antagonist to prefrontal cortex caused an increase in saccadic latency and the error end-point of saccades to contralateral targets. These effects were dose- and delay-dependent, and were specific to the D_1 receptor. They were not observed after application of D_2- or D_3-dopamine antagonists (Williams and Goldman-Rakic, 1995).

Dopamine also appears to play a role in the function of the striato-collicular pathways. The dopaminergic neurotoxin 1-methyl-4-phenyl-1,2,3,6-tetrahydropyridine (MPTP) when applied to the neostriatum produced a selective abnormality of memory-guided saccades (Kato et al., 1995; Kori et al., 1995). This may be mediated by the differential effects of D_1-dopamine and D_2-dopamine receptors on neurotransmission in direct and indirect pathways between the striatum and superior colliculus. Two distinct striato-collicular pathways have been identified: the first is a direct pathway, mediated by GABA, projecting to the internal segment of the globus pallidus and the SnPr, and the second an indirect pathway projecting to the substantia nigra via the external segment of the globus pallidus and the subthalamic nucleus (Alexander and Crutcher, 1990). Activation of the first pathway disinhibits the superior colliculus, while activation of the second pathway enhances superior collicular inhibition due to two inhibitory connections. Neuronal activity in the subthalamic nucleus related to fixation, visual stimuli and saccades may increase basal ganglia efferent activity, and thus inhibit saccades, via its excitatory projections to the SnPr (Matsumara et al., 1992); this would therefore provide an opposing mechanism to the direct striato-nigral pathway. It has been suggested that the D_1-dopamine receptor facilitates neurotransmission in the first pathway, whereas the D_2-dopamine receptor inhibits neurotransmission in the second pathway (Gerfen et al., 1990). The net outcome of

---

[2] The Goldman-Rakic group (Constantinidis et al., 2002) have recently produced further neurophysiological data strongly supporting a mechanism for inhibitory control that is, at least, partly 'housed' in the prefrontal cortex.

these dopaminergic actions releases the superior colliculus from the inhibitory effects of the caudate nucleus, and facilitates the initiation of saccades. Given that the effect of iontophoretically applied dopamine is usually inhibitory, and that the release of endogenous dopamine decreases the excitability of cortico-striatal afferents terminals (Garcia-Munoz et al., 1991) it seems likely that the effects on saccades of dopamine depletion in Parkinson's disease and dopamine antagonists, used in schizophrenia medication, are mediated by the indirect pathway.

The importance of dopaminergic mechanisms in the function of prefrontal cortex may underlie the inhibitory component of working memory deficits in schizophrenia and Parkinson's disease. Dysfunction of prefrontal dopamine is thought to be involved in schizophrenia (Liddle, 1987) and the cognitive deficits are similar to those in patients with prefrontal injury. Prefrontal dopaminergic modulation may also be involved in the cognitive deficits seen in PD. Compelling evidence came from Weinberger et al. (1988), showing that patients have reduced prefrontal blood flow during the WCST test, and that the concentration of dopamine and its metabolites in the prefrontal cortex was reduced by 45–60% compared to controls.

Gamma amino butyric acid (GABA) and inhibitory control

Lorazepam binds to the regulatory sites of the $GABA_A$ receptor. The action of $GABA_A$ receptor acts on the α-subunit and modulates allosterically, GABA-gating of the receptor-operated chloride channel. As the $GABA_A$ receptor mediates the majority of the fast inhibitory neurotransmission in the brain, it is likely to play an important role in the inhibitory control of saccades. GABAergic caudate-nigral projection to the superior colliculus is ideally suited to contribute to the gating of saccades. Iontophoretic application of muscimol (a GABA agonist) into the superior colliculus prolongs the latency of reflexive saccades that are directed into the cell's movement field. Hikosaka and Wurtz (1985) found that there was a dramatic reduction in the peak velocity and amplitude of the primary saccade; the accuracy of the final eye position with respect to the target is relatively unimpaired (Hikosaka and Wurtz, 1985). The perturbation of saccadic control with muscimol was most severe for memory-guided saccades, producing gross impairment of peak velocity, latency, primary saccade gain and final eye position. Bicucciline (a GABA antagonist) produced irrepressible, spontaneous saccades directed into the contralateral field, with difficulty maintaining fixation during the delayed (i.e. inhibition) period of the task. A functional mechanism of saccadic inhibition that is mediated by GABA is consistent with the reported abnormality of inhibitory control in early Huntington's disease (Lasker et al., 1987) where there is pathology of the caudate and external segment of globus pallidus. This mechanism may also be responsible for the reported effects of modulation of saccadic inhibition by GABAergic compounds (Thaker et al., 1989a,b) in schizophrenic patients with tardive dyskinesia. These studies suggest that GABA regulates the inhibitory nigro-collicular pathway.

Serotonin (5HT) and inhibitory control

Serotonin may affect saccades via a number of oculomotor pathways, including dense $5HT_2$ projections from the caudate nucleus to the nigro-collicular pathway (Hikosaka, 1989; Lavoie and Parent, 1990; Brandao et al., 1991) and cerebellar projections to oculomotor neurons. An important physiological role for 5HT role in the control of saccades is also consistent with the following. (1) 5HT neurons in brain stem and cerebellum project to pause cells in the region of the median raphe nuclei, which is the primary location of 5HT oculomotor neurons in the brain stem. (2) L-tryptophan (5HT precursor) medication can cause pathological disinhibition of saccades (Baloh et al., 1982). (3) Fluoxetine (an SSRI) disinhibits saccadic activity during non-REM sleep (Schenck et al., 1992), presumably via the inhibition of saccadic pause neurons in the brain stem that project from 5HT cells of the dorsal raphe nucleus. (4) Iontophoretic application of serotonin on pause cells decreases neuronal excitation and disinhibits burst cells (Ashikawa et al., 1991).

Two recent studies support the hypothesis that the $5HT_2$-binding property of atypical drugs has a beneficial effect on inhibitory control in patients with schizophrenia. Burke et al. (2002) reported that risperidone improved antisaccade errors in patients with schizophrenia, compared to patients on clozapine or sulpiride (risperidone apparently has an adverse effect on smooth pursuit eye tracking; Sweeney et al., 1997). Saccadic inhibition errors (though not clinical symptoms) were also reduced with addition of cyproheptadine (a $5HT_2$ antagonist) to the neuroleptic treatment of chronic schizophrenics (Chaudhry et al., 2002). Given the reduced affinity for the dopamine receptors compared to the $5HT_2$ receptors, novel atypical drugs may have a similar beneficial effect on inhibitory control. One study, with first-episode schizophrenic patients, found that olanzapine and resperidone had similar effects on inhibitory control in the antisaccade task (Broerse et al., 2002). In the memory-guided task the level of inhibitory errors of the patients on resperidone was similar to that of the healthy controls. However, patients on olanzapine had a significantly higher rate of inhibitory errors than the controls. The beneficial effects of $5HT_2$ antagonism upon inhibition may occur directly at the level of the superior colliculus or via inhibition of GABAergic projections from the caudate nucleus to the nigro-collicular pathway colliculus (Lavoie and Parent, 1990). $5HT_2$-binding compounds may also mediate saccadic inhibition and visual fixation through the control of spatial attention. Recent evidence supports a wider role of 5HT mechanisms in the control of response inhibition (Harrison et al., 1997; Robbins et al., 1998).

Saccadic inhibition and executive function: evidence from Parkinson's disease (PD)

Evidence on the relationship of inhibitory control, cognition and the role of dopamine has emerged from attempts to unravel the source of saccadic abnormalities in PD. The clinical triad of tremor, rigidity and akinesia are the hallmarks of idiopathic Parkinson's disease. Pathologically, there is degeneration of dopaminergic cells in the substantia nigra (SnPr), pars compacta, depleting the striatum of dopamine with more marked changes in the putamen than in the caudate. However, there is also depletion of dopamine in the prefrontal cortex (Scatton et al., 1983). Several other lines of evidence suggest that dopamine has a critical role in the functioning of the prefrontal cortex. The concentration of dopamine is higher in the prefrontal cortex than in other cortical areas and afferent dopaminergic fibres are known to terminate in the prefrontal cortex. More direct evidence comes from neuronal activity in the prefrontal cortex in relation to on working memory. These neurons increase their firing rates following local application of dopamine (see e.g. Sawaguchi and Goldman-Rakic, 1994; Sawaguchi, 2001).

Converging neurophysiological evidence suggests that the basal ganglia play an important role in the inhibitory gating of saccades. Stimulation of the SnPr is known to generate inhibition of the superior colliculus (Chevalier et al., 1981). SnPr tonically inhibits the activity of cells in the superior colliculus, and this pathway appears to have a more important role in the control of memory-guided saccades than in the control of reflexive saccades. Change in neuronal activity in the SnPr also precedes that of the superior colliculus for memory-guided saccades, but with reflexive saccades firing rates change simultaneously or after changes occur in the superior colliculus (Hikosaka and Wurtz, 1983). This pathway operates by the release of tonic inhibition of the superior colliculus and thereby reducing activity in nigro-collicular pathways which allows a burst of activity in the superior colliculus, and the initiation of a saccadic eye movement.

Although motor abnormalities are the predominant feature in Parkinson's disease, there is growing evidence that basal ganglia pathology also produces significant impairment of executive functions. The evidence of cognitive impairment in patients with Parkinson's disease comes from a range of tasks examining executive functions, including the internal control of attention, card sorting and planning tasks, memory retrieval, the manipulation of internal representation of spatial information and cognitive flexibility (Gotham et al., 1986; Taylor et al., 1986; Brown and Marsden, 1990; Cooper et al., 1991; Owen et al., 1993; Dubois and Pillon, 1997; Lees and Smith, 1983), as well as functional imaging studies (Jenkins et al., 1994). All of these cognitive operations, which are considered to be specifically sensitive to frontal lobe lesions, are disturbed in PD (Dubois and Pillon, 1997). Similar deficits of short-term spatial representational memory have been reported in patients with damage to the dorsolateral prefrontal cortex and patients with basal ganglia lesions (Partiot et al., 1996).

Studies (sometimes in the same laboratory) disagree on the effects of Parkinson's disease (PD) on psychometric parameters, including simple reaction time and saccadic eye movements. For example, some studies have reported preservation of inhibitory control and working memory (Crawford et al., 1989; Lueck et al., 1990, 1992a,b), while others have found significant impairment in some tasks (Hodgson et al., 1999).[3] However, few studies have taken in account the heterogeneity of frontal lobe impairment in Parkinson's disease. In a recent study of the somatomotor system (Berry et al., 1999) in which PDs with and without prefrontal impairment were distinguished by performance errors on the WCST, reaction times were slowed only in the PDs with prefrontal impairment. Together with previous data these results indicated that subgroups of patients with PD and schizophrenia might share a functional impairment of the prefrontal cortex and similar consequences in terms of inhibitory control (see above).

But, the evidence of frontal impairment in PD from oculomotor studies is controversial. In a brief survey of oculomotor research in PD, Briand et al. (1999) noted that 11 of 12 studies reported preserved prosaccades. However, there is conflicting evidence on the status of antisaccade performance in PD. Lueck et al. (1990) reported hypometric memory-guided saccades but were unable to find evidence of a PD impairment of antisaccades; similar findings emerged from other laboratories (Fukushima et al., 1994; Vidailhet et al., 1994). More recently, conflicting evidence of increased inhibition errors in PD has emerged (Kitagawa et al., 1994; Crevits and De Ridder, 1997). There appears to be at least two sources of variability that might account for these conflicting data: the first source concerns a stimulus factor, the second relates to the variability between patients.

Hypothesis 1: the 'GAP' determines the frequency of inhibition errors in PD

During visual fixation the resources of visual attention are 'engaged' on the target (Posner, 1980)

and saccadic eye movements are inhibited. A shift to the 'disengaged' state occurs prior to a saccade and facilitates oculomotor preparation for a saccade to a novel target (Fischer and Weber, 1993; Fischer et al., 1995). This process is facilitated by the removal of the fixation point shortly before the target is presented, a procedure known as the GAP (Fischer and Ramsperger, 1984). The GAP has a powerful disinhibitory influence on saccadic latencies and also facilitates the generation of so-called 'express saccades' by releasing visual attention and enabling a rapid transfer of attentional processing to the target (Fischer and Ramsperger, 1984; Munoz and Wurtz, 1992). The converse 'overlap' procedure, where the fixation point remains in view during the presentation of the target, generates an increase in saccadic latencies (Saslow, 1967). Parkinsonian studies can be distinguished by the presence or absence of the GAP (see Lueck et al., 1990; Vidailhet et al., 1994; Briand et al., 1999). Although this issue was recognised by Briand et al. (1999), there has been no systematic attempt to evaluate directly the significance of the GAP. This leaves open the possibility that the impairment of antisaccades in PD may be task-sensitive, although a systematic trend has not emerged across studies (cf. Kitagawa et al., 1994; Vidailhet et al., 1994; Crevits and De Ridder, 1997).[4]

Hypothesis 2: variation in PD frontal impairment can account for the antisaccade abnormality

An alternative possibility relates to the variability of cognitive impairment in PD and the possible impact

---

[3] As the estimate of memory performance (final eye position) in the saccadic task required 'accurate' fixation within a limited time period (200 ms), PD patients may have had insufficient time to generate all components in the sequence of eye movements towards the 'memorised' target.

[4] There are a number of problems with the study of Briand et al., 1999. (1) The average age of patients was 73.9, which was older than many other PD studies. (2) Patients were withdrawn from medication in order to eliminate medication confusion, therefore patients may have been unmotivated and underaroused, possibly also depressed. (3) A remarkable feature of these data are the unusual high mean error rates of 75%, which exceed those normally seen in severe patients with chronic schizophrenia. (4) Alarmingly only 55.6 of errors were spontaneously corrected, suggesting that other non-specific factors may have influenced patient performance since this correction rate shows a more severe loss of self-monitoring in comparison to patients with Alzheimer's disease, where we find mean correction rates of approximately 70% (T.J. Crawford et al., unpublished data, British Oculomotor Research meeting 2001, London, UK).

on saccadic inhibition. Variability in clinical and cognitive behaviour is well recognised in PD, both within and between patients. A recent example comes from Partiot et al. (1996), who used the averaged group score from a delayed response task as evidence for a frontal impairment in PD. However, closer inspection of the data showed that the deficit was only evident in a subgroup of PD patients, 8 out of 27. This variability indicates that Parkinson's patients are not homogeneous in their frontal impairment.

The Parkinson's disease study

Various studies have found 'frontal' lobe type impairment in patients with PD. They perform poorly in the Wisconsin Card Sort test (WCST; Paolo et al., 1995) with increased perseverative errors and erroneously maintaining the wrong cognitive set (e.g. Taylor et al., 1986). These errors have been attributed to a number of impairments that are related to functional impairment of the dorsolateral frontal lobe. However, the effects on antisaccade control of frontal impairment in PD control are unclear. Crevits and De Ridder (1997) found that PD patients made significantly more errors of omission, consisting of the failure to generate saccadic eye movements in comparison to controls, termed 'visual akinesia' (i.e. saccadic omission errors). The aim of this study was to determine whether a cognitive measure of frontal impairment would predict antisaccade inhibition errors, and to explore 'omission' and 'commission' errors in this disease.

Saccadic eye movements in the standard antisaccade tasks (see Crawford et al., 1995a) were compared in nine patients with mild to moderate PDs (7 males, 2 females, mean age = 63.3, SD = 9.66) and a group of elderly healthy controls (3 males, 5 females, mean age = 70.25, SD = 9.94). Neuropsychological impairment was assessed using the WCST. Patients and controls did not differ on measures of the saccadic parameters in the prosaccade task, nor did the groups differ in latencies across tasks. PDs showed a significant increase in antisaccade errors compared to the controls in both the GAP and NOGAP versions of the antisaccade task, which did not differ from each other ($p < 0.01$). Fig. 6 shows that the PD errors were primarily inhibition errors (IEs), that omission errors (OEs) were gener-

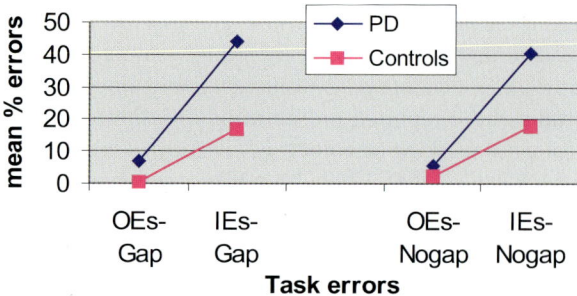

Fig. 6. Saccadic inhibition errors (IEs), but not OEs, are increased in both GAP and NO GAP antisaccade tasks in patients with Parkinson's disease. OEs, saccadic omission errors; IEs, saccadic inhibition errors.

ated infrequently. It is difficult to explain this marked absence of omission errors in terms of a memory impairment. PDs, in comparison to controls, had more perseverative ($p < 0.05$), but not categorical, errors on the WCST.

Fig. 7 shows that the antisaccade inhibition error rates were highly correlated ($r = 0.83$, $p < 0.01$) with the frequency of perseverative errors in the WCST.[5] The results are consistent with the schizophrenia data and suggest that the Parkinsonian variability in antisaccade performance can be, at least, partially explained by performance on a putative frontal lobe task. Although these results indicate that the modulation of saccadic inhibition errors and frontal lobe cognitive operations are clearly related (see Roberts et al., 1994), the results will require replication with larger numbers of patients.

In view of the neurochemical imbalance in dopaminergic neurotransmission common to Parkinson's disease and schizophrenia changes in dopaminergic tone could be considered responsible for the impairment of inhibition. However, Crawford et al. (1995b) investigated the effect of typical neuroleptics in schizophrenics and bipolar patients on a range of oculomotor tasks, including the antisaccade task. Patients who had remained unmedicated for a minimum of six months, were compared with patients who continued on their medication. The re-

---

[5] The results appear to be highly selective to the WCST. For example, a number of studies in our laboratory have shown no correlation between the antisaccade inhibition errors and performance on the Stroop task (see e.g. Crawford et al., 1996).

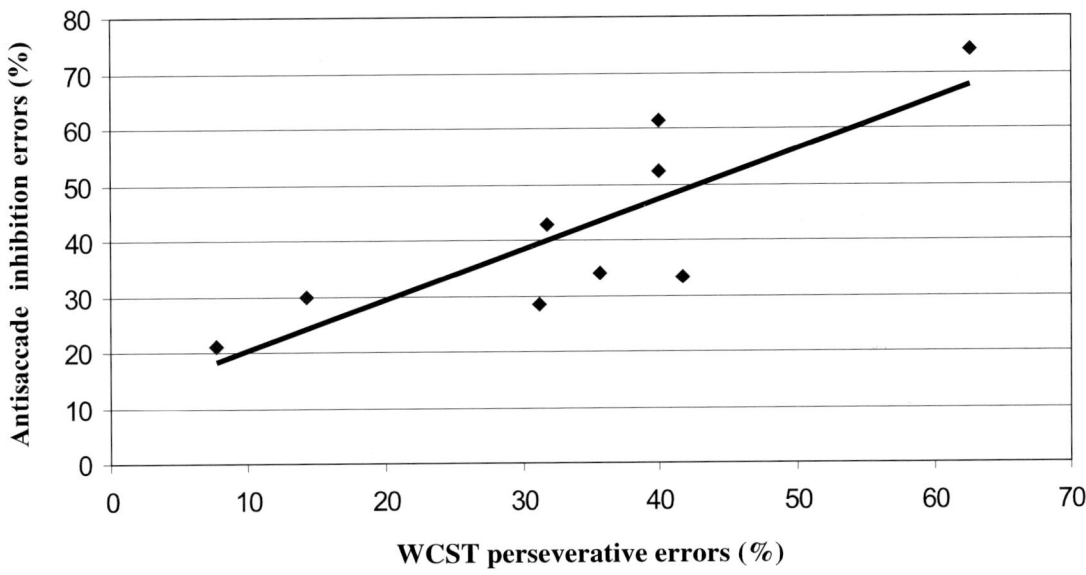

Fig. 7. Antisaccade inhibition errors are correlated with perseverative errors on the Wisconsin Card Sort Test (WCST) in Parkinson's disease.

sults showed that inhibition errors were unrelated to medication status.

Conclusions

Studies of the saccade eye movements have focussed traditionally on the fundamental sensorimotor processing to explore WHEN? and WHERE? operations primarily based on reflexive saccade paradigms (e.g. Findlay and Walker, 1999). However, complementary paradigms (Broerse et al., 2001a) have placed the study of saccadic control within a broader 'cognitive' context, to explore the higher levels of control including working memory, prediction and response selection (GO vs. NO GO and MOVE TOWARDS vs. MOVE AWAY). In contrast to the more automatic operations, this level of control ensures that behaviour is not predetermined by the most salient stimulus that is currently present. The converging evidence from neurophysiological, behavioural, neuropsychological and functional imaging studies suggests that the inhibition of reflexive operations should now be considered in models of high-level cognitive operations.

Historically, various lines of evidence have converged on the view that the brain expends much of its neural resources on inhibiting its own activity in a critical step towards the cognitive control of behaviour. Stenhouse (1974) has argued that the development of behavioural inhibition was a central factor in the 'evolution' of intelligence. Other theories have identified an important role of inhibitory control in the intellectual development of the infant (Diamond, 1996). If inhibitory control is a necessary phylogenetic and ontogenetic antecedent to high-order intelligence the further exploration of its demise in neuropsychiatric disorders is likely to yield greater insights on its cognitive impact and to contribute to development of neuropsychological theories of cognition. In our view, research on the inhibitory control of saccadic eye movement should be encouraged in this wider context of cognitive function.

A major challenge for future research will be the lack of definitional rigour and weak construct validity, given that cognitive inhibitory control is unlikely to be a homogenous construct (see Broerse et al., 2001b; Shilling et al., 2002). Recent studies have shown important dissociations in inhibitory control both across and within task domains (e.g. Shilling et al., 2002). Although the construct of cognitive inhibition is once again beginning to emerge as a useful construct in research, it currently lacks a precise definition (cf. Diamond, 1996; Barclay, 1997). Nor is it clear how the inhibitory neural circuitry that controls saccadic eye movements relates to other schemes of cognitive inhibition.

Abbreviations

DLPFC   dorsolateral prefrontal cortex
FEF   frontal eye fields
PPC   posterior parietal cortex
SC   superior colliculus

Acknowledgements

We would like to acknowledge our many colleagues and collaborators in this programme of research. J. Baxendale, A. Broerse, L. Clarke, J. Connell, M. Hawken, C. Kennard, M. Reveley, B. Haegar, L. Henderson.

References

Alexander, G.E. and Crutcher, M. (1990) Functional architecture of basal ganglia circuits: neural substrate of parallel processing. *Trends Neurosci.*, 13: 266–271.

Ashikawa, H., Furaya, N. and Yabe, T. (1991) Effects of serotonin, GABA and glycine on the activity of pause neurons during vestibular nystagmus in the cat. *Acta Otolaryngol.*, 111: 999–1005.

Bain, A. (1859) *The Emotions and the Will*. Parker, London.

Baloh, R.W., Markham, C.H. and Furuya, N. (1982) Inhibition of pontine omnipauser neurons in the cat by 5-Hydroxytryptophan. *Exp. Neurol.*, 76: 586–593.

Barclay, R.A. (1997) Behavioural inhibition, sustained attention, and executive functions: constructing a unifying theory of ADHD. *Psychol. Bull.*, 121(1): 65–94.

Basso, M.A. and Wurtz, R.H. (1997) Modulation of neuronal activity by target uncertainty. *Nature*, 389: 67–69.

Berger, B., Trotter, S., Verney, C., Gasper, P. and Alverez, C. (1988) Regional and laminar distribution of the dopamine and serotonin innervation in the macaque cerebral cortex. *J. Comp. Neurol.*, 273: 99–199.

Berry, E.L., Nicoloson, R.I., Foster, J.K., Behrmann, M. and Sagar, H.J. (1999) Slowing of reaction time in Parkinson's disease: the involvement of the frontal lobes. *Neuropsychologia*, 37: 787–795.

Brandao, M.L., Lopezgarcia, J.A., Graeff, F.G. and Roberts, M.H.T. (1991) Electrophysiological evidence for excitatory 5-HT2 and depressant 5-HT1a receptors on neurons of the rat midbrain tectum. *Brain Res.*, 556: 259–266.

Briand, K.A., Strallow, D., Hening, W., Poizner, H. and Sereno, A.B. (1999) Control of voluntary and reflexive saccades in Parkinsons's disease. *Exp. Brain Res.*, 129: 38–48.

Broerse, A., Crawford, T.J. and den Boer, J. (2001a) Parsing cognition in schizophrenia using saccadic eye movements: a selective review. *Neuropsychologia*, 39: 742–756.

Broerse, A., Holthausen, E.A., van den Bosch, R.J. and den Boer, J.A. (2001b) Does frontal normality exist in schizophrenia? A saccadic eye movement study. *Psychiatr. Res.*, 103(2–3): 167–178.

Broerse, A., Crawford, T.J. and den Boer, J. (2002) Differential effects of olanzapine and risperidone on cognition in schizophrenia? A saccadic eye movement study. *J. Neuropsychiatry. Clin. Neurosci.*, in press.

Brown, R.G. and Marsden, C.D. (1990) Cognition in Parkinson's disease: from description to theory. *Trends Neurosci.*, 13: 21–29.

Brown, R., Crane, A. and Goldman, P. (1979) Regional distribution of monamines in the cerebral cortex and subcortical structures of rhesus monkey: concentrations and in vivo synthesis rates. *Brain Res.*, 168: 133–150.

Brozoski, T., Brown, R., Rosvold, H. and Goldman, P. (1979) Cognitive deficit caused by depletion of dopamine in prefrontal cortex of rhesus monkey. *Science*, 205: 929–932.

Burke, J.G., Patel, J.K.M., Morris, P.K. and Reveley, M.A. (2002) Improved antisaccade performance with risperidone in schizophrenia. *J. Neurol. Neurosurg. Psychiatry*, 72(4): 449–454.

Chaudhry, I.B., Soni, S.D., Hellewell, J.S.E. and Deakin, J.F.W. (2002) Effects of the 5HT antagonist cyproheptadine on neuropsychological function in chronic schizophrenia. *Schizophr. Res.*, 53: 17–24.

Chen, L.L. and Wise, S.P. (1995) Neuronal activity in the supplementary eye field during acquisition of conditional oculomotor associations. *J. Neurophysiol.*, 73: 1101–1121.

Chen, L.L. and Wise, S.P. (1996) Evolution of directional preferences in the supplementary eye field during acquisition of conditional oculomotor associations. *J. Neurosci.*, 16: 3067–3081.

Chevalier, G., Deniau, J.M., Thierry, A.M. and Feger, J. (1981) The nigro-tectal pathway. An electrophysiological reinvestigation in the rat. *Brain Res.*, 213: 253–263.

Clementz, B.A. (1996) The ability to produce express saccades as a function of gap interval among schizophrenia patients. *Exp. Brain Res.*, 111: 121–130.

Clementz, B.A., McDowell, J.E. and Zisook, S. (1994) Saccadic system functioning among schizophrenia patients and their first-degree biological relatives. *J. Abnorm. Psychol.*, 103: 277–287.

Constantinidis, C., Williams, G.V. and Goldmac-Rakic, P.S. (2002) A role for inhibition in shaping temporal flow of information in prefrontal cortex. *Nat. Neurosci.*, 5(2): 175–180.

Cooper, J.A., Sagar, H.J., Jordan, N., Harvey, N.S. and Sullivan, E.V. (1991) Cognitive impairment in early, untreated Parkinson's disease and its relationship to motor disability. *Brain*, 114: 2095–2122.

Crawford, T.J., Henderson, L. and Kennard, C. (1989) Abnormalities of nonvisually-guided eye movements in Parkinson's disease. *Brain*, 112: 1573–1586.

Crawford, T.J., Haeger, B., Kennard, C., Reveley, M.A. and Henderson, L. (1995a) Saccadic abnormalities in psychotic patients, I. Neuroleptic-free psychotic patients. *Psychol. Med.*, 25: 461–471.

Crawford, T.J., Haeger, B., Kennard, C., Reveley, M.A. and Henderson, L. (1995b) Saccadic abnormalities in psychotic patients, II. The role of neuroleptic treatment. *Psychol. Med.*, 25: 473–483.

Crawford, T.J., Puri, B.K., Nijran, K.S., Jones, B., Kennard, C. and Lewis, S.W. (1996) Abnormal saccadic distractibility in patients with schizophrenia: a 99mTc-HMPAO SPET study. *Psychol. Med.*, 26: 265–277.

Crevits, L. and De Ridder, K. (1997) Disturbed striatoprefrontal mediated visual behaviour in moderate to severe parkinsonian patients. *J. Neurol. Neurosurg. Psychiatry*, 63: 296–299.

Currie, J., Joyce, S., Maruff, P., Ramsden, B., McArthur, J.C. and Malone, V. (1993) Selective impairment of express saccade generation in patients with schizophrenia. *Exp. Brain Res.*, 97: 343–348.

Diamond, A. (1996) Evidence for the importance of dopamine for prefrontal cortex functions early in life. *Philos. Trans. R. Soc. Lond. B*, 351: 1483–1494.

Diefendorf, A. and Dodge, R. (1908) An experimental study of the ocular reactions of the insane from photographic records. *Brain*, 31: 451–489.

Dubois, B. and Pillon, B. (1997) Cognitive deficits in Parkinson's disease. *J. Neurol.*, 244: 2–8.

Everling, S. and Fischer, B. (1998) The antisaccade: a review of basic research and clinical studies. *Neuropsychologia*, 36: 885–899.

Everling, S. and Munoz, D.P. (2000) Neuronal correlates for preparatory set associated with pro-saccades and anti-saccades in the primate frontal eye field. *J. Neurosci.*, 20: 387–400.

Everling, S., Dorris, M.C., Klein, R.M. and Munoz, D.P. (1999) Role of primate superior colliculus in preparation and execution of anti-saccades and pro-saccades. *J. Neurosci.*, 19: 2740–2754.

Ferrier, D. (1876) *The Functions of the Brain*. Smith, Elder, London.

Findlay, J.M. and Walker, R. (1999) A model of saccade generation based on parallel processing and competitive inhibition. *Behav. Brain Sci.*, 22: 661–674; discussion 674–721.

Fischer, B. and Ramsperger, E. (1984) Human express saccades: extremely short reaction times of goal directed eye movements. *Exp. Brain Res.*, 57: 191–195.

Fischer, B. and Weber, H. (1992) Characteristics of 'anti' saccades in man. *Exp. Brain Res.*, 89: 415–424.

Fischer, B. and Weber, H. (1993) Express saccades and visual-attention. *Behav. Brain Sci.*, 16: 553–567.

Fischer, B., Gezeck, S. and Huber, W. (1995) The 3-loop model — a neural-network for the generation of saccadic reaction-times. *Biol. Cybern.*, 72: 185–196.

Forbes, K. and Klein, R.M. (1996) The magnitude of the fixation offset effect with endogenously and exogenously controlled saccades. *J. Cogn. Neurosci.*, 8(4): 344–352.

Fukushima, J., Fukushima, K., Chiba, H., Tanaka, S., Yamashita, I. and Kato, M. (1988) Disturbances of voluntary control of saccadic eye movements in schizophrenic patients. *Biol. Psychiatry*, 23: 670–677.

Fukushima, J., Morita, N., Fukushima, K., Chiba, T., Tanaka, S. and Yamashita, I. (1990) Voluntary control of saccadic eye movements in patients with schizophrenic and affective disorders. *J. Psychiatr. Res.*, 24: 9–24.

Fukushima, J., Fukushima, K., Miyasaka, K. and Yamashita, I. (1994) Voluntary control of saccadic eye movement in patients with frontal cortical lesions and Parkinsonian patients in comparison with that in schizophrenics. *Biol. Psychiatry*, 36: 21–30.

Garcia-Munoz, M., Young, S. and Groves, P. (1991) Terminal excitability of the corticostiatal pathway, I. Regulation by dopamine receptor stimulation. *Brain Res.*, 551: 195–206.

Gaymard, B., Ploner, C.J., Rivaud, P.S. and Pierrot-Deseilligny, C. (1999) The frontal eye field is involved in spatial short-term memory but not in reflexive saccade inhibition. *Exp. Brain Res.*, 129: 288–301.

Gerfen, C., Engber, T., Mahan, L., Susel, Z., Chase, T., Monsma, J. and Sibley, D. (1990) D1 and D2 dopamine receptor-regulated gene expression of striatonigral and striatopallidal neurons. *Science*, 250: 1429–1432.

Gotham, A.M., Brown, R.G. and Marsden, C.D. (1986) Depression in Parkinson's disease; a quantitative and qualitative analysis. *J. Neurol. Neurosurg. Psychiatry*, 49: 381–389.

Green, J.F. and King, D.J. (1998) The effects of chlorpromazine and lorazepam on abnormal antisaccade and no-saccade distractibility. *Biol. Psychiatry*, 44: 709–715.

Guitton, D., Buchtel, H.A. and Douglas, R.M. (1985) Frontal lobe lesions in man cause difficulties in suppressing reflexive glances and in generating goal-directed saccades. *Exp. Brain Res.*, 58: 455–472.

Hallet, P. (1978) Primary and secondary saccades to goals defined by instructions. *Vision Res.*, 18: 1279–1296.

Harrison, A.A., Everitt, B.J. and Robbins, T.W. (1997) Central 5-HT depletion enhances impulsive responding without affecting the accuracy of attentional performance: interactions with dopaminergic mechanisms. *Psychopharmacology (Berl.)*, 133: 329–342.

Heaton, R.K. (1981) Wisconsin Card Sorting Test Manual. Psychological Resources; Odessa, FL.

Hikosaka, O. (1989) Role of basal ganglia in saccades. *Rev. Neurol.*, 145: 580–586.

Hikosaka, O. and Wurtz, R.H. (1983) Visual and oculomotor functions of monkey substantia nigra pars reticulata. I. Relation of visual and auditory responses to saccades. II. Visual responses related to fixation of gaze. III. Memory-contingent visual and saccade responses. IV. Relation of substantia nigra to superior colliculus. *J. Neurophysiol.*, 49: 1230–1301.

Hikosaka, O. and Wurtz, R.H. (1985) Modification of saccadic eye-movements by GABA-related substances, 1. Effect of muscimol and bicuculline in monkey superior colliculus. *J. Neurophysiol.*, 53: 266–291.

Hodgson, T.L., Dittrich, W.H., Henderson, L. and Kennard, C. (1999) Eye movements and spatial working memory in Parkinson's disease. *Neuropsychologia*, 37: 927–938.

Hutton, S.B., Crawford, T.J., Puri, B.K., Duncan, L.J., Chapman,

M., Kennard, C., Barnes, T.R. and Joyce, E.M. (1998) Smooth pursuit and saccadic abnormalities in first-episode schizophrenia. *Psychol. Med.*, 28: 685–692.

Jenkins, I.H., Passingham, R.E., Frackowiak, R.S.J. and Brooks, D.J. (1994) The effect of movement rate on cerebral activation: a study with positron emission tomography. *Mov. Disord.*, 9: 486.

Karoumi, B., VentreDominey, J., Vighetto, A., Dalery, J. and d'Amato, T. (1998) Saccadic eye movements in schizophrenic patients. *Psychiatr. Res.*, 77: 9–19.

Kato, M., Miyashita, N., Hikosaka, O., Matsumura, M., Usui, S. and Kori, A. (1995) Eye movements in monkeys with local dopamine depletion in the caudate nucleus, I. Deficits in spontaneous saccades. *J. Neurosci.*, 15: 912–927.

Kimberg, D.Y. and Farah, M.J. (1993) A unified account of cognitive impairments following frontal lobe damage: the role of working memory in complex, organized behavior. *J. Exp. Psychol. Gen.*, 122: 411–428.

Kimberg, D.Y. and Farah, M.J. (2000) Is there an inhibitory module in the prefrontal cortex? Working memory and the mechanism underlying cognitive control. In: S. Monsell and J. Driver (Eds.), *Control of Cognitive Processes. Attention and Performance XVIII*. MIT Press, Cambridge, MA, pp. 739–751.

Kitagawa, M., Fukushima, J. and Tashiro, K. (1994) Relationship between antisaccades and the clinical symptoms in Parkinson's disease. *Neurology*, 44: 2285–2289.

Kori, A., Miyashita, N., Kato, M., Hikosaka, O., Usui, S. and Matsumura, M. (1995) Eye movements in monkeys with local dopamine depletion in the caudate nucleus, II. Deficits in voluntary saccades. *J. Neurosci.*, 15: 928–941.

Kristjánsson, A., Chen, Y. and Nakayama, K. (2001) Less attention is more in the preparation of antisaccades, but not prosaccades. *Nat. Neurosci.*, 4(10): 1037–1042.

Lasker, A.G., Zee, D.S., Hain, T.C., Folstein, S.E. and Singer, H.S. (1987) Saccades in Huntington's disease: initiation defects and distractibility. *Neurology*, 37: 364–370.

Lavoie, B. and Parent, A. (1990) Immunohistochemical study of the serotoninergic innervation of the basal ganglia in the squirrel-monkey. *J. Comp. Neurol.*, 299: 1–16.

Lees, A.J. and Smith, E. (1983) Cognitve deficits in the early stages of Parkinson's disease. *Brain*, 106: 257–270.

Liddle, P. (1987) Schizophrenic syndromes, cognitive performance and neurological dysfunction. *Psychol. Med.*, 17: 49–57.

Lueck, C.J., Tanyeri, S., Crawford, T.J., Henderson, L. and Kennard, C. (1990) Antisaccades and remembered saccades in Parkinson's disease. *J. Neurol. Neurosurg. Psychiatry*, 53: 284–288.

Lueck, C.J., Tanyeri, S., Crawford, T.J., Henderson, L. and Kennard, C. (1992a) Saccadic eye movements in Parkinson's disease, I. Delayed saccades. *Q. J. Exp. Psychol. A Hum. Exp. Psychol.*, 45: 193–210.

Lueck, C.J., Crawford, T.J., Henderson, L., Van Gisbergen, J.A., Duysens, J. and Kennard, C. (1992b) Saccadic eye movements in Parkinson's disease, II. Remembered saccades — towards a unified hypothesis? *Q. J. Exp. Psychol. A Hum. Exp. Psychol.*, 45: 211–233.

Maruff, P., Danckert, J., Pantelis, C. and Currie, J. (1998) Saccadic and attentional abnormalities in patients with schizophrenia. *Psychol. Med.*, 28: 1091–1100.

Matsue, Y., Osakabe, K., Saito, H., Goto, Y., Ueno, T., Matsuoka, H., Chiba, H., Fuse, Y. and Sato, M. (1994) Smooth pursuit eye movements and express saccades in schizophrenic patients. *Schizophr. Res.*, 12: 121–130.

Matsumara, M., Kojima, J., Gaardiner, T. and Hikosaka, O. (1992). Visual and oculomotor functions of monkey subthalamic nucleus. *J. Neuropshysiol.*, 67: 1615–1632.

Monsell, S. and Driver, J. (2000) *Control of Cognitive Processes. Attention and Performance XVIII*. MIT Press, Cambridge, MA.

Muller, N., Riedel, M., Eggert, T. and Straube, A. (1999) Internally and externally guided voluntary saccades in unmedicated and medicated schizophrenic patients, Part II. Saccadic latency, gain, and fixation suppression errors. *Eur. Arch. Psychiatry Clin. Neurosci.*, 249: 7–14.

Munoz, D.P. and Wurtz, R.H. (1992) Role of the rostral superior colliculus in active visual fixation and execution of express saccades. *J. Neurophysiol.*, 67: 1000–1002.

Muri, R.M., Heid, O., Nirkko, A.C., Ozdoba, C., Felblinger, J., Schroth, G. and Hess, C.W. (1998) Functional organisation of saccades and antisaccades in the frontal lobe in humans: a study with echo planar functional magnetic resonance imaging. *J. Neurol. Neurosurg. Psychiatry*, 65: 374–377.

O'Driscoll, G.A., Alpert, N.M., Matthysse, S.W., Levy, D.L., Rauch, S.L. and Holzman, P.S. (1995) Functional neuroanatomy of antisaccade eye movements investigated with positron emission tomography. *Proc. Natl. Acad. Sci. USA*, 92: 925–929.

Owen, A.M., James, M., Leigh, P.N., Summers, B.A., Quinn, N. and Marsden, C.D. (1993) Fronto-striatal cognitive deficits at different stages of Parkinson's disease. *Brain*, 115: 1727–1751.

Paolo, A.M., Troster, A.I., Axelrod, B. and Koller, W.C. (1995) Construct validity of the WCST in normal and persons with Parkinson's disease. *Arch. Clin. Neuropsychol.*, 10: 463–473.

Partiot, A., Vérin, M., Pillon, B., Teixeira-Ferreira, C., Agid, Y. and Dubois, B. (1996) Delayed response tasks in basal ganglia lesions in man: further evidence for a stiato-frontal cooperation in behavioural adaptations. *Neuropsychologia*, 34(7): 709–721.

Paus, T., Petrides, M., Evans, A.C. and Meyer, E. (1993) Role of the human anterior cingulate cortex in the control of oculomotor, manual, and speech responses: a positron emission tomography study. *J. Neurophysiol.*, 70: 453–469.

Pierrot-Deseilligny, C., Rivaud, S., Gaymard, B. and Agid, Y. (1991a) Cortical control of reflexive visually-guided saccades. *Brain*, 114: 1473–1485.

Pierrot-Deseilligny, C., Rosa, A., Masmoudi, K., Rivaud, S. and Gaymard, B. (1991b) Saccade deficits after a unilateral lesion affecting the superior colliculus. *J. Neurol. Neurosurg. Psychiatry*, 54: 1106–1109.

Pierrot-Deseilligny, C., Israël, I., Berthoz, A., Rivaud, S. and Gaymard, B. (1993) Role of different frontal lobe areas in the control of the horizontal component of memory-guided saccades in man. *Exp. Brain Res.*, 95: 166–171.

Pierrot-Deseilligny, C., Rivaud, S., Gaymard, B., Muri, R. and

Vermersch, A.I. (1995) Cortical control of saccades. *Ann. Neurol.*, 37: 557–567.

Posner, M.I. (1980) Orienting of attention. *Q. J. Exp. Psychol.*, 32: 2–25.

Rivaud, S., Muri, R.M., Gaymard, B., Vermersch, A.I. and Pierrot-Deseilligny, D.C. (1994) Eye movement disorders after frontal eye field lesions in humans. *Exp. Brain Res.*, 102: 110–120.

Rizzolatti, G., Riggio, L., Dascola, I. and Umiltà, C. (1987) Reorienting attention across the horizontal and vertical meridians: evidence in favour of a premotor theory of attention. *Neuropsychologia*, 25: 31–40.

Robbins, T.W., Granon, S., Muir, J.L., Durantou, F., Harrison, A. and Everitt, B.J. (1998) Neural systems underlying arousal and attention: implications for drug abuse. *Ann. N.Y. Acad. Sci.*, 846: 222–237.

Roberts, R.J., Hager, L.D. and Heron, C. (1994) Prefrontal cognitive processes: working memory and inhibition in the antisaccade task. *J. Exp. Psychol.*, 123: 374–393.

Rosse, R.B., Schwartz, B.L., Kim, S.Y. and Deutsch, S.I. (1993) Correlation between antisaccade and Wisconsin Card Sorting Test performance in schizophrenia. *Am. J. Psychiatry*, 150: 333–335.

Saslow, M.G. (1967) Latency of saccadic eye movements. *J. Opt. Soc. Am.*, 57: 1030–1033.

Sawaguchi, T. (2001) The effects of dopamine and its antagonists on directional delay-period activity of prefrontal neurons in monkeys during an oculomotor delayed-response task. *Neurosci. Res.*, 41(2): 115–128.

Sawaguchi, T. and Goldman-Rakic, P.S. (1991) D1 dopamine-receptors in prefrontal cortex — involvement in working memory. *Science*, 251: 947–950.

Sawaguchi, T. and Goldman-Rakic, P.S. (1994) The role of D1-dopamine receptor in working memory: local injections of dopamine antagonists into the prefrontal cortex of rhesus monkeys performing an oculomotor delayed-response task. *J. Neurophysiol.*, 71: 515–528.

Sawaguchi, T., Marsmuara, M. and Kubuta, K. (1990) Effects of dopamine antagonists on neural activity related to a delayed response task in monkey prefrontal cortex. *J. Neurophysiol.*, 63: 1401–1412.

Scatton, B., Javoy-Agid, F., Rouquier, L., Dubois, D. and Agid, Y. (1983) Reduction of cortical dopamine, noradrenaline, serotonin and their metabolites in Parkinson's disease. *Brain Res.*, 275: 321–328.

Schenck, C.H., Mahowald, M.W., Kim, S.W., O'Connor, K.A. and Hurwitz, T.D. (1992) Prominent eye movements during NREM sleep and REM sleep behavior disorder associated with fluoxetine treatment of depression and obsessive–compulsive disorder. *Sleep*, 15: 226–235.

Schlag-Rey, M., Amdor, N., Sanchez, H. and Schlag, J. (1997) Antisaccade performance predicted by the neural activity in the supplementary eye field. *Nature*, 390: 398–401.

Schneider, J. and Kovelowski, C. (1990) Chronic exposure to low doses of MPTP, I. Cognitive deficits in motor asymptomatic monkeys. *Brain Res.*, 519: 122–128.

Sereno, A.B. and Holzman, P.S. (1993) Express saccades and smooth-pursuit eye movement function in schizophrenic, affective-disorder, and normal subjects. *J. Cogn. Neurosci.*, 5: 303–316.

Shilling, V.M., Chetwynd, A. and Rabbitt, P.M.A. (2002) Individual inconsistency across measures of inhibition: an investigation of the construct validity of inhibition in older adults. *Neuropsychology*, 40: 605–619.

Stenhouse, D. (1974) *The Evolution of Intelligence: A General Theory and Some of Its Implications*. Allen and Unwin, London.

Straube, A., Riedel, M., Eggert, T. and Muller, N. (1999) Internally and externally guided voluntary saccades in unmedicated and medicated schizophrenic patients, Part I. Saccadic velocity. *Eur. Arch. Psychiatry Clin. Neurosci.*, 249: 1–6.

Sweeney, J.A., Mintun, M.A., Kwee, S., Wiseman, M.B., Brown, D.L., Rosenberg, D.R. and Carl, J.R. (1996) Positron emission tomography study of voluntary saccadic eye-movements and spatial working-memory. *J. Neurophysiol.*, 75: 454–468.

Sweeney, J.A., Bauer, K.S., Keshavan, M.S., Haas, G.L., Schooler, N.R. and Kroboth, P.D. (1997) Adverse effects of risperidone on eye movement activity: a comparison of risperidone and haloperidol in antipsychotic-naive schizophrenic patients. *Neuropsychopharmacology*, 16: 217–228.

Taylor, A.E., Saint-Cyr, J.A. and Lang, A.E. (1986) Frontal lobe dysfunction in Parkinson's disease. *Brain*, 109: 845–883.

Thaker, G.K., Nguyen, J.A. and Tamminga, C.A. (1989a) Increased saccadic distractibility in tardive dyskinesia: functional evidence for subcortical GABA dysfunction. *Biol. Psychiatry*, 25: 49–59.

Thaker, G.K., Nguyen, J.A. and Tamminga, C.A. (1989b) Saccadic distractibility in schizophrenic patients with tardive dyskinesia. *Arch. Gen. Psychiatry*, 46: 755–756.

Thelen, E., Schöner, G., Scheir, C. and Smith, L.B. (2001) The dynamics of embodiment: the field theory of infant perseverative reaching. *Behav. Brain Sci.*, 24: 1–86.

Vidailhet, M., Rivaud, S., Gouider-Khouja, N., Pillon, B., Bonnet, A.M., Gaymard, B., Agid, Y. and Pierrot-Deseilligny, C. (1994) Eye movements in parkinsonian syndromes. *Ann. Neurol.*, 35: 420–426.

Volkmann, A.W. (1838) Ueber Reflexbewegungen. *Archiv für Anatomie, Physiologie n.v.*: 15–43.

Walker, R., Walker, D.G., Husain, M. and Kennard, C. (2000) Control of voluntary and reflexive saccades. *Exp. Brain Res.*, 130: 540–544.

Weinberger, D.R., Berman, K.F. and Chase, T. (1988) Mesocortical dopamine and human cognition. *Ann. N.Y. Acad. Sci.*, 537: 330–338.

Weinberger, D.R., Berman, K.F. and Daniel, D.G. (1992) Mesoprefrontal cortical dopaminergic activity and prefrontal hypofunction in schizophrenia. *Clin. Neuropharmacol.*, 15 (Suppl. 1): 568a–569a.

Williams, S.M. and Goldman-Rakic, P.S. (1993) Characterization of the dopaminergic innervation of the prefrontal-cortex using a dopamine-specific antibody. *Cereb. Cortex*, 3: 199–222.

Williams, G.V. and Goldman-Rakic, P.S. (1995) Modulation of memory fields by dopamine D1 receptors in prefrontal cortex. *Nature*, 376(6541): 572–575.

Yeterian, E. and Pandya, D. (1994) Laminar origin of striatal and thalamic projections of the prefrontal cortex in rhesus monkeys. *Exp. Brain Res.*, 39: 383–398.

Zhang, M. and Barash, S. (2000) Neuronal switching of sensorimotor transformations for antisaccades. *Nature*, 408: 971–974.

CHAPTER 31

Control of volitional and reflexive saccades in Tourette's syndrome

Douglas P. Munoz [1,2,3,*], Adrienne L. LeVasseur [1,2] and J.R. Flanagan [1,2,3]

[1] *Center for Neuroscience Studies, Queen's University, Kingston, ON, Canada*
[2] *Department of Physiology and* [3] *Psychology, Queen's University, Kingston, ON, Canada*

Abstract: We hypothesized that Tourette's syndrome (TS) patients would display abnormal control of saccades because of overlap between brain areas suspected in TS pathophysiology and those involved saccade control. Subjects were required to look toward (pro-saccade) or away from (anti-saccade) a visual target. Saccadic reaction times were elevated among TS subjects in all tasks. The occurrence of reflexive pro-saccades in the immediate anti-saccade task was normal, suggesting that the ability to inhibit reflexive saccades was not impaired in TS. However, timing errors (eye movements made prior to GO signal in delayed saccade tasks) were increased in TS indicating that ability to inhibit or delay planned motor programs is significantly impaired in TS.

Introduction

Tourette's syndrome (TS) is an inherited condition characterized by the presence of motor and phonic tics that can be worsened by anxiety or fatigue (Singer, 1997) and improved by concentration (Jankovic, 1997). Although the physiological basis for tics and TS remains unknown, a substantial amount of evidence suggests a disorder of frontal–striatal circuits (Singer, 1997). TS patients have demonstrated deficits in memory search, abstract reasoning, and verbal fluency (Bornstein, 1991), which are processes that are believed to be regulated by frontal–striatal systems (Rauch and Savage, 1997). Volumetric abnormalities of the basal ganglia have been reported (Wolf et al., 1996), as well as increased dopamine binding within the caudate nucleus of the striatum (Singer et al., 1993; Hyde et al., 1995; Wolf et al., 1996). Dopamine blockers have been most successful in treatment of the disorder (Kurlan, 1997), whereas dopaminergic drugs and CNS stimulants exacerbate tics (Hallett, 1993; Jankovic, 1997).

The saccadic system can be used effectively to investigate the neural control of movement. First, the movements can be measured relatively accurately and easily. Second, the premotor circuit controlling saccade generation is understood better than most other systems (Wurtz and Goldberg, 1989; Leigh and Zee, 1999; Munoz et al., 2000). Saccades are triggered via parallel descending pathways from the cerebral cortex to the superior colliculus and brainstem reticular formation. Saccades evoked by the sudden appearance of peripheral visual stimuli depend primarily upon direct projections from the visual and parietal cortices to the superior colliculus. Volitional saccades, made in the context of learned or remembered behavior, depend more upon the frontal cortex and its direct and indirect (via basal ganglia) projections to the superior colliculus and brainstem. In addition, regions of prefrontal cortex, the substantia nigra pars reticulata and superior colliculus may

---

* Correspondence to: D. Munoz, Department Physiology, Queen's University, Kingston, ON K7L 3N6, Canada. Tel.: +1-613-533-2111; Fax: +1-613-533-6840; E-mail: doug@eyeml.queensu.ca

provide important fixation-related signals to suppress reflexive or unwanted saccades. Patients with pathophysiology in the frontal cortex and/or basal ganglia disorders display characteristic dysfunctions in saccade suppression and the execution of volitional saccades (Guitton et al., 1985; Lasker et al., 1987; Pierrot-Deseilligny et al., 1991; Fukushima et al., 1994; Kitawaga et al., 1994; Briand et al., 1999).

It has been suggested that TS may result from over activity of the direct pathway through the basal ganglia (Hallett, 1993). Activation of the direct pathway enhances saccade initiation, while activation of the indirect pathway inhibits saccade initiation (Hikosaka et al., 2000; Sato and Hikosaka, 2002). Dopamine enhances transmission through the direct pathway and inhibits the indirect pathway, acting through D_1 and D_2 receptors, respectively. Because increased binding capacity of D_2 receptors in the caudate nucleus correlates with symptom severity in monozygotic twins with TS (Wolf et al., 1996), the movement disorder may also be related to underactivity of the indirect pathway.

Because of the overlap in brain areas linked to saccade control and pathophysiology in TS, we hypothesized that TS patients will display abnormal control of voluntary saccadic eye movements (LeVasseur et al., 2001). The main aim of this paper is to describe some of the deficits in saccade control of TS subjects in a variety of tasks. We also contrast the TS results with results collected from other patient groups to gain insight into the etiology of the disorder.

Methods

Subjects

The details of the methodology have been described previously (Munoz et al., 1998a; LeVasseur et al., 2001). All experimental procedures were reviewed and approved by the Queen's University Human Research Ethics Board. Briefly, ten subjects with Tourette's syndrome (TS), ranging between 11 and 55 years of age, were recruited along with ten age- and sex-matched control subjects (Table 1). The TS subjects met clinical criteria for diagnosis and were referred by a neurologist. Control subjects reported no history of neurological or psychiatric disorders. No performance differences were obvious between groups of medicated and non-medicated TS subjects (see Table 1). It was not possible to ask medicated subjects to cease their medication for experimental purposes given that it takes at least 1 week for clearance of these medications from the system. Such a request can be disruptive to the subject's everyday life, especially when employment is involved.

TS has a high rate of comorbidity with other neurological disorders, such as attention-deficit hyper-

TABLE 1

Subject information

Subject	Age (years)	Age of control (years)	Sex	Medication	Co-morbid symptoms
1	55	53	m	haloperidol (5 mg/day) clonidine (0.1 mg q.d.)	–
2	38	41	m	resperidone (4 mg/day)	–
3	11	12	m	luvox (50 mg/day) resperidone (4 mg/day)	ADHD
4	17	18	m	prozac (20 mg/day) pimozide (8 mg b.d.)	ADHD
5	43	45	f	pimozide (6 mg/day) luvox (50 mg/day)	developmentally delayed
6	35	35	m	pimozide (6 mg/day)	–
7	10	11	m	–	–
8	17	17	m	–	OCD
9	23	23	m	–	–
10	23	22	m	–	–

activity disorder (ADHD) and obsessive–compulsive disorder (OCD) (Freeman, 1997; Singer, 1997). Several of the TS subjects in this study had comorbid conditions (see Table 1). Subjects 3 and 4 were also diagnosed with ADHD, subject 8 was diagnosed with OCD and subject 5 was developmentally delayed. If and when the results of these subjects deviated from the other TS subjects, additional analysis was carried out in order to confirm that these extreme values were not responsible for the overall trend observed in the TS subjects.

Experimental paradigms

Subjects were required to participate in experiments on 3 separate days. Each recording session lasted no more than 60 min, and there were breaks between blocks of trials during which participants were provided with snacks and drinks to maintain alertness. On day 1, subjects performed one block (120 trials) of immediate pro-saccades (Fig. 1A, C, D), followed by two blocks (120 trials each) of immediate anti-saccades (Fig. 1B, C, D). On day 2, subjects performed three blocks (160 trials each) of randomly interleaved delayed pro- and anti-saccades (Fig. 1A,

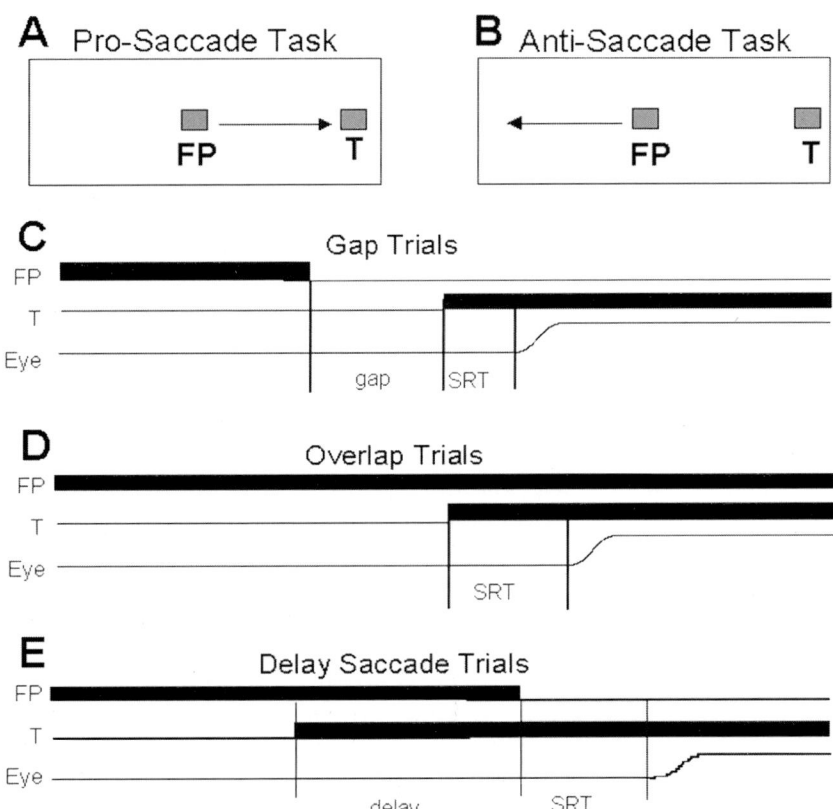

Fig. 1. Anti- and pro-saccade tasks. In the pro-saccade task (A) the subject was instructed to look from the central fixation point (FP) towards the eccentric target stimulus (T). In the anti-saccade task (B) the subject was instructed to look away from the eccentric target, towards its mirror position. In both tasks, the state of fixation prior to the saccade was manipulated. In the overlap condition (C), the FP remained on when the T appeared. In the gap condition (D), the FP disappeared 200 ms before the appearance of the target stimulus. In both conditions, the SRT was measured from the time of target appearance to the onset of eye movement. In the delayed pro/anti-saccade task (E), the target appeared while the FP remained illuminated and the subject was instructed to refrain from initiating a saccade until the FP disappeared. The delay period between T appearance and FP disappearance varied between 200 and 1000 ms. In the delayed saccade task, SRT was measured from FP disappearance to the onset of the eye movement.

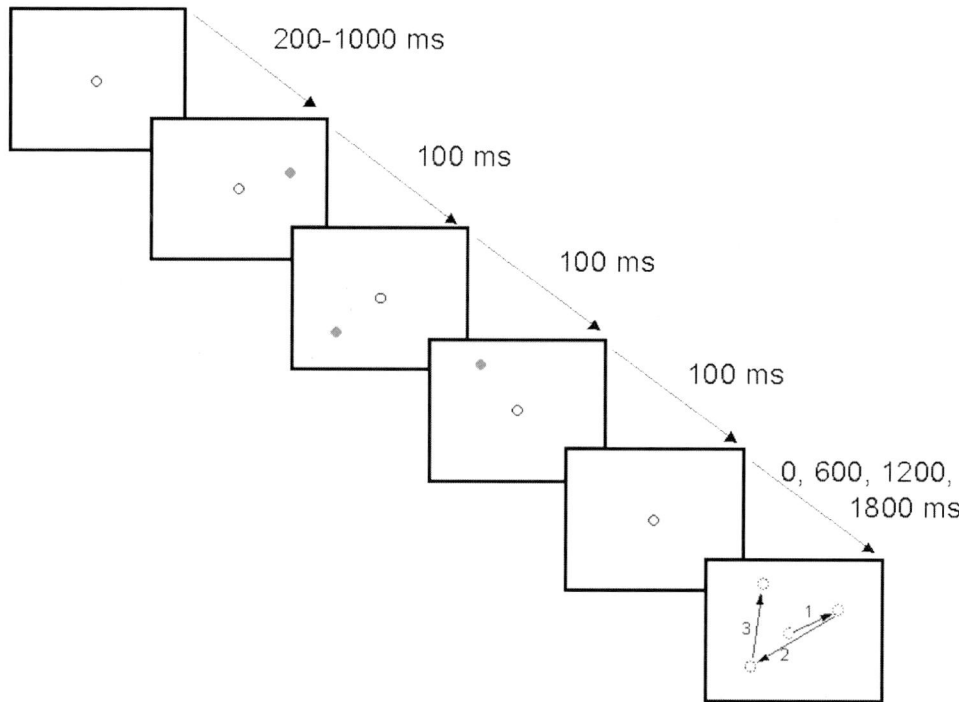

Fig. 2. Delayed memory-guided sequential saccade task. Subjects were instructed to fixate the central FP until it disappeared. On each trial, three target stimuli (1, 2, 3) were presented sequentially for 100 ms in three of the four quadrants of the visual field. Target location within each quadrant and sequence of the three targets varied randomly from trial to trial. The interval between disappearance of the final target of the sequence and disappearance of the FP was varied randomly (0, 600, 1200, 1800 ms). Subjects were instructed to move their eyes after the FP disappeared to the remembered location of each of the targets in the correct order of their appearance.

B, E). On day 3, subjects performed two blocks (96 trials each) of delayed memory-guided saccade sequences to peripheral targets (Fig. 2). Ten subjects performed the immediate and delayed anti-/pro-saccade tasks but only seven subjects performed the delayed memory-guided sequential saccade experiment.

Two separate laboratories were used for these experiments. The immediate and delayed pro- and anti-saccade tasks were performed using electro-oculography to measure eye movements (Munoz et al., 1998a). Subjects were seated upright in a dental chair equipped with a head rest, that could be adjusted for height, such that they faced the center of a translucent visual screen 100 cm away. The experiments were performed in darkness and silence except for the controlled presentation of visual stimuli, which consisted of light emitting diodes (LEDs). A red LED (2.0 cd/m^2) was back projected onto the center of the translucent screen and served as a central fixation point (FP). In the delayed saccade task, a central green LED (1.0 cd/m^2) alternated randomly with the central red FP. Eccentric red LEDs (5.0 cd/m^2) were mounted into small boxes on portable stands that were positioned 20° to the left and right of the central FP. Between trials, the screen was diffusely illuminated (1.0 cd/m^2) with background slides to reduce dark adaptation and boredom.

The delayed memory-guided sequential saccade task was performed in a separate laboratory (see Cabel et al., 2000 for details). Subjects were seated 60 cm in front of a black display monitor on which the white FP (0.2 cd/m^2) appeared. Stimuli were presented on a viewSonic 17PS monitor using an S3 VGA card. The visual display had a resolution of 640 × 480 pixels, with a frame rate of 60 Hz. Subjects wore a head-mounted infrared eye-tracking device which recorded eye movements.

In the immediate pro-saccade task (Fig. 1A), subjects were instructed to look from the central FP to an eccentric target that appeared randomly either 20° to the left or right. Each trial began when the background illumination was turned off. After 250 ms of darkness, the FP appeared. After 1000 ms, one of two events occurred. In the overlap condition, the FP remained illuminated while the target appeared (Fig. 1C). In the gap condition, the FP disappeared and after a gap period of 200 ms, the target appeared (Fig. 1D). The target remained illuminated for 1000 ms, after which all LEDs were turned off and the background illumination came on for 500 ms to signify the end of the trial. Gap trials yield shorter saccadic reaction times (SRTs) than overlap trials (Saslow, 1967) and increases the propensity of reflexive responses (Fisher and Ramsperger, 1984; Munoz and Corneil, 1995), likely due to disengagement of visual fixation prior to target appearance. Target location (20° right or left) and fixation condition (gap or overlap) were randomly interleaved within a block of trials.

In the immediate anti-saccade task (Fig. 1B), the presentation of stimuli was identical to the prosaccade task. Subjects were instructed to look at the central FP, but then to look to the opposite side of the vertical meridian after the appearance of the target. Once again, target location (20° right or left) and fixation condition (gap or overlap) were randomly interleaved within a block of trials.

In the delayed pro-/anti-saccade task (Fig. 1E), subjects were required to perform volitional saccades on every trial. Each trial began when the background illumination was turned off. After 250 ms of darkness, either the red or green FP appeared. After 1000 ms, the eccentric target appeared and remained illuminated. The FP then disappeared after a randomized delay of 200, 400, 600, 800, or 1000 ms. Subjects were instructed to remain fixated upon the visible FP until it disappeared and then look toward the target if the central FP was red and to look away from the target if the central FP was green. The target remained illuminated for 1000 ms, after which all LEDs were turned off and the background illumination came on for 500 ms to signify the end of the trial. Target location (20° right or left), color of the fixation point (red or green), and delay interval (200, 400, 600, 800, 1000 ms) were all randomly interleaved within a block of trials. Subjects were not given any practice prior to data collection. They were, however, asked to repeat the instructions to the experimenter prior to the initiation of data collection.

In the delayed memory-guided sequential saccade task (Fig. 2), performed on experimental day 3, subjects were instructed to fixate the central FP while eccentric targets were flashed sequentially in three of the four quadrants of the visual field. Within each quadrant, the target flashed at one of 25 preset locations, which were evenly spaced over a visual range of 9° eccentricity in the x and y direction at the center of the quadrant. Each target appeared in isolation for 100 ms with no temporal gap between target presentations. Subjects were instructed to wait for disappearance of the FP, and then look to the remembered location of the targets in the sequence in which they appeared. The precise sequence of target appearance and location of the target within each quadrant varied randomly between trials, and there was equal probability of the target appearing in each quadrant. The interval between disappearance of the final target of the sequence and disappearance of the FP also varied randomly (0, 600, 1200, 1800 ms). Each subject performed 20 practice trials before recording began.

Recording and analysis

Horizontal eye movements were measured using direct current electro-oculography in the immediate and delayed anti- and pro-saccade tasks. The experimental paradigms, visual displays, and storage of eye-movement data were under the control of a 486 computer running a real-time data acquisition system (REX: Hays et al., 1982). Horizontal eye position was digitized at a rate of 500 Hz. Digitized data were stored on a hard disk for subsequent off-line analysis.

Saccades were scored as correct if the first movement after target appearance was in the correct direction and if it occurred after disappearance of the FP in the delayed saccade paradigm. Saccades were classified as direction errors if the first saccade after target appearance was in the wrong direction, and as timing errors if they occurred before disappearance of the FP in the delayed saccade paradigm.

In the immediate pro- and anti-saccade tasks, SRT was measured from the time of target appearance to the onset of the first saccade. In the delayed saccade paradigm, SRT was measured from the time of FP disappearance to the onset of the first saccade. Movements in the immediate pro- and anti-saccade tasks were classified as anticipatory and were excluded from analysis if they were initiated less than 90 ms after target appearance. In the delayed pro-/anti-saccade task, saccades initiated before FP disappearance or within 90 ms after FP disappearance were excluded from analysis of SRT. Mean SRTs were computed from trials with SRTs between 90 and 1000 ms. From the data of each subject, the following values were computed for gap, overlap, right, and left trials: mean SRT for correct trials, coefficient of variation of SRTs for correct trials, percentage direction errors, percentage express saccades (saccades with latencies approaching the minimal conduction time in the oculomotor system: 90–140 ms; see Fisher et al., 1993 for review) in the anti- and pro-saccade tasks, and percentage of timing errors (saccades executed prior to disappearance of FP) in the delayed saccade task. Normally distributed data was analyzed with ANOVA tests and non-normally distributed data analyzed using non-parametric, Mann–Whitney tests, comparing results from all TS subjects to all age- and sex-matched controls.

In the delayed memory guided saccade sequence task, eye position data were collected using a video-based eyetracker (Eyelink, SR Research Ltd.) that was mounted on the subject's head with an adjustable headband (see Cabel et al., 2000 for details). The accuracy of subjects' movements to each target was measured by calculating the distance between each target location and the closest eye fixation. Eye movement sequences that were not executed in the same order as target sequences were classified as sequence errors. Eye movements occurring prior to disappearance of the FP were classified as timing errors. These movements were further analyzed to determine the direction of the first saccade in which timing error movements were made. The percentage of timing and sequence errors were calculated for each subject. Distribution of the data was reviewed. Normally distributed data was analyzed with ANOVA tests and non-normally distributed data analyzed using non-parametric, Mann–Whitney tests, comparing results from all TS subjects to all age- and sex-matched controls.

Results

Immediate pro-saccade task

Fig. 3 illustrates representative eye position traces recorded from a TS subject and an age- and sex-matched control subject in the immediate pro-saccade task. Note that both subjects were able to execute the tasks properly. In addition, the saccades of the TS subject tended to be initiated with reaction times greater than that of the control subject. The mean SRT in the immediate pro-saccade task was elevated among TS subjects ($F(1,76) = 28.15$, $P < 0.001$; see Fig. 4A). Table 2 contains mean values for SRT, the gap effect, intra-subject variance in SRT expressed as the coefficient of variation, and the percentage of express saccades for TS and control subjects in the immediate pro-saccade task. The percentage of express saccades during gap trials (Fig. 5A) was reduced among TS subjects ($U = 122.00$, $P < 0.05$). Intra-subject variance was greater in TS than control subjects ($F(1,76) = 6.22$, $P < 0.05$), and the difference in variability between the groups was consistent in both fixation conditions (gap vs. overlap) ($F(1,76) = 0.08$, $P > 0.7$), indicating that the gap effect was not altered in the TS subjects.

Immediate anti-saccade task

Due to the nature of TS, we hypothesized that TS subjects would have difficulty suppressing reflexive saccades. Fig. 3B illustrates eye position traces from a TS and control subject showing that the subject could perform the anti-saccade task correctly.

TABLE 2

Results from the immediate pro-saccade task

	SRT (ms)	Gap effect (ms)	CV	Express (%)
Patients	287 ± 12[a]	60 ± 22	30 ± 9[a]	3 ± 6[a]
Controls	225 ± 6	60 ± 7	25 ± 14	5 ± 11

Mean values (± standard error) for SRT (collapsed across direction and fixation state), gap effect (overlap SRT − gap SRT), coefficient of variation in SRT (CV) and percentage direction errors in TS and control subjects.
[a] Significant difference from controls.

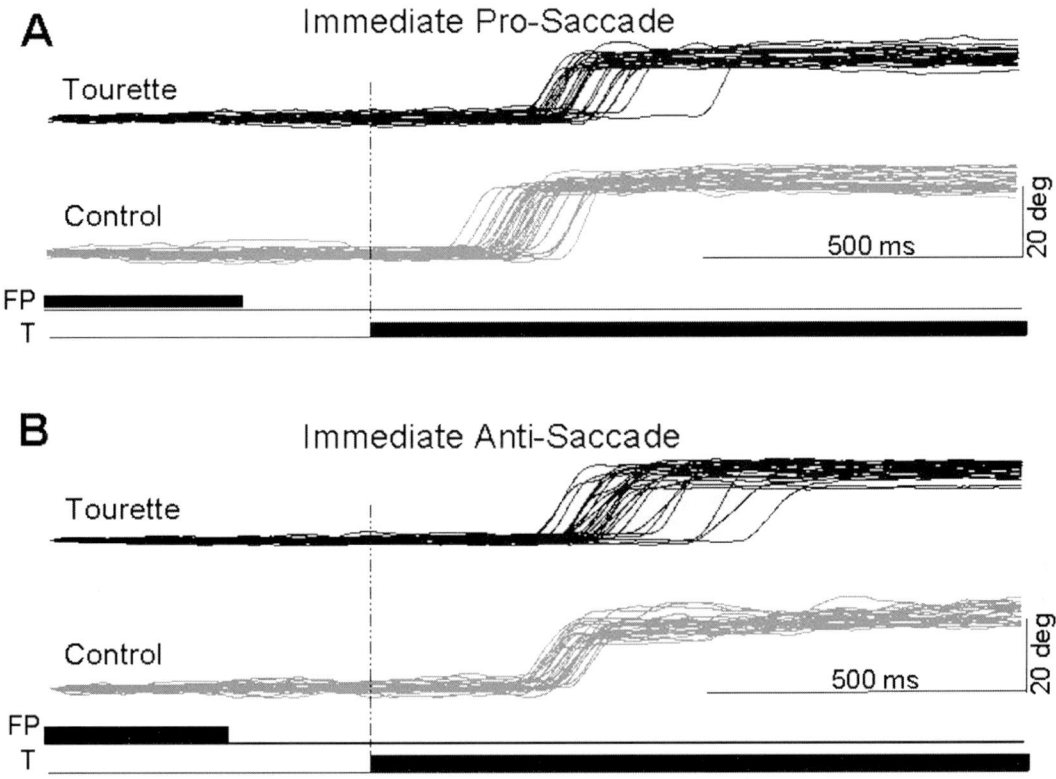

Fig. 3. Eye position traces recorded from a representative TS and control subject performing the immediate pro-saccade task (A) and immediate anti-saccade task (B).

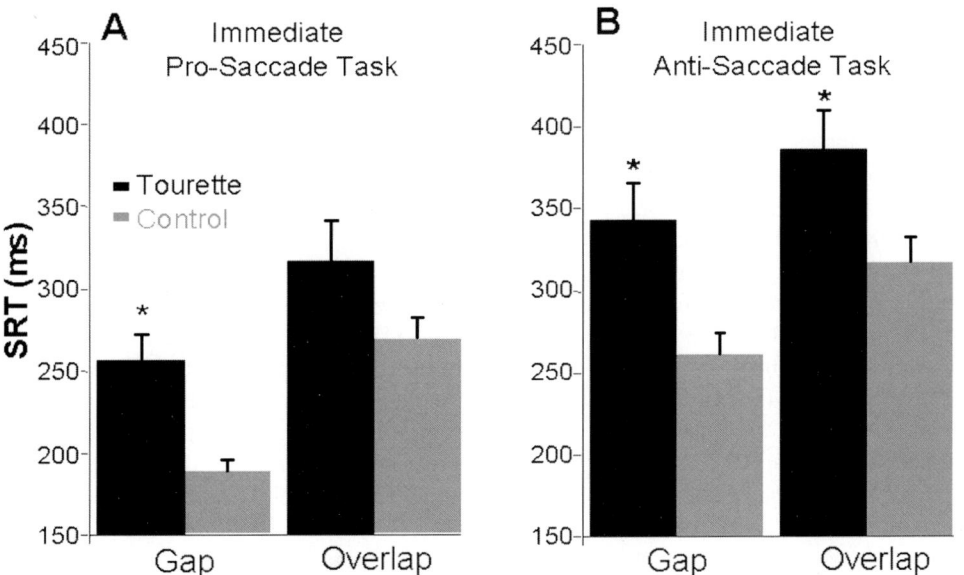

Fig. 4. Mean SRT (± standard error) for control and TS subjects in the immediate pro-saccade task (A) and anti-saccade task (B) with gap and overlap conditions. * Statistically significant difference from control subjects (t-test, $P < 0.05$).

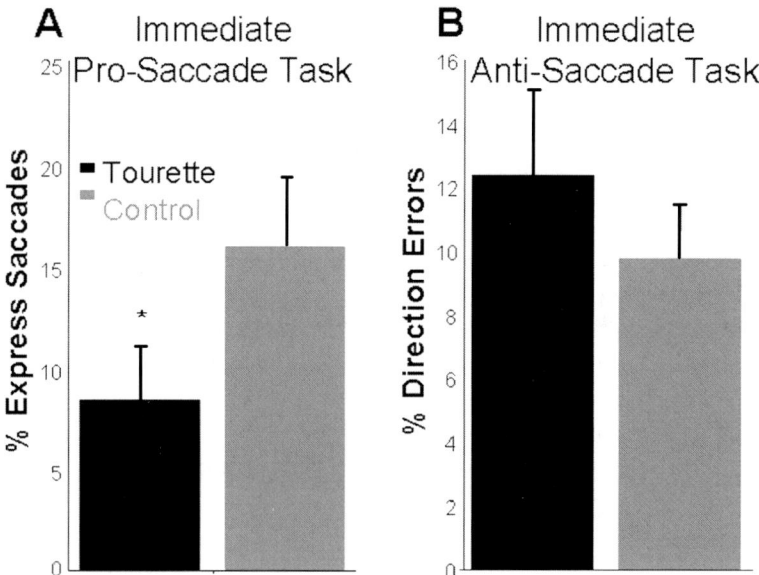

Fig. 5. (A) Percentage of express saccades elicited in the immediate pro-saccade task. (B) Percentage of direction errors made in the immediate anti-saccade task. * Significant difference between TS and control subjects ($P < 0.05$).

TABLE 3

Results from the immediate anti-saccade task

	SRT (ms)	Gap effect (ms)	CV	Direction errors (%)
Patients	365 ± 12[a]	42 ± 7	29 ± 14[a]	5 ± 16
Controls	286 ± 9	64 ± 12	20 ± 15	4 ± 17

Mean values (± standard error) for SRT (collapsed across direction and fixation state), gap effect (overlap SRT − gap SRT), coefficient of variation in SRT (CV) and percentage direction errors in TS and control subjects.

[a] Significant difference from controls.

The percentage of direction errors in the immediate anti-saccade task was not significantly greater in TS subjects than control subjects ($U = 730$, $P > 0.4$; see Figs. 3B and 5B). TS subjects did have significantly greater mean SRT than control subjects ($F(1,76) = 32.9$, $P < 0.001$; see Fig. 4B, Table 3). Intra-subject variance of SRT was significantly greater for TS subjects ($U = 426.5$, $P < 0.001$). The gap effect (mean overlap SRT − mean gap SRT) was not significantly different between TS and control subjects ($F(1,76) < 1$, $P > 0.4$).

Delayed pro-/anti-saccade task

When subjects were asked to delay saccades, TS subjects made more timing errors than control subjects on both pro-saccade ($U = 19.00$, $P < 0.05$, Fig. 6A) and anti-saccade trials ($U = 22.00$, $P < 0.05$; Fig. 6B). A timing error consisted of a saccade that was initiated before disappearance of the FP or within the first 90 ms after FP disappearance (i.e. anticipating FP disappearance). Although TS subjects did not make more direction errors than controls in the immediate anti-saccade task (Fig. 5B), they did make significantly more direction errors on anti-saccade trials in the delayed saccade task ($U = 22.00$, $P < 0.05$). Mean SRT of correct delayed saccades were significantly greater among TS subjects ($F(1,54) = 21.1$, $P < 0.001$).

To examine the influence of the delay interval (period from target appearance to FP disappearance), the percentage of each saccade type (correct, timing error, direction error, timing and direction error) was also computed independently for each delay interval employed (Fig. 7). As the duration of the delay interval increased, the percentage of correct trials decreased and the percentage of timing errors increased for TS subjects, but remained relatively constant for

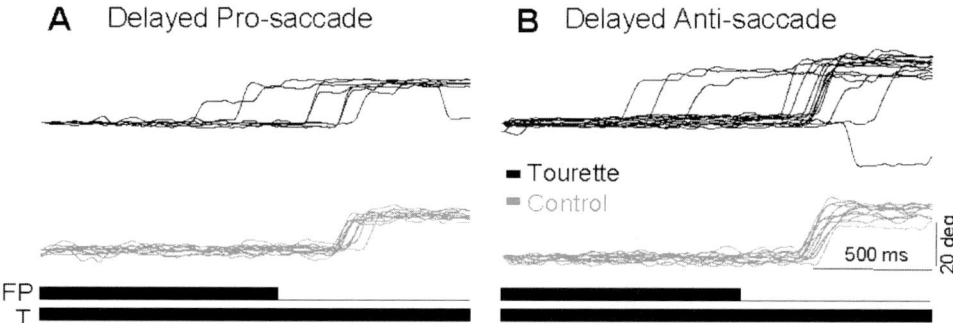

Fig. 6. Eye position traces recorded from a representative TS and control subject performing the delayed pro-saccade task (A) and delayed anti-saccade task (B).

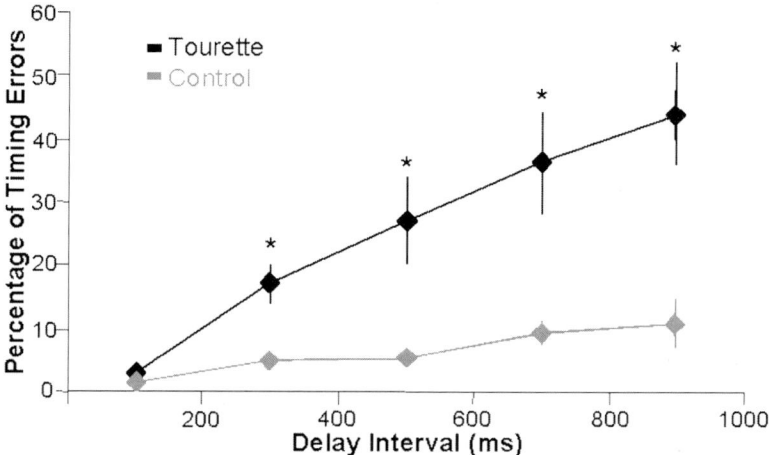

Fig. 7. Percentage (± standard error) of timing errors for each delay interval used in the delayed pro-/anti-saccade task. * Significant difference between TS and control subjects ($P < 0.05$).

controls. Among both TS and control subjects, the number of direction errors diminished with increased delay intervals (see LeVasseur et al., 2001). These results indicate that TS subjects experienced difficulty delaying the appropriate eye motor program for prolonged periods of time, rather than difficulty inhibiting the eye motor program altogether.

Delayed memory guided sequential saccade task

The data in the immediate and delayed pro- and anti-saccade tasks suggest that TS subjects are able to suppress reflexive saccades but often generate inappropriate early saccades when waiting for a delayed GO signal. To determine whether these early saccades result from an inability to suppress a movement to the most recently presented eccentric sensory stimulus or an inability to suppress a planned movement, we devised a sequential memory-delayed task (Fig. 2) in which subjects had to remember the sequence of three successive target locations and delay the initiation of the sequence of saccades to the remembered locations of the targets until the FP disappeared. If TS subjects were unable to suppress movements to the most recent stimuli during the delay interval, then timing errors should be directed to the last of the successive flashes. In contrast, if TS subjects were unable to suppress the appropriate motor plan, then the first saccade of the timing error should be directed to the location of the first flash.

As expected, the percentage of timing errors in this task was significantly greater among TS sub-

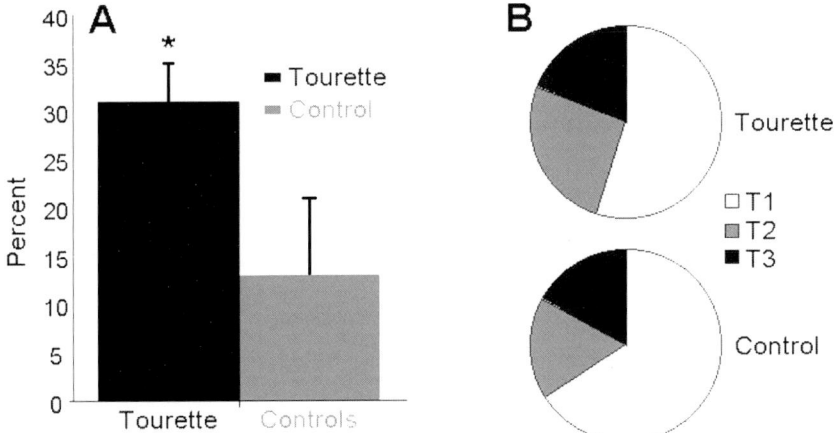

Fig. 8. (A) Percentage of timing errors in the delayed memory-guided sequential saccade task. *TS subjects made significantly more timing errors (*t*-test, $P < 0.05$). (B) Direction of timing errors. Timing errors were made in the direction of the first target (T1) more often than to the second (T2) or third (T3) target of the remembered sequence for both TS and control subjects.

jects, ($U = 11.00$, one-tailed $P < 0.05$; Fig. 8A). Post hoc pair-wise comparisons for direction of timing errors showed that both TS and control subjects ($F(1, 12) = 2.00$, $P > 0.15$) most often looked to the first target, rather that the second or third target ($F(2, 24) = 23.72$, $P < 0.001$; Fig. 8B). These findings indicate that for both TS and control subjects, timing errors result from a failure to suppress a planned motor program rather than a simple reflexive movement to the most previous sensory stimulus.

The percentage of appropriately delayed trials which had the correct sequence was also examined. On average control subjects performed the correct sequence on 67% of delayed trials, while TS subjects performed the correct sequence on 49% of delayed trials. This difference was not significant ($U = 15.5$, $P > 0.2$). The accuracy of subjects' eye movements to the three targets of the remembered sequence was also analyzed for these trials (Table 4). Accuracy of saccades to the remembered location of the first ($U = 13.0$, $P > 0.1$), second ($U = 13.0$, $P > 0.1$), and third ($U = 10.0$, $P = 0.07$) targets in the sequence was similar between TS and control subjects. These results indicate that, although TS subjects had difficulty with the timing of the sequence, they did not have significant difficulty with execution of the motor plan itself.

Medication and comorbidities

Precautions were taken in order to ensure that neither treatments nor comorbidities were responsible for the observed differences between TS and controls rather than the disease itself. After analyzing data of all subjects, statistical tests were carried out for the following subgroups of TS patients and their age- and sex-matched control subjects: medicated TS patients ($n = 6$), non-medicated TS patients ($n = 4$), TS patients without comorbidities ($n = 6$), all TS patients excluding a patient with a developmental problem ($n = 9$), all TS patients excluding a patient with OCD ($n = 9$), and all TS patients excluding patients with ADHD ($n = 8$).

Longer latencies were observed for TS compared to control subjects during all tasks in all subgroups tested with the exception of non-medicated subjects.

TABLE 4

Mean (± standard error) distance in eye position from targets T1, T2, and T3 for correct trials in the delayed memory-guided sequential saccade task in TS and control subjects

	Distance from T1 (degrees)	Distance from T2 (degrees)	Distance from T3 (degrees)
Patients	3.2 ± 3.5	3.4 ± 3.3	3.4 ± 3.0
Controls	1.9 ± 4.1	2.6 ± 1.5	2.6 ± 1.0

There were no significant differences between TS and control subjects.

However, in these cases, performance differences were consistent with significant findings; lack of significance ($P > 0.01$) was likely due to the small number of subjects in this subgroup ($n = 4$). It therefore does not appear that medication or comorbidities were responsible for the longer latencies observed in TS subjects. Similarly, the lower percentage of express saccades in TS subjects was consistent in non-medicated and non-comorbid subgroups. In all subgroups analyzed, the percentage of direction errors during the anti-saccade task remained similar in TS and control subjects, and the percentage of timing errors in the delayed saccade task remained higher in TS subjects. It can therefore be concluded that the TS disorder itself was responsible for all of the above-mentioned findings.

In contrast, it is possible that medication and/or comorbid conditions enhanced the increase in intra-subject variance observed in TS subjects. Though intra-subject variance remained higher among TS subjects in all subgroups, the difference was reduced below significance in both non-comorbid (pro-task, $P = 0.322$; anti-task, $P = 0.170$) and non-medicated (pro-task, $P = 0.196$; anti-task, $P = 0.239$) subgroups. Lack of significance cannot be attributed to a small n value in this case, since the non-comorbid group had $n = 6$. Three of the four subjects with comorbid conditions were on medication, and it is therefore possible that increased intra-subject variance was enhanced by either or both of these two factors. This indicates that medication and comorbidities are valid issues to be taken into consideration, though they were not responsible for trends observed in SRT, express saccades, direction errors, or timing errors among TS subjects.

Discussion

We have demonstrated that specific characteristics of saccade initiation are impaired in TS subjects. We emphasize three main findings. First, TS subjects demonstrated profound difficulties in delaying saccades in the delayed and memory-guided sequential saccade tasks. Second, saccadic reaction times were significantly greater in TS subjects. Third, the percentage of direction errors in the immediate anti-saccade task was unaffected in TS subjects. From these findings we conclude that TS subjects had difficulty delaying planned motor programs but not reflexive responses. We first discuss these data in relation to previous findings and then provide a new theoretical framework to consider the dysfunction of TS.

Saccadic abnormalities in TS

We observed that TS subjects experienced difficulty delaying purposeful saccades for extended periods of time in the delayed and memory tasks. These timing errors were not the result of an inability to suppress reflexive saccades. In addition, the motor programs themselves did not appear to be compromised, because timing errors were most often directed towards the first target of the sequence. Comparable results have been obtained in a study involving grasping movements in a single TS subject (Flanagan et al., 1999). Although limb and eye movements appear to be subserved by distinct corticostriatothalamic circuits, these circuits have a similar architecture (for review see Alexander et al., 1986; Rauch and Savage, 1997) and the basal ganglia may play a similar role in the control of eye and limb movements. It is therefore potentially instructive to compare deficits in TS across these motor systems. The TS subject in the study of Flanagan et al. (1999) was instructed to wait for a GO signal before lifting an object up or down with a single arm movement. Several arm tics were recorded during the delay period before the GO signal and these had the same direction and anticipatory grip force adjustments as the voluntary movements initiated after the GO signal. These results indicate that the tics represented an inability to suppress a planned and well-coordinated motor program until the appropriate time.

Previous studies have observed elevated SRTs in TS subjects. Straube et al. (1997) reported a general elevation of SRTs in TS subjects in several different oculomotor paradigms. Although Farber et al. (1999) reported significantly elevated SRTs in TS subjects during anti-saccade overlap trials, they reported normal SRTs in TS subjects during a pro-saccade task. This inconsistency between results may be related to task instruction. In the study of Farber et al. (1999), subjects were instructed to perform saccades as rapidly as possible.

The results in the present study are also consistent with the finding of Straube et al. (1997) that the ability to inhibit reflexive pro-saccades, indicated by the frequency of direction errors in the immediate anti-saccade task, is not impaired in TS subjects. Although Farber et al. (1999) reported an elevated number of direction errors in the anti-saccade task, they noted that this difference was caused by only 19% of the TS subjects, and several of their subjects had comorbid signs of ADHD or OCD. Narita et al. (1997) also reported in a case study that one TS subject was unable to perform the anti-saccade task. However, this subject was referred to their department because he had the feeling that his eyes were crossing intermittently — a condition which may have complicated performance of eye movement tasks.

The increased frequency of direction errors in TS subjects during delayed anti-saccade trials was likely caused by increased cognitive loading. Subjects were required not only to think about delaying eye movements, but also about whether to make a pro-saccade or anti-saccade on each trial. All types of errors (timing, direction, timing and direction) were significantly greater for TS subjects during anti-saccade trials in the delay task.

Comparison with other neurological/psychiatric disorders

Different disorders of the basal ganglia, such as ADHD (Ross et al., 1994; Munoz et al., 1998b, 1999), Huntington's disease (Lasker et al., 1987; Tian et al., 1991; Rubin et al., 1993; Lasker and Zee, 1997), Parkinson's disease (Crevits and DeRidder, 1997; O'Sullivan et al., 1997; Straube et al., 1998; Briand et al., 1999; Chen et al., 1999; Hodgson et al., 1999; Shaunak et al., 1999), and OCD (Sweeney et al., 1992; Tien et al., 1992; Rosenberg et al., 1997; Maruff et al., 1999) present sometimes overlapping yet distinct manifestations in terms of saccade abnormalities. ADHD subjects have difficulties suppressing reflexive pro-saccades in an immediate anti-saccade task and they also trigger an excessive number of intrusive saccades during periods of instructed fixation (Munoz et al., 1998b, 1999). ADHD subjects also respond reflexively in a memory delayed saccade (Ross et al., 1994) tasks. We hypothesize that ADHD subjects lack a saccade suppression signal.

Recent models of saccade initiation (e.g. Carpenter and Williams, 1995; Trappenberg et al., 2001) suggest that there is a threshold level of pre-saccadic activity required to initiate a saccade. Saccadic reaction times are determined by the baseline and threshold levels of activity, as well as the rate of rise of activity toward the threshold (see Fig. 9). In normal individuals performing a delayed saccade task (solid lines in Fig. 9), the appearance of the peripheral target generates a phasic activation that will not reach saccade threshold. This information can then be held in a buffer until after the FP disappears and the correct saccade is triggered.

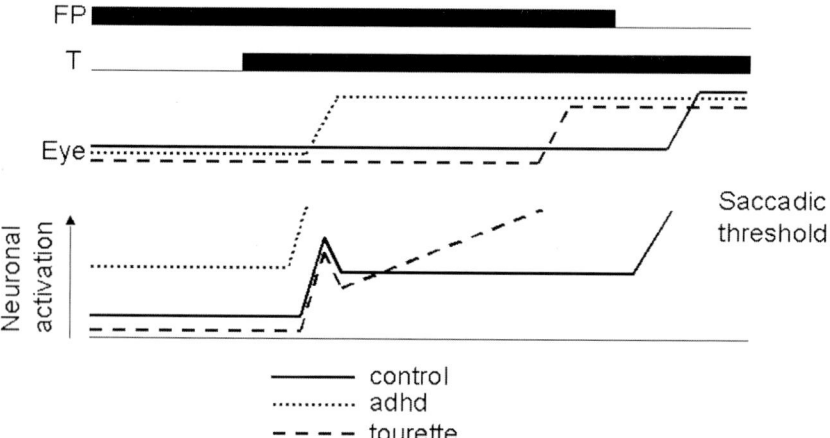

Fig. 9. Hypothetical saccade response and neural function accumulating to a threshold required for saccade initiation in control (solid line), ADHD (dotted line), and TS (dashed line) subjects. See text for additional details.

In ADHD subjects performing a delayed saccade task (dotted lines in Fig. 9), we believe that, because there is an impairment in saccade suppression, there is an elevated baseline so that it is easier to trigger a saccade immediately following the appearance of the peripheral target. The timing errors produced by TS subjects are very different; they are triggered long after target appearance (see Figs. 6 and 7). In addition, TS subjects have longer reaction times and fewer express saccades than age-matched control subjects. Therefore, we speculate that in TS subjects performing the delayed saccade task (dashed lines in Fig. 9), there is a reduced baseline so that it is harder to initiate a saccade. However, after the appearance of the saccade target, the information cannot remain in the buffer without drifting toward the saccade threshold such that a saccade can be triggered before the GO signal (FP disappearance) on long delay trials. Thus, the dysfunction in ADHD and TS is very different and suggests very different pathophysiology. The impaired saccade suppression ability in ADHD leads to an elevated baseline, while the inability to keep a motor program stored in buffer is impaired in TS.

Recent neurophysiological evidence from experiments involving non-human primates has revealed that successful suppression of reflexive saccades in the anti-saccade task is dependent on prestimulus reduction in excitability of saccade-related neurons in the superior colliculus (Everling et al., 1999) and the frontal eye fields (Everling and Munoz, 2000). Evidence from lesion studies also suggests that regions in the frontal eye fields and prefrontal cortex may be critical for suppression of reflexive pro-saccades in an anti-saccade task (Guitton et al., 1985; Heide and Kömpf, 1994; Pierrot-Deseilligny et al., 1995; Sommer and Tehovnik, 1997; Gaymard et al., 1998). We hypothesize that in ADHD, these saccade suppression signals are weaker so that reflexive saccades are triggered too easily. These pathways appear to function normally in TS.

The basal ganglia may be responsible for the difficulty TS subjects experience suppressing voluntary saccades by increasing cortical activity during delay periods. Parallel and overlapping circuits through the basal ganglia act as funneling systems, integrating information from various areas of the cortex before projecting back to single cortical areas (Alexander et al., 1986). In doing so, the direct and indirect pathways through the basal ganglia normally cooperate competitively to ensure appropriate levels of signaling. If these pathways are not balanced properly, the intensity of resulting signals may be inappropriate, leading to altered levels of excitability in pathways involved in planning motor programs. In a model of basal ganglia function, Hallett (1993) suggested that an overactive direct pathway gives rise to excessive voluntary movement, such as tics. Although several hypotheses of neurotransmitter abnormalities in TS have been proposed (see Singer, 1997 for review), the theory of a dopamine abnormality is supported by most of the evidence. Singer (1997) suggested that dopamine hyperinnervation in the striatum of TS patients may lead to increased activity of the direct pathway and decreased activity of the indirect pathway, via D_1 and D_2 receptors, respectively, which would cumulatively result in increased glutamatergic cortical excitation and inappropriate behavior. Though reports of neuroanatomical pathology in TS have varied (Demirkol et al., 1999; McAbee et al., 1999; Mostofsky et al., 1999), reports of abnormalities of the striatum (Singer et al., 1993; Hyde et al., 1995; Wolf et al., 1996) have been most consistent. It is therefore possible that an imbalance in the direct and indirect pathways through the basal ganglia result in abnormal corticostriatal circuits influencing areas which are involved in holding planned motor programs in a buffer. Although the exact identity of these areas remains to be identified, the dorsolateral prefrontal cortex (Joseph and Barone, 1987; Fuster, 1997; Hasegawa et al., 1998), the supplementary motor area (Schall, 1991a), and the frontal eye fields (Schall, 1991b), are all areas which have delay activity in oculomotor tasks, and which also receive direct feedback integrated through the basal ganglia (Alexander et al., 1986).

Conclusions

Saccadic eye movements in TS have characteristics which are significantly different from those in normal subjects and patients with other disorders with pathophysiology in the basal ganglia. TS subjects do not have difficulty with the suppression of reflexive eye movements, but they do have difficulty with the prolonged suppression of planned motor programs.

This suggests that the disorder leads directly or indirectly to significant inefficiency or overactivity of pathways or areas that hold motor programs in a buffer for later use, but does not significantly affect pathways or areas involved in the inhibition of simple motor reflexes.

Acknowledgements

This work was supported by a research grant from the Tourette syndrome Association to J.R.F. and D.P.M.

References

Alexander, G., DeLong, M. and Strick, P. (1986) Parallel organization of functionally segregated circuits linking basal ganglia and cortex. *Annu. Rev. Neurosci.*, 9: 338–357.

Bornstein, R. (1991) Neuropsychological performance in adults with Tourette's syndrome. *Psychiatry Res.*, 37: 229–236.

Briand, K., Strallow, D., Hening, W., Poizner, H. and Sereno, A. (1999) Control of voluntary and reflexive saccades in Parkinson's disease. *Exp. Brain Res.*, 129: 38–48.

Cabel, D.W.J., Armstrong, I.T., Reingold, E. and Munoz, D.P. (2000) Control of saccade initiation in a countermanding task using visual and auditory stop signals. *Exp. Brain Res.*, 133: 431–441.

Carpenter, R.H. and Williams, M.L. (1995) Neural computation of log likelihood in control of saccadic eye movements. *Nature*, 377: 59–62.

Chen, Y.F., Chen, T. and Tsai, T.T. (1999) Analysis of volition latency on antisaccadic eye movements. *Med. Eng. Phys.*, 21: 555–562.

Crevits, L. and DeRidder, K. (1997) Disturbed striatoprefrontal mediated visual behaviour in moderate to severe parkinsonian patients. *J. Neurol. Neurosurg. Psychiatry*, 63: 296–299.

Demirkol, A., Erdem, H., Inan, L., Yigit, A. and Guney, M. (1999) Bilateral globus pallidus lesions in a patient with Tourette syndrome and related disorders. *Biol. Psychiatry*, 46: 863–867.

Everling, S. and Munoz, D.P. (2000) Neuronal correlates for preparatory set associated with pro-saccades and anti-saccades in the primate frontal eye field. *J. Neurosci.*, 20: 387–400.

Everling, S., Dorris, M.C., Klein, R.M. and Munoz, D.P. (1999) Role of primate superior colliculus in preparation and execution of anti-saccades and pro-saccades. *J. Neurosci.*, 19: 2740–2754.

Farber, R.H., Swerdlow, N.R. and Clementz, B.A. (1999) Saccadic performance characteristics and the behavioural neurology of Tourette's syndrome. *J. Neurol. Neurosurg. Psychiatry*, 66: 305–312.

Fisher, B. and Ramsperger, E. (1984) Human express saccades: extremely short reaction times in the monkey. *Exp. Brain Res.*, 57: 191–195.

Fisher, B., Weber, H. and Biscaldi, M. (1993) The time of secondary saccades to primary targets. *Exp. Brain Res.*, 97: 356–360.

Flanagan, J.R., Jakobson, L.S. and Munhall, K.G. (1999) Anticipatory grip adjustments are observed in both goal-directed movements and movement tics in an individual with Tourette's syndrome. *Exp. Brain Res.*, 128: 69–75.

Freeman, R. (1997) Attention deficit hyperactivity disorder in the presence of Tourette syndrome. *Neurol. Clin.*, 15: 411–420.

Fuster, J.M. (1997) *The Prefrontal Cortex: Anatomy, Physiology, and Neuropsychology of the Frontal Lobe*, 3rd edn. Lippincott-Raven, Philadelphia, PA.

Fukushima, J., Fukushma, K., Miyasaka, K. and Yamashita, I. (1994) Voluntary control of saccadic eye movement in patients with frontal cortical lesions and parkinsonian patients in comparison with that in schizophrenics. *Biol. Psychiatry*, 36: 21–30.

Gaymard, B., Ploner, C.J., Rivaud, S., Vermersch, A.I. and Pierrot-Deseilligny, C. (1998) Cortical control of saccades. *Exp. Brain Res.*, 123: 159–163.

Guitton, D., Buchtel, H.A. and Douglas, R.M. (1985) Frontal lobe lesions in man cause difficulties in suppressing reflexive glances and in generating goal-directed saccades. *Exp. Brain Res.*, 58: 455–472.

Hallett, M. (1993) Physiology of basal ganglia disorders: an overview. *Can. J. Neurol. Sci.*, 20: 177–183.

Hasegawa, R., Toshiyuki, S. and Kubota, K. (1998) Monkey prefrontal neuronal activity coding the forthcoming saccade in an oculomotor delayed matching-to-sample task. *J. Neurophysiol.*, 79: 322–333.

Hays, A.V., Richmond, R.J. and Optician, L.M. (1982) A UNIX-based multiple process system for real-time data acquisition and control. *WESCON Conf. Proc.*, 2: 1–10.

Heide, W. and Kömpf, D. (1994) Saccades after frontal and parietal lesion. In: A.F. Fuchs, T. Brandt, U. Büttner and D.S. Zee (Eds.), *Contemporary Ocular Motor and Vestibular Research: a Tribute to David A. Robinson*. Thieme, Stuttgart, pp. 225–227.

Hikosaka, O., Takikawa, Y. and Kawagoe, R. (2000) Role of the basal ganglia in the control of purposive saccadic eye movements. *Physiol. Rev.*, 80(3): 953–978.

Hodgson, T.L., Dittrich, W.H., Henderson, L. and Kennard, C. (1999) Eye movements and spatial working memory in Parkinson's disease. *Neuropsychologia*, 37: 927–938.

Hyde, T.M., Stacey, M.E., Coppola, R., Handel, S.F., Rickler, K.C. and Weinberger, D.R. (1995) Cerebral morphometric abnormalities in Tourette's syndrome: a quantitative MRI study of monozygotic twins. *Neurology*, 45: 1176–1182.

Jankovic, J. (1997) Phenomenology and classification of tics. *Neurol. Clin.*, 15: 267–275.

Joseph, J.P. and Barone, P. (1987) Prefrontal unit activity during a delayed oculomotor task in the monkey. *Exp. Brain Res.*, 67: 460–468.

Kitawaga, M., Fukushima, J. and Tashiro, K. (1994) Relationship between antisaccades and the clinical symptoms in Parkinson's disease. *Neurology*, 44: 2285–2289.

Kurlan, R. (1997) Treatment of tics. *Neurol. Clin.*, 15: 403–409.

Lasker, A.G. and Zee, D.S. (1997) Ocular motor abnormalities in Huntington's disease. *Vision Res.*, 37: 3639–3645.

Lasker, A., Zee, D., Hain, T., Folstein, S. and Singer, H. (1987) Saccades in Huntington's disease: initiation defects and distractibility. *Neurology*, 37: 364–370.

Leigh, R. and Zee, D. (1999) *The Neurology of Eye Movements*, 3rd edn. Oxford University Press, Oxford.

LeVasseur, A.L., Flanagan, J.R., Riopelle, R.J. and Munoz, D.P. (2001) Control of volitional and reflexive saccade's in Tourette's syndrome. *Brain*, 124: 2045–2058.

Maruff, P., Purcell, R., Tyler, P., Pantelis, C. and Currie, J. (1999) Abnormalities of internally generated saccades in obsessive–compulsive disorder. *Psychol. Med.*, 29: 1377–1385.

McAbee, G.N., Wark, J.E. and Manning, A. (1999) Tourette syndrome associated with unilateral cystic changes in the gyrus rectus. *Pediatr. Neurol.*, 20: 322–324.

Mostofsky, S.H., Wendlandt, J., Cutting, L., Denckla, M.B. and Singer, H.S. (1999) Corpus callosum measurements in girls with Tourette syndrome. *Neurology*, 53: 1345–1347.

Munoz, D.P. and Corneil, B.D. (1995) Evidence for interactions between target selection and visual fixation for saccade generation in humans. *Exp. Brain Res.*, 103: 168–173.

Munoz, D.P., Broughton, J.R., Goldring, J.E. and Armstrong, I.T. (1998a) Age-related performance of human subjects on saccadic eye movement tasks. *Exp. Brain Res.*, 121: 391–400.

Munoz, D.P., Hampton, K.A., Moore, K.D. and Armstrong, I.T. (1998b) Control of saccadic eye movements and visual fixation in children and adults with attention deficit hyperactivity disorder. *Soc. Neurosci. Abstr.*, 24: 671.

Munoz, D.P., Hampton, K.A., Moore, K.D. and Goldring, J.E. (1999) Control of purposive saccadic eye movements and visual fixation in children with attention deficit and hyperactivity disorder. In: W. Becker, H. Deubel and T. Mergner (Eds.), *Current Oculomotor Research: Physiological and Psychological Aspects*. Plenum, New York, pp. 415–423.

Munoz, D.P., Dorris, M.C., Paré, M. and Everling, S. (2000) On your mark, get set: brainstem circuitry underlying saccade initiation. *Can. J. Physiol. Pharm.*, 78: 934–944.

Narita, A.S., Shawkat, F.S., Lask, B., Taylor, D.S. and Harris, C.M. (1997) Eye movement abnormalities in a case of Tourette syndrome. *Dev. Med. Child Neurol.*, 39: 270–273.

O'Sullivan, E.P., Shaunak, S., Henderson, L., Hawken, M., Crawford, T.J. and Kennard, C. (1997) Abnormalities of predictive saccades in Parkinson's disease. *NeuroReport*, 8: 1209–1213.

Pierrot-Deseilligny, C., Rivaud, S., Gaymard, B. and Agid, Y. (1991) Cortical control of reflexive visually guided saccades. *Brain*, 114: 1473–1485.

Pierrot-Deseilligny, C., Rivaud, S., Gaymard, B., Müri, R. and Vermersch, A.-I. (1995) Cortical control of saccades. *Ann. Neurol.*, 37: 557–567.

Rauch, S.L. and Savage, C.R. (1997) Neuroimaging and neuropsychology of the striatum: bridging basic science and clinical practice. *Psychiatry Clin. North Am.*, 20: 741–768.

Rosenberg, D.R., Dick, E.L., O'Hearn, K.M. and Sweeney, J.A. (1997) Response-inhibition deficits in obsessive–compulsive disorder: an indicator of dysfunction in frontostriatal circuits. *J. Psychiatry Neurosci.*, 22: 29–38.

Ross, R.G., Hommer, D., Breiger, D., Varley, C. and Radant, A. (1994) Eye movement task related to frontal lobe functioning in children with attention deficit disorder. *J. Am. Acad. Child Adolesc. Psychiatry*, 33: 869–874.

Rubin, A.J., King, W.M., Reinbold, K.A. and Shoulson, I. (1993) Quantitative longitudinal assessment of saccades in Huntington's disease. *J. Clin. Neuroophthalmol.*, 13: 59–66.

Sato, M. and Hikosaka, O. (2002) Role of primate substantia nigra pars reticulata in reward-oriented sccadic eye movement. *J. Neurosci.*, 22(6): 2363–2373.

Saslow, M.G. (1967) Effects of components of displacement-step stimuli on latency for saccadic eye movements. *J. Opt. Soc. Am.*, 57: 1024–1029.

Schall, J.D. (1991a) Neuronal activity related to visually guided saccadic eye movements in the supplementary motor area of rhesus monkeys. *J. Neurophysiol.*, 66: 530–556.

Schall, J.D. (1991b) Neuronal activity related to visually guided saccades in the frontal eye fields of Rhesus monkeys: comparison with supplementary eye fields. *J. Neurophysiol.*, 66: 559–579.

Shaunak, S., O'Sullivan, E., Blunt, S., Lawden, M., Crawford, T. and Henderson, L. (1999) Remembered saccades with variable delay in Parkinson's disease. *Mov. Disord.*, 14: 80–86.

Singer, H.S. (1997) Neurobiology of Tourette syndrome. *Neurol. Clin.*, 15: 357–379.

Singer, H.S., Reiss, A.L., Brown, J.E., Aylward, E.H., Shih, B. and Chee, E. et al. (1993) Volumetric MRI changes in basal ganglia of children with Tourette's syndrome. *Neurology*, 43: 950–956.

Sommer, M.A. and Tehovnik, E.J. (1997) Reversible inactivation of macaque frontal eye field. *Exp. Brain Res.*, 116: 229–249.

Straube, A., Mennicken, J.B., Riedel, M., Eggert, T. and Muller, N. (1997) Saccades in Gilles de la Tourette's syndrome. *Mov. Disord.*, 12: 536–546.

Straube, A., Ditterich, J., Oertel, W. and Kupsch, A. (1998) Electrical stimulation of the posteroventral pallidum influences internally guided saccades in Parkinson's disease. *J. Neurol.*, 245: 101–105.

Sweeney, J.A., Palumbo, D.R., Halper, J.P. and Shear, M.K. (1992) Pursuit eye movement dysfunction in obsessive–compulsive disorder. *Psychiatry Res.*, 42: 1–11.

Tian, J.R., Zee, D.S., Lasker, A.G. and Folstein, S.E. (1991) Saccades in Huntington's disease: predictive tracking and interaction between release of fixation and initiation of saccades. *Neurology*, 41: 875–881.

Tien, A.Y., Pearlson, G.D., Machlin, S.R., Bylsma, F.W. and Hoehn-Saric, R. (1992) Oculomotor performance in obsessive compulsive disorder. *Am. J. Psychiatry*, 149(5): 641–646.

Trappenberg, T.P., Dorris, M.C., Munoz, D.P. and Klein, R.M. (2001) A model of saccade initiation based on the competitive integration of exogenous and endogenous signals in the superior colliculus. *J. Cogn. Neurosci.*, 13: 1–16.

Wolf, S.S., Jones, D.W., Knable, M.B., Gorey, J.G., Lee, K.S. and Hyde, T.M. et al. (1996) Tourette syndrome: prediction of phenotypic variation in monozygotic twins by caudate nucleus D2 receptor binding. *Science*, 273: 1225–1227.

Wurtz, R. and Goldberg, M. (1989) *The Neurobiology of Saccadic Eye Movements*. Elsevier, Amsterdam.

CHAPTER 32

Oculomotor control in a group of very low birth weight (VLBW) children

David Newsham * and Paul C. Knox

Division of Orthoptics, Department of Allied Health Professions, University of Liverpool, Thompson Yates Building, Brownlow Hill, Liverpool L69 3GB, UK

Abstract: VLBW infants are at risk of lesions including intraventricular haemorrhage and periventricular leucomalacia. Those with normal IQ still present with reading difficulties. Oculomotor performance was assessed on 14 VLBWs (IQ > 85) and 15 full-term age-matched controls. Anti-saccade errors were significantly higher for the VLBWs (78%) compared to full terms (62%) ($P = 0.02$). Smooth pursuit latency was longer for the VLBWs compared to the full terms. Greater anti-saccade errors may be indicative of a lesion affecting the frontal cortex or developmental delay. Oculomotor deficits in VLBW children may be associated with the higher incidence of reading difficulties that have been reported.

Introduction

Premature infants with very low birth weight (VLBW) are commonly defined in the literature as those who were born before 32 weeks' gestation, weighing less than 1500 g. Advances in medical technology over the past 20 years have meant that the chance of survival of VLBW infants has dramatically increased (Kiely et al., 1981; Stewart et al., 1981). The survivors, however, are at increased risk of suffering from a number of cerebral lesions, often resulting from haemorrhage or ischaemia. It is not surprising therefore that when compared to full-term (FT) controls, VLBW children have consistently higher levels of problems in areas such as attention deficit and hyperactivity (McCormick et al., 1996; Sommerfelt et al., 1996), cognitive ability and academic achievement (Klebanov et al., 1994; Horwood et al., 1998), language and social skills (Hack et al., 1992, 1994) and psychomotor skills (Pharoah et al., 1994; Powls et al., 1995). Teachers, parents and caregivers have also expressed concerns about the academic potential of these children at school age (Desmond et al., 1986). We wished to investigate the development of the oculomotor system in VLBW children in order to assess whether oculomotor deficits might be contributing to their problems.

Very low birth weight children and reading difficulties

Typically, severe impairment affects 14% of VLBW children (Whitfield et al., 1997) and 23% of extremely low birth weight (ELBW) children (<1000 g) (Saigal et al., 1991). When children with neurosensory impairments (cerebral palsy, hydrocephalus, microcephaly, blindness, and deafness) and abnormal IQ are excluded, it remains the case that mean IQ for VLBW infants is significantly lower than that of matched full-term control children (Michelsson et al., 1984; Rickards et al., 1993; Lloyd et al., 1988). Reading ability has been shown to be impaired in

---

* Correspondence to: D. Newsham, Division of Orthoptics, Department of Allied Health Professions, University of Liverpool, Thompson Yates Building, Brownlow Hill, Liverpool L69 3GB, UK. Tel.: +44-151-794-5737; Fax: +44-151-794-5781; E-mail: newts@liv.ac.uk

VLBW children in many studies often together with other academic abilities and in conjunction with a poor IQ (<85) (Klein et al., 1989; The Scottish Low Birthweight Study Group, 1992; Marlow et al., 1993; Pharoah et al., 1994; Horwood et al., 1998). Typically it has been reported that 45% of VLBW children have difficulty in one or more academic subjects (Marlow et al., 1993) and 27% require learning support (Horwood et al., 1998) compared with only 19% and 9%, respectively, for full-term matched controls. These educational difficulties do not appear to reduce as the children get older, with little difference between the level of disability at the initial detection at 6 years of age, and upon reassessment at 12 years of age (Botting et al., 1998). Many VLBW children who are free from major neurological impairments are educated in mainstream schools. However there is evidence that a significant proportion of VLBW children with IQs within the normal range still exhibit reading problems (Aram et al., 1991; Saigal et al., 1992; Hall et al., 1995; O'Callaghan et al., 1996; Whitfield et al., 1997; Botting et al., 1998; Johnson and Breslau, 2000; Saigal et al., 2000). For the purposes of our investigation and in line with previous research, we take normal IQ to be 85 or above, falling within one standard deviation of the mean score of 100. The prevalence of specific learning disorder in VLBW children has generally been quoted at between 28% purely with reading difficulties (Saigal et al., 1992) to 47% in one study in which arithmetic and reading disorders were grouped together (Whitfield et al., 1997).

Brain insults in VLBW children

One of the main deficiencies of preterm neonates is that they have a limited ability to autoregulate cerebral blood flow. Cerebral perfusion is therefore susceptible to changes resulting from differences in arterial blood pressure. An abrupt increase in the arterial pressure can often lead to an intraventricular haemorrhage either limited to the germinal matrix or rupturing into the lateral ventricles. The germinal matrix is a structure that is most prominent between 24 and 34 weeks of gestation and has almost regressed by term. Germinal matrix tissue is abundant over the head of the caudate nucleus and can also be found in the periventricular region. The first studies using CT and ultrasound between 1979 and 1983, reported the incidence of all forms of intracranial haemorrhage affecting VLBW infants to be between 40% and 50% (Burstein et al., 1979; Dolfin et al., 1983). More recently a decline in the incidence of haemorrhage has been reported with the incidence of intraventricular and intraparenchymal haemorrhage at about 20% (Batton et al., 1994). The reduction in the reported incidence of haemorrhage during the 11–15 years between the studies may well reflect the advances in neonatal care that occurred during this period.

A reduction of systemic blood pressure in conjunction with impaired autoregulation of cerebral blood flow leads to hypoxic–ischaemia affecting the vulnerable periventricular white matter. This resulting white matter atrophy, scar formation and occasional cysts are collectively known as periventricular leucomalacia. The reported incidence ranges from 3% to 10% for bilateral cystic leucomalacia (Trounce et al., 1986; De Vries et al., 1988) and if non-cystic periventricular leucomalacia is included, up to 28% (Trounce et al., 1986). Perhaps of more direct relevance to oculomotor control, an older study found 21% of VLBW newborns had cerebellar haemorrhages (either macroscopic or microscopic) when examined at autopsy (Martin et al., 1976). There have also been reports of lesions affecting the thalamus, occurring in 50% of preterm children (with the pulvinar being affected in 43% of cases) associated with periventricular leucomalacia, all of whom had spastic cerebral palsy (Yokochi, 1997).

Oculomotor abnormalities might obviously result from damage to areas of the brain involved in oculomotor control. The white matter lesions that occur next to the trigonal area in periventricular leucomalacia could compromise fibre bundles connecting the striate cortex with the cortical motion processing area (middle temporal visual area, MT/V5) (Miller and Fine, 1977; Tusa and Ungerleider, 1988; Dutton et al., 1996). The cerebellar damage mentioned above might also cause oculomotor abnormalities (Buttner and Straube, 1995). One study has also shown choroid plexus haemorrhages in the region of the caudate nucleus in 41% of a group of VLBW children (Reeder et al., 1982). The caudate nucleus has also been reported to suffer lesions from an infarct of the lenticulostriate branch of the middle cerebral artery (De Vries et al., 1997) and a rat model for hypoxic–ischaemic lesions in premature infants demonstrated oedema and neuronal loss in the caudate nucleus (Sheldon et al., 1996). Lesions affecting the thalamus, particularly the pulvinar might also lead to saccadic deficits (Straschill and Takahashi, 1981). Thus a number of structures known to be involved in the control of eye movement are indeed prone to damage in VLBW children.

Binocular and visual anomalies in VLBW children

VLBW children are at greater risk of ocular defects than full-term children, not only as a result of retinopathy of prematurity, but also due to intraventricular haemorrhage and periventricular leucomalacia (Gibson et al., 1990). A high incidence of visual impairment including reduced visual acuity, refractive errors, strabismus, and nystagmus, varying between 15% and 33% has been reported (Keith and Kitchen, 1983; Gibson et al., 1990). The incidence of visual impairment in the general population of preschool children is reported to be between 5% and 10% and between 2% and 5% for amblyopia (Schmitt, 1987). By the time children reach 7 years of age, up to 13% will have some defect of visual function (Peckham, 1986). A more recent study examined 137 VLBW children in comparison to controls and found in the VLBW group 9.5% had strabismus, 50% had abnormal stereopsis, 17% had abnormal visual acuity, 48% had poor contrast sensitivity and one child had nystagmus (Powls et al., 1997). Overall in this study reduced visual function was present in 63.5% of the VLBW children compared with only 36% of the full-term controls. The study also reported an association between contrast sensitivity and reading ability as well as mathematics ability and IQ. The rate of development of various aspects of visual and binocular function has also been examined in preterm infants compared to full-term infants (Weinacht et al., 1999). Ocular alignment, convergence, fusion, grating acuity and OKN were all tested. No significant differences were found between the development of these functions between the two groups. However patients were excluded from the study if they had neurological disorders or ocular disease or if the gestation was less than 31 weeks leading to an unusually low risk sample.

Oculomotor control in VLBW children

Jacobson et al. (1998) reported that some VLBW children with periventricular leucomalacia did not appear to be able to execute voluntary saccades and had difficulty with smooth pursuit. Unfortunately no quantitative data were reported. Langaas et al. (1998) examined eye movements in children born prematurely with developmental co-ordination disorder. They examined smooth pursuit and found a significantly reduced gain in the children who were born prematurely compared to full-term controls. However only eight subjects were included in each group, and the nature of insults affecting premature children makes this population very heterogeneous. We are not aware of any published data on the performance of VLBW children in anti-saccade tasks.

In one study, the effect of visual and eye movement anomalies on reading in a small VLBW group was assessed (Jacobson, 1998). All four subjects had strabismus, impaired motility and nystagmus. Eye movement assessment involved recording fixational behaviour using an infrared reflection technique whilst viewing a spot centrally and analysis of eye movements during reading. The study found that none of the subjects made normal eye movements during reading and compensated with head movements. It was concluded, however, that none of the individual factors that were found could be predictive of reading ability. Also as there was no control group for comparison and given the very small sample size, firm conclusions are difficult to draw.

From the evidence reviewed it is clear that VLBW children may often have reading difficulties in the presence of normal IQ indicating that the reading difficulty is not wholly due to a global cognitive deficit. These reading difficulties could therefore be referred to as a specific learning disorder. While the precise cause remains unclear, VLBW children are a high risk group for various deficits affecting behavioural, cognitive, and motor areas. Given the nature of the numerous cerebral insults that often affect VLBW children they also appear to be a high-risk group for developing eye movement defects, including saccadic disorders, which might affect reading. Very little research has been conducted on eye movements in VLBW children and the studies that have included some form of assessment have had methodological weaknesses. It has been well documented, however, that VLBW children have an increased incidence of visual and binocular problems, encompassing many areas of visual function. Research in other groups of individuals has shown that saccadic deficits can compromise the reading process and lead to reading difficulties.

Saccade deficits and reading difficulty

Research using single case reports has shown that both cerebellar lesions such as spinocerebellar degeneration and basal ganglia lesions such as Huntington's chorea, can compromise saccades and affect reading ability (Pirozzolo and Rayner, 1979). The case of the cerebellar lesion resulted in saccadic dysmetria and the patient attempted to use compensatory head movements during reading. The case of Huntington's chorea was found to cause a reduction in saccadic velocity to about one third of normal and again the patient attempted to make compensatory head movements during reading. Both of the case reports showed that the patients had impaired reading as a result of the saccadic disorders, in the presence of normal cognitive abilities in other areas. Research involving the effect of saccadic abnormalities on reading in patients with neurological disorders is often based on single patient case reports, and may be considered to have less scope than larger studies. Despite this, the research above does demonstrate that poor saccadic control of eye movements can lead to poor reading ability.

Dyslexia is an area where the control of eye movements has been extensively investigated. Dyslexia is a distinct form of reading disorder different to the complex nature of problems encountered by VLBW children (where actual oculomotor defects may be present in conjunction with, or in the absence of, general cognitive difficulties). However, a comparison between the two groups would be useful as there is a sub-group of VLBW subjects who have a specific reading disorder in the presence of a normal IQ. Given the lack of published literature on eye movement control and reading in VLBW subjects, it would be helpful to review the extent to which eye movements may contribute to the reading difficulties in dyslexia. Currently there is still some controversy as to the role eye movements may play in contributing to dyslexia. Dyslexic subjects with subtle cerebellar dysfunction have been investigated (Raymond et al., 1988). The dyslexic group showed significantly worse fixational stability and control than the control group but the study still lacked evidence to prove that the fixational problems were the cause of the reading difficulties. Whilst the early research into the contribution of eye movements to dyslexia undertaken by Pavlidis (1981, 1983, 1985) has not been replicated, other research in this area has compared various aspects of saccadic eye movements, including saccadic reaction time, saccadic latency, anticipatory saccades, and regressive saccades, for normal and dyslexic subjects. Significant differences were shown to be present and a significant correlation was found between abnormal saccadic control and reading disability (Biscaldi et al., 1998). Recently, the control of anti-saccades has been investigated in dyslexic subjects in relation to controls.

Anti-saccade errors and reading difficulty

The anti-saccade task as described by Hallett (1978) requires subjects to suppress a reflexive saccade towards a target and then generate a voluntary saccade to the opposite side at approximately the same distance from the fixation target. The ability to perform this task has been shown to be compromised in disorders involving the frontal cortex such as schizophrenia (Clementz et al., 1994) and attention deficit hyperactivity disorder (Munoz et al., 1999). The extent of anti-saccade control has been shown to develop with age. Children below the age of 10 years often have high error rates in the region of 60%, which reduce rapidly to the age of 15 years reaching a level of about 15% by 20 years (Fischer and Weber, 1997). A similar reduction in anti-saccade errors between the ages of 6 and 15 years, has also been reported by Munoz et al. (1996) and Fukushima et al. (2000). It is important, therefore, to use appropriately age-matched controls in research involving children, in order to conclude that any increase in error rate is typical of a disorder as opposed to the normal differences expected with different age groups. The ability to execute anti-saccades has also been investigated in dyslexia. Biscaldi et al. (2000) found up to 50% of dyslexics had control of anti-saccades at a level 1.5 standard deviations below the mean of controls.

In light of the reported cerebral lesions affecting VLBW children and the growing concern regarding the educational outcomes (including specific reading difficulties) of a large proportion of the children in mainstream education who were free from major neurological incident, we decided to investigate a cohort of VLBW children to explore any deficits of oculomotor function. Thus the aim of our research was to investigate the oculomotor control in a group of VLBW children in relation to full-term controls and to identify any oculomotor anomalies that could contribute to the increased incidence of reading difficulties.

Methods

With informed consent and local ethical approval, fourteen VLBW children aged 8–9 years with a gestation of 32 weeks or less were recruited from a geographically defined cohort. VLBW children with less than normal IQ (<85), gross ocular motility or neurological deficits, or with less than 0.3 LogMAR acuity in the better eye, were excluded. The VLBW children were matched for sex and age with full-term controls from the same geographical region. The VLBW children and controls were tested on a number of standard saccade, anti-saccade and pursuit paradigms. Subjects sat, with their head stabilised, 57 cm from a visual display, which they viewed monocularly with their left eye; the right eye was occluded. Occlusion of one eye enabled amblyopic subjects to be included and in such an event the amblyopic eye would be occluded to ensure that the target could still be viewed adequately. For all tasks the fixation, saccade and pursuit targets were small dark squares ($0.3 \times 0.3°$) presented on a light background (contrast 90%) and each trial commenced with a fixation target appearing in the centre of the display for a random period of 0.5–1.5 s. In saccade and anti-saccade tasks, targets appeared randomly 5° to the left or right of fixation; in pursuit tasks, targets stepped 5° to the left or right, then moved at 14 deg/s back trough the centre of the display. Saccades of 5° amplitude were chosen as this more closely reflects the size of saccades used in everyday life compared to larger amplitude saccades of 10° or 20°, but it is acknowledged that 5° saccades will only provide a snapshot of the main sequence.

Movement of the left eye was recorded by infrared oculography, using the Skalar Iris Eye Tracker (spatial and temporal resolution of 0.1° and 1 ms). The output from the eye-tracker was digitised with 16-bit precision at 1 kHz, and data written to hard disk for off-line analysis. Subjects were exposed to 52 trials in each experimental run for visually guided saccade and pursuit tasks, and 96 trials for the anti-saccade task. At the end of each run a set of 24 calibration trials was collected and the subject allowed to rest before the next task.

Saccade and pursuit parameters were measured for trials that were not contaminated by blinks or head movements. We measured saccade amplitude, latency, peak velocity and duration. Anti-saccade error rates were calculated by dividing the number of trials on which a pro-saccade error was made by the number of valid trials. Smooth pursuit latency was measured using a regression technique from trials in which the first eye movement after target appearance was a smooth eye movement i.e. for presaccadic smooth pursuit. A regression of eye velocity on time was calculated from approximately 50 ms before to 50 ms after the target appearance, where the velocity would be expected to be zero. A second regression was calculated for the acceleration phase of the pursuit response. The intercept between the two regression functions was taken as the time of pursuit initiation. Eye velocity was measured by averaging over 20-ms epochs from 0 to 20 ms and 80 to 100 ms from the time of target appearance, from 80 to 100 ms after pursuit initiation (at the end of the open loop period) and finally 20 ms centred on the peak smooth eye movement velocity. At the 0–20- and 80–100-ms epochs after the target appeared the eye should not be moving. As little prediction or anticipation was expected in these tasks, the presence of velocity would give an indication of the stability of fixation. The velocities at these epochs could occur in either a leftward or rightward direction irrespective of the direction of the pursuit target. Mean velocities were therefore calculated for all eye movements to the left and all movements to the right, irrespective of the direction of the pursuit target. This provides a more accurate representation of the stability of fixation and avoids misleading results arising from the leftward and rightward velocities canceling each other out.

Results

Currently 14 VLBW subjects and 15 full-term controls have been recruited. Saccades were analyzed on all 29 children. Anti-saccade data were collected on all children except for one control and one VLBW child. Both children were unable to continue with the task as a result of becoming distressed and testing was abandoned in both cases. Smooth Pursuit analysis was conducted on all data collected, except for one control. The timing data in this case had been lost due to a technical problem with the equipment. All other children performed all the tests without difficulties. The mean age of the VLBW group was 9 years 1 month (range 8 years 5 months to 9 years 11 months) compared to 9 years 3 months (range 8 years 4 months to 10 years 0 months). There were no significant differences between the groups in terms of age when tested ($P > 0.05$). The mean gestation for the VLBW group was 29.7 weeks (range 24–32 weeks) with a mean birth weight of 1358 g (range 512–1860 g).

Saccade analysis

Mean saccade amplitudes were calculated for both groups for leftward and rightward saccades (Fig. 1). The mean amplitudes for the VLBW group (left $-5.2°$, 95% CI, $-5.7°$ to $-4.7°$; right $5.3°$, 95% CI, $4.7°$ to $5.9°$) were not statistically significantly different ($P > 0.05$) to those of the full-term group (left $-5.3°$, 95% CI, $-5.7°$ to $-4.9°$; right $5.1°$, 95% CI, $4.8°$ to $5.5°$). There was more variability in amplitude in the VLBW group (SD left 0.9, right 1.1) compared to controls (SD left 0.7, right 0.6), with the variance reaching significance for rightward saccades in the VLBW group (Levene's test, $P = 0.02$). Comparison of individual mean saccade amplitudes against the pooled mean full-term saccade amplitude revealed that for leftward saccades two VLBW children, and for rightward saccades four VLBW children, were more than 1.5 standard deviations away from the 'normal' amplitude (Fig. 2). There were no significant differences in mean saccade latency ($P > 0.05$) between the groups for

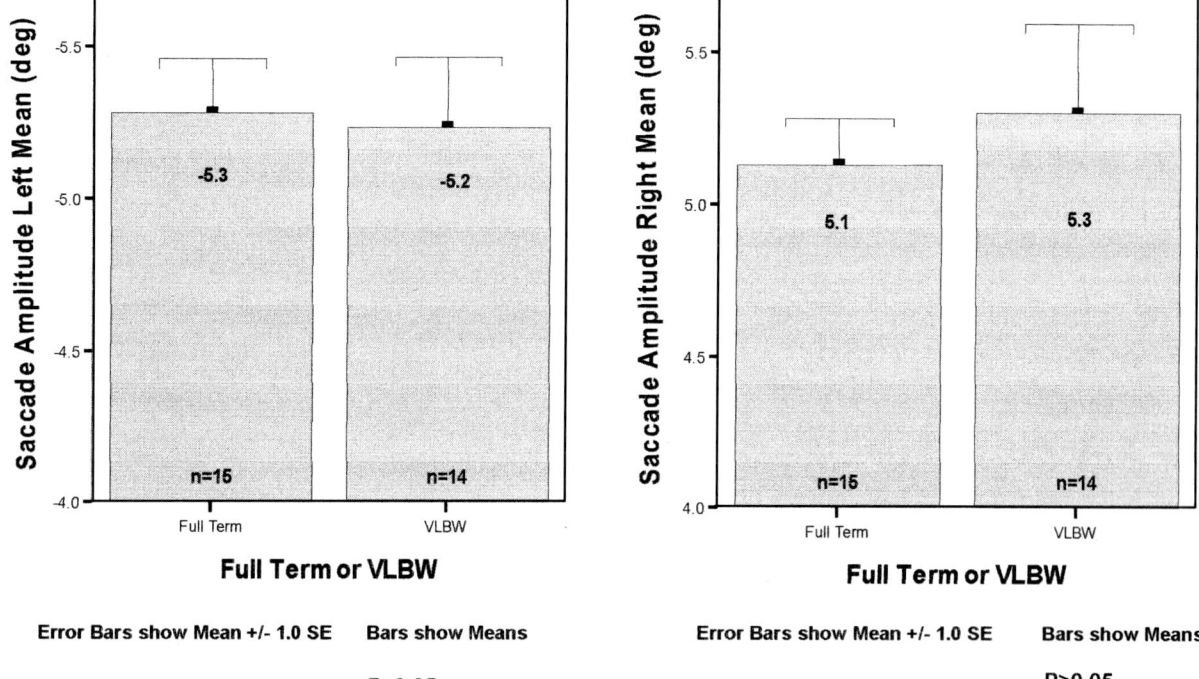

Fig. 1. Comparison of mean leftward and rightward saccade amplitude between VLBW and full-term children.

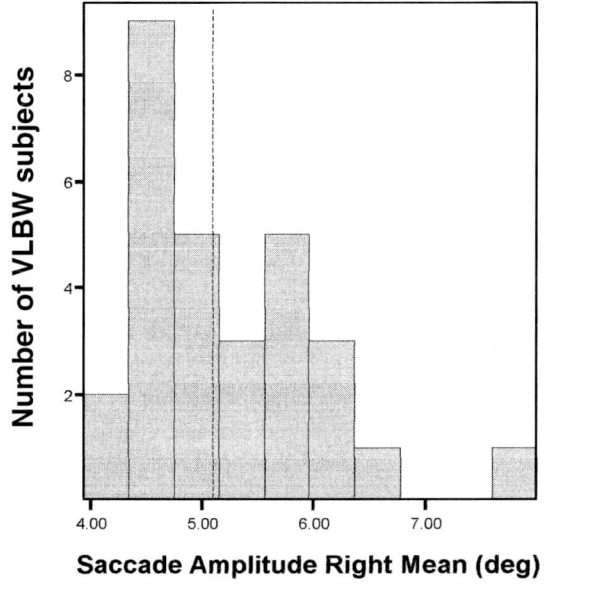
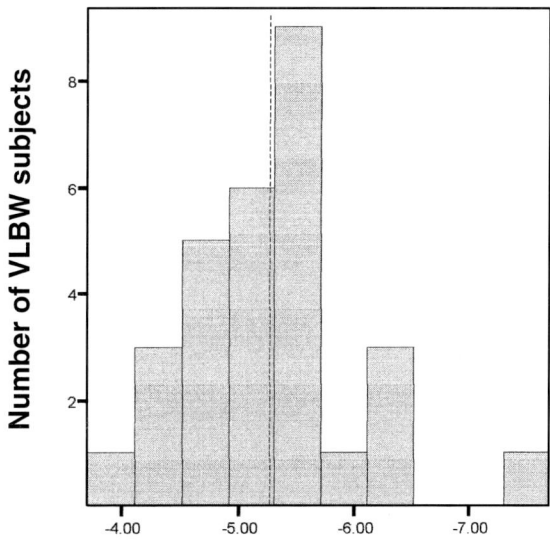

Fig. 2. Variability of saccade accuracy among individuals within the VLBW group.

either leftward (VLBW 201.1 ms, 95% CI, 179.2–223.0 ms; FT 202.1 ms, 95% CI, 185.2–219.0 ms) or rightward saccades (VLBW 207.4 ms, 95% CI, 188.0–226.8 ms; FT 204.5 ms, 95% CI, 185.7–223.3 ms) (Fig. 3). The relationship between peak velocity and amplitude (main sequence) was compared for both leftward and rightward saccades for both groups (Fig. 4). While a clear representation of a relationship is difficult to achieve as only 5° saccades were tested, there was some indication that the velocities were similar when accurate 5° saccades were made, but lower than expected in VLBW children for hypermetric saccades. When comparing mean duration, no significant difference could be found between the groups during leftward (VLBW 45.0 ms, 95% CI, 41.1–48.9 ms; FT 44.0 ms, 95% CI, 41.5–46.5 ms) or rightward (VLBW 44.6 ms, 95% CI, 41.6–47.7 ms; FT 43.4 ms, 95% CI, 41.2–45.6 ms) saccades (Fig. 5).

Anti-saccade analysis

The mean proportion of rejected trials was similar for both groups (VLBW 8.1%, FT 10.6%) and the difference was not significant ($P > 0.05$). The VLBW children made significantly more errors on the anti-saccade task compared to the full-term controls (Fig. 6). The mean percentage of anti-saccade errors for the VLBW groups was 78.3% (95% CI, 68.8–87.7) compared to 62.1% (95% CI, 51.4–72.9) for the full terms ($P = 0.02$).

Pursuit analysis

Smooth pursuit latency was longer for the VLBW group compared to the controls (Fig. 7). The mean latency for leftward pursuit was longer for the VLBW group (221.4 ms, 95% CI, 205.4–237.4) compared to the full terms (201.4 ms, 95% CI, 181.8–220.9) though this did not reach significance ($P = 0.099$). The difference was significant for rightward pursuit (VLBW 203.8 ms, 95% CI, 190.1–217.5; FT 177.3 ms, 95% CI, 161.1–193.5) ($P = 0.01$). Smooth pursuit acceleration was not markedly different between the groups with the full-term group having pursuit with greater acceleration in a rightward direction (221.8 deg/s/s, 95% CI, 169.7–273.9) compared to VLBWs (202.9 deg/s/s, 95% CI, 156.4–249.3) ($P > 0.05$), but in a leftward direction the VLBW group had greater pursuit

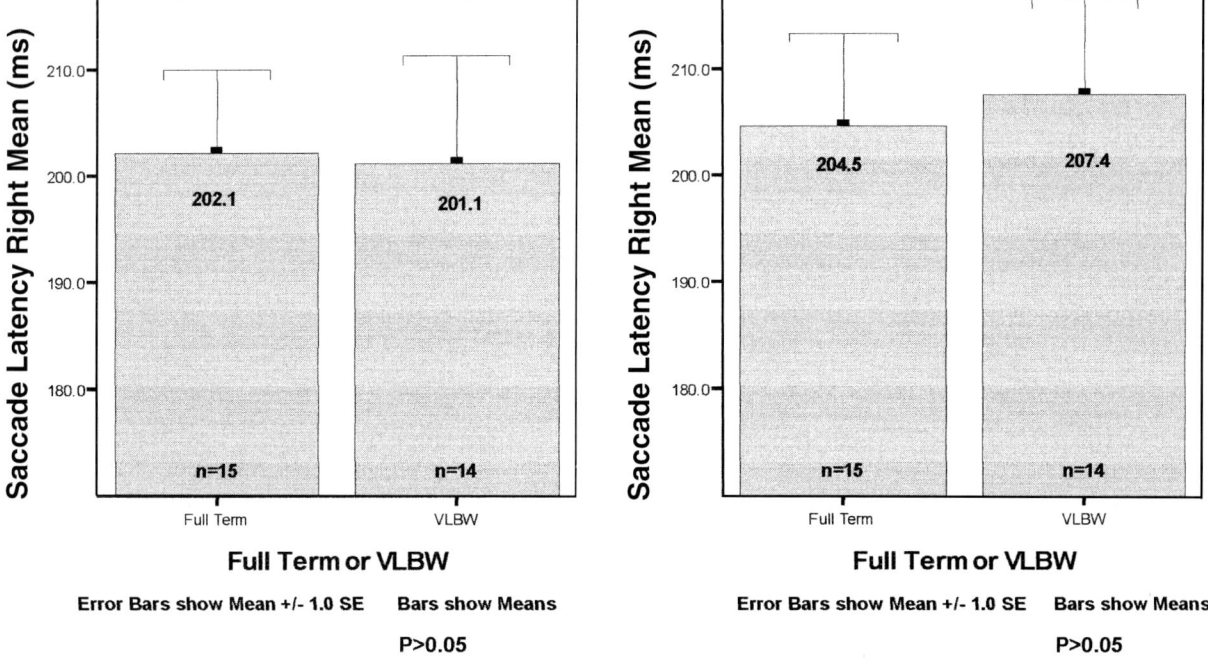

Fig. 3. Comparison of mean leftward and rightward saccade latency between VLBW and full-term children.

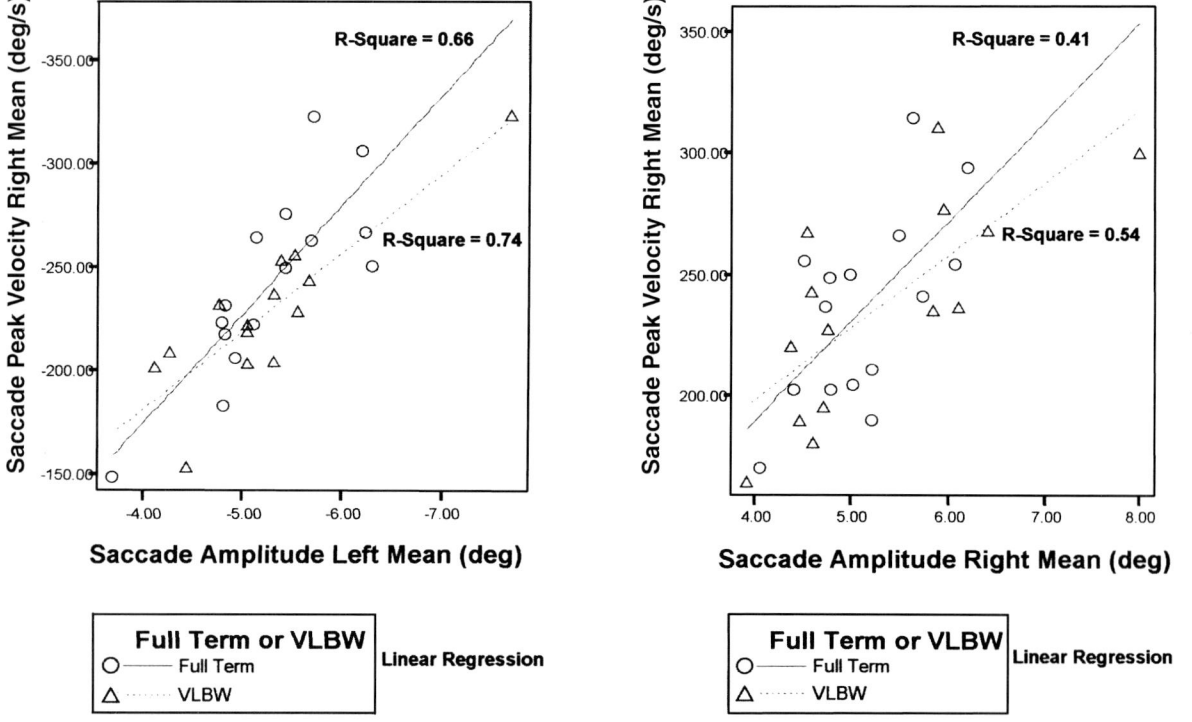

Fig. 4. Relationship of peak velocity vs. saccade amplitude (main sequence) (leftward and rightward), with linear regression, between VLBW and full-term children.

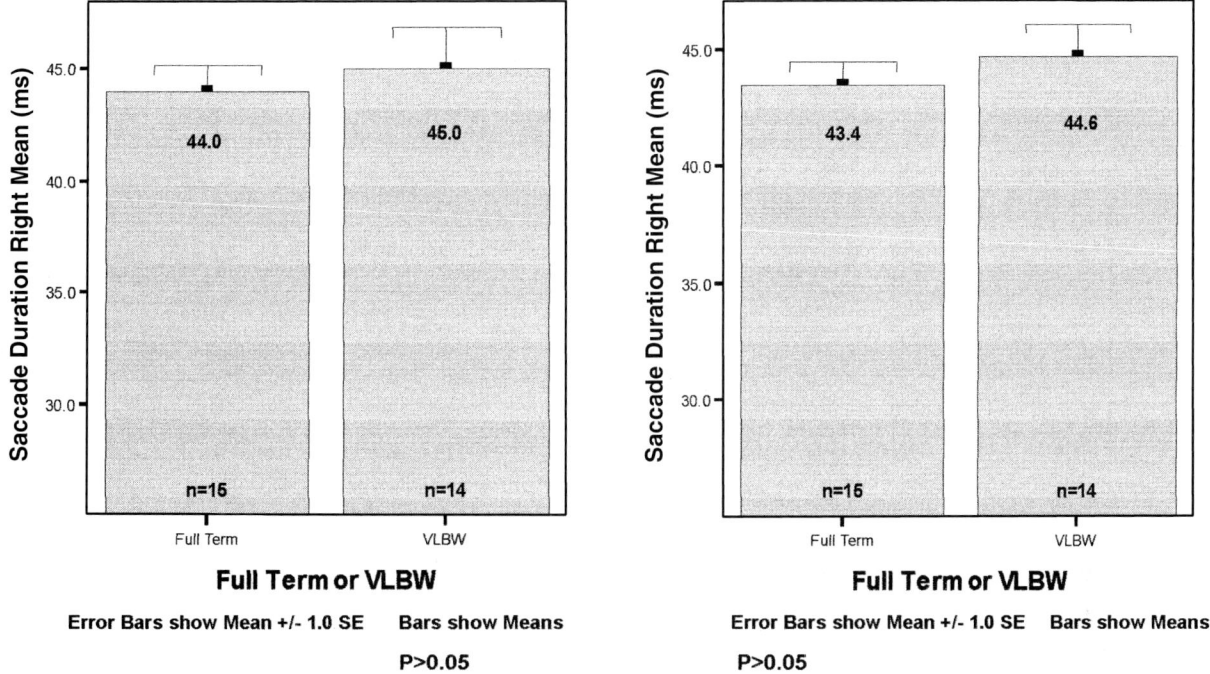

Fig. 5. Comparison of mean leftward and rightward saccade duration between VLBW and full-term children.

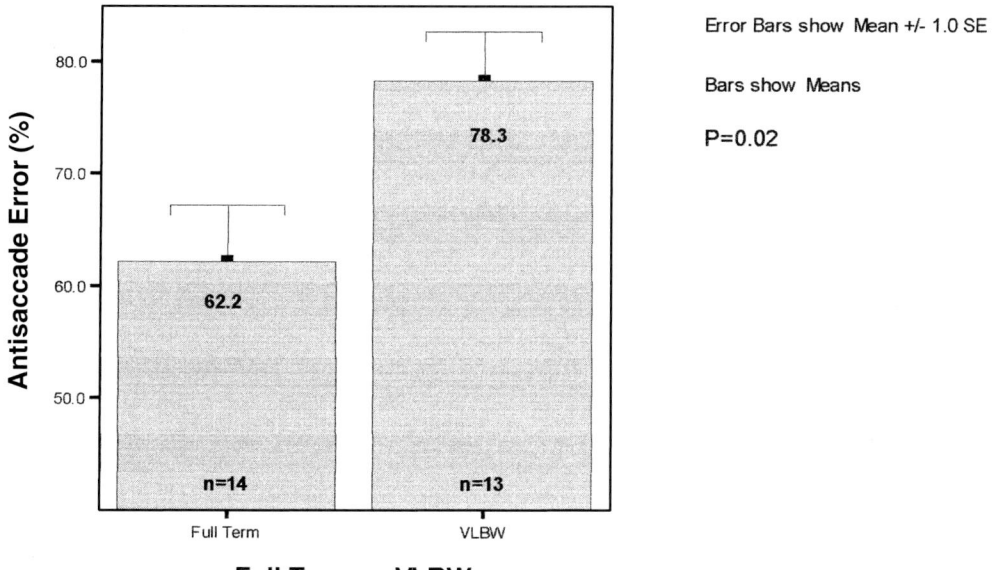

Fig. 6. Comparison of anti-saccade error rate between VLBW and full-term children.

acceleration (220.6 deg/s/s, 95% CI, 160.1–281.2) compared to the controls (164.1 deg/s/s, 95% CI, 136.1–192.2) ($P > 0.05$).

Measurement of eye velocity from 0 to 20 ms and 80 to 100 ms after target appearance allows us to estimate the stability of fixation (Figs. 8 and 9). With

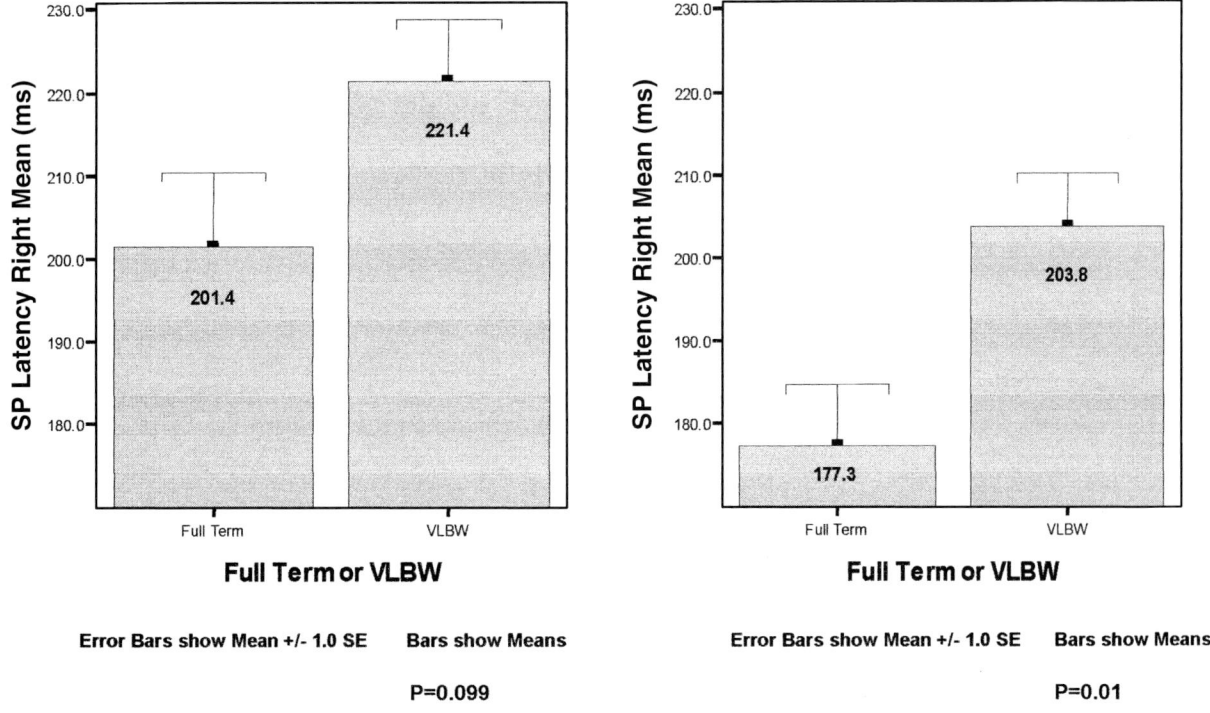

Fig. 7. Comparison of mean leftward and rightward smooth pursuit latency between VLBW and full-term children.

the type of tasks we employed in these experiments, we would expect little anticipation or prediction, therefore during these two epochs the eye should not be moving. Comparison of the velocities from 0 to 20 ms and 80 to 100 ms after the target appeared revealed a tendency for fixation to be less stable in the VLBW group but this only reached significance for leftward pursuit at the 80–100-ms epoch. At 0–20 ms after the target appeared the mean velocity for the VBLW group was −1.4 deg/s (leftward pursuit) and 1.5 deg/s (rightward pursuit), compared to −1.0 deg/s (leftward pursuit) ($P > 0.05$) and 1.1 deg/s (rightward pursuit) ($P = 0.07$) for the full terms. At 80–100 ms after the target appeared the mean velocity for the VLBW group was −1.4 deg/s (leftward pursuit) and 1.6 deg/s (rightward pursuit), compared to −0.9 deg/s (leftward pursuit) ($P = 0.02$) and 1.3 deg/s (rightward pursuit) ($P > 0.05$) for the full terms. At 80–100 ms after pursuit began (at the end of the open loop period) the mean velocities were very similar for both groups with no significant differences in either direction. The mean velocity for the VLBW group was −8.4 deg/s (leftward) and 8.2 deg/s (rightward) compared to −8.8 deg/s (leftward) ($P > 0.05$) and 8.7 deg/s (rightward) ($P > 0.05$) for the full terms. Finally the mean peak slow eye velocities were also similar for both groups. The mean peak slow eye velocities for the VLBW group were −14.7 and 16.1 deg/s, compared to −16.0 and 18.3 deg/s for the full terms (leftward and rightward, respectively) ($P > 0.05$).

Discussion

Saccade amplitudes were not statistically significantly different between the VLBW and full-term groups. However, there was more variability in amplitude in the VLBW group (SD left 0.9, right 1.1) compared to controls (SD left 0.7, right 0.6). Given the expected heterogeneity of the VLBW group we compared individual mean VLBW amplitudes to the pooled mean full-term amplitude to determine the number of individuals that were substantially different (1.5 SD) from controls. While some individual full-term children were 1.5 standard deviations away from the pooled mean amplitude this was true for

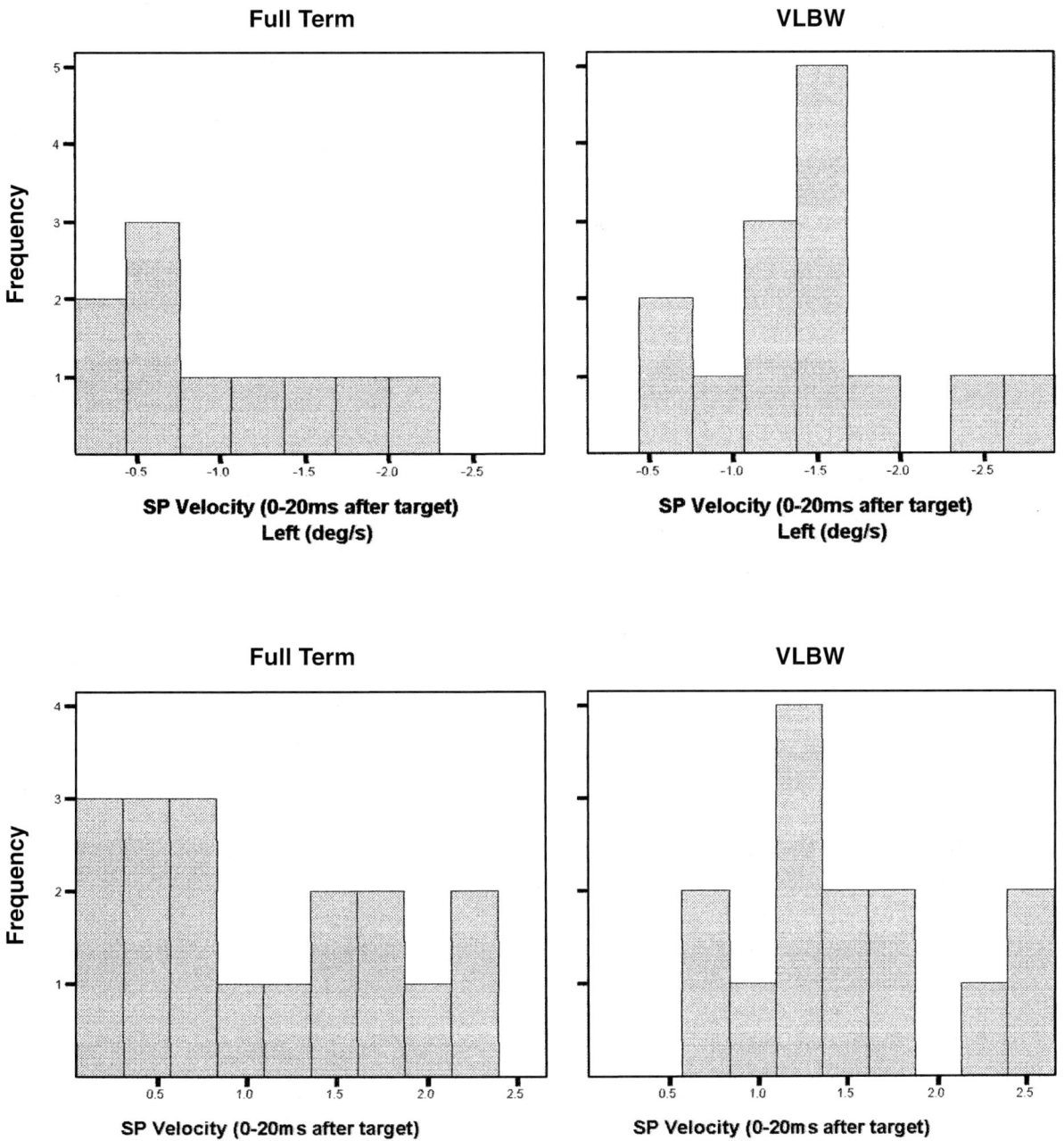

Fig. 8. Distribution of smooth pursuit velocity (leftward and rightward) at 0–20-ms epoch after appearance of the target in VLBW and full-term children.

twice as many VLBWs than controls (leftward, 2 vs. 1; rightward, 4 vs. 2). While not a marked dysmetria, this might be suggestive of diffuse or subtle damage relatively low in the hierarchy of oculomotor control circuits in a proportion of the VLBWs — perhaps in the cerebellum (see discussion of brain lesions

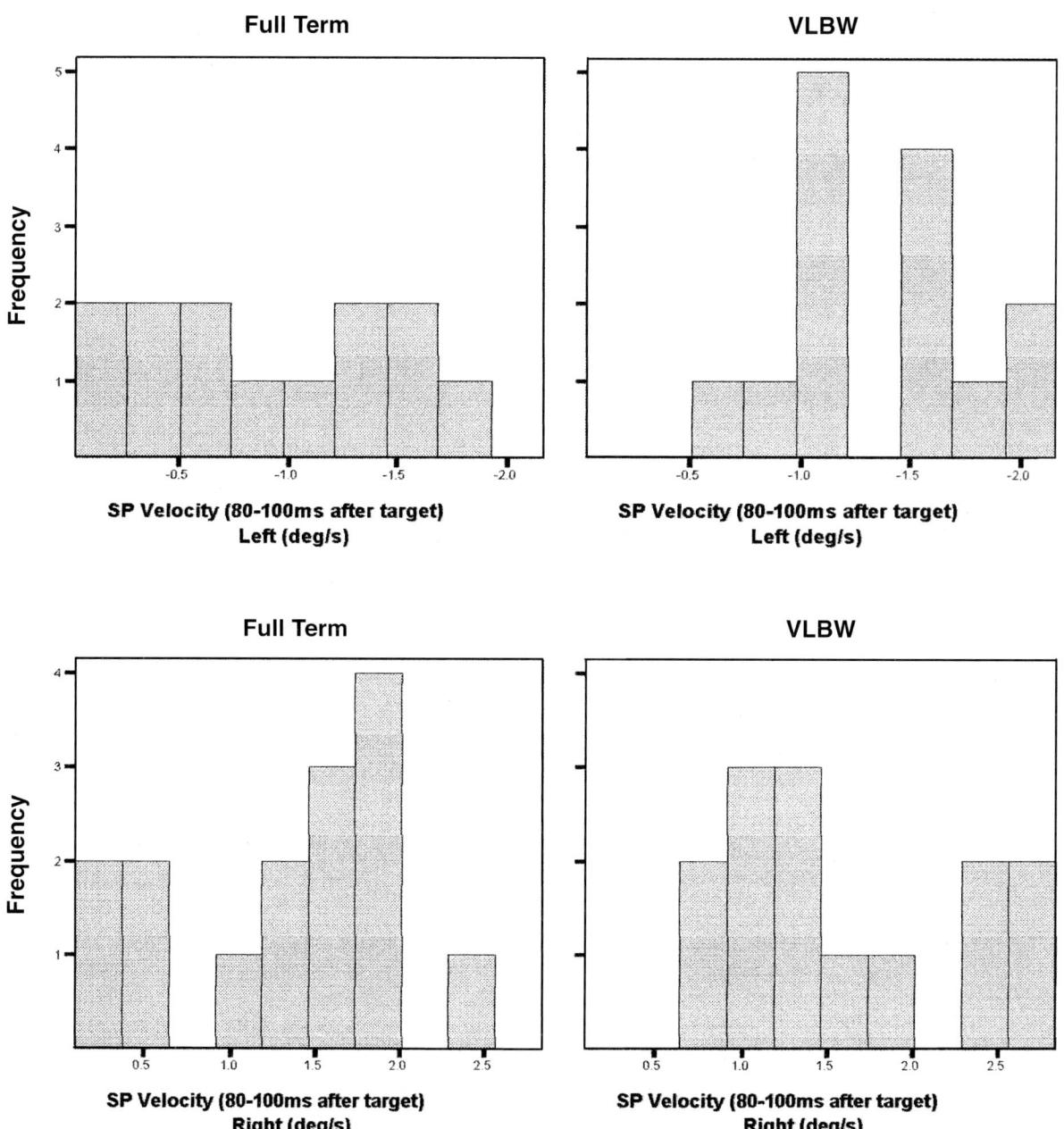

Fig. 9. Distribution of smooth pursuit velocity (leftward and rightward) at 80–100-ms epoch after appearance of the target in VLBW and full-term children.

above). There was little difference between the two groups in terms of either saccade latency or main sequence relationships. This suggests the most of the saccade circuitry, including both cortical and subcortical structures must be reasonably intact. This is interesting given the certain structures such as the caudate nucleus and the pulvinar have been reported to be at risk in VLBWs. However, we have examined only a relatively small proportion of what is a heterogeneous group. It remains to be seen whether our findings are typical of the group as a whole. Unfortunately it is not possible to compare our findings with those of others, as the only other study that we have found which investigated the control of saccades in VLBW children did not present any quantitative data (Jacobson et al., 1998).

We found a significantly higher error rate in the anti-saccade task in the VLBW group (78.3%) compared to the full-term controls (62.2%). It has been shown that the anti-saccade error rate improves rapidly with age (Munoz et al., 1996; Fukushima et al., 2000) and it should be noted that our groups were carefully matched for age. It is thought that the inverse relationship between anti-saccade error and age is due to delayed maturation of the frontal cortex (Munoz et al., 1996). The increased error rate in the VLBW group is consistent with a number of possibilities. It is possible that the VLBWs have diffuse or subtle damage to the frontal cortex, which is being picked up with the anti-saccade task. Continued testing with this task will allow us to investigate whether there is an improvement. An alternative is that there is a developmental delay, which manifests itself in the snapshot of performance we have presented here as an increased error rate. Again, further testing should reveal an improvement. Whether we eventually see error rates decline to normal levels will reveal whether there is a lingering deficit, which cannot be compensated for.

The increased rate of anti-saccade errors in the VLBW group may be associated with the increased incidence of specific reading difficulties that has been reported in VLBW children. The control of anti-saccades has recently been linked with dyslexia (Biscaldi et al., 2000; Fischer et al., 2000). Biscaldi et al. (2000) confirmed that the anti-saccade performance increases with age, but dyslexics had significantly poorer performance in comparison to controls above the age of 8 years. Fifty percent of dyslexics failed to execute an anti-saccade (or reverse the pro-saccade with a corrective saccade) at a level of 1.5 standard deviations below the mean of the controls. The authors conclude that the findings indicate the functional deficits in the region of the frontal cortex can be associated with dyslexic symptoms. It should be noted, however, that functional neuroimaging studies have demonstrated that a variety of brain regions are involved in the generation of anti-saccades. Increased regional cerebral blood flow has been shown in the areas of the cingulate gyrus, insula, globus pallidus, striatum and thalamus, during anti-saccades (Anderson et al., 1994; O'Driscoll et al., 1995; Petite et al., 1995; Sweeney et al., 1996). Involvement of the caudate nucleus and substantia nigra pars reticulata in the generation of anti-saccades is also supported due to patients with progressive supranuclear palsy showing increased error rates (Blin et al., 1995). Clinical studies suggest that the globus pallidus and putamen are not essential in order to perform the task (Vermesch et al., 1996). It is also possible that anti-saccade deficits are linked with deficits of the magnocellular system (Fischer et al., 2000), as the cortical areas involved in saccade preparation receive the visual information via the magnocellular pathway from the retinal ganglion Y-cells and lateral geniculate nucleus.

Smooth pursuit latency and acceleration was broadly similar for both groups with a slightly longer latency for the VLBW group but significant in one direction only. These findings differ to those of Langaas et al. (1998) who reported no increase in pursuit latency in eight children born prematurely in comparison to controls. However there are methodological differences between the studies, as Langaas et al. (1998) used sinusoidal pursuit tasks. Analysis of eye velocity over the 0–20- and 80–100-ms epochs revealed some evidence that fixation was less steady in the VLBWs. While this assessment of fixation only provides an estimate of stability over short epochs, it is presumably precisely problems over this sort of timescale, which would cause reading difficulties. However, we also intend to investigate fixation over longer epochs in future experiments. Experiments of this type were conducted by Raymond et al. (1988), who discovered fixational instability in a group of children with subtle cerebellar dysfunction born full-term, suffering from dyslexia. It is interesting to compare our findings with this study, as whilst the subjects were not VLBW children, the authors did investigate fixational control in a group suffering from subtle lesions affecting the cerebellum, a lesion that may affect VLBW children, and an attempt was also made to determine if the fixational instability could lead to the reading difficulties. The method used to assess stability of fixation involved a target much larger than used in our research and the fixation was assessed during a period of 4 s. Despite the methodological differences, and although the authors did not suggest that the fixational instability was causative of reading problems, it does demonstrate that lesions of the cerebellum can lead to reduced fixational control.

The velocities at the end of the open loop period (80–100 ms after pursuit began) and the peak slow eye velocity were similar for both groups. This suggests that if the VLBWs have a pursuit deficit, it is not a general one and is perhaps specific to pursuit initiation. Our results contrast to Langaas et al. (1998) who found that VLBW children have a reduced pursuit gain in comparison to controls. However, there are a number of important differences between the two studies, not only in the type of pursuit task as mentioned earlier, but also in the age range of the subjects. The mean age of their subjects was 5 years 8 months compared to 9 years 1 month for the subjects in our cohort. It is therefore possible that with time there is some recovery or further development.

Overall, the VLBW children show some deficits of oculomotor control in comparison to full-term controls. This is not surprising given the nature and variety of lesions that can affect VLBW children. There appear to be mild deficits in the areas of pursuit initiation and control of fixation, with some individuals showing saccade dysmetria. Fixational control will be explored in future research using a specific fixation task. The most notable deficit appears to be in the control of anti-saccades, which is interesting given the recent reports of similar errors in dyslexic subjects (Biscaldi et al., 2000). It is possible that the impaired control of anti-saccades in VLBW children is associated with the increased incidence of reading difficulties that affect this group and further research is required in this area. Further longitudinal research will also help to determine if the anti-saccade errors improve in the VLBW group at the same rate as normal individuals, and whether the rate eventually reaches a normal level.

Having examined monocular control we are now examining the coordination of the eyes in VLBWs. Currently we are examining binocular saccades and investigating dynamic alignment and also vergence changes during saccades to targets in depth. Finally, we intend to look at correlations between oculomotor performance and other data that have been collected on these subjects, which include MRI scans, ADHD assessments, perinatal data and other aspects of motor function (fine and gross motor function using the movement ABC test, the developmental test of visual motor integation, deep tendon reflexes and assessment of subtle motor co-ordination difficulties using tests comprising the clinical observations of motor postural skills — COMPS) that have been assessed by an Occupational Therapist.

Abbreviations

FT   full term
VLBW   very low birth weight

Acknowledgements

The authors would like to thank Prof. R Cooke, Department of Child Health, University of Liverpool, for his help and advice in undertaking this research.

References

Anderson, T.J., Jenkins, I.J., Brooks, D.J., Hawken, M.B., Frackowiak, R.S. and Kennard, C. (1994) Cortical control of saccades and fixation in man: a PET study. *Brain*, 117: 1073–1084.

Aram, D., Hack, M., Hawkins, S., Weissman, B. and Borawski-Clark, E. (1991) Very low birth weight children and speech and language development. *J. Speech Lang. Hear. Res.*, 34: 1169–1179.

Batton, D.G., Holtrop, P., Dewitte, D., Pryce, C. and Roberts, C. (1994) Current gestational age-related incidence of major intraventricular hemorrhage. *J. Pediatr.*, 125: 623–625.

Biscaldi, M., Gezeck, S. and Stuhr, V. (1998) Poor saccadic control correlates with dyslexia. *Neuropsychologia*, 36: 1189–1202.

Biscaldi, M., Fischer, B. and Hartnegg, K. (2000) Voluntary saccadic control in dyslexia. *Perception*, 29: 509–521.

Blin, J., Mazetti, P., Mazoyer, B., Rivaud, S., Ben-Ayed, S. and Malapani, C. (1995) Does the enhancement of cholinergic neurotransmission influence brain glucose kinetics and clinical symptomatology in progressive supranuclear palsy? *Brain*, 118: 1485–1495.

Botting, N., Powls, A., Cooke, R.W. and Marlow, N. (1998) Cognitive and educational outcome of very low birthweight children in early adolescence. *Dev. Med. Child Neurol.*, 40: 652–660.

Burstein, J., Papile, L. and Burstein, R. (1979) Intraventricular hemorrhage in premature newborns: a prospective study with CT. *Am. J. Radiol.*, 132: 631–635.

Buttner, U. and Straube, A. (1995) The effect of cerebellar midline lesions on eye movements. *Neuro-Ophthalmology*, 15: 75–82.

Clementz, B.A., McDowell, J.E. and Zisook, S. (1994) Saccadic system functioning among schizophrenia patients and their first-degree biological relatives. *J. Abnorm. Psychol.*, 103: 277–287.

Desmond, M.M., Williamson, W.D. and Wilson, G.S. (1986) School failure in prematurely born children: can it be prevented? *J. Perinatol.*, 6: 309–315.

De Vries, L.S., Wigglesworth, J.S., Regev, R. and Dubowitz, L.M.S. (1988) Evolution of periventricular leukomalacia during the neonatal period and infancy: correlation of imaging and post mortem findings. *Early Hum. Dev.*, 17: 205–219.

De Vries, L.S., Groenendaal, F., Eken, P., van Haastert, I.C., Rademaker, K.J. and Meiners, L.C. (1997) Infarcts in the vascular distribution of the middle cerebral artery in preterm and fullterm infants. *Neuropediatrics*, 28: 88–96.

Dolfin, T., Skidmore, M.B., Fong, K.W., Hoskins, E.M. and Shannon, A.T. (1983) Incidents, severity and timing of subependymal and intraventricular hemorrhages in preterm infants born in a perinatal unit as detected by serial real-time ultrasound. *Pediatrics*, 71: 541–546.

Dutton, G., Ballantyne, J. and Boyd, G. (1996) Cortical visual dysfunction in children: a clinical study. *Eye*, 10: 302–309.

Fischer, B. and Weber, H. (1997) Effects of stimulus conditions on the performance of antisaccades in man. *Exp. Brain Res.*, 116: 191–200.

Fischer, B., Hartnegg, K. and Mokler, A. (2000) Dynamic visual perception of dyslexic children. *Perception*, 29: 523–530.

Fukushima, J., Hatta, T. and Fukushima, K. (2000) Development of voluntary control of saccadic eye movements. I. Age-related changes in normal children. *Brain Dev.*, 22: 173–180.

Gibson, N.A., Fielder, A.R., Trounce, J.Q. and Levene, M.I. (1990) Ophthalmic findings in infants of very low birthweight. *Dev. Med. Child Neurol.*, 32: 7–13.

Hack, M., Breslau, N., Aram, D., Weissman, B., Klein, N. and Borawski-Clark, E. (1992) The effect of very low birthweight and social risk on neurocognitive abilities at school age. *J. Dev. Behav. Pediatr.*, 13: 412–420.

Hack, M., Taylor, H.G., Klein, N., Eiben, R., Schatschneider, C. and Meruri-Minich, N. (1994) School age outcomes in children with birthweights under 750 g. *N. Engl. J. Med.*, 331: 753–759.

Hall, A., McLeod, A., Counsell, C., Thomson, L. and Mutch, L. (1995) School attainment, cognitive ability and motor function in a total Scottish very-low-birthweight population at eight years: a controlled study. *Dev. Med. Child Neurol.*, 37: 1037–1050.

Hallett, P.E. (1978) Primary and secondary saccades to goals defined by instructions. *Vision Res.*, 20: 329–339.

Horwood, L.J., Mogridge, N. and Darlow, B.A. (1998) Cognitive, educational and behavioural outcomes at 7–8 years in a national very low birthweight cohort. *Arch. Dis. Child Fetal Neonatal Ed.*, 79: 12–20.

Jacobson, L. (1998) *Visual Dysfunction and Ocular Signs Associated with Periventricular Leukomalacia in Children Born Preterm.* PhD Thesis.

Jacobson, L., Ygge, J. and Flodmark, O. (1998) Nystagmus in periventricular leukomalacia. *Br. J. Ophthalmol.*, 82: 1026–1032.

Johnson, E.O. and Breslau, N. (2000) Increased risk of learning disabilities in low birth weight boys at age 11 years. *Biol. Psychiatry*, 47: 490–500.

Keith, C.G. and Kitchen, W.H. (1983) Ocular morbidity in infants of very low birthweight. *Br. J. Ophthalmol.*, 67: 302–305.

Kiely, J.L., Paneth, N., Stein, Z. and Susser, M. (1981) Mortality and neurological impairment in low birthweight infants. *Dev. Med. Child Neurol.*, 23: 650–659.

Klebanov, P.K., Brooks-Gunn, J. and McCormick, M.C. (1994) School achievement and failure in very low birthweight children. *J. Dev. Behav. Pediatr.*, 15: 248–256.

Klein, N.K., Hack, M. and Breslau, N. (1989) Children who were very low birthweight: development and academic achievement at nine years of age. *J. Dev. Behav. Pediatr.*, 10: 32–37.

Langaas, T., Mon-Williams, M., Wann, J.P., Pascal, E. and Thompson, C. (1998) Eye movements, prematurity and developmental co-ordination disorder. *Vision Res.*, 38: 1817–1826.

Lloyd, B.W., Wheldall, K. and Perks, D. (1988) Controlled study of intelligence and school performance of very low birthweight children from a defined geographical area. *Dev. Med. Child Neurol.*, 30: 36–42.

Marlow, N., Roberts, L. and Cooke, R. (1993) Outcome at 8 years for children with birthweights of 1250 g or less. *Arch. Dis. Child*, 68: 286–290.

Martin, R., Roessman, U. and Fanaroff, A. (1976) Massive intracerebellar hemorrhage in low birthweight infants. *J. Pediatr.*, 89: 290–293.

McCormick, M.C., Workman-Daniels, K. and Brooks-Gunn, J. (1996) The behavioural and emotional wellbeing of school age children with different birthweights. *Pediatrics*, 97: 18–25.

Michelsson, K., Lindahl, E., Parre, M. and Helenius, M. (1984) Nine-year follow-up of infants weighing 1500 g or less at birth. *Acta Paediatr.*, 73: 835–841.

Miller, N.R. and Fine, S.L. (1977) The ocular fundus in neuro-ophthalmological diagnosis. In: *Sights and Sounds in Ophthalmology.* CV Mosby, St Louis, pp. 50–53.

Munoz, D.P., Goldring, J.E., Hampton, K.A. and Moore, K.D. (1996) Age-related performance of human subjects on pro- and anti-saccade tasks. *Soc. Neurosci. Abstr.*, 22: 1688.

Munoz, D.P., Hampton, K.A., Moore, K.D. and Goldring, J.E. (1999) Control of purposive saccadic eye movements and visual fixation in children with attention-deficit hyperactivity disorder. In: Becker et al. (Eds.), *Current Oculomotor Research.* Vol. 58, Plenum Press, New York, pp. 415–423.

O'Callaghan, M.J., Burns, Y.R., Gray, P.H., Harvey, J.M., Mohay, H., Rogers, Y.M. and Tudehope, D.I. (1996) School performance of ELBW children: a controlled study. *Dev. Med. Child Neurol.*, 38: 917–926.

O'Driscoll, G.A., Alpert, N.M., Matthysse, S.W., Levy, D.L., Rauch, S.L. and Holzman, P.S. (1995) Functional neuroanatomy of antisaccade eye movements investigated with positron emission tomography. *Proc. Natl. Acad. Sci. USA*, 92: 925–929.

Pavlidis, G.T. (1981) Do eye movements hold the key to dyslexia? *Neuropsychologia*, 19: 57–64.

Pavlidis, G.T. (1983) The 'dyslexia syndrome' and its objective diagnosis by erratic eye movements. In: K. Rayner (Ed.), *Eye Movements in Reading: Perceptual and Language Processes*. Academic Press, New York, NY, pp. 441–466.

Pavlidis, G.T. (1985) Eye movement differences between dyslexics, normal and slow readers while sequentially fixing digits. *Am. J. Optom. Physiol. Optics*, 62: 820–822.

Peckham, C.S. (1986) Vision in childhood. *Br. Med. Bull.*, 42: 150–154.

Petite, L., Tzourio, N., Orssaud, C., Pietrzyk, U., Berthoz, A. and Mazoyer, B. (1995) Functional neuroanatomy of the human visual fixation system. *Eur. J. Neurosci.*, 7: 169–174.

Pirozzolo, F.J. and Rayner, K. (1979) Eye movements and reading disorders. In: H. Whittaker and H.A. Whittaker (Eds.), *Studies in Neurolinguistics*. Academic Press, New York, pp. 104–107.

Pharoah, P.O.D., Stevenson, C.J., Cooke, R.W.I. and Stevenson, R.C. (1994) Clinical and subclinical deficits at 8 years in a geographically defined cohort of low birthweight infants. *Arch. Dis. Child.*, 70: 264–270.

Powls, A., Botting, N., Cooke, R.W.I. and Marlow, N. (1995) Motor impairment in children 12–13 years old with a birthweight of less than 1250 g. *Arch. Dis. Child, Fetal Neonatal Ed.*, 72: 62–66.

Powls, A., Botting, N., Cooke, R.W.I., Stephenson, G. and Marlow, N. (1997) Visual impairment in very low birthweight children. *Arch. Dis. Child, Fetal Neonatal Ed.*, 76: 82–87.

Raymond, J.E., Ogden, N.A., Fagan, J.E. and Kaplan, B.J. (1988) Fixational instability and saccadic eye movements of dyslexic children with subtle cerebellar dysfunction. *Am. J. Optom. Physiol. Optics*, 65: 174–181.

Rickards, A.L., Kitchen, W.H., Doyle. L.W., Ford, G.W., Kelly, E.A. and Callanan, C. (1993) Cognition, school performance and behaviour in very low birthweight and normal birth weight children at 8 years of age: A longitudinal study. *J. Dev. Behav. Pediatr.*, 14: 363–368.

Reeder, J.D., Kaude, J.V. and Setzer, E.S. (1982) Choroid plexus hemorrhage in premature neonates: recognition by sonography. *Am. J. Neuroradiol.*, 3: 619–622.

Saigal, S., Szatmari, P., Rosenbaum, P., Campbell, D. and King, S. (1991) Cognitive abilities and school performance of extremely low birth weight children and matched term control children at age 8 years — A regional study. *J. Pediatr.*, 118: 751–760.

Saigal, S., Szatmari, P. and Rosenbaum, P. (1992) Can learning disabilities in children who were extremely low birthweight be identified at school entry? *Dev. Behav. Pediatr.*, 13: 356–361.

Saigal, S., Hoult, L.A., Streiner, D.L., Stoskopf, B.L. and Rosenbaum, P.L. (2000) School difficulties at adolescence in a regional cohort of children who were extremely low birthweight. *Pediatrics*, 105: 325–331.

Schmitt, B.D. (1987) Ambulatory pediatrics. In: C.H. Kempe, H.K. Silver, D. O'Brien and A. Fulginiti (Eds.), *Current Pediatric Diagnosis and Treatment*, 9th edn. Appleton and Lange, Norwalk, pp. 153–180.

Sheldon, R.A., Chuai, J. and Ferriero, D.M. (1996) A rat model for hypoxic-ischemic brain damage in very premature infants. *Biol. Neonate*, 69: 327–341.

Sommerfelt, K., Troland, K., Ellertsen, B. and Markestad, T. (1996) Behavioural problems in low birthweight preschoolers. *Dev. Med. Child Neurol.*, 38: 927–940.

Stewart, A.L., Reynolds, E.O.R. and Lipscomb, A.P. (1981) Outcome for infants of very low birth weight: survey of the world literature. *Lancet*, i: 1038–1041.

Straschill, M. and Takahashi, H. (1981) Changes of EEG and single unit activity in the human pulvinar associated with saccadic gaze shifts and fixation. In: A.F. Fuchs and W. Becker (Eds.), *Progress in Oculomotor Research*. Elsevier, Amsterdam, pp. 225–231.

Sweeney, J.A., Mintun, M.A. and Kwee, S. (1996) Positron emission tomography study of voluntary saccadic eye movements and spatial working memory. *J. Neurophysiol.*, 75: 454–468.

The Scottish Low Birthweight Study Group (1992) The Scottish low birthweight study: II Language attainment, cognitive status and behavioural problems. *Arch. Dis. Child*, 67: 682–686.

Trounce, J.Q., Rutter, N. and Levene, M.I. (1986) Periventricular leukomalacia and intraventricular haemorrhage. *Arch. Dis. Child*, 61: 1196–1202.

Tusa, R.J. and Ungerleider, L.G. (1988) Fiber pathways of cortical areas mediating smooth pursuit eye movements in monkeys. *Ann. Neurol.*, 23: 174–183.

Vermesch, A.I., Muri, R.M., Rivaud, S., Vidailhet, M., Gaymard, B., Agid, Y. and Pierrot-Deseilligny, C. (1996) Saccade disturbances after bilateral lentiform nucleus lesions in humans. *J. Neurol. Neurosurg. Psychiatry*, 60: 179–184.

Weinacht, S., Kind, C., Monting, J.S. and Gottlob, I. (1999) Visual development in preterm and full-term infants: a prospective masked study. *Invest. Ophthalmol. Vis. Sci.*, 40: 346–353.

Whitfield, M.F., Grunau, R.V.E. and Holsti, L. (1997) Extremely premature (<800 g) school children: multiple areas of hidden disability. *Arch. Dis. Child, Fetal Neonatal Ed.*, 77: 85–90.

Yokochi, K. (1997) Thalamic lesions revealed by MR associated with periventricular leukomalacia and clinical profiles of subjects. *Acta Paediatr.*, 86: 493–496.

CHAPTER 33

A new framework for investigating both normal and abnormal eye movements

Richard A. Clement [1,*], Richard V. Abadi [2], David S. Broomhead [3] and Jonathon P. Whittle [4]

[1] *Visual Sciences Unit, Institute of Child Health, University College London, 30 Guilford Street, London WC1N 1EH, UK*
[2] *Department of Optometry and Neuroscience, UMIST, P.O. Box 88, Manchester M60 1QD, UK*
[3] *Department of Mathematics, UMIST, P.O. Box 88, Manchester M60 1QD, UK*
[4] *The University of Sheffield, Department of Ophthalmology and Orthoptics, Royal Hallamshire Road, Sheffield S10 2JF, UK*

Abstract: Any comprehensive framework for understanding eye movements has to include both normal and abnormal eye movement behaviour. One approach which is applicable to the entire range of oculomotor behaviour is provided by the techniques of nonlinear dynamics. The stability of models of the oculomotor system can be analysed in terms of the characteristics of their fixed points and periodic orbits, and the method of delays can be used to recover such parameters from measurements of eye position. Within this framework, quantitative comparisons can be made between the predictions of different models, and both normal and clinical eye movement recordings.

Introduction

The normal oculomotor system behaves in a remarkably machine-like way. Saccadic eye movements have characteristic relationships between peak velocity and amplitude and duration and amplitude, which hold throughout life (Bahill et al., 1975; Lebedev et al., 1996). By comparison, abnormal eye movements show a variety that is both rich and strange. There are hypo- and hyper-metric saccades, post-saccadic drifts, square-wave jerks, macrosaccadic oscillations, ocular flutter, nystagmus and opsoclonus to name just some of the disorders of fixation (Leigh and Zee, 1999). Not surprisingly, oculomotor researchers are continually seeking the appropriate framework for investigating both normal and abnormal eye movements.

* Correspondence to: R.A. Clement, Visual Sciences Unit, Institute of Child Health, University College London, 30 Guilford Street, London WC1N 1EH, UK. E-mail: r.clement@ich.ucl.ac.uk

One approach is to adopt a framework which has been used successfully with limb movements. In his teaching video on supranuclear disorders, Daroff (1990) illustrates a number of nystagmus rhythms by moving his hands from side to side in parallel. This in itself is an interesting movement, because if the hand movements are made in time with a metronome 180° out of phase, instead of in synchrony, then as the metronome beats faster the hand movements suddenly switch from being out of phase to being in phase (Kelso, 1995). It is just this abrupt switch from one sort of behaviour to another that a framework for investigating both normal and abnormal eye movements needs to be able to explain. In the case of hand movements, the techniques of dynamical systems theory have been used to explore the abrupt changes in behaviour, and in this paper we outline the application of such techniques to the characterisation of eye movements, using congenital nystagmus as an example of an abnormal eye movement.

The nonlinear dynamics approach

The nonlinear dynamics approach is directed towards describing the way in which the oculomotor system changes from one state to the next. A geometric picture of the state changes can be made by treating each of the variables which specify the state as a coordinate in a vector space, referred to in this context as a phase or state space. The successive states of the oculomotor system form a trajectory in state space, and the behaviour of the system can be described in terms of the geometric properties of the trajectory.

For instance, if the oculomotor system is in equilibrium, then the equilibrium state corresponds to a single point in phase space, referred to as a fixed point, because if a trajectory reaches this point, it will not move from the point unless the system is perturbed. We began with the assumption that normal fixation corresponds to the behaviour of the oculomotor system at a stable fixed point, and that pathological fixation conditions correspond to an unstable fixed point. Mathematically, the stability of a fixed point can be quantified by studying the evolution of nearby states. Close to a fixed point, the behaviour of a system is approximately linear, and can be characterised in terms of the eigenvalues and eigenvectors. Eigenvectors are special trajectories of the linear model that converge to, or diverge from the fixed point at a rate determined by the eigenvalues. These concepts are illustrated by the behaviour shown in Fig. 1 of a simple model of the saccadic pulse generator. Examples of other applications of these techniques to neurophysiological systems are given by Kaplan and Glass (1995), Wilson (1999) and Dayan and Abbott (2001).

Modelling of normal and abnormal eye movements

A model of the behaviour of the normal oculomotor system can be readily constructed from standard dynamic components such as the slow/fast component illustrated in Fig. 1, which exhibits an alternation of a slowly varying and a rapidly varying behaviour, and the mutual inhibition component, which typically shows 'winner-takes-all' behaviour.

For example, consider a simple model of the saccadic system, which is shown schematically in Fig. 2. The burst of innervation is produced by a bilaterally symmetric slow/fast system in which the left and right burst cells are mutually inhibitory (Broomhead et al., 2000). The pause cells fire steadily when the

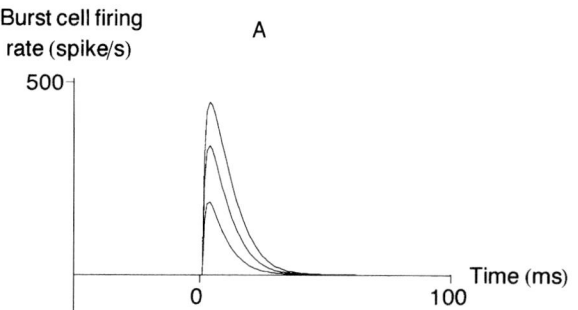
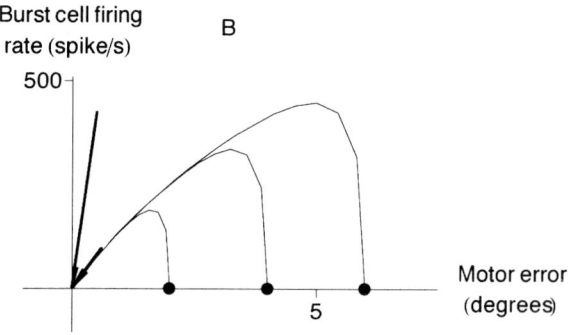

Fig. 1. A dynamical systems description of the saccadic burst generator. The behaviour of the system is described by a pair of differential equations: $\varepsilon db/dt = -b + f(m)$ and $dm/dt = -b$, where b is the burst cell firing rate in spikes per second, m is the difference between the current eye position and the target eye position, $f(m)$ is a sigmoidal function which describes how the burst cell firing rate depends on the motor error (Van Gisbergen et al., 1981) and ε is a small number. (A) Burst cell firing during 2°, 4° and 6° saccades, plotted as a function of time. (B) The corresponding trajectories in the two-dimensional phase space of the system are shown by continuous lines. The initial states are marked by dots, and in each case the trajectories end up at the origin, which is a stable fixed point of the system. The directions of the eigenvectors associated with the fixed point are marked by arrows, and the ratio of the lengths of the arrows is equal to the ratio of the eigenvalues. This ratio depends on the value of ε. With the value of 0.001 used in these simulations there is a larger eigenvalue, which forces the trajectory rapidly onto the curve defined by $f(m)$, and a smaller eigenvalue which constrains the trajectory to move along this curve towards the origin. By convention, the larger eigenvalue is known as the fast eigenvalue and the smaller eigenvalue is known as the slow eigenvalue.

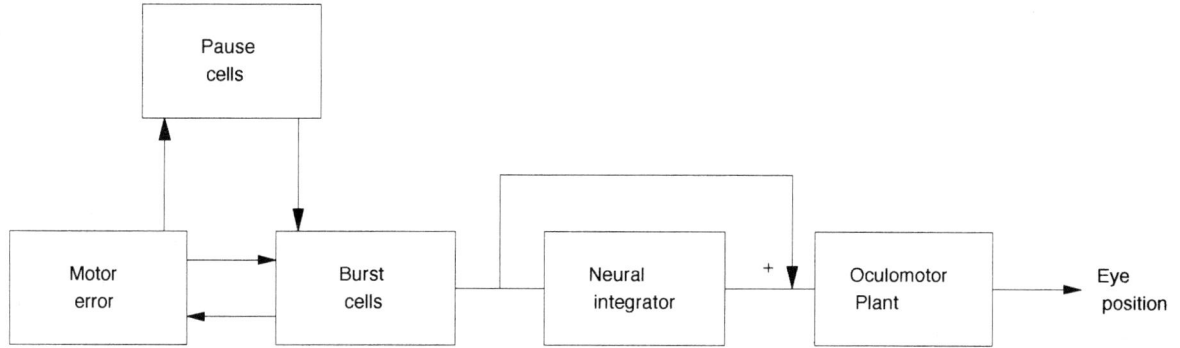

Fig. 2. Diagram of the flow of signals in a model of the saccadic eye movement system, which was used to produce the simulated eye movements shown in Fig. 3.

eye is fixating the target, and inhibit the burst cells. The behaviour of the neural integrator is described by a low pass filter with a time constant Tn, which is equal to 25 s in the normal oculomotor system, and the behaviour of the oculomotor plant is described by two low pass filters in series. The model can be easily extended to include a more sophisticated model of the plant which generates more realistic descriptions of the tensions in the muscles (Abadi et al., 2000). Appendix A gives the seven equations which describe the model, which can be solved numerically to simulate normal saccadic eye movements.

Quantitative modelling of the oculomotor system shows that a number of parameters, such as the integrator time constant and pause cell weighting, have to be set correctly for stable fixation. In our model the slow/fast ratio parameter ε determines how closely the burst cell firing follows the normal curve of burst cell firing against motor error. When this is slightly lower than normal dynamic overshoot occurs (Abadi et al., 2000), and when it is considerably lower than normal, macrosaccadic oscillations occur. The activity of the pause cells is modulated by both colliculus and frontal eye field fixation cells (Munoz, 2002), and one possibility is that the abnormal fixation patterns arise when the pause cells do not fire when the target image lies directly on the fovea. If the peak of the pause cell firing is offset from the foveal direction then different nystagmus waveforms are obtained, depending on the size of the offset. If the offset is 0.75° then an accelerating slow phase (typical of congenital nystagmus) is generated, whereas if the offset is 1°, then a decelerating slow phase (typical of manifest latent nystagmus) is produced. These predictions are illustrated in Fig. 3. The significance of these simulations is that they show that a wide range of saccadic disorders are inherent in the dynamics of the normal saccadic system.

Analysis of eye movement recordings

The changes in the state of the oculomotor system can be recovered from a recording of eye position using the method of delays (Takens, 1981; Sauer et al., 1991) in which a sliding window of n samples is moved through the data, generating a sequence of n-dimensional vectors. The dynamics of the oculomotor system and the dynamics of the delay vectors are closely related. Specifically, quantities which are independent of coordinates — for example, eigenvalues — can be computed using delay vectors and theory tells us that they will be the same as if we had calculated them using direct knowledge of the equations governing the behaviour of the oculomotor system.

The method of delays can be used to characterise the stability of fixation in oculomotor disorders such as congenital nystagmus, in which fixation is disrupted by predominantly jerky horizontal eye movements (Harris, 1997; Dell'Osso and Daroff, 1999; Gottlob, 2001). It is usually possible to identify a foveation period in each nystagmus cycle, during which the deviation and rate of deviation of the line of fixation from the target are least. We found that in congenital nystagmus the behaviour of the oculomotor system during the foveation period is linear, and that the stability of the fixed point can

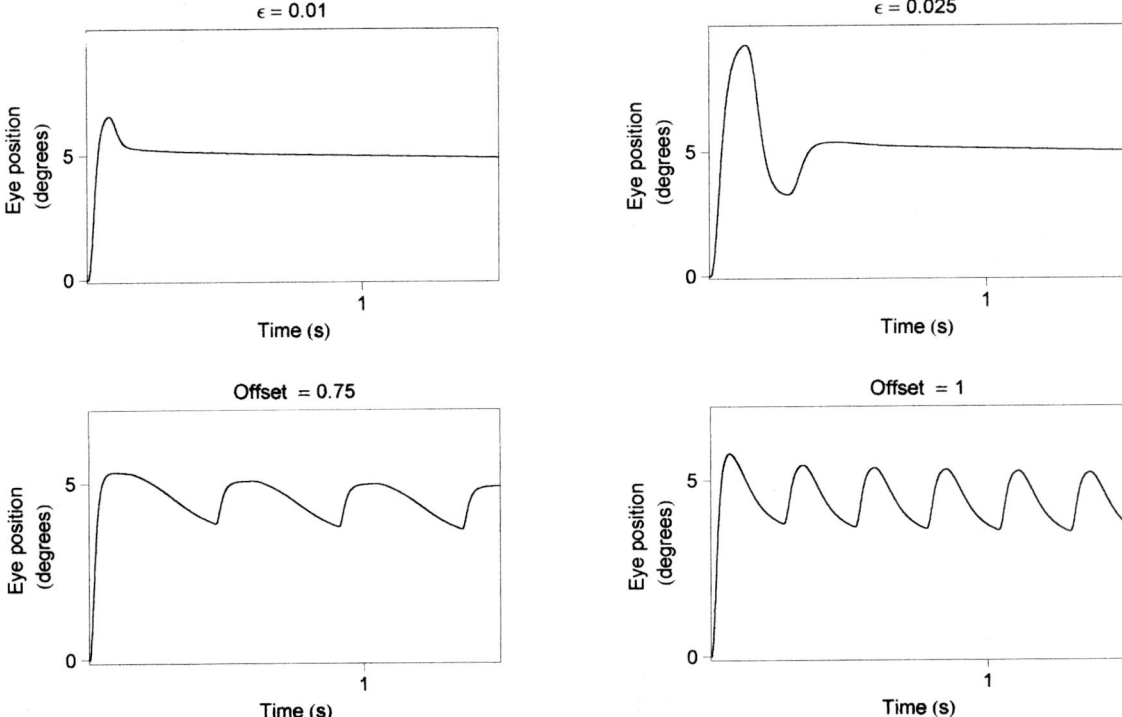

Fig. 3. Simulations of various types of eye movement disorders. The upper two figures show the saccadic dysmetria which results from changing the slow/fast ratio parameter ε in the model from its normal value of 0.005. The lower two figures show the nystagmus which results from moving the peak of the pause cell firing rate away from the center of the fovea. In the model this was simulated by adding an offset to the normal pause cell function of motor error.

be characterised by three eigenvalues; a small positive eigenvalue, which describes the unstable drift away from the fixation direction, a large negative eigenvalue, which characterises the stable corrective movement back to the point of fixation and a neutral eigenvalue, which implies that rather than a single fixed point there is a line of fixed points (Abadi et al., 1997).

Recent work in dynamical systems theory has shown that the behaviour of a deterministic system can be understood in terms of a limited number of fundamental cycles and so identification of such cycles, generally, unstable, low period periodic orbits, provides a method of characterising a deterministic system. The fixed point technique for finding periodic orbits in noisy experimental data involves taking a section through the phase space that cuts all the trajectories transversally, so that each cycle of the nystagmus waveform is represented by a single point, and then transforming the data so that it is concentrated on the periodic orbits, which can then be easily identified by sharp peaks in a histogram of the transformed data (So et al., 1997). This technique can be used to show that, despite the variability of the waveform, there is a single underlying oscillation in congenital nystagmus. Furthermore, the technique can be extended to identify the waveform shapes most closely associated with the periodic orbits, which any deterministic model of congenital nystagmus must be capable of reproducing. This procedure is illustrated in Fig. 4.

Discussion

The framework provided by nonlinear dynamics provides new insights into the oculomotor system at both the theoretical and experimental levels. Although any model can be implemented within a

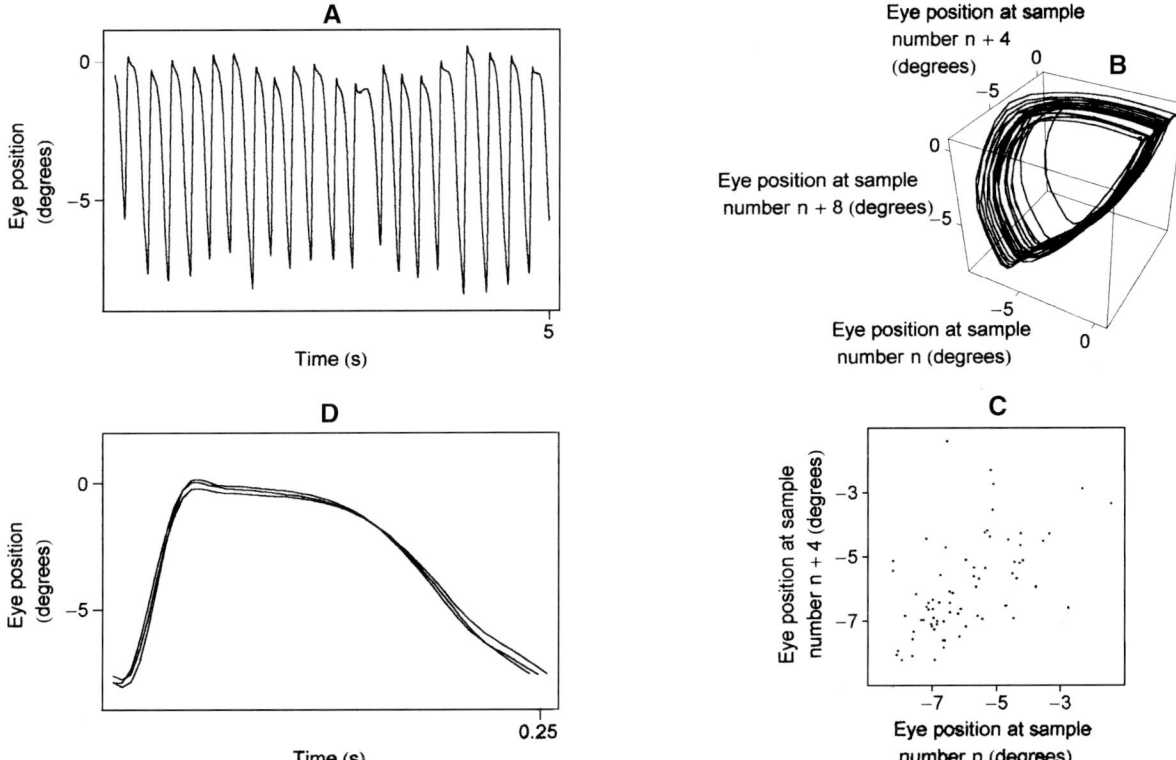

Fig. 4. Application of the method of delays to a recording of congenital nystagmus eye movements. (A) Eye movements, sampled at 5-ms intervals, measured from a subject with idiopathic congenital nystagmus during steady fixation of a stationary target. (B) Phase space trajectory for the waveform shown in A, reconstructed from the data by using the method of delays. The delay vectors were formed by taking three position measurements spaced four sampling intervals apart. A complete cycle of nystagmus, consisting of a slow phase followed by a quick phase, corresponds to clockwise circuit of the plot of trajectories. The fixed point in phase space associated with fixation of the target is located on the crease in the top right hand corner of the plot. The stability of this fixed point is characterized by three eigenvectors. The end of the quick phase of nystagmus approaches the crease along the direction of a stable eigenvector and the start of the slow phase leaves the crease along the direction of an unstable eigenvector. The third neutral eigenvector lies along the crease. (C) Section through the phase space obtained by calculating the points where the portions of the trajectories corresponding to the fast phases intersect with a level surface defined by fixing the position at sampling point $n+8$ to be equal to -4. Each point now represents a complete cycle of the nystagmus waveform. This section of the trajectories defines a map from one cycle of the nystagmus to the next and a fixed point of this map corresponds to periodic orbit of the nystagmus. Transformation of the data by technique of So et al. (1997) revealed a fixed point at $(-6, -6)$ in the section. (D) Cycles of nystagmus which are transformed most closely to the underlying periodic orbit.

powerful enough control system simulation package, this formulation will often lead to the inclusion of components which may not be necessary. For example, it is possible to produce a comprehensive model of the saccadic burst generator which does not require a resetable integrator, if the nonlinear interactions between the pause, long lead burst cells and short lead burst cells are taken into account (Gancarz and Grossberg, 1998). This point is especially important when explaining the origin of eye movement disorders, which may not involve structural damage to some putative component in a block diagram, but may arise from structurally intact components interacting outside their normal behavioural range.

At the experimental level, the techniques based on the method of delays provide new ways of characterising the behaviour of the oculomotor system. For instance, the underlying periodicity of congenital nystagmus is well established from spectral analysis of eye movement time series (Reccia et al., 1990), but a longstanding criticism of clinical classifications of congenital nystagmus waveforms is that they do not directly relate to the mechanism of the condition (Abadi and Dickinson, 1986). The advantage of the nonlinear dynamics approach is that it enables identification of the portions of the waveforms where the system is closely following a periodic orbit, which is useful clinically, because it enables one to isolate the characteristic waveforms from out of the range of oscillatory behaviour shown by any one subject.

Identification of the waveforms associated with periodic orbits within nystagmus recordings provides a challenge for models of the underlying ocular motor mechanism (Dell'Osso, 1967; Optican and Zee, 1984; Broomhead et al., 2000), which must be able to generate similar periodic orbits, if they are to be considered realistic. Several models have been produced which explain the different congenital nystagmus waveform shapes, but currently no model of the normal ocular motor system has been extended to produce a typical nystagmus time series. We believe it is important to have a framework which accommodates both normal and clinical eye movements, because our work with congenital nystagmus shows that many quantitative explanations of normal eye movements do not readily extend to clinical findings.

Conclusion

The nonlinear dynamics approach provides a framework both for characterising experimental data in terms of fixed points and periodic orbits, and for explaining a diverse range of abnormal eye movements in terms of established oculomotor physiology. The approach holds out the possibility of directly relating models to experimental data by comparing the fixed points and periodic orbits found experimentally with those predicted by models.

Appendix

Let p = eye position, v = eye velocity, n = neural integrator firing rate, l = left burster firing rate, r = right burster firing rate, m = motor error and a = pause cell firing rate. Then seven equations can be used to model the behaviour of the normal oculomotor system.

Muscle plant:
$$dp/dt = v \qquad (1)$$

$$dv/dt = -(1/T1 + 1/T2)v \\ + (-p + n + (T1 + T2)(r - l))/T1T2 \qquad (2)$$

Neural integrator:
$$dn/dt = -n/Tn + (r - l) \qquad (3)$$

Burst cells and motor error:
$$\varepsilon(dl/dt) = -l + f(-m - r - 2.5a) \qquad (4)$$
$$\varepsilon(dr/dt) = -r + f(m - l - 2.5a) \qquad (5)$$
$$dm/dt = -(r - l) \qquad (6)$$

Pause cells:
$$\varepsilon(da/dt) = -a + g(m) \qquad (7)$$

where $T1 = 0.15$ s, $T2 = 0.012$ s, $Tn = 25$ s and

$f(x) = $ If $x > 2$,
then $x = 840(x + 2)^2/(50 + (x + 2)^2)$
and $x = 0$ otherwise

$g(x) = 1 - (x + \alpha)^2/(1 + (x + \alpha)^2)$

In the normal system gain of the saccadic system $\varepsilon = 0.005$ and the offset of the peak of the pause cell firing from the foveal direction $\alpha = 0$. In the simulations, the initial conditions of all variables were set to zero, except for the motor error m, which was set to 5°.

References

Abadi, R.V. and Dickinson, C.M. (1986) Waveform characteristics in congenital nystagmus. *Doc. Ophthalmol.*, 64: 153–167.

Abadi, R.V., Broomhead, D.S., Clement, R.A., Whittle, J.P. and Worfolk, R. (1997) Dynamical systems analysis: a new method of analysing congenital nystagmus waveforms. *Exp. Brain Res.*, 117: 335–361.

Abadi, R.V., Scallan, C. and Clement, R.A. (2000) The characteristics of dynamic overshoots in square-wave jerks, and in congenital and manifest latent nystagmus. *Vis. Res.*, 40: 2813–2829.

Bahill, A.T., Clark, M.R. and Stark, L. (1975) The main sequence, a tool for studying human eye movements. *Math. Biosci.*, 24: 191–204.

Broomhead, D.S., Clement, R.A., Muldoon, M.R., Whittle, J.P., Scallan, C. and Abadi, R.V. (2000) Modelling of congenital nystagmus waveforms produced by saccadic system abnormalities. *Biol. Cyb.*, 82: 391–399.

Daroff, R.B. (1990) Eye Movement Disorders. Tape 4. Miscellaneous Ocular Oscillations, Professional Information Library. P.O. Box 795129, Dallas, TX 75379, USA.

Dayan, P. and Abbott, L.F. (2001) *Theoretical Neuroscience: Computational and Mathematical Modelling of Neural Systems*. MIT Press, Cambridge, MA.

Dell'Osso, L.F. (1967) A model for the horizontal tracking system of a subject with nystagmus. Visual and Vestibular responses. *20th Annu. Conference Engineering Med.*, USA.

Dell'Osso, L.F. and Daroff, R.B. (1999) Nystagmus and saccadic intrusions and oscillations. In: J.S. Glaser (Ed.), *Neuro-Ophthalmology*. Williams and Wilkinson Lippincott, Baltimore, MD, pp. 369–401.

Gancarz, G. and Grossberg, G. (1998) A neural model of the saccade generator in the reticular formation. *Neural Networks*, 11: 1159–1174.

Gottlob, I. (2001) Nystagmus. *Curr. Opin. Ophthalmol.*, 12: 378–383.

Harris, C.M. (1997) Nystagmus and eye movement disorders. In: D. Taylor (Ed.), *Paediatric Ophthalmology*. Blackwell Press, Oxford, pp. 869–896.

Kaplan, D. and Glass, L. (1995) *Understanding Nonlinear Dynamics*. Springer Verlag, New York.

Kelso, J.A.S. (1995) *Dynamic Patterns: The Self Organisation of Brain and Behaviour*. Bradford, Cambridge, MA.

Lebedev, S.L., Van Gelder, P. and Tsui, W.H. (1996) Square-root relations between main saccadic parameters. *Invest. Ophthalmol. Vis. Sci.*, 37: 2750–2758.

Leigh, R.J. and Zee, D.S. (1999) *The Neurology of Eye Movements*. Oxford University Press.

Munoz, D.P. (2002) Commentary: saccadic eye movements: overview of neural circuitry. In: J. Hyönä, D.P. Munoz, W. Heide and R. Radach (Eds.), *The Brain's Eye: Neurobiological and Clinical Aspects of Oculomotor Research. Progress in Brain Research*, Vol. 140. Elsevier, Amsterdam, pp. 89–96.

Optican, L.M. and Zee, D.S. (1984) A hypothetical explanation of congenital nystagmus. *Biol. Cyb.*, 50: 119–134.

Reccia, R., Roberti, G. and Russo, P. (1990) Computer analysis of ENG spectral features from patients with congenital nystagmus. *J. Biomed. Eng.*, 12: 39–45.

Sauer, T., Yorkem, J.A. and Casdagli, M. (1991) Embedology. *J. Stat. Phys.*, 65: 579–616.

So, P., Ott, E., Sauer, T., Gluckman, B.J., Grebogi, C. and Schiff, S.J. (1997) Extracting unstable periodic orbits from chaotic time series data. *Phys. Rev. E*, 55: 5398–5417.

Takens, F. (1981) Detecting strange attractors in turbulence. In: D.A. Rand and L.S. Young (Eds.), *Lecture Notes in Mathematics 898 'Dynamical Systems and Turbulence'*. Springer Verlag, Berlin, pp. 366–381.

Van Gisbergen, J.A.M., Robinson, D.A. and Gielen, S. (1981) A quantitative analysis of generation of saccadic eye movements by burst neurons. *J. Neurophysiol.*, 45: 417–442.

Wilson, H.R. (1999) *Spikes, Decisions and Actions*. Oxford University Press, New York.

CHAPTER 34

Commentary: Eye movement research with clinical populations

John A. Sweeney [1,*], Deborah Levy [2] and Margret S.H. Harris [1]

[1] *Center for Cognitive Medicine, Departments of Psychiatry, Neurology and Psychology, University of Illinois at Chicago, Chicago, IL, USA*
[2] *Department of Psychiatry, Harvard University, Boston, MA, USA*

Abstract: The preceding set of chapters span the disciplines of neurology and psychiatry, and provide a diverse introduction to clinical eye movement research. They illustrate how oculomotor paradigms can be used to learn about acute and chronic perturbations in brain function, disturbances in brain development, disturbances in sensorimotor as well as cognitive systems, and the effects of therapeutic and illicit drugs on brain function. This commentary discusses these contributions, provides an overview of broad methodological issues involved in applying eye movement studies to psychiatric populations using the antisaccade task as an exemplar, and considers the potential of collaborations between eye movement and brain imaging researchers to advance understanding of clinical eye movement abnormalities and of what they reveal about the organization of the oculomotor system.

Introduction

Recent decades have seen far reaching advances in the understanding and treatment of brain disorders. A significant proportion of this progress stems from multidisciplinary collaboration, and from the utilization of novel, previously unavailable approaches for investigating brain structure and function. New methodological approaches for studying the brain 'in vivo' have included magnetic resonance imaging (MRI), positron emission tomography (PET) and single photon emitted computed tomography (SPECT) brain imaging methodologies that localize where brain activity occurs with high spatial resolution, high density electro-encephalography (EEG) and magneto-encephalography (MEG) that monitor when brain activity occurs with high temporal resolution, and the development of vastly improved behavioral paradigms to probe brain function developed through cognitive neuroscience. Together, these advances have dramatically altered and improved the clinical and research evaluation of brain anatomy, neurochemistry, and physiology.

In parallel with these methodological advances, and at times using these methods, considerable research has been conducted to evaluate brain function in clinical disorders investigating abnormalities in eye movement control. Investigators have used oculomotor paradigms to localize brain pathology, to identify familial endophenotypes for genetically transmitted disorders, to track disease progression and treatment effects, to assist in the differential diagnosis of clinically similar disorders, and to model failures in brain maturation.

There are many reasons why clinical investigators have relied on oculomotor paradigms to investigate brain disorders. Most, if not all, are obvious to most

---

*Correspondence to: J.A. Sweeney, Center for Cognitive Medicine, Department of Psychiatry, MC 913, 912 S. Wood St., The Neuropsychiatric Institute, University of Illinois at Chicago, Chicago, IL 60612, USA. Tel.: +1-312-413-9205; Fax: +1-312-413-8837; E-mail: jsweeney@psych.uic.edu

neurologists and clinical eye movement researchers, but they merit review to provide an intellectual context for other readers.

First, there is a long tradition of utilizing clinical assessments of eye movements in standard bedside neurological examinations. Thus, the analysis of eye movement activity to learn about brain function is a natural strategy for clinicians interested in brain disorders (Leigh and Zee, 1999). As clinical psychologists and psychiatrists became interested in cortical dysfunctions in severe mental illnesses such as schizophrenia, they began to utilize cognitively demanding oculomotor paradigms to investigate neurophysiological abnormalities of neocortical function. Similar efforts to use eye movement paradigms to investigate effects of neocortical tumors, strokes and lobectomies were pursued by neurologists and cognitive psychologists (Pierrot-Deseilligny et al., 1995; Heide and Kömpf, 1998; Walker et al., 1998).

Second, neurophysiologists recording activity from single neurons in behaving non-human primates began to monitor changes of neuronal activity in neocortex and basal ganglia while monkeys performed oculomotor paradigms, providing critical knowledge about multiple brain regions involved in the control of visual attention and eye movements (Bruce and Goldberg, 1985; Hikosaka, 1989; Munoz and Wurtz, 1992; Colby et al., 1996; Schall and Bichot, 1998). This extended prior unit recording work that primarily focused on brainstem and cerebellum. Notable in this regard have been efforts to investigate the role of prefrontal cortex in holding representations of spatial location information and plans for eye movements 'on-line' over time (Goldman-Rakic, 1987; Joseph and Barone, 1987). In particular, work by Patricia Goldman-Rakic and colleagues has helped establish the neurophysiology of spatial working memory systems in the primate brain relying heavily on eye movement paradigms, including an extensive delineation of the role of a number of neurotransmitters in its normal function (Sawaguchi and Goldman-Rakic, 1994; Rao et al., 2000).

Third, functional brain imaging studies with healthy human subjects have shown a general homology of function between human and non-human primates in the control of eye movement activity, establishing an important bridge for taking knowledge from the monkey laboratory to the clinic (Luna and Sweeney, 1999). Functional neuroimaging, by monitoring brain activity during specific cognitive tasks, also provides a set of techniques for directly investigating and delineating neurophysiological abnormalities in brain disorders. However, such efforts require the selection of good behavioral paradigms to probe regional brain function. For this purpose, eye movement tasks have several ideal characteristics. They robustly elicit brain activation and permit the probing of multiple widely distributed brain regions simultaneously. Patients can perform simple eye movement tasks adequately even with significant compromise to their cognitive function. There is also a large body of literature demonstrating eye movement impairments in many clinical disorders that can guide the selection of specific paradigms useful for studying brain function in particular patient populations of interest.

Fourth, human studies have begun to delineate developmental profiles of the control of eye movements throughout the life span. The ability to voluntarily control eye movement activity continues in significant ways through childhood into late adolescence. In addition to being useful for monitoring disturbances in the maturation of brain systems needed for eye movement control in pediatric patients, other investigators have documented a gradual reduction in performance of eye movement tasks in late life that is massively accelerated in dementing conditions (Fischer et al., 1997; Munoz et al., 1999; Sweeney et al., 2001).

Relying on the simultaneous parallel advances in these interrelated lines of research, clinicians began to utilize eye movement paradigms to investigate the pathophysiology and sequelae of a variety of neurological and psychiatric disorders. Advances were also made in using eye movement monitoring to advance understanding of the effects of pharmacotherapy on brain function, and to establish oculomotor endophenotypes for familial/genetic disorders.

In the chapters comprising this section of the text, investigators report summaries of their findings in studies using eye movement tasks to investigate brain disorders. The variety of clinical populations represented in this effort reflects the rapid and diverse translation of eye movement research into the clinical arena. The aim of this commentary is to discuss those contributions, to consider various broad strategic issues related to conducting clinical eye movement research especially as it pertains to psychiatry, and to point to what will likely be new directions for work in this area.

Neurological disorders

Historically, most clinical investigations of eye movement abnormalities have been conducted with neurological disorders. Most early work was done with patients presenting with brainstem or cerebellar pathology. But, paralleling the expansion of basic eye movement research into investigations of neocortical function, there has been an increasing effort to use eye movement studies to clarify important aspects of disorders of neocortex and the basal ganglia. This increasingly diverse focus is reflected in the chapters included in this section devoted to neurological disorders.

The chapter by Sprenger et al. describes an eye movement study conducted to investigate the phenomenon of visual neglect (Sprenger et al., 2002, this volume). Visual hemineglect is a dramatic clinical phenomenon involving inattention to one hemifield, usually the left hemifield after damage to the right/contralateral hemisphere. The investigation by Sprenger and colleagues is important, because prior studies have not clarified how disturbances in visual search and other cognitive/perceptual deficits may be related to this abnormality. Their study shows that in addition to unilateral neglect, affected patients also demonstrate a disruption of visual orienting throughout visual displays when the neglect is caused by right parietal damage, a general reduction in the efficiency of serial visual search, and impairments in spatial working memory in the ipsilateral hemifield. These findings are intriguing because they provide a much richer and more comprehensive understanding of the complexity of perceptual and cognitive deficits associated with the clinical presentation of visual neglect. Their findings also highlight the need for future studies investigating the broader perceptual competence of patients presenting with neglect, and of how specific lower-level cognitive deficits may combine to lead to their clinically observed perceptual disturbances.

MacAskill et al. (2002, this volume) provide an excellent review of mechanisms of neuronal and behavioral plasticity in the control of saccadic eye movements. These investigators review the phenomenon of saccade adaptation, by which subjects learn to alter the metrics of saccades when past experience shows that saccades have a consistent postsaccadic error. The clinical importance of this phenomenon is evident when patients need to change the neural commands for saccades when eye muscle atrophy or neurological disease cause a consistent directional error in final eye position in saccadic eye movements. The oculomotor vermis in the cerebellum is believed to be especially important for this process. Further work with this phenomenon is clinically important because this task is useful for separating eye movement problems related to cerebellar dysfunction from disorders involving other brain regions. It is also essential as part of broader efforts to learn about basic mechanisms of neuronal plasticity in the cerebellum.

In their contribution, Heitger et al. (2002, this volume) report findings from eye movement studies conducted following closed head injury. Closed head injuries are a common cause of emergency medical care, and are known to have persistent adverse cognitive consequences in a considerable number of individuals. Head injuries more often have clinical significance when associated with a loss of consciousness, and when followed by post-traumatic amnesia and neurological signs and symptoms. Diffuse axonal damage caused by shearing forces on the brain at the time of the head trauma is believed to account for many persistent neurobehavioral deficits. In their chapter on this topic, Heitger and colleagues point out that because of the multiple functionally integrated brain regions involved in eye movement control and their wide spatial distribution throughout the brain, oculomotor control may be especially vulnerable to such trauma.

Few studies have been conducted to determine whether eye movement function is altered after closed head injury. Thus, the chapter by Heitger et al. reporting abnormal execution of memory-guided saccade sequences in patients within two days of head trauma is a novel effort to bring quantitative eye movement studies into the clinic. Importantly, with a demanding eye movement paradigm and quantitative measurements, these investigators were able to document abnormalities when bedside examination of eye movement activity did not reveal deficits. Further work is needed to more broadly characterize the types and prevalence of oculomotor deficits that occur in this patient group. It also will be important to determine whether these deficits are only acute effects seen in the period immediately after the head trauma, or whether they become chronic impairments. If the latter is the case, it will be useful to further validate the findings with additional oculomotor tests, as they may be beneficial for monitoring effects of cognitive rehabilitation and pharmacological interventions with these patients.

The chapter by Crawford and colleagues represents a far-reaching theoretical effort to establish the importance of inhibitory cortical systems for general adaptive behavior, and the independence of these processes from working memory operations (Crawford et al., 2002, this volume). The use of antisaccade paradigms to examine voluntary inhibition capacities, and the oculomotor delayed response paradigm to investigate spatial working memory, provide an opportunity to use well established paradigms for investigating the association and dissociation of these two key executive mental operations. These investigators utilized clinical eye movement data from schizophrenia and Parkinson's disease, and results of studies demonstrating a differential impact of a typical antipsychotic medication and a benzodiazepine on working memory and response inhibition, to begin to establish a functional independence of inhibitory capacities from working memory processes. As the authors point out, the importance of the capacity to voluntarily inhibit context-inappropriate responses is a key requirement for adaptive behavior in complex environments. It is often most adaptive to attend and respond to information based on its relevance for the context of the moment rather than its immediate perceptual salience. The mechanisms through which such choices are implemented remain poorly understood. Inhibitory processes in attention and behavior urgently need more careful investigation, more sophisticated theoretical delineation, and better differentiated research methodologies to facilitate research in this area. The work reported by Crawford and colleagues provides several advances along these lines.

Neuropsychiatric disorders

Between the fields of psychiatry and neurology are a group of border-zone disorders cared for by both disciplines. Such disorders often have received especially modest research attention, and their pathophysiological mechanisms often remain poorly characterized. In this context, eye movement studies may be able to provide useful non-invasive approaches for gaining a deeper understanding about regional brain dysfunction in these disorders.

Munoz and colleagues conducted a thorough investigation of prosaccades, antisaccades and delayed saccades in a group of individuals with Tourette's syndrome (Munoz et al., 2002, this volume). The results indicate an interesting dissociation of inhibitory failures rarely seen in other disorders. While the Tourette's patients were able to suppress saccades to peripheral targets on an antisaccade task, they had difficulty delaying saccades to remembered target locations. This interesting set of findings suggests a difficulty suppressing the enactment of internally generated motor plans rather than a difficulty suppressing responses to sensory cues. These findings provide an excellent demonstration of the potential for using well-chosen oculomotor paradigms to clarify distinctive cognitive and neurophysiological disturbances in brain disorders. Further studies with unmedicated patients, studies of treatment effects on this pattern of deficit, studies relating oculomotor deficits to clinical severity of the illness, and studies linking this inhibitory disturbance to other cognitive manifestations of a difficulty inhibiting action are needed to establish the full range of implications of this potentially very important set of observations.

Developmental studies

The chapter by Newsham and Knox constitutes an important contribution to this series of papers for several reasons. First, the data provide documentation for the potential of non-invasive oculomotor studies to identify cognitive deficits in individuals born prematurely with low birth weight. Second, more generally, the data highlight the potential of eye movement studies to investigate neurodevelopmental difficulties (Newsham and Knox, 2002, this volume).

As with most successful studies of new clinical populations, one feels a sense of opportunity for the potential to help diagnose patients and understand clinical problems using new diagnostic procedures such as these eye movement paradigms. But, at the same time, many questions are raised about the implications of the study. First, one wonders about the immediate clinical relevance of the observed impairments in eye movement control in these patients. Further studies are needed to establish the linkage of these oculomotor findings to the behavioral and academic problems that often bring this subject population to clinical attention in childhood. For example, studies are necessary to directly clarify the functional significance of the oculomotor abnormalities to reading and other academic problems observed in these individuals, and perhaps to conduct attentional problems seen in this population as well. Second, additional research is needed to more thoroughly assess eye movement systems to clarify the full range of oculomotor deficits associated with this condition. For example, studies using a larger range of target step amplitudes for saccade tasks are needed to fully evaluate the integrity of the main sequence for saccadic eye movements.

The developmental implications of the observed oculomotor abnormalities also need additional delineation. Children continue to show improvement in eye movement abilities through mid-adolescence and early adulthood. Some clinical populations show delayed development, gradually catching up to healthy subjects in task performance, while others show developmental failures with gradually increasing disparity from healthy subjects through adolescence. While it was a sound experimental strategy to begin investigations in this area with a narrowly defined age group (9 year olds), examining low birth weight children across the age span, especially longitudinally, could provide additional useful information regarding the functional impact of low birth weight on brain maturation and cognitive development.

Another relatively novel application of eye movement research related to developmental disturbances is provided in the chapter by Huestegge and colleagues reporting long-term adverse effects of substance abuse (Huestegge et al., 2002, this volume). There is a large body of literature using eye movement measurements to monitor and document acute effects of drug treatment. This is especially the case for benzodiazepines and barbiturates, which have sedative properties and slow the velocity and increase the latency and duration of saccades. In contrast, the long-term effects of drug treatments have received little systematic attention.

One example where more information is needed about the long-term effects of CNS-active substances pertains to the potential long-term consequences of drug abuse on brain function. Drug abuse is well known to be an international epidemic, and documentation of its adverse effects is important for educational efforts to reduce illicit drug abuse, especially in children and adolescents. Knowledge about the specific enduring negative effects of drug abuse is also important for educational and occupational planning for those who have abused drugs regularly, and to provide better understanding of persistent adverse cognitive effects of different types of drug abuse.

The chapter by Huestegge and colleagues reports findings documenting that cannabis abuse causes cognitive deficits in subjects who began their pattern of abuse in mid-adolescence, and adds to the growing body of literature documenting persistent adverse consequences resulting from drug abuse. Their finding that persistent cognitive problems occur more prominently in those who begin their drug abuse prior to age 17 years suggests that drug abuse may interfere with normal brain maturation in a way that causes enduring adverse cognitive deficits measurable with the visual search task used by the investigators. Importantly, monitoring eye movement activity during their complex scanning task revealed problems in attentional control and use of higher-order executive search strategies rather than in motor execution of eye movements per se.

Mathematical modeling of oculomotor deficits

Because the eye movement system behaves in a remarkably consistent manner over time, mathematical models of eye movement activity have been developed to characterize the normal operation of eye movement control systems. Such approaches may be useful for better understanding abnormalities of eye movement control seen in clinical populations. The chapter by Clement and colleagues discusses an overall mathematical approach from non-linear systems theory for developing such models (Clement et al., 2002, this volume). Importantly, the paper addresses issues related to the neocortical control of eye movement. Most mathematical models of eye movement control were developed to explain brainstem and cerebellar function. Models will be needed to formally understand interactions of neocortex with the superior colliculus as they pertain to eye movement control in order to fully understand the origins of disturbances in eye movement control in brain disorders.

Eye movement research in psychiatry

The role of eye movement research has a somewhat different role to play in the investigation of psychiatric and neurological disorders. Rather than serving the purpose of delineating effects of relatively well characterized brain pathology in neurology research, in psychiatric research, eye movement studies are needed to provide objective quantitative documentation about the nature of poorly understood brain dysfunctions.

While several eye movement tasks have been used in studies of psychiatric disorders, the most commonly employed one is certainly visual pursuit tracking (Holzman, 2000). Pursuit tracking abnormalities in schizophrenic patients were first reported by Diefendorf and Dodge (1908), in what was one of the first studies in which measurements of eye movements were obtained to study abnormalities in cognitive and brain function in a clinical condition. Philip Holzman 'rediscovered' this deficit in a series of studies reported in the mid-1970s (Holzman et al., 1973, 1974). Insightfully, he not only demonstrated the high prevalence of this deficit and its relative specificity for schizophrenia, but also recruited unaffected family members of schizophrenic patients and demonstrated that they commonly demonstrated this deficit as well. Various aspects of this abnormality have been studied extensively in several laboratories since that time (Iacono and Koenig, 1983; Sweeney et al., 1994; Trillenberg et al., 1998; Thaker et al., 1999), and reviews of this literature are available (Clementz and Sweeney, 1990; Levy and Holzman, 1997).

Psychiatric investigators gradually refined their measurement approaches to characterize the pursuit deficit from early qualitative ratings to a quantitative evaluation of pursuit and saccadic eye movements during visual tracking. Eye tracking deficits in disorders other than schizophrenia including affective disorders and obsessive–compulsive disorders have been studied (Iacono and Koenig, 1983; Sweeney et al., 1992, 1994), as have the concordance of tracking deficits in twin samples (Holzman et al., 1980; Iacono, 1982) and the prevalence of pursuit impairment in larger samples of families with a schizophrenic proband (Clementz et al., 1990; Thaker et al., 1998). Genetic linkage to the tracking deficit was established in one study (Arolt et al., 1995), and several efforts to replicate and extend that observation are underway.

Since then, oculomotor research with psychiatric disorders has used eye movement paradigms to investigate other sensorimotor systems. Several groups have investigated the integrity of visually guided saccades (Iacono et al., 1981) and the adverse effects of certain pharmacological treatments for schizophrenia on saccade metrics (Sweeney et al., 1997).

Other investigators have moved to employ more complex eye movement paradigms to investigate neocortically mediated deficits. Progress in this work has benefited from investigations of the neural substrate of working memory and other cognitive functions in behaving non-human primates (Joseph and Barone, 1987; Funahashi et al., 1989), and studies using similar tasks to investigate the effects of focal lesions related to stroke and tumors in clinical populations (Pierrot-Deseilligny et al., 1997). One paradigm used in these research protocols has been the oculomotor delayed response task (also called the memory-guided saccade task). It has been used to investigate spatial working memory deficits in several psychiatric illnesses (Park and Holzman, 1992; Sweeney et al., 1998).

A second task used to investigate cognitive deficits in psychiatric illnesses is the antisaccade task. As discussed in the chapters by Munoz et al. and by Crawford et al., this task requires the subject to inhibit a reflexive saccade to a novel peripheral stimulus, and instead to make a voluntary saccade to the mirror image location at which no target is visible. Failure to inhibit reflexive saccades (looking toward rather than away from the peripheral target as instructed) is defined as a prosaccade error. Originally developed by Hallett (1978) to explore the metrics of non-visually guided saccades, the antisaccade task was introduced as a clinical research tool by Guitton et al. (1985), who used this paradigm to probe the frontal cortical circuitry subserving both the inhibition of reflexive saccades and the generation of voluntary saccades. An excellent overview of basic and clinical antisaccade studies can be found in Everling and Fischer (1998). We will discuss this task below in more detail in order to illustrate general themes and research strategies involved in bringing such cognitive oculomotor tasks into the psychiatric clinic.

At face value, the antisaccade task provides an oculomotor counterpart to other neurobehavioral indices of disinhibition encountered in patients with frontal lobe pathology in that correct performance requires inhibition of reflexive responses. In this context, failures to inhibit prosaccades would seem to implicate compromised control over reflexive but context-inappropriate responding. Guitton et al. (1985) reported that patients with frontal lobe lesions showed profound impairments in performing the antisaccade task. In contrast, patients with temporal lobe lesions did not differ from a healthy control group, suggesting some degree of specificity for the task in tapping dorsolateral prefrontal dysfunction. Although Guitton et al. (1985) described a more complex pattern of performance deficits in patients with frontal lobe lesions than the mere failure to inhibit reflexive saccades on a high proportion of trials administered, error rate is the measure of performance that has been most widely adopted in clinical studies.

Performance on the antisaccade task was subsequently studied in patients with a wide variety of neurological disorders. Not only patients with lesions in various regions of frontal cortex (Pierrot-Deseilligny et al., 1991; Fukushima et al., 1994), but also patients with Huntington's disease (Leigh et al., 1983; Lasker et al., 1988; Tian et al., 1991), progressive supranuclear palsy (Pierrot-Deseilligny et al., 1989), and Parkinson's disease (Kitagawa et al., 1994; Crevits and De Ridder, 1997; Briand et al., 1999; but for contradictory results see Lueck et al., 1990; Fukushima et al., 1994; Vidailhet et al., 1994) have been shown to demonstrate increased error rates on this task relative to healthy individuals. It should be noted in this regard that the poor performance of some patients with basal ganglia disease extends the potential usefulness of the antisaccade task to serve as a probe of frontal–striatal circuitry rather than solely of the intrinsic integrity of prefrontal cortex. Imaging studies in healthy individuals performing this task are consistent with the involvement of both frontal and striatal regions, but as part of a much more widely distributed network that subserves voluntary eye movements and spatial attention (Paus et al., 1993; O'Driscoll et al., 1995; Sweeney et al., 1996; Doricchi et al., 1997; Luna et al., 2001).

Performance on the antisaccade task has been extensively studied in psychiatric patient populations, particularly in schizophrenia patients. Every study of schizophrenia patients of which we are aware has reported that individuals affected by this illness make significantly more reflexive saccade errors than do non-psychiatric controls (Fukushima et al., 1988, 1990a,b, 1994; Thaker et al., 1989; Rosse et al., 1993; Clementz et al., 1994; Matsue et al., 1994; Crawford et al., 1995b, 1998; Sereno and Holzman, 1995; Allen et al., 1996; Tien et al., 1996; Katsanis et al., 1997; McDowell and Clementz, 1997; Hutton et al., 1998, 2002; Karoumi et al., 1998, 2001; Levy et al., 1998; Maruff et al., 1998; Ross et al., 1998; McDowell et al., 1999; Muller et al., 1999; Curtis et al., 2001a; Gooding and Tallent, 2001; Brownstein et al., 2002). The consistency of this finding is all the more remarkable, because it transcends the specific antisaccade paradigms used (standard, gap and overlap), variations in experimental procedures across studies (e.g. number of trials, number of peripheral target eccentricities, timing parameters) and clinical differences in the patient samples (acutely psychotic, remitted, first-episode, and chronically ill). Treatment with antipsychotic medication does not seem to be responsible for this deficit in that error rates are significantly elevated in chronically unmedicated (Crawford et al., 1995b) and chronically medicated schizophrenics (Crawford et al., 1995a), as well as in neuroleptic-naïve first-episode schizophrenics (Hutton et al., 1998; Muller et al., 1999). Moreover, error rate is generally not significantly related to daily dose of antipsychotic medication (Fukushima et al., 1990b; Clementz et al., 1994; Curtis et al., 2001a; Gooding and Tallent, 2001; Brownstein et al., 2002; but see Karoumi et al., 2001). Other features of performance on the antisaccade tasks that are of interest, such as latency of correct antisaccades, have not been as consistent in distinguishing schizophrenia patients from healthy controls. Some investigators reported that antisaccade latency is slowed in schizophrenic patients relative to healthy controls (Thaker et al., 1989; Fukushima et al., 1990a,b, 1994; Matsue et al., 1994; McDowell and Clementz, 1997; Crawford et al., 1998; Hutton et al., 1998; Karoumi et al., 1998, 2001; Maruff et al., 1998; Brownstein et al., 2002), and others found no difference in latency between these two groups (Clementz et al., 1994; Crawford et al., 1995b; Katsanis et al., 1997; McDowell and Clementz, 1997; Hutton et al., 1998; Levy et al., 1998).

Poor performance on the antisaccade task has not been as consistently associated with any other psychiatric disorder. Conflicting findings have been reported for patients with bipolar disorder (Fukushima et al., 1990b; Clementz et al., 1994; Crawford et al., 1995b; Sereno and Holzman, 1995; Tien et al., 1996; Katsanis et al., 1997; McDowell and Clementz, 1997; Curtis et al., 2001a; Gooding and Tallent, 2001), major depression (Fukushima et al., 1990b; Clementz et al., 1994; Katsanis et al., 1997; Sweeney et al., 1998; Curtis et al., 2001a), obsessive–compulsive disorder (Tien et al., 1992; McDowell and Clementz, 1997; Rosenberg et al., 1997), and attention-deficit hyperactivity disorder (Rothlind et al., 1991; Aman et al., 1998; Munoz et al., 1999). The one comparison of patients with 'anxiety neurosis' and healthy controls yielded no difference in error rate (Crawford et al., 1995b). Some of the issues relevant to the variability in findings in bipolar disorder and major depression, for which the most data are available, are discussed below. This literature raises the important issue of establishing diagnostic specificity for oculomotor deficits in psychiatric research. Unlike the case of many neurologic disorders in which pathophysiologic models of disease processes are established, psychiatric investigators are still working to develop valid neurobiological models of mental disorders. It therefore becomes crucial to establish that a pattern of neurobehavioral deficits observed in a disorder of interest is specific to that disorder, and is not, for example, a secondary result of general social and biological stresses associated with having a major psychiatric illness.

The elevated error rates of bipolar patients compared with healthy individuals in some studies (Sereno and Holzman, 1995; Tien et al., 1996; Katsanis et al., 1997; McDowell and Clementz, 1997; Curtis et al., 2001a; Gooding and Tallent, 2001) suggests that compromised control over inhibitory processes may be characteristic of this disorder as well. This finding would fit with the overly energetic impulsive pattern of behavior that is a cardinal clinical feature of mania. In other studies, however, no group difference in error rate was observed (Fukushima et al., 1990b; Clementz et al., 1994; Crawford et al., 1995b). Two features of sample composition complicate the attempt to reconcile these conflicting findings: in some studies, bipolar patients were part of larger groups of affective disorder and/or non-schizophrenic patients (Fukushima et al., 1990b; Clementz et al., 1994; Sereno and Holzman, 1995) and clinical state varied within the bipolar group or the larger group of affective disorder patients (Fukushima et al., 1990a; Sereno and Holzman, 1995; Tien et al., 1996). A somewhat clearer but still incomplete understanding of the variability in findings emerges if one considers only those studies in which bipolar patients constituted an independent sample and were in a uniform clinical state (Crawford et al., 1995b; Katsanis et al., 1997; McDowell and Clementz, 1997; Curtis et al., 2001a; Gooding and Tallent, 2001). Poor performance in bipolar patients does not seem to be strictly a function of clinical state, because both currently psychotic bipolar patients (Katsanis et al., 1997; Curtis et al., 2001a) and non-acutely ill bipolar patients (McDowell and Clementz, 1997; Gooding and Tallent, 2001) have been demonstrated to show elevated error rates compared with healthy individuals. On the other hand, the partially remitted bipolar patients in the study of Crawford et al. (1995b) did not make significantly more errors than controls. In addition, the poorer performance of bipolar patients in the McDowell and Clementz (1997) study, most of whom had previously been psychotic, seemed to be a function of a subgroup (three of their 15 patients) whose high error rates were somewhat uncharacteristic of the rest of the sample. No study, however, has reported normal antisaccade performance in acutely psychotic bipolar patients.

A more definitive resolution of the effects of clinical state on antisaccade performance in bipolar patients awaits longitudinal data on patients who are tested during a period of acute psychosis and during remission. Should such data be forthcoming, they would be valuable for several reasons. First, the data could show that the persistent trait-like performance deficits on the antisaccade task associated with schizophrenia are more clinically state-dependent in bipolar disorder, and therefore result from a different type of disease process. Second, they could provide an important clinical tool for documenting treatment effects and change of illness-state in this serious mental illness. Longitudinal studies tracking patients through periods of acute treatment, especially if they are medication free prior to baseline testing, are needed to provide important information about the impact of acute exacerbation of illness and pharmacological treatments on the functional integrity of frontostriatal circuits in major mental disorders. Eye movement tasks, by virtue of providing a non-invasive quantitative tool for investigating these brain systems, may prove especially valuable in this regard.

Although most studies have reported that patients with major depression do not show elevated error rates on antisaccade tasks compared with healthy subjects (Fukushima et al., 1990b; Clementz et al., 1994; Katsanis et al., 1997; Curtis et al., 2001a), such a conclusion must be tempered by two considerations. First, all of the negative results were obtained in studies that used a single peripheral eccentricity. In the one study that used multiple eccentricities, error rate was increased in patients with major depression, but only for more eccentric (and not for less eccentric) targets (Sweeney et al., 1998). Thus, it is possible that the use of a single predictable target eccentricity masked the presence of an abnormality that would have been evident with a different experimental design.

Paradigm variations (e.g. gap, standard and overlap), in addition to number of eccentricities of possible target locations within a specific paradigm, also affect error rate and latency of correct antisaccades (Fischer and Weber, 1992, 1997; McDowell and Clementz, 1997). One can see such effects when contrasting the results of an overlap condition using two eccentricities in relatives of schizophrenia patients (McDowell et al., 1999) with the results when one eccentricity is used (Curtis et al., 2001b).

The effects of these methodological aspects of the antisaccade testing procedure and their relation to clinical impairment in different disorders need to be more fully explored before definitive conclusions about antisaccade task performance in major depression — and perhaps other disorders — can be made. This reflects an important issue for clinical research. How patterns of impairment in spatial attention, motor control and the voluntary regulation of behavior characterizing different brain disorders might interact with different task manipulations on the antisaccade tasks requires more exploration. As illustrated in the chapter by Munoz and colleagues, analyzing and specifying the precise task conditions that reveal reduced inhibitory capacity can provide important insights into specific brain abnormalities in neuropsychiatric disorders.

Second, in the studies reporting negative results, the sample sizes of groups of patients with major depression were consistently smaller than those of the psychiatric patients who did show elevated error rates in the same studies (with the exception of Curtis et al. (2001a)). In one study, patients with major depression were part of a group of non-schizophrenic patients (Clementz et al., 1994), making it difficult to separate their performance from that of the group as a whole, which was overall also comparatively small. In contrast, the one study that did find increased errors on an antisaccade task in patients with major depression had the largest sample of patients with major depression (Sweeney et al., 1998). This raises the possibility that a milder deficit in depressed patients performing the antisaccade task might only be detected with larger samples, or possibly with relatively severely ill patients as were recruited by Sweeney and colleagues. Whether the varying results in studies with depressed patients reflect reduced power to detect abnormal performance secondary to small samples, differences in experimental methods, or clinical state-related factors remain unresolved issues.

The consistent finding of increased antisaccade errors in schizophrenia patients raised the possibility that similar deficits in performance may also occur in their clinically unaffected relatives as has been shown to be the case with pursuit tracking abnormalities. This possibility led several researchers to investigate whether high error rates on this task might be associated with genetic liability to schizophrenia or to dysfunctions in the same brain regions that were implicated in the patients themselves. Antisaccade task performance in relatives of schizophrenia patients has been compared to that of controls on standard, gap, and overlap versions of the antisaccade task. On the standard antisaccade task, unaffected relatives of schizophrenic patients made significantly more errors than healthy subjects in some studies (Clementz et al., 1994; Katsanis et al., 1997; McDowell and Clementz, 1997; Curtis et al., 2001a; Karoumi et al., 2001), but not in others (Thaker et al., 1996, 2000; Crawford et al., 1998; Brownstein et al., 2002). The substantial overlap in the lower 95% confidence limits of the 'positive' studies and the upper 95% confidence limits of the 'negative' studies indicates that all of the results for the standard antisaccade task could be consistent with a small difference in error rate between unaffected relatives and healthy subjects, but not with a large difference. If poor performance on the antisaccade task taps processes related to genetic vulnerability, unaffected relatives of schizophrenic patients as a group would be expected to have both a higher mean error score and a larger variance than controls, but this is not consistently the case. It is possible that a different antisaccade paradigm may be more useful in discriminating relatives from controls, but the literature does not consistently support the superiority of any specific alternative paradigm. Relatives of schizophrenic patients also make increased errors on gap (Ross et al., 1998) and overlap (McDowell and Clementz, 1997; McDowell et al., 1999) versions of the antisaccade task. Some data suggest that the overlap paradigm, especially the 'far-overlap' condition, yields the larger effect size in distinguishing relatives (and patients) from healthy controls (McDowell et al., 1999), but replications of that effect are needed. In an independent sample of relatives, the overlap condition minimized the difference between relatives and controls (Curtis et al., 2001b). Additional studies are needed to clarify which experimental paradigms yield the most robust differences between relatives and healthy controls, as well as the potential usefulness of this task in genetic studies of schizophrenia.

While eye movement tasks such as the antisaccade paradigm offer promising approaches for investigating cognitive and neurophysiologic aspects of psychiatric disorders, this review illustrates the complexity of this effort. Importantly, details of tasks and their relation to differential performance deficits in different disorders need to be examined. Also, the large majority of research in this area has used medicated patients with varying levels of illness severity in study protocols. This has left the potential utility of eye movement tasks for evaluating the neurophysiology of acute episodes of illness relatively unexplored. Further, because psychopharmacologic treatments target the brain and have been shown to affect motor and cognitive processes, it is crucial that more patient samples be recruited who are not currently receiving pharmacologic treatment so that the linkage of oculomotor deficits to disease processes can be more definitively established.

Other neuropsychiatric disorders

As discussed in several chapters in this book, there are various disorders in Psychiatry and Neurology for which the use of eye movement studies have been active and productive for some time. The application of eye movement procedures to the study of neurological disorders is thoroughly and expertly reviewed by Leigh and Zee (1999). However, it is important to note that there are disorders at the interface of these two medical disciplines, an area which is starting to be defined as the domain of Neuropsychiatry, which have received much less attention. One of the regions of interest within this new discipline is the domain of head trauma as discussed in the chapter by Heitger and colleagues. Another example is HIV infection (Currie et al., 1988; Sweeney et al., 1991). A third example is autism, for which despite the high prevalence and severity of this disorder and its documented neocortical and cerebellar pathology, few studies have used eye movement or other neurobehavioral methods to study the illness. Eye movement deficits in autism have been reported (Minshew et al., 1999), and eye movement investigations appear to be a promising approach for investigating brain disturbances characteristic for this disorder. Lastly, it is important to note that developmental studies of eye movement control in healthy individuals document progressive improvement in performance on eye movement tasks up through mid-adolescence

(Fischer et al., 1997). A developmental delay in the ability to perform an antisaccade task was demonstrated by Rosenberg et al. (1997), suggesting that eye movement tasks may be useful for investigating brain dysmaturation in multiple neuropsychiatric illnesses (Luna and Sweeney, 2001).

Functional brain imaging

Laboratory studies of eye movement control offer many advantages as approaches for learning about cognitive and brain disturbances. They are simple, non-invasive, quantitative and informative. However, direct linkage of a particular eye movement deficit to a specific regional brain dysfunction is often difficult, because above the brainstem and perhaps cerebellum, oculomotor control is not maintained by discrete regions serving clearly discrete functions, but by partially redundant systems performing their role in integrated widely distributed brain circuitry.

Functional brain imaging, first using positron emission tomography and more often now using functional magnetic resonance imaging, provides an approach for localizing specific regions in the brain where neurons become active when a particular task of interest is performed. A general summary of issues related to conducting eye movement research using functional magnetic resonance imaging is available (Luna and Sweeney, 1999). In situations where disturbances in multiple brain regions can cause similar disturbances in eye movement control, localization information of functional imaging can be especially useful.

Functional neuroimaging studies have now documented the roles not only of the frontal and parietal eye fields in the control of eye movements, but of the supplementary eye fields, the pre-supplementary motor area, precuneus, posterior and anterior cingulate, dorsolateral prefrontal cortex as well as the striatum, thalamus and superior colliculus. One general conclusion from functional imaging studies of eye movement control has been a close homology of the organization of the human and non-human primate brain in the control of eye movements. Not only is this seen at the level of a gross similarity in the topology of cortical regions involved in eye movement control, but in levels of detail such as the separation of pursuit and saccadic subregions of the frontal eye fields with a saccade region being seen along the rostral wall of the arcuate sulcus (monkey) and precentral sulcus (human) and a pursuit region being seen closer to the fundus of both sulci (Rosano et al., 2002).

A second general conclusion from functional imaging studies has been that when tasks are more dependent on cognitive than sensorimotor systems, such as when responses are made to remembered rather than visual targets, or during the performance of an antisaccade task, more activity is seen not only in the cortical eye fields, but also rostral to them (Sweeney et al., 1996; Petit et al., 1998; Heide et al., 2001; Luna et al., 2001). For example, in a study by Merriam et al. (2001), when saccades were made based on a decision about sensory cues rather than simply toward visual targets, activation was seen rostral to the frontal eye fields in the dorsolateral prefrontal cortex, rostral to the supplementary motor area in the pre-supplementary motor area, and rostral to the parietal eye field in the anterolateral aspect of the intraparietal sulcus.

With a growing and generally consistent literature from functional neuroimaging studies of healthy individuals, developing experience with the technique, general standardization of approaches for the analysis of functional imaging data, and with technology now available to permit monitoring of eye movement activity in MRI scanners (Kimmig et al., 1999), there is growing interest in using functional neuroimaging to explore the neuronal basis of eye movement abnormalities in clinical populations. Some early studies associated resting brain activity levels with pursuit deficits observed in schizophrenic patients in the laboratory (Ross et al., 1995). More recent studies examining brain activity during performance of eye movement tasks have been conducted with relatives of schizophrenic patients using pursuit tasks (O'Driscoll et al., 1999) and with schizophrenic patients performing antisaccade tasks (McDowell et al., 2002; Raemaekers et al., 2002).

There is great promise for utilizing functional brain imaging to learn about brain dysfunctions causing eye movement abnormalities in psychiatric and neurologic disorders. It will complement and depend upon laboratory studies of eye movement activity in several ways. First, extensive laboratory testing with different tasks and task parameters is needed to select the appropriate paradigms for neuroimaging studies. Second, laboratory and neuroimaging studies almost always need to be done in parallel to establish the range of eye movement abnormalities associated with an abnormal pattern of brain activation seen in imaging studies with clinical populations. Last, laboratory and imaging studies provide different information. Imaging data provide detailed information about the localization of brain regions in which activity is increased during task performance as well as where it is differentially increased or decreased in patient populations relative to healthy subjects. Currently available imaging approaches provide limited information about how activity is changed in regions of interest. Unlike laboratory studies where samples of eye movement activity are typically acquired every 1 or 2 ms, in fMRI studies images of each brain area of interest are typically acquired every 1 or 2 s. As a result, the temporal resolution needed to determine how brain activity changes or is altered during task performance is limited. These issues can be dealt with in 'event-related' approaches to fMRI studies that can tease apart the multiple operations required by the antisaccade task (fixation, inhibiting a saccade, generating an antisaccade without sensory guidance), and perhaps eventually by sophisticated approaches for merging EEG and fMRI data sets with high precision. Further, and most importantly, even if these issues were addressed by technical advances, sophisticated laboratory studies are the only approach that can document the types of eye movement abnormality that exist under different task conditions in different clinical populations. Thus, one of the future directions for clinical studies of eye movement abnormalities will be to establish collaborations between laboratory and imaging investigators to combine their resources to advance knowledge about the brain disorders causing eye movement abnormalities in psychiatric and neurological disorders.

General conclusions

There is considerable potential for the investigation of eye movement abnormalities in clinical populations. This potential includes efforts to learn about the pathophysiology of poorly understood conditions and to better understand the neurobehavioral effects of better known disorders, to monitor disease progression, to study patterns of abnormal developmental trajectories in pediatric and geriatric populations, to define endophenotypes for heritable brain disorders, and to investigate the short term and chronic effects of therapeutic medications and drugs of abuse. Over the past decade, clinical investigators have made considerable strides in efforts to investigate eye movement abnormalities resulting from pathology above the level of the brainstem and cerebellum. Further advances in this line of work are likely by utilizing functional neuroimaging to localize regions of abnormal brain function and by using a growing array of oculomotor paradigms to investigate not only sensorimotor systems but processes of attention, working memory, implicit or procedural learning of sequential responses, and the voluntary inhibition of context inappropriate behavior.

Abbreviations

CNS	central nervous system
EEG	electro-encephalography
fMRI	functional magnetic resonance imaging
HIV	human immunodeficiency virus
MRI	magnetic resonance imaging
PET	positron emission tomography
SPECT	single photon emitted computed tomography

References

Allen, J.S., Lambert, A.J., Johnson, F.Y., Schmidt, K. and Nero, K.L. (1996) Antisaccadic eye movements and attentional asymmetry in schizophrenia in three Pacific populations. *Acta Psychiatr. Scand.*, 94: 258–265.

Aman, C.J., Roberts Jr., R.J. and Pennington, B.F. (1998) A neuropsychological examination of the underlying deficit in attention deficit hyperactivity disorder: frontal lobe versus right parietal lobe theories. *Dev. Psychol.*, 34: 956–969.

Arolt, V., Purmann, S., Nolte, A., Lencer, R., Leutelt, J., Muller, B., Schurmann, M. and Schwinger, E. (1995) Possible linkage of ETD and markers on chromosome 6p. *Psychiatr. Gen.*, 5: S33.

Briand, K.A., Strallow, D., Hening, W., Poizner, H. and Sereno, A.B. (1999) Control of voluntary and reflexive saccades in Parkinson's disease. *Exp. Brain Res.*, 129: 38–48.

Brownstein, J., Krastoshevsky, O., McCollum, C., Kundamal, S., Matthysse, S., Holzman, P.S., Mendell, N.R. and Levy, D.L. (2002) Antisaccade performance is abnormal in schizophrenia patients but not in their biological relatives. Manuscript under review.

Bruce, C.J. and Goldberg, M.E. (1985) Primate frontal eye fields. I. Single neurons discharging before saccades. *J. Neurophysiol.*, 53: 603–635.

Clement, R.A., Abadi, R.V., Broomhead, D.S. and Whittle, J.P. (2002) A new framework for investigating both normal and abnormal eye movements. In: J. Hyönä, D.P. Munoz, W. Heide and R. Radach (Eds.), *The Brain's Eye: Neurobiological and Clinical Aspects of Oculomotor Research. Progress in Brain Research*, Vol. 140. Elsevier, Amsterdam, pp. 499–505.

Clementz, B.A. and Sweeney, J.A. (1990) Is eye movement dysfunction a biological marker for schizophrenia? A methodological review. *Psychol. Bull.*, 108: 77–92.

Clementz, B.A., Sweeney, J.A., Hirt, M. and Haas, G.L. (1990) Pursuit gain and saccadic intrusions in first-degree relatives of probands with schizophrenia. *J. Abnorm. Psychol.*, 99: 327–335.

Clementz, B.A., McDowell, J.E. and Zisook, S. (1994) Saccadic system functioning among schizophrenia patients and their first-degree biological relatives. *J. Abnorm. Psychol.*, 103: 277–287.

Colby, C.L., Duhamel, J.R. and Goldberg, M.E. (1996) Visual, presaccadic, and cognitive activation of single neurons in monkey lateral intraparietal area. *J. Neurophysiol.*, 76: 2841–2852.

Crawford, T.J., Haeger, B., Kennard, C., Reveley, M.A. and Henderson, L. (1995a) Saccadic abnormalities in psychotic patients. II. The role of neuroleptic treatment. *Psychol. Med.*, 25: 473–483.

Crawford, T.J., Haeger, B., Kennard, C., Reveley, M.A. and Henderson, L. (1995b) Saccadic abnormalities in psychotic patients. I. Neuroleptic-free psychotic patients. *Psychol. Med.*, 25: 461–471.

Crawford, T.J., Sharma, T., Puri, B.K., Murray, R.M., Berridge, D.M. and Lewis, S.W. (1998) Saccadic eye movements in families multiply affected with schizophrenia: the Maudsley family study. *Am. J. Psychiatry*, 155: 1703–1710.

Crawford, T.J., Bennett, D., Lekwuwa, G. and Shaunak, S. (2002) Cognition and the inhibitory control of saccades in schizophrenia and Parkinson's disease. In: J. Hyönä, D.P. Munoz, W. Heide and R. Radach (Eds.), *The Brain's Eye: Neurobiological and Clinical Aspects of Oculomotor Research. Progress in Brain Research*, Vol. 140. Elsevier, Amsterdam, pp. 449–466.

Crevits, L. and De Ridder, K. (1997) Disturbed striatoprefrontal mediated visual behaviour in moderate to severe parkinsonian patients. *J. Neurol. Neurosurg. Psychiatry*, 63: 296–299.

Currie, J., Benson, E., Ramsden, B., Perdices, M. and Cooper, D. (1988) Eye movement abnormalities as a predictor of the acquired immunodeficiency syndrome dementia complex. *Arch. Neurol.*, 45: 949–953.

Curtis, C.E., Calkins, M.E., Grove, W.M., Feil, K.J. and Iacono, W.G. (2001a) Saccadic disinhibition in patients with acute and remitted schizophrenia and their first-degree biological relatives. *Am. J. Psychiatry*, 158: 100–106.

Curtis, C.E., Calkins, M.E. and Iacono, W.G. (2001b) Saccadic disinhibition in schizophrenia patients and their first-degree biological relatives: a parametric study of the effects of increasing inhibitory load. *Exp. Brain Res.*, 137: 228–236.

Diefendorf, A.R. and Dodge, R. (1908) An experimental study of the ocular reactions of the insane from photographic records. *Brain*, 31: 451–489.

Doricchi, F., Perani, D., Incoccia, C., Grassi, F., Cappa, S.F., Bettinardi, V., Galati, G., Pizzamiglio, L. and Fazio, F. (1997) Neural control of fast-regular saccades and antisaccades: an investigation using positron emission tomography. *Exp. Brain Res.*, 116: 50–62.

Everling, S. and Fischer, B. (1998) The antisaccade: a review of basic research and clinical studies. *Neuropsychologia*, 36: 885–899.

Fischer, B. and Weber, H. (1992) Characteristics of 'anti' saccades in man. *Exp. Brain Res.*, 89: 415–424.

Fischer, B. and Weber, H. (1997) Effects of stimulus conditions on the performance of antisaccades in man. *Exp. Brain Res.*, 116: 191–200.

Fischer, B., Biscaldi, M. and Gezeck, S. (1997) On the development of voluntary and reflexive components in human saccade generation. *Brain Res.*, 754: 285–297.

Fukushima, J., Fukushima, K., Morita, N. and Yamashita, I. (1990a) Further analysis of the control of voluntary saccadic eye movements in schizophrenic patients. *Biol. Psychiatry*, 28: 943–958.

Fukushima, J., Morita, N., Fukushima, A.K., Chiba, T., Tanaka, S. and Yamashita, I. (1990b) Voluntary control of saccadic eye movements in patients with schizophrenic and affective disorders. *J. Psychiatry Res.*, 24: 9–24.

Fukushima, J., Fukushima, K., Miyasaka, K. and Yamashita, I. (1994) Voluntary control of saccadic eye movement in patients with frontal cortical lesions and parkinsonian patients in comparison with that in schizophrenics. *Biol. Psychiatry*, 36: 21–30.

Fukushima, J., Fukushima, K., Chiba, T., Tanaka, S., Yamashita, I. and Kato, M. (1988) Disturbances of voluntary control of saccadic eye movements in schizophrenic patients. *Biol. Psychiatry*, 23: 670–677.

Funahashi, S., Bruce, C.J. and Goldman-Rakic, P.S. (1989) Mnemonic coding of visual space in the monkey's dorsolateral prefrontal cortex. *J. Neurophysiol.*, 61: 331–349.

Goldman-Rakic, P.S. (1987) Circuitry of primate prefrontal cortex and regulation of behavior by representational memory. In: V.B. Mountcastle (Ed.), *Handbook of Physiology, Section 1. The Nervous System. Vol. V. Higher Functions of the Brain, Part 1.* American Physiology Society, Bethesda, MD, pp. 373–417.

Gooding, D.C. and Tallent, K.A. (2001) The association between antisaccade task and working memory task performance in schizophrenia and bipolar disorder. *J. Nerv. Ment. Dis.*, 189: 8–16.

Guitton, D., Buchtel, H.A. and Douglas, R.M. (1985) Frontal lobe lesions in man cause difficulties in suppressing reflexive glances and in generating goal-directed saccades. *Exp. Brain Res.*, 58: 455–472.

Hallett, P.E. (1978) Primary and secondary saccades to goals defined by instructions. *Vision Res.*, 18: 1279–1296.

Heide, W. and Kömpf, D. (1998) Combined deficits of saccades and visuo-spatial orientation after cortical lesions. *Exp. Brain Res.*, 123: 164–171.

Heide, W., Binkofski, F., Seitz, R.J., Posse, S., Nitschke, M.F., Freund, H.-J. and Kömpf, D. (2001) Activation of fronto-parietal cortices during memorized triple-step sequences of saccadic eye movements: an fMRI study. *Eur. J. Neurosci.*, 13: 1177–1189.

Heitger, M.H., Anderson, T.J. and Jones, R.D. (2002) Saccade sequences as markers for cerebral dysfunction following mild closed head injury. In: J. Hyönä, D.P. Munoz, W. Heide and R. Radach (Eds.), *The Brain's Eye: Neurobiological and Clinical Aspects of Oculomotor Research. Progress in Brain Research*, Vol. 140. Elsevier, Amsterdam, pp. 433–448.

Hikosaka, O. (1989) Role of basal ganglia in saccades. *Rev. Neurol.*, 145: 580–586.

Huestegge, L., Radach, R., Kunert, H.-J. and Heller, D. (2002) Visual search in long-term cannabis users with early age of onset. In: J. Hyönä, D.P. Munoz, W. Heide and R. Radach (Eds.), *The Brain's Eye: Neurobiological and Clinical Aspects of Oculomotor Research. Progress in Brain Research*, Vol. 140. Elsevier, Amsterdam, pp. 377–394.

Holzman, P.S. (2000) Eye movements and the search for the essence of schizophrenia. *Brain Res. Rev.*, 31: 350–356.

Holzman, P.S., Proctor, L.R. and Hughes, D.W. (1973) Eye tracking patterns in schizophrenia. *Science*, 181: 179–181.

Holzman, P.S., Proctor, L.R., Levy, D.L., Yasillo, N.J., Meltzer, H.Y. and Hurt, S.W. (1974) Eye-tracking dysfunctions in schizophrenic patients and their relatives. *Arch. Gen. Psychiatry*, 31: 143–151.

Holzman, P.S., Kringlen, E., Levy, D.L. and Haberman, S.J. (1980) Deviant eye tracking in twins discordant for psychosis: a replication. *Arch. Gen. Psychiatry*, 37: 627–631.

Hutton, S.B., Crawford, T.J., Puri, B.K., Duncan, L.J., Chapman, M., Kennard, C., Barnes, T.R.E. and Joyce, E.M. (1998) Smooth pursuit and saccadic abnormalities in first-episode schizophrenia. *Psychol. Med.*, 28: 685–692.

Hutton, S.B., Joyce, E.M., Barnes, T.R.E. and Kennard, C. (2002) Saccadic distractability in first-episode schizophrenia. *Neuropsychologia*, 40: 1729–1736.

Iacono, W.G. (1982) Eye tracking in normal twins. *Behav. Genet.*, 12: 517–526.

Iacono, W.G. and Koenig, W.G.R. (1983) Features that distinguish the smooth-pursuit eye-tracking performance of schizophrenic, affective disorder, and normal individuals. *J. Abnorm. Psychol.*, 92: 29–41.

Iacono, W.G., Tuason, V.B. and Johnson, R.A. (1981) Dissociation of smooth-pursuit and saccadic eye tracking in remitted schizophrenics. *Arch. Gen. Psychiatry*, 38: 991–996.

Joseph, J.P. and Barone, P. (1987) Prefrontal unit activity during a delayed oculomotor task in the monkey. *Exp. Brain Res.*, 67: 460–468.

Karoumi, B., Ventre-Dominey, J., Vighetto, A., Dalery, J. and d'Amato, T. (1998) Saccadic eye movements in schizophrenic patients. *Psychiatry Res.*, 77: 9–19.

Karoumi, B., Saoud, M., d'Amato, T., Rosenfeld, F., Denise, P., Gutknecht, C., Gaveau, V., Beaulieu, F.E., Dalery, J. and Rochet, T. (2001) Poor performance in smooth pursuit and antisaccadic eye-movement tasks in healthy siblings of patients with schizophrenia. *Psychiatry Res.*, 101: 209–219.

Katsanis, J., Kortenkamp, S., Iacono, W.G. and Grove, W.M. (1997) Antisaccade performance in patients with schizophrenia and affective disorder. *J. Abnorm. Psychol.*, 106: 468–472.

Kimmig, H., Greenlee, M.W., Huethe, F. and Mergner, T. (1999) MR-eyetracker: a new method for eye movement recording in functional magnetic resonance imaging. *Exp. Brain Res.*, 126: 443–449.

Kitagawa, M., Fukushima, J. and Tashiro, K. (1994) Relationship between antisaccades and the clinical symptoms in Parkinson's disease. *Neurology*, 44: 2285–2289.

Lasker, A.G., Zee, D.S., Hain, T.C., Folstein, S.E. and Singer, H.D. (1988) Saccades in Huntington's disease: slowing and dysmetria. *Neurology*, 38: 427–431.

Leigh, R.J. and Zee, D.S. (1999) *The Neurology of Eye Movements*, 3rd edn. Oxford Univ. Press, New York.

Leigh, R.J., Newman, S.A., Folstein, S.E., Lasker, A.G. and Jensen, B.A. (1983) Abnormal ocular motor control in Huntington's disease. *Neurology*, 33: 1268–1275.

Levy, D.L. and Holzman, P.S. (1997) Eye tracking dysfunction and schizophrenia: an overview with special reference to the genetics of schizophrenia. *Int. Rev. Psychiatry*, 9: 365–371.

Levy, D.L., Mendell, N.R., LaVancher, C., Brownstein, J., Shorrock, K., Krastoshevsky, O., Teraspulsky, L., Lo, Y., Bloom, R., Matthysse, S. and Holzman, P.S. (1998) Disinhibition in antisaccade performance in schizophrenia. In: M.F. Lenzenweger and R. Dworkin (Eds.), *Origins and Development of Schizophrenia: Advances in Experimental Psychopathology*. American Psychological Association Press, Washington, DC, pp. 185–210.

Lueck, C.J., Tanyeri, S., Crawford, T.J., Henderson, L. and Kennard, C. (1990) Antisaccades and remembered saccades in Parkinson's disease. *J. Neurol. Neurosurg. Psychiatry*, 53: 284–288.

Luna, B. and Sweeney, J.A. (1999) Cognitive functional magnetic resonance imaging at very-high-field: eye movement control. *Top. Magnet. Reson. Imaging*, 10: 3–15.

Luna, B. and Sweeney, J.A. (2001) Studies of brain and cognitive maturation through childhood and adolescence: a strategy for testing neurodevelopmental hypotheses. *Schizophr. Bull.*, 27: 443–455.

Luna, B., Thulborn, K.R., Munoz, D.P., Merriam, E.P., Garver, K.E., Minshew, N.J., Keshavan, M.S., Genovese, C.R., Eddy, W.F. and Sweeney, J.A. (2001) Maturation of widely distributed brain function subserves cognitive development. *Neuroimage*, 13: 786–793.

MacAskill, M.R., Anderson, T.J. and Jones, R.D. (2002) Saccadic adaptation in neurological disorders. In: J. Hyönä, D.P. Munoz, W. Heide and R. Radach (Eds.), *The Brain's Eye: Neurobiological and Clinical Aspects of Oculomotor Research. Progress in Brain Research*, Vol. 140. Elsevier, Amsterdam, pp. 417–431.

Maruff, P., Danckert, J., Pantelis, C. and Currie, J. (1998) Saccadic and attentional abnormalities in patients with schizophrenia. *Psychol. Med.*, 28: 1091–1100.

Matsue, Y., Saito, H., Osakabe, K., Awata, S., Ueno, T., Matsuoka, H., Chiba, H., Fuse, Y. and Sato, M. (1994) Smooth pursuit eye movements and voluntary control of saccades in the antisaccade task in schizophrenic patients. *Jpn. J. Psychiatry Neurol.*, 48: 13–22.

McDowell, J.E. and Clementz, B.A. (1997) The effect of fixation condition manipulations on antisaccade performance in schizophrenia: studies of diagnostic specificity. *Exp. Brain Res.*, 115: 333–344.

McDowell, J.E., Myles-Worsley, M., Coon, H., Byerley, W. and Clementz, B.A. (1999) Measuring liability for schizophrenia using optimized antisaccade stimulus parameters. *Psychophysiology*, 36: 138–141.

McDowell, J.E., Brown, G.G., Paulus, M., Martinez, A., Stewart, S.E., Dubowitz, D.J. and Braff, D.L. (2002) Neural correlates of refixation saccades and antisaccades in normal and schizophrenia subjects. *Biol. Psychiatry*, 51: 216–223.

Merriam, E.P., Colby, C.L., Thulborn, K.R., Luna, B., Olson, C.R. and Sweeney, J.A. (2001) Stimulus–response incompatibility activates cortex proximate to three eye fields. *Neuroimage*, 13: 794–800.

Minshew, N.J., Luna, B. and Sweeney, J.A. (1999) Oculomotor evidence for neocortical systems but not cerebellar dysfunction in autism. *Neurology*, 52: 917–922.

Muller, N., Riedel, M., Eggert, T. and Straube, A. (1999) Internally and externally guided voluntary saccades in unmedicated and medicated schizophrenic patients: Part II. Saccadic latency, gain, and fixation suppression errors. *Eur. Arch. Psychiatry Clin. Neurosci.*, 249: 7–14.

Munoz, D.P. and Wurtz, R.H. (1992) Role of the rostral superior colliculus in active visual fixation and execution of express saccades. *J. Neurophysiol.*, 67: 1000–1002.

Munoz, D.P., Hampton, K.A., Moore, K.D. and Goldring, J.E. (1999) Control of purposive saccadic eye movements and visual fixation in children with attention-deficit hyperactivity disorder. In: W. Becker, H. Duebel and T. Mergner (Eds.), *Current Oculomotor Research: Physiological and Psychological Aspects*. Plenum Press, New York, NY, pp. 415–423.

Munoz, D.P., Commentary: saccadic eye movements: overview of neural circuitry. In: J. Hyönä, D.P. Munoz, W. Heide and R. Radach (Eds.), *The Brain's Eye: Neurobiological and Clinical Aspects of Oculomotor Research. Progress in Brain Research*, Vol. 140. Elsevier, Amsterdam, pp. 89–96.

Newsham, D. and Knox, P.C. (2002) Oculomotor control in a group of very low birth weight (VLBL) children. In: J. Hyönä, D.P. Munoz, W. Heide and R. Radach (Eds.), *The Brain's Eye: Neurobiological and Clinical Aspects of Oculomotor Research. Progress in Brain Research*, Vol. 140. Elsevier, Amsterdam, pp. 483–498.

O'Driscoll, G.A., Alpert, N.M., Matthysse, S.W., Levy, D.L., Rauch, S.L. and Holzman, P.S. (1995) Functional neuroanatomy of antisaccade eye movements investigated with positron emission tomography. *Proc. Natl. Acad. Sci. USA*, 92: 925–929.

O'Driscoll, G.A., Benkelfat, C., Florencio, P.S., Wolff, A.L., Joober, R., Lal, S. and Evans, A.C. (1999) Neural correlates of eye tracking deficits in first-degree relatives of schizophrenic patients: a positron emission tomography study. *Arch. Gen. Psychiatry*, 56: 1127–1134.

Park, S. and Holzman, P.S. (1992) Schizophrenics show spatial working memory deficits. *Arch. Gen. Psychiatry*, 49: 975–982.

Paus, T., Petrides, M., Evans, A.C. and Meyer, E. (1993) Role of the human anterior cingulate cortex in the control of oculomotor, manual, and speech responses: a positron emission tomography study. *J. Neurophysiol.*, 70: 453–469.

Petit, L., Courtney, S.M., Ungerleider, L.G. and Haxby, J. (1998) Sustained activity in the medial wall during working memory delays. *J. Neurosci.*, 18: 9429–9437.

Pierrot-Deseilligny, C.H., Rivaud, S., Pillon, B., Fournier, E. and Agid, Y. (1989) Lateral visually-guided saccades in progressive supranuclear palsy. *Brain*, 112: 471–487.

Pierrot-Deseilligny, C., Rivaud, S., Gaymard, B. and Agid, Y. (1991) Cortical control of reflexive visually-guided saccades. *Brain*, 114: 1473–1485.

Pierrot-Deseilligny, C., Rivaud, S., Gaymard, B., Muri, R. and Vermersch, A.I. (1995) Cortical control of saccades. *Ann. Neurol.*, 37: 557–567.

Pierrot-Deseilligny, C., Gaymard, B., Muri, R. and Rivaud, S. (1997) Cerebral ocular motor signs. *J. Neurol.*, 244: 65–70.

Raemaekers, M., Jansma, J.M., Cahn, W., Van der Geest, J.N., van der Linden, J.A., Kahn, R.S. and Ramsey, N.F. (2002) Neuronal substrate of the saccadic inhibition deficit in schizophrenia investigated with 3-dimensional event-related functional magnetic resonance imaging. *Arch. Gen. Psychiatry*, 59: 313–320.

Rao, S.G., Williams, G.V. and Goldman-Rakic, P.S. (2000) Destruction and creation of spatial tuning by disinhibition: $GABA_A$ blockade of prefrontal cortical neurons engaged by working memory. *J. Neurosci.*, 20: 485–494.

Rosano, C., Krisky, C.M., Welling, J.S., Eddy, W.F., Luna, B., Thulborn, K.R. and Sweeney, J.A. (2002) Pursuit and saccadic eye movement subregions in human frontal eye field: a high-resolution fMRI investigation. *Cereb. Cortex*, 12: 107–115.

Rosenberg, D.R., Averbach, D.H., O'Hearn, K.O., Seymour, A.B., Birmaher, B. and Sweeney, J.A. (1997) Oculomotor response inhibition abnormalities in pediatric obsessive compulsive disorder. *Arch. Gen. Psychiatry*, 54: 831–838.

Ross, D.E., Thaker, G.K., Holcomb, H.H., Cascella, N.G., Medoff, D.R. and Tamminga, C.A. (1995) Abnormal smooth pursuit eye movements in schizophrenic patients are associated with cerebral glucose metabolism in oculomotor regions. *Psychiatry Res.*, 58: 53–67.

Ross, R.G., Harris, J.G., Olincy, A., Radant, A., Adler, L.E. and Freedman, R. (1998) Familial transmission of two independent saccadic abnormalities in schizophrenia. *Schizophr. Res.*, 30: 59–70.

Rosse, R.B., Schwartz, B.L., Kim, S.Y. and Deutsch, S.I. (1993) Correlation between antisaccade and Wisconsin Card Sorting Test performance in schizophrenia. *Am. J. Psychiatry*, 150: 333–335.

Rothlind, J.C., Posner, M.I. and Schaughency, E.A. (1991) Lateralized control of eye movements in attention deficit hyperactivity disorder. *J. Cogn. Neurosci.*, 3: 377–381.

Sawaguchi, T. and Goldman-Rakic, P.S. (1994) The role of D1-dopamine receptor in working memory: local injections of dopamine antagonists into the prefrontal cortex of rhesus monkeys performing an oculomotor delayed-response task. *J. Neurophysiol.*, 71: 515–528.

Schall, J.D. and Bichot, N.P. (1998) Neural correlates of visual and motor decision processes. *Curr. Opin. Neurobiol.*, 8: 211–217.

Sereno, A.B. and Holzman, P.S. (1995) Antisaccades and smooth pursuit eye movements in schizophrenia. *Biol. Psychiatry*, 37: 394–401.

Sprenger, A. Kömpf, D. and Heide, W. (2002) Visual search in patients with left visual hemineglect. In: J. Hyönä, D.P. Munoz, W. Heide and R. Radach (Eds.), *The Brain's Eye: Neurobiological and Clinical Aspects of Oculomotor Research. Progress in Brain Research*, Vol. 140. Elsevier, Amsterdam, pp. 395–416.

Sweeney, J.A., Brew, B.J., Keilp, J.G., Sidtis, J.J. and Price, R.W. (1991) Pursuit eye movement dysfunction in HIV-1 seropositive individuals. *J. Psychiatry Neurosci.*, 16: 247–252.

Sweeney, J.A., Palumbo, D.R., Halper, J.P. and Shear, M.K. (1992) Pursuit eye movement dysfunction in obsessive–compulsive disorder. *Psychiatry Res.*, 42: 1–11.

Sweeney, J.A., Clementz, B.A., Haas, G.L., Escobar, M.D., Drake, K. and Frances, A.J. (1994) Eye tracking dysfunction in schizophrenia: characterization of component eye movement abnormalities, diagnostic specificity, and the role of attention. *J. Abnorm. Psychol.*, 103: 222–230.

Sweeney, J.A., Mintun, M.A., Kwee, S., Wiseman, M.B., Brown, D.L., Rosenberg, D.R. and Carl, J.R. (1996) Positron emission tomography study of voluntary saccadic eye movements and spatial working memory. *J. Neurophysiol.*, 75: 454–468.

Sweeney, J.A., Bauer, K.S., Keshavan, M.S., Haas, G.L., Schooler, N.R. and Kroboth, P.D. (1997) Adverse effects of risperidone on eye movement activity: a comparison of risperidone and haloperidol in antipsychotic-naive schizophrenic patients. *Neuropsychopharmacology*, 16: 217–228.

Sweeney, J.A., Strojwas, M.H., Mann, J.J. and Thase, M.E. (1998) Prefrontal and cerebellar abnormalities in major depression: evidence from oculomotor studies. *Biol. Psychiatry*, 43: 584–594.

Sweeney, J.A., Rosano, C., Berman, R.A. and Luna, B. (2001) Inhibitory control of attention declines more than working memory during normal aging. *Neurobiol. Aging*, 22: 39–47.

Thaker, G.K., Nguyen, J.A. and Tamminga, C.A. (1989) Increased saccadic distractibility in tardive dyskinesia: functional evidence for subcortical GABA dysfunction. *Biol. Psychiatry*, 25: 49–59.

Thaker, G.K., Cassady, S., Adami, H.M., Moran, M. and Ross, D.E. (1996) Eye movements in spectrum personality disorders: comparison of community subjects and relatives of schizophrenic patients. *Am. J. Psychiatry*, 153: 362–368.

Thaker, G.K., Ross, D.E., Cassady, S.L., Adami, H.M., Laporte, D., Medoff, D.R. and Lahti, A. (1998) Smooth pursuit eye movements to extraretinal motion signals: deficits in relatives of patients with schizophrenia. *Arch. Gen. Psychiatry*, 55: 830–836.

Thaker, G.K., Ross, D.E., Buchanan, R.W., Adami, H.M. and Medoff, D.R. (1999) Smooth pursuit eye movements to extraretinal motion signals: deficits in patients with schizophrenia. *Psychiatry Res.*, 88: 209–219.

Thaker, G.K., Ross, D.E., Cassady, S.L., Adami, H.M., Medoff, D.R. and Sherr, J. (2000) Saccadic eye movement abnormalities in relatives of patients with schizophrenia. *Schizophr. Res.*, 45: 235–244.

Tian, J.R., Zee, D.S., Lasker, A.G. and Folstein, S.E. (1991) Saccades in Huntington's disease: predictive tracking and interaction between release of fixation and initiation of saccades. *Neurology*, 41: 875–881.

Tien, A.Y., Pearlson, G.D., Machlin, S.R., Bylsma, F.W. and Hoehn-Saric, R. (1992) Oculomotor performance in obsessive–compulsive disorder. *Am. J. Psychiatry*, 149: 641–646.

Tien, A.Y., Ross, D.E., Pearlson, G. and Strauss, M.E. (1996) Eye movements and psychopathology in schizophrenia and bipolar disorder. *J. Nerv. Ment. Dis.*, 184: 331–338.

Trillenberg, P., Heide, W., Junghanns, K., Blankenburg, M., Arolt, V. and Kömpf, D. (1998) Target anticipation and impairment of smooth pursuit eye movement in schizophrenia. *Exp. Brain Res.*, 120: 316–324.

Vidailhet, M., Rivaud, S., Gouider-Khouja, N., Pillon, B., Bonnet, A.M., Gaymard, B., Agid, Y. and Pierrot-Deseilligny, C. (1994) Eye movements in Parkinsonian syndromes. *Ann. Neurol.*, 35: 420–426.

Walker, R., Husain, M., Hodgson, T.L., Harrison, J. and Kennard, C. (1998) Saccadic eye movement and working memory deficits following damage to human prefrontal cortex. *Neuropsychologia*, 36: 1141–1159.

Subject Index

abstract representation, 142, 149, 153, 155–157, 160, 167
adverse effects, 377–379, 391, 435, 436, 458, 511, 512
age of onset, 380, 382, 383, 391
allocation of attention, 103, 121, 257, 262, 267–269, 271, 276, 402
allocentric, 182, 352, 355, 395
anticipation, 52, 171, 205, 247, 256, 260, 262, 290, 291, 487, 492
antisaccade (anti-saccade), 13, 15–18, 435, 436, 444, 450–452, 459, 510, 514, 515
aperture problem, 230, 231, 234
attention, 9, 51, 52, 58, 63, 100–105, 107–109, 112–115, 119–121, 129, 134, 146, 147, 153, 159, 169, 170, 177, 182, 184–186, 190–194, 197–202, 204–206, 212, 226, 235, 242, 255–258, 260–264, 267–271, 274, 279, 280, 286, 287, 291, 292, 319, 350, 351, 360, 361, 378–380, 382, 395–400, 402, 403, 406, 410, 411, 413, 433–435, 449, 450, 452, 458, 483, 510, 511, 513, 515, 516, 518
attention deficit hyperactivity disorder (ADHD), 268, 468, 469, 476, 478, 479, 486, 496
auditory targets, 51–55, 58, 319, 320, 370
autism, 516
awareness, 99–105, 108, 109, 111, 114, 115, 200, 201, 396, 399, 427

basal ganglia, 3, 89, 90, 94, 95, 112, 377, 400, 424, 428, 456, 458, 467, 468, 477–479, 486, 508, 509, 513
bipolar disorder, 453, 514, 515
blanking, 76–78, 122, 165, 169–174, 176, 177, 181, 185–187, 189–194, 204, 205, 251, 429
blanks, 79, 99–101, 105–107, 119–122, 124, 127–129, 167, 170–172, 175, 176, 184–186, 188–193, 197, 198, 202, 205, 206, 242, 248, 349
blinks, 99, 119, 120, 122, 124, 127–129, 150, 202, 214, 487

body-centered, 331, 355, 395, 400
brainstem, 3, 28, 40, 62, 70, 85, 89–95, 211, 317, 390, 424, 434, 435, 443, 467, 508, 509, 512, 517, 518
buildup neurons, 10–16, 38
burst neurons, 10, 11, 21, 28, 36, 38, 41, 91, 92, 443

cannabis, 377–380, 382–388, 390–392, 511
central processing, 51, 55, 57–59
cerebellar lesion, 422, 486
cerebellum, 3, 26, 28, 34, 38–41, 44, 46, 89, 90, 93–95, 112, 211, 292, 313, 317, 369, 370, 377, 421–424, 444, 457, 493, 495, 496, 508, 509, 517, 518
change blindness, 102, 105, 108, 110, 112, 114, 119–122, 124, 127–129, 133, 134, 147, 150, 184, 185, 197–200, 202, 349, 350, 361
change detection, 99–103, 105, 106, 109–113, 119–121, 127–129, 134–136, 149, 150, 152, 153, 159, 160, 169, 181–183, 185, 203
children, 70, 268, 423, 483–496, 499, 511
closed head injury (CHI), 417, 423, 433–436, 438–444, 509
cognitive, 3, 4, 13, 68, 69, 111–113, 121, 128, 140, 147, 221, 234, 250, 255–257, 260–264, 279, 280, 290, 295, 319, 351, 378–380, 395–398, 402, 413, 421, 423, 434, 435, 438, 443, 444, 449, 450, 452, 453, 457–462, 478, 483, 485, 486, 507–513, 516, 517
coherence field, 199, 201–203
coherence theory, 199
congenital nystagmus, 499, 501–504

delayed saccade task, 315, 467, 469, 470, 472, 474, 477–479
depression, 70, 383, 514, 515
diffuse axonal injury (DAI), 442, 443
distractor (distracter), 8, 9, 105, 140, 169, 170, 176–178, 212–223, 226, 227, 256, 268, 287, 341–347, 354, 355, 367, 381, 402
dopamine, 456–458, 467, 468, 479

dorsolateral prefrontal cortex (DLPFC), 4, 90, 92, 94, 95, 252, 274, 424, 435, 442, 443, 450–452, 458, 479, 517
dual task paradigm, 382
dyslexia, 486, 495

efference copy, 166, 177, 288, 306, 317, 319, 322, 413
egocentric, 182, 321, 323, 329, 395, 396, 400, 413
eigenvalues, 500–502
eigenvectors, 500, 503
episodic representation, 133–136, 145–147
event-related potential (ERP), 104, 113, 379
excitatory burst neurons (EBN), 21, 26, 28, 29, 32–35, 38, 40, 41, 43–47, 91–94
expectation, 107, 129, 155, 250, 272, 283, 290, 293, 397
express saccade, 9, 12, 14, 18, 61, 62, 64, 67–70, 355, 452, 472, 474, 477, 479
extraretinal signals, 166, 170, 177, 367
eye-centered, 301–303, 306, 307, 309, 332, 333, 335, 337, 338, 357, 368
eye position, 9, 22, 24, 26, 38, 39, 41, 43, 44, 52, 54, 57–59, 91, 92, 121, 124, 126, 158, 166, 213, 216, 248, 257, 259, 280, 282–285, 290, 301, 302, 313–315, 318, 321–323, 329–332, 335, 336, 349, 352–354, 357, 359, 366–368, 403, 407, 409, 418, 433, 436, 437, 439–441, 454–457, 459, 471–473, 475, 476, 499–501, 504, 509
eye velocity, 46, 91, 165, 213, 216, 221, 230, 233, 240–249, 251, 271, 279, 283–285, 287–292, 425, 487, 491, 495, 496, 504

fastigial nucleus (FN), 5, 7, 21, 26, 27, 38–41, 46, 93, 94, 422
first-order motion, 281, 283, 285
fixation, 3–18, 22, 26, 28, 36, 38, 39, 52–59, 61–65, 67–70, 75, 89, 90, 92–95, 110, 119–129, 134, 146, 149–152, 157–160, 167–171, 174, 178, 181–186, 188–194, 204, 205, 211–217, 220–223, 229, 245, 251, 267, 268, 279, 280, 283–288, 290, 302, 313, 314, 316, 319, 322, 323, 330, 331, 337, 349, 351–358, 360, 361, 367, 380–384, 386, 388, 390, 391, 397, 398, 400, 403, 407, 409–411, 419, 426, 437, 450, 451, 456–459, 469–472, 474, 478, 486, 487, 491, 492, 495, 496, 499–503, 518
fixation neurons, 4, 5, 7, 9–12, 14–16, 36, 61, 65, 67–70, 93
fixational instability, 495, 496
Fourier motion, 282, 283, 285
fovea, 17, 21, 22, 89, 90, 93, 119, 126–128, 149, 150, 157–159, 165, 225, 229, 239, 242, 279, 285, 293, 322, 330, 331, 367, 411, 419, 501, 502
frame of reference, 280, 288, 293–295, 301–303, 307, 309, 314, 368
frontal cortex, 93–95, 251, 313, 369, 424, 443, 467, 468, 483, 486, 495, 513
frontal eye field (FEF), 4, 27, 29, 58, 59, 62, 68–70, 90, 92, 94, 95, 251, 252, 274, 347, 358, 399, 400, 402, 404, 406, 412, 413, 422, 435, 442, 443, 450, 451, 501
frontal lesion, 395, 397, 399, 401, 404, 406, 410, 412
functional magnetic resonance imaging (fMRI), 112, 379, 399, 517
functional neuroimaging, 495, 508, 517, 518

gamma amino butyric acid (GABA), 456, 457
gap effect, 10, 12, 18, 55, 61, 211, 212, 214, 217, 220–223, 284, 472, 474
gap saccade task, 9–12, 14, 61–65, 68, 70, 94
global effect, 341–347

haloperidol, 454–456, 468
hand movements, 103, 302–307, 309, 311–315, 323, 330, 341–347, 349, 352, 355–358, 361, 362, 365–371, 499
head movements, 38, 124, 171, 293–295, 336, 337, 400, 403, 418, 421, 437, 485–487
head position, 75, 295, 331, 336, 359
head-centered, 331, 332, 355, 395
hemi-spatial neglect, 395–399, 401, 402, 413
high-level vision, 295
Huntington's disease, 457, 513
hypermetria, 422, 423, 433, 439–442
hypometria, 400, 418, 423–425, 427, 428, 435, 442

iconic memory, 151, 204
implicit perception, 104, 200, 202, 206
implicit processing, 104, 107, 109, 111

inhibition, 5, 7, 16, 21, 26, 28, 29, 33, 34, 36, 38, 44–47, 70, 73, 74, 76–85, 92, 94, 128, 346, 347, 382, 435, 449–462, 480, 510, 513, 518
inhibition of return, 382, 397, 398, 401, 402, 412, 413
inhibitory burst neurons (IBN), 26, 28, 34, 44–46, 91–93
initial eye acceleration, 230, 286–288, 292
initiation of smooth pursuit, 225, 229, 256, 258, 260, 279, 285, 291
intracortical microstimulation (ICMS), 287, 290, 293
intraparietal sulcus (IPS), 112, 252, 357, 401, 443, 517

latency, 12, 16, 22, 36, 39, 51–59, 61, 64, 73, 74, 76–85, 122, 128, 182, 190, 191, 211–223, 230, 232, 258, 262, 268–276, 283–288, 292, 305, 341, 342, 344, 345, 354–356, 358, 359, 425, 450, 452, 457, 483, 487–490, 492, 494, 495, 511, 514, 515
lateral intraparietal cortex (LIP), 4, 70, 90, 92, 94, 178, 231, 313, 315, 322, 452
learning, 104, 252, 279, 280, 292, 336, 417, 418, 423, 429, 434, 443, 444, 484, 485, 517, 518
limb movements, 274, 301, 302, 306, 307, 309, 311, 314, 315, 435, 477, 499
local motion signals, 225, 229, 233, 234
lorazepam, 454–457
low-level vision, 295

macrosaccadic oscillations, 499, 501
magnetic misreaching, 318, 319, 321–323, 369–371
magnocellular, 78, 167, 232, 495
main sequence, 22, 23, 25, 26, 33, 43, 46, 385, 386, 390, 487, 489, 490, 494, 511
marijuana, 377, 378, 392
medial rectus paresis, 418
medial superior temporal (MST), 226, 231, 268, 287, 292–295
memory-guided saccades, 95, 152, 421, 424, 427–429, 435, 436, 440–444, 452, 456–459
method of delays, 499, 501, 503
middle temporal (MT), 212, 215, 221, 226–228, 230, 231, 233–235, 268, 286, 287, 290–293, 435, 484
monkey, 4, 5, 7–9, 13, 28, 29, 33, 43, 58, 61–65, 68, 85, 178, 212, 226, 229–231, 252, 256, 279, 282, 286, 290, 291, 293–295, 313–315, 321, 355, 358, 368–370, 411, 419–421, 443, 452, 508, 517
motion integration, 225, 226, 228, 231, 233, 234, 281
motion perception, 167, 229, 263, 287
motion processing, 211, 212, 215, 221–223, 225, 226, 251, 268, 279–283, 285–288, 290, 293, 295, 484
motion signals, 167, 212, 221, 223, 226–228, 230, 232, 234, 283, 285–287
motoneurons (MN), 26, 28, 34, 43, 91, 92, 94, 292
motor control, 89, 111, 245, 311, 323, 429, 515
motor learning, 245, 251, 292, 429
multiple-object tracking (MOT), 134–136, 140, 202
mutual inhibition, 500
myasthenia gravis, 417–419

natural behavior, 350, 351, 355, 358, 359, 361
natural scenes, 74, 110, 149, 154, 155, 159, 168, 169, 350, 399
neurology, 112, 341, 365, 395, 417, 507, 510, 512, 516
non-visual attention, 256
nonlinear dynamics, 499, 500, 502, 504
nystagmus, 288, 417, 485, 499, 501–504

object files, 135, 136, 144–146, 194
object perception, 142, 181–183, 186, 193, 221
obsessive-compulsive disorder (OCD), 469, 476, 478
ocular dominance, 329, 333, 334
ocular following, 226, 229, 230, 232, 233
oculocentric, 317, 321, 322, 329, 332, 395
oculomotor control, 51, 281, 311, 317, 435, 484, 487, 493, 496, 509, 517
oculomotor plant, 21, 22, 24, 25, 39–41, 43, 45, 46, 501
omnipotent neurons (OPN), 26, 28, 33, 34, 36, 43, 44, 46, 91, 92, 94
opsoclonus, 417, 423, 428, 499
optic ataxia, 316–319, 321–323, 369, 370

paramedian pontine reticular formation, 21, 69, 70, 92
parietal cortex, 313, 314, 322, 347, 444
parietal eye field (PEF), 443, 517
parietal lesion, 392, 399, 402, 403, 413

parietal reach region (PRR), 301, 313, 315, 322, 333, 337, 368
parieto-temporal, 396, 397, 399, 401, 404, 412, 413
Parkinson's disease (PD), 243, 244, 417, 419, 420, 424, 426–428, 435, 442, 449, 452, 457–461, 510, 513
parvocellular, 78, 232
peak velocity, 22, 23, 39, 43, 45, 52, 241, 243, 244, 365, 385, 386, 421, 450, 457, 487, 489, 490, 499
pop-out effect, 395, 398, 402, 403, 406, 407, 410–413
positron emission tomography (PET), 252, 370, 421, 443, 507, 517
post-concussion syndrome (PCS), 62, 403, 434, 444
post-saccadic enhancement, 284, 285, 287, 292
post-traumatic amnesia (PTA), 433–436, 441, 509
posterior parietal cortex (PPC), 69, 94, 95, 274, 279, 293, 295, 301, 302, 305–307, 309, 323, 368–370, 401, 435, 442, 443, 451
prediction, 108, 240–242, 244, 249, 279–281, 290, 381, 454, 461, 487, 492
prefrontal cortex (PFC), 61–65, 67–70, 252, 443, 450, 452–454, 456–459, 467, 479, 508, 513
premotor cortex (PMC), 301, 313, 314, 337, 368, 369
preparatory neurons, 61, 65, 67, 68
priming, 104, 105, 146, 350
proprioceptive, 306, 316, 319, 320, 322, 367, 370, 396
proto-objects, 199–201, 203–205
psychiatry, 255, 507, 509, 510, 516
psychological refractory period, 257–260
Purkinje cells, 26, 27, 38, 39, 46, 93
pursuit deficit, 268, 496, 512, 517
pursuit initiation, 211, 226, 228, 230, 232, 233, 268, 283–288, 487, 496
pursuit velocity, 250, 267, 271, 493, 494

reaction time (RT), 7, 53, 95, 109, 122, 125, 126, 128, 189, 240, 263, 271, 272, 312, 384, 417, 451, 459 reading, 3, 21, 73–76, 82–84, 90, 110, 152, 167, 181, 193, 194, 354, 381, 382, 386, 388, 391, 396, 483–486, 496, 511
reading difficulties, 483–487, 495, 496
reference object, 168, 173, 176–178
refixations, 412, 413, 418
reflexive saccades, 61, 70, 94, 95, 421–424, 426–429, 435, 441, 444, 450–453, 456–458, 461, 467, 472, 475, 477, 479, 486, 512, 513
reinspections, 377, 381, 382, 390, 391
retina, 22, 26, 36, 78, 85, 89, 94, 151, 205, 225, 239, 242, 251, 293, 301, 302, 313, 314, 321, 322, 330, 335, 355, 357, 358
retinal image, 120, 149, 151, 152, 157, 159, 165, 166, 211, 221, 279, 283, 287, 288, 290, 293, 294, 329, 335, 336
retinal signals, 177, 293, 321, 332
retinotopic, 5, 17, 36, 38, 51, 53, 55, 146, 152, 193, 205, 313, 314, 332, 333, 355, 370

saccade, 4, 5, 7–10, 12–17, 21–24, 26–29, 32–36, 38–41, 43–47, 51–59, 61–65, 67–70, 73–77, 79–85, 90–95, 99, 104, 110, 111, 119, 120, 122–124, 127–129, 134, 146, 149–152, 165–178, 181–194, 197, 198, 202–206, 211, 212, 214, 216, 220, 223, 239, 240, 248, 252, 262, 263, 267–269, 274, 279–281, 283–288, 290–292, 301, 302, 304–309, 311–315, 322, 323, 329, 341–344, 346, 349, 350, 354, 355, 357–361, 365–369, 381–386, 388–392, 397–402, 406, 407, 409–413, 418–429, 433–444, 449–459, 461, 467–472, 474–479, 485–492, 494–496, 499, 500, 509–513, 517, 518
saccade gain, 40, 422, 423, 426, 427, 439–441, 457
saccade initiation, 36, 62, 426, 468, 477, 478
saccadic accuracy, 93, 342
saccadic adaptation, 366, 370, 419–424, 428, 444
saccadic dysmetria, 419–421, 428, 486, 502
saccadic inhibition, 73, 74, 76–85, 95, 450, 453–455, 457, 458, 460
saccadic latency, 272, 283, 305, 456, 486
saccadic neurons, 4–10, 13, 16, 93
saccadic reaction time (SRT), 8, 61, 64, 172, 284, 469, 471–474, 477, 486
saccadic suppression, 85, 95, 120, 165–167, 169, 170, 178, 182, 287, 428
saccadic targeting, 355
scan path, 380–382, 387, 388, 390, 391, 396–404, 406, 409, 412, 413
scanning strategy, 121, 392, 409
scene perception, 153, 159

scene representation, 134, 184, 186, 350, 353
schizophrenia, 70, 268, 449, 452, 453, 457, 459, 460, 486, 508, 510, 512–516
scotoma, 419
second-order motion, 281, 283, 286
sequences of memory-guided saccades, 433, 436, 438, 441–444
sequential saccade task, 470, 471, 476, 477
serial search, 381, 397–399, 401, 402, 407, 412, 413
serotonin, 457
single photon emitted computed tomography (SPECT), 507
smooth pursuit (SP), 21, 211–223, 225, 226, 229, 240, 242, 245, 252, 255–264, 267–269, 279, 280, 283, 286, 289, 290, 292, 437, 444, 458, 483, 485, 487–489, 492, 495
space constancy, 165, 166, 170, 172, 173, 176–178
spatial averaging, 341
spatial frequency, 73, 74, 78–81, 83, 84, 167, 257, 287, 292
spatial working memory, 395–397, 401, 402, 406, 407, 412, 413, 443, 451, 455, 456, 508–510, 512
spatiotopic, 152, 167, 182, 183, 193, 205
superior colliculus (SC), 3–5, 7, 10, 21, 22, 26, 28, 29, 33–41, 46, 57–59, 61, 62, 68–70, 85, 89, 90, 92–95, 178, 267, 284, 313, 314, 317, 347, 355, 369, 370, 422, 424, 435, 443, 450, 451, 456–458, 467, 479, 512, 517
supplementary eye field (SEF), 4, 69, 70, 90, 92, 94, 251, 252, 314, 369, 452
supplementary motor area (SMA), 252, 435, 443

thalamus, 3, 38, 39, 69, 89, 90, 94, 95, 423, 435, 443, 484, 485, 495, 517
theta motion, 232, 234, 282, 285, 286
time optimal control, 21, 33, 40, 43
Tourette's syndrome, 435, 467, 468, 510
transcranial magnetic stimulation (TMS), 62, 301, 303–309, 323, 368–370, 443
transient, 12, 22, 65, 73, 74, 76, 77, 79–85, 102, 104, 108, 112, 120, 129, 182, 185, 197, 198, 215, 221, 262, 263, 304, 349, 353
transsaccadic integration, 110, 150, 165, 171, 177, 178, 182, 183, 193
transsaccadic memory, 133, 134, 146, 147, 154, 156, 165–169, 177, 181–183, 205

useful field of view (UVF), 381, 398

very low birth weight (VLBW), 483–496
virtual environment, 349, 351, 359, 361
visual analog, 151, 181, 184–186, 190–194, 205, 206
visual attention, 102, 112, 134, 169, 197, 206, 255, 256, 259–264, 267, 316, 400, 413, 459, 508
visual buffer, 101, 151, 159, 193, 352
visual exploration, 398, 399, 410, 413
visual index, 135, 136, 145, 202
visual memory, 104, 129, 151, 153, 169, 204, 349, 350, 358–360
visual scanning, 377, 380, 382, 383, 386, 390, 391
visual search, 73–76, 82–84, 90, 95, 102, 105, 112, 114, 256, 269, 350, 360, 377, 380–382, 390–392, 395–404, 411–413, 509, 511
visual short-term memory, 134, 168, 174, 184, 185, 194, 205, 353, 361, 377, 391, 392
visual stability, 134, 147, 165, 167–170, 177, 178
visual working memory (VWM), 133–136, 144–147, 380, 382
visually evoked potential (VEP), 74, 77–79, 84, 85
visually guided reaching, 368
visually guided saccades, 58, 95, 422–424, 450, 451, 487, 512
visuomotor transformation, 329, 331, 332, 335
volitional control, 239, 250
volitional saccades, 424, 450, 467, 468, 471

Wisconsin card sort test (WCST), 452, 453, 457, 459–461
working memory, 113, 134, 140, 142, 169, 252, 349, 350, 380, 398, 401, 406, 412, 413, 449, 453–459, 461, 510, 512, 518